Handbuch der experimen

Handbook of Experime

Heffter Heubner

XXXI

Herausgeber   Editorial Boar

O. Eichler, Heidelberg · A. Farah, Renss

H. Herken, Berlin · A. D. Welch, New Bru

Beirat   Advisory Board

G. Acheson · E. J. Ariëns · Z. M. Bacq · P. Calabresi

E. G. Erdös · V. Erspamer · U. S. von Euler · W. F

R. Furchgott · A. Goldstein · G. B. Koelle · O. Krayer ·

M. Rocha e Silva · F. Sakai · P. Waser · W. Wilbr

Antianginal Drugs

Pathophysiological, Haemodynamic, Methodological,
Pharmacological, Biochemical and Clinical Basis for
Their Use in Human Therapeutics

By

R. Charlier

With 54 Figures

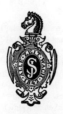

Springer-Verlag Berlin · Heidelberg · New York 1971

Robert Charlier, Director of the Pharmacological Research Department,
LABAZ Research Center. Lecturer, Faculty of Medicine,
University of Liege, Belgium

ISBN 3-540-05365-4 Springer-Verlag Berlin · Heidelberg · New York

ISBN 0-387-05365-4 Springer-Verlag New York · Heidelberg · Berlin

Druck: Joh. Roth sel. Ww., München

Contents

Introduction 1

Coronary Atherosclerosis: General Considerations 7
Epidemiology of Coronary Atherosclerosis 7
Clinical Manifestations of Coronary Atherosclerosis 8
General Therapeutic Measures in Angina Pectoris 8
Physical Training in Angina Pectoris 8
Treatment of Determining Factors of Atherosclerosis
— of Formed Anatomical Lesions: Surgery 10
— of Predisposing Factors 14
a) Hypercholesterolaemia and Hypertriglyceridaemia 14
b) High Blood Pressure 16
c) Metabolic Diseases 16
d) Tobacco 16
— of the Anginal Syndrome 17

I. Pathophysiology of Angina Pectoris 19
1. Pathophysiology of the Anginal Attack 23
Imbalance Between Myocardial Oxygen Consumption and Coronary Blood Flow 23
Lactate Production 25
Myocardial Electrolyte Balance 26
Robinson's Index 29
2. Cardiac Dynamics during the Anginal Attack 30
3. Part Played by Hypersympathicotony in the Anginal Attack 35
4. Trends in Pharmacological Research for the Development of Antianginal Medications 39
4.1. Coronary Vaso-Dilation 39
4.2. Reduction in Cardiac Work 40
4.3. Inhibition of Monoamineoxydase 41
4.4. Blockade of Hypersympathicotony 42
4.5. Blockade of the Adrenergic β-Receptors 42
4.6. Overall Inhibition of Hypersympathicotony 43
4.7. Dilatation of the Coronary Conductance Vessels 44
4.8. Improvement of Functional Coronary Microcirculation 45
4.9. Development of a Collateral Coronary Circulation 45
4.10. Potentiation of the Endogenous Mediators of the Coronary Autoregulation . . 47
4.11. Prophylaxis of Myocardial Necrosis 48
4.12. Inhibition of Platelet Aggregation or Adhesiveness 49

II. Haemodynamic Basis for Coronary Pharmacology 52
General Considerations 52
Blood Pressure 55
Myocardial Oxygen Consumption 55
Cardiac Work 56
Cardiac Output 56
Heart Rate 56
Regulation of Coronary Circulation 58
Hypoxaemia 59
Vasomotor Metabolites 59
CO_2 59
Lactic Acid 59

pH   59
Histamine   60
Potassium   60
Adenosine   60
"Sympathine"   62
Bradykinine   63
Hyperemine   64

III. Pharmacological Methodology for Testing Antianginal Drugs   65

Coronary Blood Flow   65
Isolated Heart   65
Heart *in situ*   68

1. *Measurement of Coronary Outflow*   68
1.1. Morawitz Technique   70
1.2. Heart-Lung Preparation   70
1.3. Rodbard Technique   70
1.4. Busch Technique   71
1.5. Catheterization of the Coronary Sinus without Thoracotomy   71

2. *Measurement of Coronary Inflow*   72
2.1. Techniques with Extra-Arterial Cannulation   72
2.1.1. Melville Technique   72
2.1.2. Schofield Technique   72
2.2. Techniques with Intra-Arterial Cannulation.   73
2.2.1. Gregg Technique   73
2.2.2. Pieper Technique   74
2.2.3. Berne Technique   74
2.3. Techniques without Arterial Cannulation   75
2.3.1. Direct Methods   75
2.3.1.1. The Thermostromuhr   76
2.3.1.2. The Calorimetric Method   76
2.3.1.3. Method Using the Electromagnetic Flow Transducer   77
2.3.1.4. Method Using the Ultrasonic Flowmeter   78
2.3.2. Indirect Methods   79
2.3.2.1. The Nitrous Oxide Technique   79
2.3.2.2. Methods Based on the Employment of Radioactive Substances   81
2.3.2.2.1. Non-diffusible Substances   81
2.3.2.2.2. Diffusible Substances   81
2.3.2.2.3. Diffusible Inert Gases   83

3. *Nutritional Myocardial Micro-Circulation*   85

4. *Collateral Coronary Circulation*   85
4.1. Acute Experiment   85
4.1.1. Linder Technique   85
4.1.2. Rees Technique   85
4.1.3. McGregor Technique   85
4.2. Chronic Experiment   86
4.2.1. Meesmann Technique   86
4.2.2. Schmidt Technique   86
4.2.3. Schaper Technique   86

5. *Experimental Chronic Coronary Insufficiency*   87

Measuring Cardiac Output   90
Measuring Cardiac Work   92
Measuring Myocardial Oxygen Consumption   92

IV. Clinical Methods for Assessment of the Therapeutic Value of Antianginal Medications   95

Diagnosis of Angina Pectoris   95
Clinical Assessment of Antianginal Drugs 101

1. Objective Methods 102
1.1. Russek Method 102
1.2. Levy Method 106

1.3. Riseman Method 106
1.4. Solvay Method 108
1.5. Rookmaker Method 109
1.6. Frick Method 109

2. Subjective Methods 109
Greiner Method 111

3. Conclusions on Methods of Clinical Assessment 116

V. Pharmacological and Clinical Features of Antianginal Drugs 118

Nitrites 118

1. Nitroglycerin 120
   — Effect on Coronary Flow in Dogs 123
   — Effect on Coronary Flow in Humans 125
   — Haemodynamic Effects in Humans 126
   — Haemodynamic Effects in the Case of the Angina Patient Suffering an Attack 128
   — Mechanisms of the Antianginal Effect 129
   — Therapeutic Effect of Nitroglycerin 135
   — Special Galenic Preparations 137

2. Triethanolamine Trinitrate 138

3. Erythrityl Tetranitrate 140

4. Pentaerythritol Tetranitrate 140

5. Mannitol Hexanitrate 143

6. Amyl Nitrite 143

7. Octyl Nitrite 144

8. Sodium Nitrite 145

9. Isosorbide Dinitrate 146

10. Nilatil 148

11. Etrynit 149

12. Propanediol Dinitrates 149

Papaverine 150
Xanthines 152

1. Aminophylline 153

2. Choline Theophyllinate 155

3. Various Theophylline Derivatives 155

Khellin 157
Carduben 159
Diacromone 159
Phenyl-chromone 160
Recordil 160
Monoamineoxydase Inhibitors (Maoi) 160
Irrigor 164
Segontin 165
Amplivix 168
Isoptin 172
Persantine 181
Intensaine 188
Ustimon 192
Ildamen 196
Clinium 199
β-Adrenergic Blocking Drugs 205

1. Inderal 206
   — Primary Cardiac Effect 207
   — Effect on Coronary Flow 208
   — Effect on Cardiac Output 210
   — Antianginal Effect 211
   — Mechanisms of the Antianginal Effect 214
   — Effect on the Cardiac Function 215
   — Recommendations for the Treatment of Angina Pectoris 217

— Ineffectiveness of Inderal in Acute Myocardial Infarction 217
— The Use of Inderal in Cardiac Arrhythmia 218
  2. Trasicor 222
      Clinical Application 227
  3. Aptin 229
  4. Eraldin 235
  5. ICI 45763 or Kö 592 (doberol) 245
  6. Visken (LB 46) 246
  7. Ro 3-3528 248
  8. INPEA 248
  9. Sotalol (M.J. 1999) 249
  10. Recetan 252
  11. PhQA 33 253
  12. AH 3474 253
  13. D 477 A 254
  14. USVC 6524 254
  15. S-D/1601 254
  16. Bunolol 255
Cordarone 255
  1. Pharmacological Properties 256
  1.1. Intrinsic Effects 256
  1.2. Antiadrenergic Effects 262
  1.2.1. α-antiadrenergic Effects 262
  1.2.2. β-antiadrenergic Effects 263
  1.3. Action Mechanisms and Therapeutic Deductions 266
  1.3.1. Intrinsic Effects 266
  1.3.2. Antiadrenergic Effects 271
  1.4. Anti-Arrhythmic Properties 276
  2. Therapeutic Properties 276
  2.1. Antianginal Effects in Open Tests 276
  2.2. Antianginal Effects in Double-Blind Tests. 279
  2.3. Effects on the Symptomatology of the Cardiac Overload Tests 280
  2.3.1. Hypoxia Test 280
  2.3.2. Ergometric Bicycle Test. 280
  2.3.3. Master Type Effort Test. 284
  2.4. Effects on Pathological Electrocardiogram in Coronary Angina. 285
  2.5. Anti-Arrhythmic Effects 285
  2.6. Clinical Tolerance and Side Effects 286

Miscellaneous 288

Section no. 1 288
Adenylocrat 288
Aminocetone 288
Anginin 289
Baralgin 289
Baxacor 289
Eucilat 291
Griseofulvine 291
Mederel 292
Opticardon 293
Pexid 293
Piridoxilate 294
Polarising Solutions 295
Sandolanid 296
Surheme 297
Terodiline 297
Tromcardin 298
Vastarel 298
Vialibran 298

Section no. 2 299
Morphine 299
Barbiturates 299
Ethyl Alcohol 300
Valium 301
Phenothiazines 302
    Chlorpromazine 302
    Mepazine 303
    Chloracizine 303
Diphenylhydantoin 303
Cinchona Alcaloids 303
Daucarine 304
Vitamin E 305
Hexoestrol 305
Adenosine and Related Substances 305
Thyroxine 306

Section no. 3 307
Phenoxy-Isopropyl-Norsuprifen 307
Phenyl-Isobutyl-Norsuprifen 307
Cyclospasmol 308
Vasculat 308
Reserpine 308
Padutin 309
Recosen 309
Cortunon 310
Heparin 310
Dicoumarol 311
Ilidar 312
Priscol 312
Hydergine 312
Ronicol 313
Poly-Methoxyphenol Derivatives 313
Triparanol 314
Varia 314
Carotid Sinus Nerve Stimulation 315
Prospects of future research 316

Table of Side Effects in Man 320

References 323

Author Index 372

Subject Index 431

Introduction

If the numerous therapeutic acquisitions of the past few years have enriched very different fields of human pathology, it does seem that coronary pathology has been given very special attention, as witness the wide variety of antianginal medications placed at the disposal of the medical profession. There are various explanations for this state of affairs, one of them probably being that the medications successively proposed do not fully satisfy the practitioner and another that the total number of individuals suffering from the clinical manifestations of coronary heart disease offers, by its size, a vast profit potential for the pharmaceutical industry. This field of applications opens up such prospects that it has encouraged a prolific amount of competition between various research laboratories, and it is no exaggeration to say that every major firm has its individual antianginal drug in its therapeutic catalogue.

A further factor has also contributed enormously to this proliferation of medicinal preparations intended for the treatment of angina pectoris: this is the rapid advance in our knowledge of the physiopathology of angina, which in turn has produced original concepts of pharmacological and biochemical research. As a result, there have emerged new substances whose action mechanisms have claimed to be best suited to the cardiovascular disorders responsible for cardiac pain. These constantly changing trends in biological research have of necessity called for ever more diversified methodological development which has made it possible to investigate and measure biological parameters hitherto unobtainable, especially in humans. Even more specialised and polyvalent equipment has thus been perfected, making it possible to combine in a single exploration a whole mass of data which, up to now, could only be gathered separately. Whereas only a short time ago, the various haemodynamic parameters were registered, so to speak, individually and often under diverse experimental conditions and then compared in an attempt to arrive at a synthesis, necessarily handicapped by variations in sensitivity of the preparations used and by the lack of homogeneousness in experimental conditions, the technical equipment currently available makes it possible to gather in a single test the desired information which, because of its diverse character, gives an overall picture of the variations in the parameters investigated under identical experimental conditions for each of those parameters. We thus get more effective comparison of information gathered at the same time as increased knowledge. A striking example of this development is the study of the action mechanisms of nitroglycerin on the angina subject. Long tackled from the angle of fragmental exploration of the multiple haemodynamic disturbances which this medication entails, it has recently been possible to do this on an all-in basis with the result that a coherent synthesis of the cardiovascular changes occurring could be arrived at, and certain action mechanisms put forward (see p. 129).

Still in the field of apparatus, many animal and human exploration methods have been perfected. Regarding the problem of angina, methodological advances have been especially marked in the measurement of myocardium blood irrigation and its metabolism. We have only to compare the technical conditions of the isolated heart methods with the highly physiological methods formulated, for example, by GREGG in 1965 in the case of the unanaesthetised dog with its coronary circulation restricted at will by controllable pneumatic occlusive cuff (see p. 90), to appreciate the progress made within a few decades. It goes without saying that a technological evolution of this nature has made for accuracy of experimental observations. Concurrently, methods have been developed for measuring the coronary flow in humans which in 1966 culminated in the development of bloodless techniques applicable to angina pectoris subjects and allowing accurate and reproducible results to be rapidly obtained (see p. 82).

A new and comparatively recent branch of activity has similarly contributed to the development of new treatments: clinical pharmacology, which by an objective functional assessment of the reactions of the human subject provides the necessary link between animal pharmacology and subjective symptomatology in man.

The discovery of antianginal drugs of ever-increasing diversity as regards chemical structure and action mechanisms has also been stimulated by the change in fundamental clinical notions as to the angina syndrome. Over the past ten years, our knowledge of the physiology of angina pectoris has been much enriched, and consequently that of the way in which various medications used for this syndrome exert their action.

There is no doubt whatsoever that it is the development of more and more sophisticated and ingenious techniques for exploring the cardiovascular system that has contributed to the achievement of such progress. Of these techniques, first place undoubtedly goes to cardiac catheterisation since from this derive directly all the techniques of intravascular investigation. The original Forssman and Cournand method, *catheterisation of the right cavities*, has already for a long time made it possible to measure the cardiac output from the Fick principle by enabling the sampling of mixed venous blood in the pulmonary artery, and also the pulmonary arterial "wedge" pressure.

Its first variant was the *catheterisation of the coronary sinus* which makes it possible to collect the myocardium venous drainage and thereby measure the coronary flow and myocardial oxygen consumption, and at the same time to study the metabolism of the various energy-producing substrates of the cardiac muscle. *Left catheterisation* then supplied a reading of the left systolic and end-diastolic ventricular pressures, followed by that of its first derivative (dp/dt) which expresses the maximum rate at which the ventricular pressure rises [671, 1511], this maximum being directly proportionate to the maximum tension potential of the ventricle at the start of contraction [1511], and then, quite recently [1111], its second derivative (d^2p/dt^2) which expresses the acceleration of ventricular pressure, a function whose maximum changes occur at the initial phase of the isometric ventricular contraction. It also makes it possible to measure, from the inner heart surface, the degree and velocity of shortening of the myocardial fibres with the aid of a new type catheter [1206].

Cardiac catheterisation has also to its credit the following further attainments:

— the production of experimental myocardial infarction in a dog with its thorax closed by blockade of the anterior interventricular artery [1507], a method which avoids any handling of the heart and its innervation, and enables the subsequent measurement as required of the anastomotic coronary blood flow during the recovery period [1505];

— the measurement, in humans, of the contractile state of the left ventricle [580] expressed by the contractility index:

$$\frac{\text{maximum rate of rise in left ventricular pressure}}{\text{maximum isovolumetric pressure} \times 2\pi\, r}$$

whose decrease is strictly linked to the degree of left decompensation;

— the quantification of the ventricular function in the angina subject by measuring the response of the end-diastolic left ventricular pressure to intravenous infusion of angiotensine [1152, 1154];

— the demonstration of depressed left ventricular function associated with the attack of angina pectoris (see p. 30);

— the so-called intracardiac oximetry, i.e. the instantaneous and continuous measurement of oxygen saturation in the cardiac chambers, without withdrawal of blood samples, by using a special intracardiac catheter (see p. 91);

— several significant advances in the understanding of intracardiac conduction and of cardiac arrhythmia:

a) studies of the mechanisms of intra-atrial conduction, three bipolar leads being obtained from the high right atrium, low right atrium, and mid-left atrium, led to the conclusion that currently accepted mechanisms of intra-atrial conduction in man need reevaluation [57 c]

b) the atrial electrocardiogram enabled the pattern of onset and spontaneous cessation of atrial fibrillation complicating myocardial infarction to be studied [23 c]

c) the capacity of the human atrio-ventricular conduction to sustain 1:1 ventriculo-atrial conduction has been assessed by means of transvenous electrodes which were placed in the right atrium and ventricle, the ventricle being paced at several rates, each in excess of the sino-atrial rate [117 c]

d) special forms of supraventricular tachycardia have been differentiated from ventricular tachycardia [75 c]

e) recording of His bundle electrograms made contribution to the understanding of atrio-ventricular conduction disturbances in patients with bilateral bundle-branch block [288 c]

f) recording of His bundle activity confirmed the hypothesis [112 c] that the recurrent supraventricular tachycardia without Wolff-Parkinson-White syndrome may frequently be caused by a reciprocal mechanism of atrial origin [116 c]. The mechanisms of such tachycardias in patients with Wolff-Parkinson-White syndrome have also been precised [58 c]

g) direct His bundle recordings supported clinical observations that Mobitz II A—V blocks are associated with bilateral bundle-branch block as well as with His bundle lesions [216 c, 230 c]

h) recording of the electrical activity of both branches of His bundle has been made possible [259 c]

i) measurement, in humans, of the refractory period of the atrio-ventricular node [1151], together with the electrical activity of the His bundle [387, 388, 1665] has been made, the latter reading providing an accurate picture of the morphology of the QRS ventricular complex [389] and showing, amongst other things: a) that in auricular fibrillation, this complex is preceded by a single and isolated deflection originating in the His bundle and which is not found in auricular flutter [1081]; and b) that in the nodal rhythms, it is not the atrio-ventricular node which is the pacemaker, but the top part of the His bundle itself [30a];

— the catheterisation at will of the two coronary arteries in humans, enabling selective coronary cine-arteriography [1788] which provides a unique opportunity of comparing the clinical symptoms and physiopathological data with the vascular morphological anomalies (atherosclerotic lesions) found to be present at the same time;

— selective monitoring of the heart rate by the atrial pacing method [1798] (which also makes it possible, by permanently fitting a catheter, to avoid thoraco-tomy for the insertion of an intrathoracic pacemaker intended to treat certain rhythm disorders, [68a]), together with the possibility of speeding it up experi-mentally to high and stable levels, as for instance in the case of angina pectoris cases in order to trigger off the cardiac attack for the purpose of physiopathological investigation [592].

This experimental reproduction of angina attacks in coronary patients has, incidentally, aroused the interest of clinicians and led them to induce cardiac pain in coronary subjects so as to get an accurate picture of the clinical physiopathology. For this purpose they have used not only the normal and standard angina-produc-ing exertion tests, but also pharmacological substances placed at their disposal by organicists, such as isoprenaline, since this catecholamine in intravenous injection produces in dogs [1257] and in humans [1034] cardiovascular overloading charac-terised by similar haemodynamic disturbances to those occurring in a man doing exercises, namely an increase in cardiac frequency, output and work, and in coronary flow and myocardial oxygen consumption, and a drop in peripheral and coronary vascular resistances. Because of this, isoprenaline induces in the angina patient myocardial ischaemia which reproduces the clinical symptomatology of the heart attack [345].

Clinical researchers have also made good use of the synthesis of other pharma-cological substances, such as for instance the specific antagonists of the adrenergic α- or β-receptors for the purpose of neutralising, as required, certain cardiovascular disturbances and so dissect the adrenergic system at its various effectors.

Finally, the use of radio-active tracers has led to the clarification of various ideas regarding haemodynamics, which it had hitherto only been possible to in-vestigate by less physiological and less accurate methods open to highly debatable interpretation. This is particularly the case for the measurement of coronary flow in animals, and even more so in humans, where it will be seen that their use has at last made it possible to perfect, by successive approximations, a method which provides in 30 seconds correct and perfectly reproducible coronary flow values both in the case of a healthy man and a coronary subject.

The development of new experimental techniques has likewise contributed to advances in our knowledge. Such techniques include polarographic electrodes pro-viding continuous readings of the blood and tissue oxygen content, special isotopic methods recently used in investigations into the myocardial microcirculation [2010], the manufacture of vascular rings of the Ameroid type [1212] which, when inserted on a temporary and/or long-term basis, make it possible to reduce as required, in a permanent and measurable manner, the blood irrigation of a given area of the myocardium, the development of catheters incorporating an electro-magnetic flow transducer [1015, 1956], and last but not least the development of new methods for inducing myocardial infarction [900] which offer, amongst other things, the possibility, by using radio-active xenon, of measuring simultaneously the blood irrigation in the infarcted area, the area immediately adjacent and an area which has remained unaffected [1508].

The latest antianginal medications answer to different research concepts from the chemical angle and, ipso facto, to highly diverse pharmacological action mechanisms. These drugs have been subjected not only to often much more elaborate pharmacological investigations than in the past, but also to biochemical exploration aimed at controlling the behaviour of the metabolism of the myocardium. Here again, the technical progress made over the past few years has made it possible in most cases to change from *in vitro* to *in vivo* research, both on animals and humans.

There has thus been built up in the field of chemico-therapeutic preventive treatment of the clinical manifestations of angina pectoris a sum total of knowledge scattered throughout written publications which it is sometimes difficult to put in a coordinated form. Very often the position is not clear. As MODELL says [1307, p. 364], information of any given antianginal drug abounds in contradictions, and this is especially true as regards its therapeutic potential. Many clinical publications are manifestly scant, and to complicate matters there are recent reports which suggest that the efficacy of certain nitrites, long accepted, could be brought into question [597, 53a, 11c].

In this area of therapeutics, there is therefore very copious material which has seemed to us to be deserving ofgeneral review, an attempt at a monograph intended to gather together the information spread over a mass of continually proliferating periodicals and to draw up a synthesis of existing acquisitions.

Thus there will be shown the advances in our knowledge of angina pectoris since 1847 when LATHAM expressed himself as follows [894]:

"Our knowledge then of angina pectoris stops short at its symptoms. Its concept cannot be made to lie in any definite form of disease beyond them. We are sure of what it is as a collection of symptoms. We are not sure of what it is as a disease."

At the present time, many contradictions persist, many points still remain unknown. But the facts learned in this field over more than a century and which are summarised in this general survey provide the guarantee of the favourable outcome of future research efforts.

Whilst underlining the essentials of what is known, the subject matter gives the promise of many things to come. In our view, therefore, it is cheering document likely to mitigate somewhat the pessimism which emerges for example from the remark in 1967 by SONNTAG [1792] who, in his desire to express the many shortcomings in our existing state of knowledge, wrote 120 years after LATHAM:

"At times, our present understanding of angina pectoris seems as imperfect as it was in 1847."

The final purpose of our survey is also to give the doctor a clear idea as to the knowledge of the various medicaments which he might be called upon to handle, and in so doing guide him in his choice. Obviously our attempt is only an interim measure since the subject is continually changing.

Since we wanted to make this work as up to date as possible, we included in the galley proofs the publications that came to our attention after submission of the manuscript. They are designated by reference numbers followed by letters (a) or (b) or (c) or (d) or (e) and are listed in an additional bibliography. The bibliography includes publications that came to our attention up to the end of December 1970.

As will be seen, we relate some personal pharmacological observations, which have formed the subject of several publications. It is notably the case as regards a

recent antianginal drug which has been perfected in the Research Center of
LABAZ. These experimental investigations are the result of team-work carried out
under the inspiring and competent direction of Dr. G. DELTOUR for more than
15 years on the synthesis and experimental exploration of original chemical structures which are based on the benzofuran nucleus, some of them having resulted
in medications which are endowed with valuable therapeutic properties [406].

I would like to express my gratitude to the entire Management of LABAZ who
placed unreservedly at our disposal both the technical and financial means which
are required for good quality pharmacological investigation.

I would also express my appreciation of the help given by those of my immediate collaborators who have assisted in the technical work.

My warmest thanks go to Mr. M. COLOT for preparing the illustrations used
in this work and to my son for the drawings and graphs he provided.

I desire to thank Prof. Z.M. BACQ who has contributed over many years to
what is best in my scientific development and has been kind enough to read through
the manuscript and to suggest that it be submitted to the Editors of the Handbook
of Experimental Pharmacology.

Coronary Atherosclerosis: General Considerations

The therapeutic aspects of coronary heart disease are of the utmost importance because human atherosclerosis is electively localized in the coronary vessels, and also because atherosclerosis results in a type of cardiopathy which is, at the present time, the main cause of death for man.

World statistics relating to causes of death emphasize the growing importance of coronary disease and its consequences in general mortality [237, 321, 720, 1985, 1986]. In a report which was submitted to the executive board of the World Health Organization during the February 1969 session held in Geneva, the following important warning appeared [253]: "L'ischémie cardiaque, ou maladie coronarienne, atteint des proportions fantastiques et s'étend à des groupes d'âge toujours plus jeunes. Il faut s'attendre à la voir augmenter et prendre les proportions d'une des plus désastreuses épidémies[1] que l'humanité ait connues, à moins que nous ne trouvions le moyen de renverser la tendance par des recherches intensives sur la cause et la prévention de cette maladie".

A reasonable estimate made for the United States in 1956 by GREGG and SABISTON [732] indicates that, among patients who die from heart disease, one-third do so from a primary coronary insufficiency related mainly to atherosclerosis, one-third die from primary coronary insufficiency associated with cardiac hypertrophy and increasing cardiac work arising from valvular lesions and arterial hypertension, and one-third as a result of a primary myocardial insufficiency. At least two-thirds of all cardiopathies and cardiac decompensations in man originate, therefore, from a disease of the coronary arteries which manifests itself functionally by relative deficiency in the quantity of arterial blood, and therefore of oxygen, supplied to the cardiac muscle by the coronary vascular system [720]. In the United States alone [1946], the incidence of coronary heart disease on mortality increased from 2195 to 2746 units per million between 1951 and 1961.

The great majority of cases of coronaropathy are associated with a more or less advanced state of coronary atherosclerosis [513, 104c], so that the incidence of coronary heart disease in man, particularly in those who have passed the age of forty, seems intimately linked with the progressive increase in arteriosclerotic disorders. The arterial degenerative process does not, however, spare young people since 77% of American male subjects under forty were found to present at autopsy asymptomatic atherosclerotic lesions involving one coronary artery [496, 497, 1786].

---

1 A comparison of male and female mortality trends in Ontario over the past few decades provides strong additional evidence for the belief that the present high death rate from ischaemic heart disease in middle-aged men constitutes a "modern epidemic" [7c]. Since about 1925, the death rate from all causes in females aged 45—64 has declined to half its previous level, while the corresponding male death rate has remained stationary, due largely to an almost threefold increase in male deaths ascribed to diseases of the heart. As, during the same period, the male and female death rates from cerebrovascular disease have remained approximately equal and stationary, it is suggested that the rise in the male death rate from ischaemic heart disease has been due to an increased tendency of the myocardium to infarction, rather than to an increased prevalence of atherosclerosis, or to an increased tendency to intravascular thrombosis.

During the last decade, the mortality rate due to coronary atherosclerosis increased steadily, exceeding by a wide margin the cancer rate, so that LENEGRE could report in 1966 that coronary heart disease was responsible for almost 100,000 deaths yearly in France [1101], the corresponding figure being 500,000 for the United States [386, 1259]. It has been estimated that human mortality due to coronaropathy exceeds a total of one million yearly for all the industrialized countries [918]. Paradoxically, despite the undeniable gravity of the problem and notwithstanding constant efforts on the part of biologists and clinicians striving for improved knowledge as to the various aspects of coronary insufficiency, the doctor is still very poorly equipped as regards coronary atherosclerosis since the therapeutic means at his disposal to combat coronary heart disease at all its stages are, on the whole, inadequate. The fundamental reason for this lies in the fact that the clinical symptoms are extremely belated as compared with the onset of the pathological process. It is only when the two major clinical manifestations occur, myocardial infarction and the anginal syndrome, that the doctor must of necessity take appropriate therapeutic measures, of which a certain number are, even at this late stage, genuinely effective.

Of the two, infarction and the anginal syndrome, the latter is, if not the most spectacular, the most frequent and the most chronically disabling of clinical manifestations of coronary heart disease. Although medicinal therapy has an unquestioned place in the treatment of angina pectoris, general measures must *first* be adopted. The best attitude for the patient to take is that he must adjust his activities to reduce the painful attacks to the minimum. It is up to the patient to assess the limits of his tolerance to exertion and not to exceed those limits. These must provide the guide-lines governing such restrictions on physical activity as the doctor may need to prescribe for the patient and the latter's capacity for continuing his professional activities.

Once these limits of tolerance to exertion have been accurately defined, careful rationalisation of daily activity may be sufficient to reduce to a considerable extent the number and severity of the painful attacks. Weight reduction, the lowering of high blood pressure, the correction of anaemia, treatment of thyrotoxicosis or myxoedema are general measures which may be advantageous in view of the fact that they are likely to increase tolerance to exertion. The use of an hypnotic may be necessary to ensure adequate sleep; the use of sedatives or tranquillisers is helpful in combatting anxiety.

The most debated question is that relating to what physical exercise may be permitted for the angina subject. Whereas up to a short time ago the medical tendency was towards voluntary restriction, daily physical exercise whose intensity and progression must be adapted to each individual case has been increasingly advocated over the past few years. Since this attitude does not meet with general acceptance, although it is based on suggestive experimental and clinical research, we propose giving the biological bases justifying this change in opinion.

The advantages of physical exercises for angina subjects find their essential experimental arguments in ECKSTEIN's work [473]. Subjecting 117 dogs to varying and more or less "controlled" degrees of constriction of the circumflex coronary artery, he recovers them and splits them into two groups: one he allows to rest, the other he exercises four times a day on an endless belt for 6—8 weeks. At the end of this period, he anaesthetises them and proceeds to two rheological examinations: firstly, the measurement of the retrograde coronary blood flow (which he showed in a previous experiment to be in excellent correlation with the development of anastomoses [472]) and then of the blood flow at the partly ligatured artery. Following this, a coloured substance is injected into this coronary artery, downstream of the constriction, and microscopic examinations are carried out for the purpose of assessing the extent and scale of such anastomoses as may have developed. The basic results show that the retrograde blood flow (and so collateral) is more considerable as the arterial constriction is severe, that the retrograde flow at a given constriction is greater in the animals which have been exercised, and finally that the exercise prescribed for animals with *moderate* arterial constriction induces a more extensive development of collateral circulation than a *severe* arterial constriction not followed by exercise. On the basis of his experiments, ECKSTEIN suggested that continuous and judicious exercise should increase the collaterals in the angina subject and minimise the clinical manifestations of coronary heart diseases.

Following upon this work, certain clinicians [1922] have assessed in angina patients the haemodynamic and metabolic changes, both at rest and during an ergometric test, occurring as a result of physical exercise consisting of a daily stint for 4—6 weeks on an ergometric bicycle lasting for 30 min. They find that the work capacity increases, that the clinical condition improves, that the amount of work required to cause the cardiac pain increases considerably, and that the cardiac output and work are reduced. KATTUS and McALPIN [948] show that a training programme consisting of daily walking leads to an improvement in physical condition, shown by an increase in capacity for exercise and by the possibility of carrying out a given exercise at a lower cardiac frequency [946]. This improvement in physical condition, which has been pointed out by others [808], is always accompanied by an improvement in the angina clinical condition which, in some cases, can go as far as the disappearance of the pain symptoms and of the electrocardiographic impairment [948]. The lessening of the exertion tachycardia thus achieved is similar, incidentally, to that found with exercising in a healthy person [397, 1875].

Both CLAUSEN et al. [334] and FRICK [593] thus arrive at the conclusion that physical exercise by the angina subject leads to an increase in the systolic output [43a] and a reduction in cardiac work which they attribute to a lessening of the generalised sympathetic vasoconstriction. In their case also, the haemodynamic changes which they note constitute a rational physiological basis in favour of physical exercise for the coronary subject. In further clinical studies carried out on patients after several months of physical training, the following changes were observed upon exertion compared to similar patients without any physical training: a decrease in heart rate, an increase in stroke volume, a decrease in tension-time index and better left and right ventricular functions [62c, 102c]. CLAUSEN considers that an increased oxidative metabolic capacity in the trained muscles reduces the demand for sympathetic stimulation during exercise and, in consequence, induces a redistribution of cardiac output and the observed reduction in tension-time index [63c]. Specifically after myocardial infarction, the haemodynamic evidence is suggestive that the circulatory response to training is superior to the change occurring as the natural reparative process [102c].

A detailed summary of the clinical developments which justify the recommending of physical activity on the part of patients suffering from coronary heart disease has been prepared by SCHWALB [1699], who stresses the fact, however, that although this activity certainly improves the heart condition it only applies to the functional condition since it has not been demonstrated that it has a beneficial incidence on the atherosclerotic process itself.

Thus we find objectified from the clinical and physiopathological angles the decision of cardiologists who advocate continuous and judicious exercise for angina sufferers with the object of improving the myocardial irrigation conditions, probably through the development of coronary anastomoses [95, 807, 854, 1341, 1757], although no new collaterals were visualised in any of ten subjects who were examined following physical training [209 c]. This attitude has led, in the countries of Eastern Europe, to a veritable explosion of centres for the treatment and prevention of coronary diseases by reeducation and muscular training [1378]. Whatever the biological reason may be, whether it involves the psychological effects of group therapy, generally improved aptitudes, or even a genuine improvement in the irrigation of the cardiac muscle, there no longer remains any doubt that the angina sufferer benefits from this recent reversal in the medical attitude to exercise [1897].

Although supervised exercise programmes should help in preventing severe complications or death, cautions must be taken to adapt the amount of permitted efforts since exercise in excess of cardiac capabilities may result in serious heart disorders. Two patients suffered severe heart complications while jogging in organised exercise programmes, an acute myocardial infarction developing in one while the other had a cardiac arrest [21a]. A third case has been reported, the subject falling to the floor with cardiac stand-still during simple calisthenics and under direct medical supervision [101a]. According to RESNEKOV [105a], subjects should always be screened by a physician to determine the level of exercise to be used and the rate of increase in the exercise loads to be undertaken. Supervised physical conditioning can be used safely in selected subjects with atherosclerotic heart disease [145 c].

Although all these general measures are unquestionably advantageous for the angina subject, the proper administration of medicaments can enable him to undertake certain activities without being restricted by the distressing pain which would occur in their absence.

These therapeutic steps, whether medicinal or otherwise, can apply to different stages and various causes, direct or predisposing, of atherosclerosis and its clinical manifestations. With LENEGRE [1101], we can briefly sum up the weapons in the existing therapeutic arsenal.

There are none for combatting the *determining factors* since these are unknown.

We are also completely powerless as regards *formed anatomical lesions*, since it would be necessary to be able either to regenerate the arterial scar tissue into sound tissue or remove the damaged myocardial tissue. Although myocardial infarctectomy is now considered as an acceptable risk in acute infarction with cardiogenic shock unresponsive to medical management [129c], and resection of a chronic infarct has been successful in some patients [143c], effective action is still in the realms of the future.

One of the most effective palliative methods would appear to be the grafting of the internal mammary artery into the myocardium as suggested by VINEBERG [1941]. This operation ensures the provision of a considerable amount of blood [376] and when the cases are carefully selected it brings significant symptomatic improvement [535]. It can only be effective in cases which have been rigourously controlled from the clinical angle and where the coronarography has revealed arterial lesions of such a nature that their symptomatic manifestations cannot within reason benefit from exclusively medical treatment [918]. The selection of patients suited to this operation must necessarily be made on the basis of a selective coronarography [533], preferably associated with a left ventriculography whose result provides the surgeon with an incontestable guide in that it shows him the immobile areas of the ventricular wall (fibrous scar or aneurism) which must definitely be excluded for the site of the graft [174]. It is desirable to add to these a physiological assessment of the left ventricular function, as for instance a measurement of the end-diastolic ventricular pressure and a scrutiny of its behaviour during an intravenous infusion of angiotensine [1152], any abnormal rise reflecting the precarious nature of the cardiac function.

The merits of other methods, notably coronary endarterectomy, were reviewed in 1967 by SABISTON [1624] and in 1969 by BAUE [111]; they are of the opinion that we are still at the investigation stage and that the results of these operative techniques call a greater degree of appraisement, particularly as regards the long-term benefits. FRIEDBERG [597] and GRISWOLD [743] add that the need for controlled experiments is a must and that they have not yet been carried out. GORLIN and TAYLOR [701], however, claim that, from a series of 100 patients followed up for a period of 2 years following the grafting of the internal mammary artery, they were in possession of objective criteria showing that angina had decreased in 75% of cases, that the incidence of further infarction had been reduced by 50% as compared with a series of check-patients, but that the vital prognosis did not appear to be significantly improved. In their view, angina pectoris is the main indication for this surgical procedure, which should be rejected where there is severe decompensation, diffuse atherosclerosis and poor physical condition. SPENCER [1805] has recently produced a fully documented survey on revascularisation of the myocardium by systemic artery transplant.

Some twenty years since he first proposed his technique for internal mammary artery implantation in the cardiac muscle, VINEBERG has given, in 1970, a general survey of the results obtained and the experience acquired with 450 cases operated on and subsequently followed up during this period [326c]. He has also shown that a single mammary artery properly implanted is capable of permanent revascularisation when half left ventricle is viable [327c].

The long-term functional benefit arrived at in patients who underwent implantation of the internal mammary artery by VINEBERG's procedure has been assessed last year in several biological and haemodynamic studies, which led to some conflicting results.

In dogs, the metabolic and physiologic contributions of an implanted internal mammary artery have been assessed 24—34 months following internal mammary artery implantation and concomitant ameroid constrictor application to coronary arteries [167c]. All implants were patent angiographically prior to evaluation by right heart bypass and continual assessment of myocardial oxygen, pyruvate, and lactate extraction. Control internal mammary artery flow averaged 17.5 ml/min per 100 g of left ventricle. Occlusion of the internal mammary artery failed significantly to alter myocardial extraction of oxygen, pyruvate and lactate or ventricular function, nor did these patent implants prevent significant changes in oxygen, pyruvate, and lactate extraction and ventricular function during and following occlusion of a remaining patent left coronary artery. These results indicate that demonstration of angiographic patency of an internal mammary artery implant does not necessarily indicate significant metabolic or functional contribution of this extracardiac blood supply to the heart.

In man, blood flow measurements of internal mammary artery implant were performed on 13 patients 2—5 years after a single implant for coronary artery disease [76c]. These flows were found to be relatively low, averaging 8.1 ml/min (ranging from 4 to 19 ml/min). Occlusion of the implants for 5 minutes failed to produce a significant change in the electrocardiogram. Such observations in angiographically patent and well-functioning implants demonstrate that implant contribution to resting myocardial blood flow seems to be modest and may be inconsequential. In another clinical investigation, twenty-three subjects with angiographically documented coronary heart disease were studied by means of arterial and coronary sinus catheterization before and one year after internal mammary artery implantations [174c]. The pre- and postoperative patterns of lactate extraction at rest and after isoproterenol stress have been determined and correlated with clinical improvement and angiographic patency of the implant. In a first group, 13 subjects had implants that were angiographically seen to fill some portion of the coronary circulation. Eight of 11 who produced lactate preoperatively reverted to normal lactate extraction. Two extracted lactate at both studies. All but two had clinical improvement. No deaths occurred over a mean follow-up period of 40 months. In a second group, ten subjects had implants with no visible connection to the coronary circulation. Only one subject had reversion of lactate production to extraction and two from extraction to production. Seven of ten did not improve clinically. Three deaths occurred over a mean follow-up period of 39 months. Agreement has been found between reversion to normal lactate metabolism, angiographic patency, and clinical improvement following internal mammary artery implantation.

In a third clinical study, left ventricular haemodynamics at rest and during supine exercise were assessed before and one year after internal mammary artery implantation in 24 patients with severe coronary artery disease and angina pectoris [217c]. Fourteen patients had evidence of one or more implants providing collaterals to coronary arteries, and ten had no evidence of collaterals from the implant. Only two patients, both with functioning implants, showed a return to normal of left ventricular end-diastolic pressure at rest and during exercise (see p. 31 for the significance of these results). There was no correlation between clinical improvement and haemodynamics at the time of the postoperative study. The conclusion is that left ventricular haemodynamics may return to normal after internal mammary artery implantation but this is uncommon.

A variation of the technic of VINEBERG has been recently proposed [124c]. Postmortem studies suggesting that distal segments of the left anterior descending coronary artery measuring 1.5 mm are normal in most patients with myocardial ischaemia (a fact which has been confirmed pathologically and clinically by JOHNSON et al. [164c]), anastomosis of the internal mammary artery to such distal segments has been performed in 31 patients. Twenty-eight patients have had immediate and complete elimination of the anginal syndrome and marked increase in exercise capacity.

From 1967 onwards, newer procedures by means of autogenous saphenous vein bypass grafts have been proposed for the revascularisation of the ischaemic myocardium. Such procedures include those from the aorta to the right coronary artery, to the left anterior descending coronary artery, to both, as well as to both and the circumflex artery. A total of 677 vein grafts were performed in less than three years by FAVALORO and his group [97c]. Other investigators reported 114 aorta-to-coronary artery saphenous vein bypass grafts in 70 patients [3c]. Thirty-four single, 28 double, and 8 triple bypass grafts were used. They were taken to the right coronary artery (38 times), to the left anterior descending coronary artery (60 times), and to the circumflex coronary artery (16 times). There were 28 patients with three-vessel coronary disease (stenosis greater than 75%) and 15 with two-vessel disease. In spite of this, the operative mortality was only 10%. Relief of symptoms, which occurs without delay, has continued in 81% of the patients.

A third group of surgeons implanted autogenous vein bypass grafts in 75 patients from the aorta to the distal unobstructed coronary arteries [59c]. All experienced exertional angina, 50% with rest or nocturnal angina. All were under medical coronary programs with incomplete control of symptoms. Duration of symptoms ranged from three months to six years. One-third had electrocardiographic evidence of a prior myocardial infarction. One-third had elevated left ventricular end-diastolic pressure. Postoperative course was remarkably uneventful. All living patients with patent grafts experienced complete or marked improvements in symptoms from time of surgery with follow-up to one year.

Recently, JOHNSON and associates [164c and 333c] have been inserting vein bypass grafts into coronary arteries as small as 1.5 mm. Ninety of their 216 patients who have undergone surgery had double or triple vein grafts simultaneously inserted into all areas of the heart. 116 patients have been restudied for angiographic evidence of vein graft patency, from 2 weeks to 14 months after surgery: all vein grafts were patent in 104 and at least one was open in 110. The most important determinant of patency was the size of the recipient vessel: anastomoses to arteries of 2 mm or more were most likely to remain open. None of 30 cases studied later than 5 months after surgery had occluded. Intra-operative flow in the vein graft was measured in 88 cases towards the end of surgery, once the blood pressure had stabilized. Mean flow in each vein ranged from 0 to 185 (mean 63) ml per minute. Size of flow depended mainly upon the size of the vascular bed: by and large, the highest flows were recorded in the grafts to the left anterior descending artery, if the septal and diagonal branches were perfused. Immediate relief of angina occurred in all patients, and in more than 80 % of those who have been recatheterized the patency rate was 90%. Early physiologic evaluation using exercise ergometry and atrial pacing has shown functional improvement consistent with the improvement in the clinical state. The death rate in this series which included a number of very sick people was 14%.

In the opinion of surgeons, the use of aorta-to-coronary artery saphenous vein bypass grafts is widely applicable, very effective, and the safest procedure available for the surgical treatment of coronary artery occlusive disease. This procedure offers the most positive approach to enhancement of the coronary circulation in appropriately selected patients that is yet available. A vein bypass graft to a suitable distal coronary artery provides immediate and prolonged blood supply to ischaemic myocardium, the estimated flow being far greater than that expected from indirect procedures.

The view of cardiologists on revascularisation surgical procedures of the myocardium which are now currently used may be summarized as follows. Although some consider that it becomes increasingly difficult to ignore surgical myocardial revascularisation because it offers not only relief for angina but also the hope of preventing recurrence of infarction [224c], FRIEDBERG [103c] is of the opinion that internal mammary artery implantation is an experimental operation of unproven value with a considerable risk of complications and surgical mortality. The claim that chest pain is relieved in 70—80% of patients is essentially similar to that claimed for a host of previous revascularization procedures which have now been abandoned. There is no convincing evidence of substantial blood flow through the implant and it is doubtful that the flow through the implant significantly benefits the metabolism or function of the ischaemic area. Angiographically patent implants in the dog with experimental coronary occlusion and similar implants for clinical coronary disease were found to contribute little to myocardial blood flow. Studies on myocardial extraction of lactic acid before and after implantation fail to supply specific measurement data or to indicate that determinations were made under identical haemodynamic circumstances, and no formal confirmatory reports from other laboratories have been published. Neither exercise electrocardiographic tests nor exercise performance following implantation showed the benefits claimed by other criteria. Myocardial infarction remains the most important complication reported to be as high as 25% in various series [125c], and implantation may accelerate rather than protect against myocardial infarction. There is no indication that the operation increases longevity. At present, direct reconstructive coronary surgery (aorta-to-coronary vein grafts) appears more promising, but the procedure has not been performed in sufficient numbers over a long enough period of time to enable proper evaluation to be made. Controlled studies, further experience, and longer follow-ups are essential.

With the *factors predisposing* to atherosclerosis, the doctor enters the domain of certain therapeutic possibilities.

a) In the forefront of these factors comes *hypercholesterolaemia* which increases tenfold the risk of coronary atherosclerosis with effect from a proportion of 220 mg % [935, 1101]. Certain people are of the opinion that *hypertriglyceridaemia* is more correlated than hypercholesterolaemia to the frequency and gravity of coronary diseases [212, 1668]. It has in fact been shown that not only the presence but also the severity of coronary atherosclerosis are significantly correlated to the rise in blood triglycerides level [527]. Others [1655] dissociate hypercholesterol-aemia and hypertriglyceridaemia. They consider as hyperlipidaemic those subjects who have either a total cholesterol level exceeding 350 mg % or a triglycerides level exceeding 222 mg % or a *simultaneous* rise in total cholesterol above 300 mg % and in triglycerides above 126 mg %. These hyperlipidaemic subjects are open to the risk of ischaemic heart disease to an extent of 3.5—5 times greater than subjects whose blood levels in these lipides are normal.

Disturbances in the lipido-glucidic metabolism probably constitute the predisposing factor for which therapeutic resources are least effective since they call for constant application if a rapid return to the initial blood cholesterol levels is to be avoided. These therapeutic measures are mainly a diet poor in lipides, and hypocholesterolaemia-inducing medicaments.

Among therapeutic measures intended to combat the symptoms of coronary affections, ever-increasing efforts are, in fact, being made to introduce dietetic and drug treatments with the object of modifying the atherosclerotic terrain by action on the factors, still for the most part little known, responsible for arterial sclerosis; even now, however, the justification for these therapeutic measures still rests on frail experimental evidence. These dietetic conceptions[2] are, in effect, based on the still unproved assumption that reduction of a raised blood cholesterol level could prevent the development of coronary atherosclerotic lesions and even cause regression of such lesions. This assumption rests on experimental and epidemio-logical arguments which suggest a direct relationship between the blood cholesterol level and the extent of atherosclerotic lesions [976, 1861]. The aetiological signific-ance of hypercholesterolaemia is still, however, extremely problematical. In the case of man, no one has so far been able to prove that a diet designed to reduce the level of blood cholesterol is capable of causing arrest or regression of the lesions in atherosclerosis [498]. There is not yet any evidence that the diets and medications which effectively lower high blood cholesterol levels do modify the natural course of atherosclerosis in man [365, 1170]. However, it has been recently shown that a special diet in which a large proportion of saturated fats have been replaced by polyunsaturated fats lowers significantly the incidence of coronary manifestations compared to a control group [327, 1527]. Such conclusions were confirmed when the frequency of coronary modifications of the electrocardiogram and the mortality due to coronaropathy were considered [1906]. It was incidentally demonstrated that this type of diet provokes a very significant drop of the cholesterol blood levels, triglycerides being reduced to a lesser extent.

---

2 Some detailed rules have been recently outlined [1878].

Another important clinical study which has been performed in double blind over a period of 8 years on a group of 846 male subjects [399] demonstrated that a diet rich in unsaturated fats, providing only 60% of ingested cholesterol compared to a control group, not only induced a quick, appreciable and sustained reduction of the blood cholesterol level but was also accompanied by a statistically significant decrease in those clinical complications linked to atherosclerosis which have been considered, namely: myocardial infarction (asymptomatic or evident), sudden death due to coronaropathy, cerebral haemorrhage, sudden death due to cardiac infarction, although the incidence of the last complication taken by itself was not significantly reduced. However, the authors consider that these results do not warrant at this stage a radical change in diet to only polyunsaturated fats, since the effect of these is not clear-cut and their possible harmful effects not established [398].

PAGE and STAMLER [1403] summarized the present consensus as follows: "There are two extremes: diet is nonsense; and diet is crucial. No-one has irrefutable evidence of either. Thus, human beings currently are presented the choice of following a daily special pattern of living, which is far from easy, or forgetting the whole thing. A great majority of people follow the latter choice". And "Lancet" added in a recent editorial [1913]: "Except for reduction of excess weight, the facts at present indicate that they may well be right".

Blood cholesterol level is certainly not the only possible atherogenic factor [906, 976]. A hereditary element is certain [1886, 1987]; obesity [1636] and diet [1391] enter into the picture; emotional stresses [1604, 1606, 1808], a markedly sedentary mode of life, and possibly also tobacco[3] [1803] and alcohol are predisposing factors, but it is extremely difficult at present to assess the part played by these various elements [1596]. Neither blood cholesterol, nor any single dietary factor is solely or mainly responsible for the development of coronary heart disease which is a multifaceted disease of multiple aetiology in which dietary factors, obesity, high blood cholesterol, triglyceride and other lipid levels, heredity, hypertension, diabetes mellitus, mental stress, and physical inactivity are predisposing factors [214c]. Recently published results, based on the definition of coronary heart disease by cinecoronary arteriography, show that definite relationships existed among incidence of coronary heart disease, age, total cholesterol and total triglycerides, with less definite ones between free cholesterol and phospholipids, for a specific group of 450 male patients referred to hospital because of suspected coronary heart disease [241c].

Even medication to reduce high blood cholesterol levels will still require many more years of investigation before a decision can be reached on its ultimate usefulness as an anti-atherogenic agent [1401].

There has been alternate praise for inhibitors of biosynthesis of endogenous cholesterol, such as phenyl acetic acid [368, 370, 626, 1238], benzmalacene [135, 870, 1402], and MER-29 (abandoned because of its toxic effects), for inhibitors of intestinal absorption of cholesterol (e. g. the vegetable sterols including β-Sitosterol), for cholesterol catabolism accelerators, notably the thyroxine-analogues such as DT_4 or dextrothyroxine [340, 64c][4], triiodothyro-acetic acid or Triac and triiodothyro-propionic acid or Triopron [152, 1060, 1092], for cholesterol excretion accelerators (choleretics, resins) or for lipoprotein modifying agents (heparinoids, unsaturated fatty acids). It would seem in order to base certain hopes on Atromid-S or clofibrate, a hypocholesterolaemia- and hypotriglyceridaemia — inducing substance

---

3 See also Cigarette smoking and cardiovascular diseases in *Circulation*, 1960, **22**, 160.
4 Known under the names Dethyron and Choloxin.

[809] which, at the daily dose of 1.5—2 g, effectively controls hyperlipidaemia [796, 1388, 1389] without involving side-effects or any major counter-indications [1625].Two- to five-year monitoring of clofibrate use reveals no serious adverse effects [324 c]. BENDER [21 c] emphasises that clofibrate therapy is more suitable for patients with types III, IV and V hyperlipoproteinaemia who have failed to respond to dietary measures than in other forms. The actual effect of this form of therapy on the incidence of atherosclerosis and its morbid and lethal consequences will probably emerge from extensive clinical investigations being currently carried out.

Despite the considerable and ever-increasing number of recent investigations devoted to this major problem [298 c], we are driven to the conclusion that research into the triggering and predisposing factors in coronary atherosclerosis, although promising [369,1635,1733], is nevertheless only at its initial stage [298 c].Unfortu- nately, it is not yet proved that medication which is genuinely effective in reducing hypercholesterolaemia reduces to any significant degree the advance of atheros- clerosis, and even less that it can prevent its appearance. MODELL [1307, p. 369] recalls that 5 years clinical research has shown that the effective reduction, by oestrogens, in the cholesterol level and in the cholesterol-phospholipide ratio does not make any difference in morbidity and mortality over a large group of patients who have had an infarction. He therefore considers that further clinical proof will have to be awaited before the atherosclerotic or predisposed patient is put on an unpleasant diet or given drugs of dubious effect.

b) The second predisposing factor to coronary atherosclerosis in order of impor- tance is *high blood pressure* which contributes undeniably to the risk of coronary atherosclerosis [1704, 55c], being able according to some authors to go so far as to quadruple it [1101]. Here the doctor has at his disposal, besides the salt-free diet, an impressive choice of antihypertensive medications, too many perhaps but generally of an active nature.

c) In third place come the *metabolic diseases* such as gout, hyperuricaemia, diabetes, obesity and even the hypothyroid condition [101], all of them dysfunc- tions whose incidence on coronary risk is less convincing, although that of hyper- glycaemia would seem obvious to certain observers [499] and that of obesity would appear marked by others [935, 20b]. These predispositions can be com- batted by constantly developing therapeutic means. Prime choice should be given, in the case of the hyperlipidaemic diabetic, to phenformine [1655] since this hypoglycaemia-inducing agent considerably lowers the high percentages of serum lipids in these patients.

d) In fourth place would come *tobacco*, in cigarette form only, which, according to a survey lasting 4.5 years on 3000 subjects, would appear to treble coronary risk as compared with non-smokers [896]. Atherosclerotic involvement of aorta and coronary arteries is greatest in heavy smokers and least in nonsmokers [305 c][5].

---

5 It is not without interest to point out the fact that, for an angina patient who smokes, to smoke a filter-tip cigarette with a high nicotine content shortens by 24% the duration of a standard exercise on a cycloergometer required to trigger off a heart attack [6a]. If the nicotine content is very low, this duration is still shortened by 14% [5a]. Simultaneously, the tension- time index level at which the cardiac pain is triggered off is reduced by 36 and 17% respec- tively [6a]. Conversely, if the exercise is carried out after smoking a nicotine-free cigarette, the anginal pain occurs within the same periods as after an exercise done by the same subjects without smoking a cigarette [7a].

In the same context, it has been reported that smoking two cigarettes during a 5—6 min period, inhaling deeply, aggravates the existing ischaemia in cases with severe coronary artery obstruction [121a].

When the doctor finally finds himself faced with the obvious clinical symptoms of coronary atherosclerosis, that is to say, in the very great majority of cases, the *anginal syndrome*, his role becomes cheering.

To counter the acute attack he has nitroglycerin which up to now has still not found any substitute.

He can use the anticoagulants of the anti-vitamin K type to ward off coronary thrombosis: their long-term effectiveness has not yet been *expressly* proved [451, 597, 743]. As stated by JAFFE [158c], it is not possible at present to definitely conclude from the various published papers exactly what is the true value of anticoagulant therapy in the treatment of coronary ischaemic disease because the majority of reports are not of controlled investigations. While earlier studies indicated a significant decrease in mortality in patients given anticoagulants, later studies have shown no such definite value. This could be due to earlier ambulation of patients more recently which has decreased the risk of pulmonary embolism and infarction even in those patients who do not receive anticoagulants. Whether anticoagulants can also prevent thrombosis in coronary arteries is also now disputed, as thrombosis is initiated by platelet agglutination, which is not affected by anticoagulants. Therefore, the dogmatic opinion that anticoagulant treatment ought to be applied to every person suffering from angina pectoris is not justified, particularly in the light of the risks inherent in this type of therapy [451]. As for heparin, this is particularly effective in cases of emergency.

Finally there remains the wealth of anti-anginal medications administered, in a more or less episodical fashion, in the hope of reducing the number of angina attacks, whatever the mechanisms with which these drugs act, and it will be seen that they can be very different.

Most of these medications have been offered to the doctor on the grounds of their effects as discovered by the pharmacologist, effects to which the latter automatically ascribes the property of improving the conditions for oxygenation of the cardiac muscle. It is in this field that increasing rivalry between applied research laboratories takes on concrete form in the development of drugs whose alleged clinical efficacy does not always carry conviction, far from it.

Despite the many uncertainties which burden both certain biological concepts on the basis of which they have been developed and their clinical benefit, the anti-anginal medications retain a dominant position in the treatment of the angina syndrome. Although many medications have been recommended, few of them have undergone the test of meticulously controlled and multi-centre clinical trials. New medications are submitted periodically to practitioners, which shows how inadequately armed they are to modify to advantage the course of this syndrome.

In this monograph, we are trying to strike the balance of our existing knowledge of the pharmacological effects, the mechanisms which dictate those effects, and the therapeutic advantages of the anti-anginal medications, conventional and modern, even though amongst the latter there are some for which experimental and/or clinical investigations are still too few to enable proper judgment to be passed.

The very great majority, but not all, of these medications have a pharmacological property in common, that of increasing the coronary blood flow in animals and, as a direct consequence, of increasing the amount of oxygen which is made available to the cardiac muscle. This in no way means, as will be seen again and again, that this pharmacological property is at the root of their anti-anginal effect.

2*

This being so, two vital questions arise:

— does the angina patient suffer from myocardial hypoxia in a state of rest and during his painful attack ?

— can the coronary vessels of the angina subject accept any speeding up of blood flow ? If so, and as a corollary, is there any advantage from the therapeutical angle in trying to increase this flow ?

A reply which is probably consistent with reality can be provided to these two questions on the basis of the most up-to-date physiopathological findings as to the haemodynamic and biochemical disturbances which characterise the patient suffering from coronary insufficiency and which are dealt with in Chapter I.

The outline of the pharmacological characteristics and therapeutic properties of the various medications dealt with, which forms the subject matter of Chapter V, should rationally be based on a brief reminder of the essential aspects of cardiovascular physiology in general and of coronary physiology in particular: these make up Chapter II. Chapter III groups the experimental techniques currently used in cardiovascular pharmacology, with a critical essay on their potentials and their limitations. The methods which clinicians advocate and apply in assessing the efficacy of anti-anginal medications for the patient seem just as fundamental: these form the subject of Chapter IV.

Chapter I

Pathophysiology of Angina Pectoris

An extensive amount of fundamental and clinical works have been devoted to the patho-physiological mechanisms which underly the anginal attack. Many conflicting opinions have been put forward since 1809 when Allen BURNS correlated anginal pain and coronary sclerosis and suggested that precordial pain is due to myocardial ischaemia, rather to relative inadaptation of myocardial irrigation to cardiac work.

No formal proof that cardiac ischaemia is the cause of angina pectoris has ever been produced but, on analogy with what happens in skeletal muscle, this logical conception is accepted without discussion. In normal man, pain is produced in voluntary muscles if their blood supply is reduced and the pain recedes again when the arterial circulation is reestablished [1134].

It can readily be admitted that the causative factor in cardiac pain is ischaemia (absolute or relative) developing in the myocardium [965, 1858, 1984]. The best qualified authorities [191, 217, 721, 953, 1102, 1530, 1591] are unanimous in considering that the production of pain arises not necessarily from ischaemia, even relative, of the myocardium, but rather from imbalance in the heart between the supply and demand of oxygen elicited by various causal factors. This means that anginal pain is not necessarily due to reduction in the coronary arterial blood flow but rather to insufficiency of the flow in relation to metabolic requirements or, in other words, non-adaptation of the oxygen supply to the needs of the heart.

Thus, the term "coronary insufficiency" has a functional connotation. It is synonymous with cardiac hypoxia. It is applied to a variety of pathological conditions which do not necessarily involve an alteration of the coronary arteries, although by far the most frequent type of coronary insufficiency is that caused by coronary atherosclerosis ending in vascular obstruction, temporary or permanent [1530]. At this point, it may be interesting to dwell briefly on those cases of angina without coronary disease i.e. individuals with chest pain in whom no arteriographic evidence of coronary disease can be demonstrated, which are discussed by JAMES [159c]. This author, when dealing with this problem, intentionally omits the differential consideration of pain due to other causes than ischaemic heart disease. He considers that some alleged cases of angina without coronary disease are wrong diagnoses of cardiac pain. He draws attention to the fact that in most coronary arteriograms it is not possible to make any interpretations at all concerning small coronary arteries which may be involved by the atherosclerotic process. From his own experience based on examination of coronary arteriograms in cases of angina "without coronary disease", which he was subsequently able to look at post mortem, he has formed the opinion that the most frequent explanation for angina without coronary disease is an incorrect interpretation of the coronary arteriogram, the apparent paradox being most often explained by the presence of abnormal large coronary arteries despite so called normal coronary arteriograms.

There may also be coronary insufficiency in severe anaemia as a result of considerable reduction in the oxygen content of the arterial blood; hyperthyroidism can also engender coronary insufficiency as the excessive and prolonged effort made by the heart increases the work of the myocardium to an extent disproportionate to the increase in coronary blood flow. LEVINE [1117] rightly emphasizes that the conception of myocardial hypoxia as the primary cause of the anginal attack, no matter how brought about, does give support to a number of current clinical observations which would be difficult to explain satisfactorily on the assumption of other mechanisms: first of all, the over-whelming frequency of angina in disease of the coronary arteries; then the occurrence of the anginal syndrome in some cases of severe pernicious anaemia with comparatively normal coronary arteries, the cardiac hypoxia here being referable to a severe reduction in haemoglobin; and thirdly, the disappearance of the anginal syndrome associated with certain cases of severe hyperthyroidism when, as a result of adequate treatment, the oxygen requirements of the heart are reduced in consequence of the lowering of general metabolism [1480]; one might add the impressive improvements that follow radioactive iodine application in euthyroid patients suffering from intractable angina and which are consequent on the reduced functioning of the thyroid [187, 188, 189, 489, 1713]. There are very few authors indeed [341] who do not hold the view that angina pectoris indicates cardiac ischaemia.

Anginal pain can, of course, be provoked or precipitated by all the factors which increase the work of the heart [24], and therefore its oxygen requirements, such as physical exercise, emotions, digestion, generalized hypoxia and so on.

Whether this ischaemia is due, as some believe [1269, 1305], to a functional cause, that is, temporary coronary arteriospasm[1] or, as others believe, more to an anatomical factor (partial or total obstruction of the vascular lumen), or again to the two processes in association, the exact mechanism whereby the hypoxia, acting upon the sensory endings of the cardiac nerves, produces the pain is still unknown[2]. At most one can reasonably assume that the hypoxia or ischaemia does not act by itself as hypoxia induces a considerable increase in the coronary blood flow [833]. It is probable that stimulation of the sensory nerve endings[3] is the work of metabolites of unknown nature which accumulate in the cardiac muscle when it functions in hypoxic conditions [1526]. Called "P factor" by LEWIS, this biochemical stimulus shares with lactic acid some characteristics: it

---

1 This conception of vascular spasm has recently received serious anatomical support in the observations of SCHERLIS and PROVENZA [1472, 1473, 1666] who demonstrated the existence in man and in the dog of muscle sphincters at the level of the arterial capillary circulation in the heart, provided with a nerve supply, which reacted by constriction to adrenaline and noradrenaline, and by relaxation to nitroglycerin. The hypothesis of coronary spasm has been evoked particularly to explain cases of angina pectoris and sudden death in which definite disease of the coronary arteries could not be found at autopsy [1b]. Sphincter-like muscles have been described at the orifice of the right coronary artery in man [4b], and it is conceivable that their contraction could markedly impair blood flow in the myocardium supplied by this vessel. Coronary arteriospasm has been proposed as a mechanism whereby angina might arise without atherosclerotic coronary disease. Spasm of a major coronary vessel seems to offer a logical explanation for attacks of angina pectoris that occurred at rest and were not associated, as it is commonly the case, with tachycardia, elevation of the blood pressure or other evidences of decreased coronary blood flow or increased cardiac work [1b]. In such cases, the sudden occurrence and prompt subsidence of the episodes and the quick relief afforded by vasodilator drugs seemed to support the theory of spasm. It is possible that spasm could result from the direct effect of catecholamines or other circulating humoral substances on the smooth muscle of the arteries or that it could be induced by vasomotor reflex impulses. However, spasm of the coronary arteries has not been consistently associated with the occurrence of anginal pain in patients with either diseased or normal vessels [1b].

2 The intensity of the anginal pain may be explained by the extreme richness of the coronary capillaries in nerve elements, which may also be provided with centripetal axone nerves which are in direct contact with the capillary wall [988].

3 See RINZLER [1526] and particularly the reviews by WHITE [1983] and by GORLIN [696] for the anatomy of the nerve paths traversed by cardiac pain.

is acid, is destroyed by both alcalis and oxydation, and it is formed the most rapidly in conditions of anoxia and of carbonic acid accumulation [191]. The present concept of pain holds that with ischaemia, various pain-producing substances or substances akin to or identical with the plasma kinins, are activated, possibly by kallikrein released from ischaemic or inflamed tissue [754]. Concentration of such substances is intensified by stagnation of blood flow, and their action to produce pain is augmented by heightened local concentration of H^+ or K^+ [479], a likely interstitial consequence of cellular hypoxia. However, GORLIN [696] points out that this theory does not answer three discrepancies:

a) pain is uncommon with acute myocarditis as opposed to myocardial ischaemia, and inflammation is notorious in releasing pain-producing substances;

b) generalized ischaemia of the heart as a whole may not necessarily cause pain, and yet a small area of ischaemia may result in major discomfort;

c) similar degrees of chemical ischaemia (seen in the same patient) may or may not initiate pain. Moreover, it has been recently demonstrated that pain is not due to the activation of bradykininogen, by muscular ischaemia, which would release bradykinine [172].

Others suggest that adenosine (which probably plays an important role in the autoregulation of coronary circulation, see p. 60) or ADP (which induces a severe thoracic pain when injected in man [391]) could be the substance which is responsible of the alarm pain [1253].

In the opinion of some investigators, the cause of anginal pain is most likely electrical in nature and the electricity is created at the plane of contact between ischaemic and non-ischaemic muscle [278c]. While uniformity of blood supply is not painful and electrical formation is stable, lack of uniformity is painful and electrical formation is unstable. Although these data are based upon experiments performed in open chest dogs under anaesthesia, and the relationship between the experiment and the human is therefore only speculative, the authors think that their data deserve consideration.

Myocardial hypoxia is associated with certain characteristic changes in the electrocardiogram; there is depression of the S-T segment with, additionally, depression or inversion of the T wave.

In angina these electrocardiographic alterations can often be produced by physical exercise[4], by an experimentally controlled hypoxia, and sometimes even by a simple emotion [257]. In animals, large doses of pituitrine, which induce coronary vasoconstriction, lead to electrocardiographic changes similar to those seen in man in angina [1268].

These pathophysiological considerations have a logical therapeutic corollary. The anginal syndrome is of course amenable to ordinary analgesic treatment and anginal pain can be effectively controlled with drugs devoid of increasing effects upon coronary blood flow [1591], such as analgesics (e.g. morphine), central sedatives (e.g. alcohol), tranquillizers (e.g. meprobamate), euphoretics (e.g. MAOI) or purely psychological remedies (e.g. a placebo). Rational angina therapy must, however, aim to increase the quantity of blood supplied to the myocardium (see p. 27). Again, it is essential that the action of the desired coronary vasodilator should be unaccompanied by stimulating effects on the myocardium which are liable to increase the oxygen consumption of the heart at a rate equal to or greater than the increase in coronary blood flow, or by general hypotensive

---

4 A close relationship exists between magnitude of exercise S—T segment depression and indices (tension-time index or Robinson's index) expressing myocardial oxygen requirements [81c]. Thus, like onset of exercise induced-angina, magnitude of S—T depression is usually related to haemodynamic factors influencing myocardial oxygen needs.

effects which could reduce the coronary perfusion pressure. It is not sufficient that a drug to be used in angina improves the coronary flow; it is essential that this favourable effect should not be marred by cardiac or systemic effects leading to any considerable increase in the oxygen requirements.

The functional role of the coronary circulation is to adapt itself to the needs of the myocardium and what matters is not so much the absolute value of the increase of coronary flow produced by a particular substance as the manner in which both the coronary flow and at the same time the oxygen requirements of the myocardium are modified.

The essential point in favour of a substance as a coronary vasodilator must be the coronary efficiency, now the relation between the blood supply to the myocardium and the oxygen required by the heart to enable it to perform its work. The coronary efficiency will only be improved if, when the arterial blood supply increases, the nutritional requirements are reduced, unchanged or only slightly increased. As it will be seen in the following chapter, assessment of changes in the coronary supply alone is not an adequate criterion by which to judge the coronary balance. It is therefore mandatory, when it is desired to make an accurate assessment of the potential therapeutic importance of a substance, that at least simultaneous changes in coronary flow and in myocardial metabolism should be considered [953, 957, 1269].

Since anginal pain does not necessarily reflect reduction in coronary arterial blood flow, one of the most fundamental deductions which derives therefrom is that myocardial irrigation is not necessarily impaired in coronary atherosclerosis, when the patient is at rest and during the acute anginal attack. As a matter of fact, although JOHNSON and SEVELIUS [903] found in 1960, by using a radioisotopic method, that the coronary blood flow was only half of normal in coronary patients at rest, it seems that these data do not correspond with reality because, by using more precise methods, it has been showed since then, on several occasions, that coronary blood flow is, at rest *absolutely normal* in the anginous patient [698, 1288, 1953]. Although the report of this fact surprised both clinicians and investigators, this finding was confirmed in 1968 by BING [167], who, by using a new isotopic method of clinical determination of coronary blood flow in man that provides accurate and reproducible results (see p. 82), measured a mean coronary blood flow of 222 ± 17 ml/min for 31 normal subjects and of 245 ± 17 ml/min for 17 patients with coronary artery disease. If such results seem astonishing at first sight, this should not however surprise on further consideration since all evidence points to the strict dependence of flow on the oxygen needs of the myocardium, and the haemodynamic factors which govern this are unchanged in anginous patients, even with severe coronary atherosclerosis [281, 1578]. Moreover, as pointed out by ROWE et al. [1578], the real resistance to flow lies peripherally in the coronary arterioles and precapillary sphincters, which are not affected by the degenerative process, rather than in the region of the atherosclerotic plaques.

However, according to a very recent report published in late 1969 by BING himself [27a], a new dimension might be given to this important physiological problem. Measuring the coronary blood flow with his coincidence counting technique and using rapid bolus injections of Rb^{84} (see p. 82) instead of Rb^{84} intravenous infusion at a constant rate for a prolonged period of time which gave him the abovementioned results, he found that there was a significant difference ($p < 0.001$) in resting myocardial blood flow between normal and coronary patients: flow was 28.7 per cent less in coronary heart disease patients than in normal subjects, the figures being respectively for two groups of 24 subjects: 237 ± 14.3 ml/min and 169 ± 9.0 ml/min. The mean values for myocardial blood flow in paired determinations being reproducible within 2.1% under control conditions in another group of 13 patients, it could be considered that the impairement of the myocardial state caused by coronary atherosclerosis is accompanied by a significantly reduced coronary blood flow.

At the last world congress of cardiology (London, Sept. 1970) two reports have confirmed that resting coronary blood flow is reduced in human coronary artery disease. The first one was by KLOCKE et al. [181c]. Since conventional inert gas measurements of coronary blood flow have shown no difference between patients with and without coronary artery disease, the possibility that a difference exists but has been masked by methodological difficulties was evaluated using multiple gas tracers, variable saturation periods and chromatographic measurements of blood tracer concentrations. Arterial and coronary sinus desaturation curves were obtained after 2—20 minute exposures to various combinations of helium, neon, hydrogen, methane, argon, krypton and nitrous oxide. It was found that the ability to detect prolonged venous-arterial differences reflecting localized areas of abnormally low flow was directly related to duration of saturation, sensitivity of chromatographic techniques and duration of observation during desaturation. When prolonged venous-arterial differences were included, resting coronary blood flow was found to be significantly lower in 23 patients with arteriographically proven coronary artery disease than in 17 patients with arteriographically normal coronary arteries, values being respectively 55 ± 9 ml/min/100 g and 77 ± 16 ml/min/100 g ($p < 0.01$). This difference was not apparent when the same curves were analyzed using conventional criteria. Reduced coronary blood flow in coronary patients at rest was also found by DI MATTEO et al. [83c], by direct measurement from intracardiac dilution curves of two isotopes (Rubidium and Technecium) which were simultaneously injected into the sub-clavian vein, the two dilution curves being recorded by the same scintillation detector connected with two different electronic systems, and the coronary blood flow being obtained as the difference between the two left peak surfaces of the dilution curves.

Facing these conflicting reports, the divergences arising probably from the different methodological procedures which have been used, it is hoped that subsequent investigations will throw more light on this fundamental question and give a consistent answer to this aspect of the physiopathology of the coronary circulation.

1. Pathophysiology of the Anginal Attack

What happens at the moment when the anginal subject has his attack? The balance which exists, when at rest, between the oxygen requirements of the myocardium and the amount of oxygen supplied to it is abruptly upset, thus creating the conditions of coronary insufficiency in the functional sense of the term.

It has been possible to show that this balance is upset *more by the fact of an increased demand for oxygen* than because of any incapacity of the coronary circulation to increase its output, i.e. supply of oxygen.

It is during angina-inducing effort that the physiological differences between the coronary circulation of the normal subject and that of the angina patient have been able to be clearly demonstrated. It is known that effort increases the work of the heart and its oxygen requirements by the combined action of three phenomena: increase in cardiac output, the speeding up of the heart rate, and the rise in blood pressure.

During exertion, the normal subject and the angina subject react very differently as shown in Fig. 1 drawn along lines indicated by MESSER [1288]. In the case of the normal subject, myocardial oxygen consumption increases, the coronary flow increases, but the oxygen content in the coronary *venous* blood remains remarkably *unchanged*. This stability of the coronary venous oxygen content means that the increase in the oxygen requirements of the heart is fully met by the rise in arterial flow *without the extraction of oxygen by the myocardium becoming more pronounced*. It will be seen in Chapter II that, in the case of the normal subject, there is a remarkable linear relation between the myocardial oxygen consumption and the coronary flow, and that this can increase as much as fivefold under conditions of violent exertion, a fact which demonstrates the existence of a large reserve of myocardial hyperirrigation by vasodilatation (see p. 56).

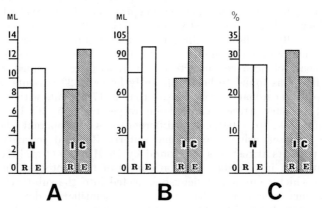

Fig. 1. Effect of exercise on: A: myocardial oxygen consumption (ml/100 g). B: coronary blood flow (ml/100 g). C: oxygen content of coronary venous blood (% of saturation). N: normal subjects. I.C.: patients with coronary insufficiency. R: values at rest. E: values during exercise. (MESSER and NEILL, 1288)

Patients presenting coronary insufficiency reveal the following characteristics during effort: myocardial oxygen consumption increases to a greater extent than in the case of normal subjects[5]. Coronary flow increases largely in the same manner as for healthy subjects, a fact important in itself which has since been confirmed [855] and which, according to certain authors [695], is in fact characterised by a greater increase than is the case for normal subjects[6].

But, and this more than anything else distinguishes the anginal from the healthy subject, *the oxygen content of the coronary venous blood is over 20% less* [1288, 1842, 1953]. This fact is of capital importance since it means that, unlike

---

5 This fact has been confirmed in late 1970 by CONTI et al. [3d] in patients with coronary artery disease in whom artificial tachycardia induced by atrial pacing resulted in a typical anginal attack: whereas myocardial oxygen consumption increased from an average of 6.31 ml/min/100 g at rest to 8.93 ml/min/100 g during pacing (non-significant difference) in patients who did not develop angina, it rose from an average of 6.4 ml/min/100 g at rest to 11.03 ml/min/100 g during pacing (significant difference at $p < 0.01$) in patients who presented angina.

6 Again, this phenomenon has been confirmed in late 1970 by CONTI et al. [3d] in patients with coronary artery disease in whom angina was provoked by pacing-induced tachycardia: during pacing, myocardial blood flow (which was measured by the selective injection of ^{133}Xe into the left coronary artery) increased by an average of 12 ml/min/100 g in patients who did not develop angina while it rose by 32 ml/min/100 g in patients who presented angina.

what occurs in the healthy subject, the extraction of oxygen by the myocardium, already at a very high level in the resting state (see Chap. II), is increased in cases of coronary insufficiency during exertion. This phenomenon is indicative of an inadequate coronary reserve and of the exhaustion of the reserve of arterial dilatation, this despite the presence of an increased flow, this not being sufficient to satisfy fully the increase in oxygen demands. COHEN et al. [346] have also shown that, during the angina episode brought on by exercise, the cardiac output and the stroke volume increase significantly less than is the case with the healthy subject. This lowered efficiency of cardiac contraction would appear to be due to a relative insufficiency of oxygen supply.

Another major characteristic of the angina patient relates to the metabolism of lactic acid. We know that the normal heart uses lactic acid as an energy-producing substrate [1667] and that during exercise its percentage increases in the arterial blood. The heart of the normal person extracts it to a greater extent but without every producing any, since its function is entirely aerobic. The reaction of the anginal subject to effort is quite different. His myocardium *produces lactate* [1033], as indicated by the fact that the latter is present in greater quantity in the coronary venous blood than in the arterial blood [345]. This phenomenon proves that the increase in oxygen extraction is not sufficient to meet the extra requirement in oxygen. The metabolism of the myocardium becomes partly anaerobic, and for this reason part of the glycolysis is diverted to the production of lactic acid [488, 1667][7]. It has also been shown that this production of lactate on the part of the anginal patient is greater as the arterial lesions are more serious, so much so that the measurement of the increase in lactic acid content of the coronary venous blood during effort provides a means for quantifying the functional metabolic deviation of the myocardium caused by coronary disease[8]. Advantage has been taken of this fact to get an indication of the extent of coronary functional capacity, in other words of the marginal state of myocardial oxygenation which results therefrom.

With the quantitative determination of excess lactic acid, the clinician is able for the first time, and this notion is a recent one since it dates from late 1966 [488, 696], to carry out a biological examination which makes it possible to assess the gravity of coronary lesions, the extent of lactate production being bound up with the morphological severity and location of the lesions [345]. It does however call for the application of an exploration method which is not yet currently used: the catheterisation of the coronary sinus of an angina patient subjected to a form of exercise. It should be pointed out that it is preferable to use the expression "standardized angina-inducing stress" rather than "exercise" since quite recent research would indicate that it does not seem immaterial what method is adopted for stimulating the myocardium to see lactate production occur in an angina patient during an attack. Indeed, PARKER et al. [1417] consider that if physical exercise is used to bring on an anginal attack, lactate production is very variable.

---

7 There is a striking analogy with observation on a dog: myocardial ischaemia generalised at the left ventricle is accompanied by accelerated glycolysis as testified by an increase in glucose consumption and the production of lactate [209]. Similarly, very localised ischaemia caused by the ligature of a small branch of the anterior interventricular artery is reflected in a discharge of lactic acid into the venous blood coming from this zone, with a considerable increase in the lactate/pyruvate ratio and a reduction in glucose level [1394].

8 Since accurate measurement of the small changes which occur in the coronary sinus blood should allow a more objective assessment of the presence and severity of ischaemia than can be made by other existing methods, an improvement on the conventional enzymatic method for lactate determinations has been recently proposed, the recovery of lactate being virtually 100%, and linear over a range of prepared lactate standards [207c].

Although the cardiac pain brought on by the intravenous injection of iso-prenaline more frequently leads to lactate production than does physical effort [73, 346, 817], PARKER et al. [1414] find that it is tachycardia caused by atrial pacing by the BALCON and FRICK method (see p. 99) which most frequently sets up lactate production during the angina pain which thus occurs. NEILL [1354] arrives at an identical conclusion, since if the oxygen requirements of the myo-cardium are increased not by muscular exercise but by artificially speeding up the heart rate by sinus pacing, it is found that, unlike what occurs in the case of the healthy subject where the lactate/pyruvate ratio in the coronary venous blood does not vary, this ratio increases sharply in the angina patient by a rise in lactate content, which indicates the presence of myocardial hypoxia without oxygen desaturation of the coronary venous blood necessarily becoming more pronounced.

The evidence that anaerobic metabolism characterises subjects developing angina pectoris during right atrial pacing has been recently confirmed by HEL-FANT et al. [60a] under convincing conditions. When pacing was performed in 39 patients with coronary heart disease, 18 developed angina. When data collected from these anginal patients were compared with their own rest state and also with the group which did not develop angina, it was found that there was highly significant difference in lactate metabolism: in the anginal group, mean extraction of 18.4% dropped to become 13.2% production, but no marked change occurred in the other group. When angina was relieved by stopping pacing, lactate meta-bolism returned to the at-rest levels in 4 subjects within a comparable period of time. Furthermore, the cardiac index fell significantly during pacing in the anginal group, but did not alter in the non-anginal group.

Myocardial electrolyte balance and lactate metabolism were studied in 30 pa-tients before, during, and after a period of atrial pacing [243c]. Eight patients with coronary artery disease who had no symptoms during pacing and four normal subjects demonstrated myocardial potassium loss but no abnormalities in lactate metabolism, the electrocardiogram, and haemodynamics during pacing. Myocar-dial potassium loss was correlated with increments in heart rate and was followed by potassium uptake during the post-pacing period. Eighteen subjects developed angina during pacing associated with haemodynamic and electrocardiographic abnormalities. This ischaemic group showed significantly greater myocardial potassium loss during pacing than the non-ischaemic group, and this was closely associated with myocardial lactate production at a ratio of 1 mEq of potassium being lost for each 2 millimoles of lactate produced. Increased acidity of coronary sinus blood also accompanied potassium loss during ischaemia. No significant changes were seen in sodium balance in either group during the study. These investigations show that potassium is lost by the heart during tachycardia induced by atrial pacing in man. This loss appears abruptly after an increase in heart rate and decreases progressively during the period of tachycardia. Whatever the mechanism of potassium loss during tachycardia, the abrupt uptake of potas-sium with the return to a normal rate is of considerable interest. This prompt uptake also occurred in the ischaemic group following cessation of pacing. This rapid restoration of potassium loss insures an early return to a normal intracellular concentration of potassium.

The greater and more sustained increase of potassium levels in coronary sinus blood in the ischaemic group than in the non-ischaemic patients suggests that myocardial ischaemia leads to potassium loss in addition to that due to an increase in heart rate. The possibility that anoxic red blood cells might contribute to the high coronary sinus concentration of potassium should be ruled out because this factor was measured in experimental ischaemia [56c] and was found not to be of significance. The net potassium loss may have been even greater than that suggested by the arterial-coronary sinus difference since coronary blood flow increases by approximately 32 ml/min/100 g of left ventricle in patients with pacing-induced ischaemia [67c]. These changes in potassium balance due to inadequate oxygen supply are probably the result of interference with the ATP-dependent cation exchange mechanism [292c].

The reasons for the differences which exist, as regards the rate of lactate production by the myocardium, between muscular exercise, atrial pacing of the heart rate and the injection of isoprenaline as artificial methods of triggering an anginal pain in a coronary subject are not yet clear, and warrant the additional research which PARKER proposes to carry out. He does point out however that the increase in the level of lactate in the coronary venous blood resulting from the induced tachycardia occurs very rapidly and before the cardiac pain, which would suggest that, under myocardial hypoxia conditions, the lactate passes freely through the membrane of the cardiac cell [1414], contrary to what occurs under satisfactory oxygenation conditions [670].

It is interesting to point out that the mean resting transmyocardial lactic dehydrogenase difference in coronary heart disease patients does not differ significantly from non-coronary subjects [112a]. Furthermore, no correlation was observed in coronary patients during isoproterenol infusion or stress-induced angina between transmyocardial lactic dehydrogenase and lactate levels, despite significant stress-induced lactate production. It was therefore concluded that transmyocardial lactic dehydrogenase levels do not distinguish coronary from non-coronary subjects, and have no value in quantifying the severity of coronary artery disease [112a].

To return then to the question of the diagnosis of coronary diseases by artificial inducement of anginal pain, whatever the method used, this type of clinical examination still deserves to be introduced into cardiological clinics — particularly in the form of atrial pacing of the heart rate which, in the Anglo-Saxon countries, is assuming an increasingly important role in methods for cardiac exploration (see p. 99) — when we bear in mind the inaccuracy of the quantitative functional diagnosis suggested by certain people on the basis of purely clinical criteria [944]: the carrying out of a "maximum" exercise on an endless track would enable a distinction to be made between the normal subject and a clinical coronary case by the fact that the capacity for exercise, maximum tachycardia and maximum systolic blood pressure are "less" in the coronary subject, the two latter phenomena reflecting the weakening of the chronotropic and inotropic cardiac reserves. As for the angina subject, he is "significantly more weakened" than the asymptomatic coronary subject. As regards the functional assessment of the gravity of coronary disease, we should point out here that, without resorting to intracardiac exploration, SOLVAY [1775] advocates another original technique whose details will be outlined later since it comes better under the methods for diagnosing anginal pain (see p. 97).

All the features of the physiological behaviour of the anginal subject which we have just mentioned provide a clear reply to the two fundamental questions propounded at the end of the preceding Section "Coronary Atherosclerosis: General Considerations" (see p. 18).

a) There is in fact an advantage in increasing oxygenation of the angina subject's myocardium, either *directly* by increasing arterial irrigation, or *indirectly* by reducing its oxygen requirements, or better still by combining the two effects. It follows that, from the medicinal viewpoint, any substance which reduces the workload of the heart, and thereby its oxygen requirements, is in theory likely to be effective for the angina pectoris subject [1571]. Even so, this effect must stem from cardiovascular changes (e.g. reduction in peripheral arterial resistance, slowing up of the heart rate) which lessen the work of the heart without impairing its haemodynamic performance, and not from biochemical processes which result in inhibiting myocardial cellular respiration. The potential advantages of such a medicament are increased if myocardial blood irrigation is increased simultaneously, since the oxygen supply to the cardiac muscle is thereby raised.

b) As far as the answer to the second question is concerned, it is obvious that the coronary flow of the angina subject can in fact increase under certain conditions. This is primarily the case during exercise, as we have just seen. It is also the case under other circumstances. For instance, it has been shown that, as with the healthy subject, the intravenous infusion of adrenaline at the dose of 2.5 μg/min for 15—20 min causes in the coronary patient with significant stenotic or occlusive lesions disclosed by coronary arteriography (whose indications are in excellent correlation with post-mortem anatomical lesions, 1854), an increase in cardiac output and myocardial oxygen consumption, together with a 37% rise in coronary flow, secondary to the increase in the metabolic needs of the myocardium [1854]. Since the increase in coronary flow is not accompanied by changes in blood pressure, adrenaline may thus be considered as a vaso-dilator according to the commonly accepted criteria [732]. These cardiovascular effects of adrenaline are virtually identical to the changes in coronary circulation occurring during exercise.

It has also been shown that the *intracoronary* injection of nitroglycerin increases by 50% the coronary flow of the angina patient where a coronarography has revealed the presence of advanced stenotic atherosclerosis [146]. Again in the case of nitroglycerin, BING [27a] has shown very recently that in 24 patients with coronary heart disease (clinical myocardial infarction in 14, or typical angina pectoris with appropriate resting electrocardiographic changes or abnormal post-exercise electrocardiograms in 10, coronary involvement being confirmed by coronary arteriography in 12 patients), the *sublingual* administration of nitroglycerin significantly increased the myocardial blood flow by 21% after 45 sec and by 11.4% after 90 sec (see p. 126).

Finally, CONTI et al. [3d] published in 1970 an interesting report dealing with the behaviour of myocardial blood flow during angina which was provoked in patients with coronary artery disease by speeding up the heart rate by atrial pacing. Myocardial blood flow was determined by the selective injection of radioactive ^{133}Xe into the left coronary artery. While it seems logical to expect that patients with myocardial ischaemia produced by pacing would not be able to increase coronary blood flow to balance increased oxygen requirements, a totally unexpected finding was the significantly greater increase in myocardial blood flow in patients who presented angina during pacing compared to that of patients who did not develop cardiac pain: blood flow increased by an average of 12 ml/min/100 g in patients who did not develop angina whereas, in patients who presented angina during pacing, myocardial blood flow increased by an average of 32 ml/min/100 g, which represents an average augmentation of 50%. This finding is best explained by a vasodilator response to acute ischaemia.

These many examples of increase in myocardial flow in the patient suffering from coronary atherosclerosis do show that the opinion of those clinicians who claim the *fixed character* of the sclerosed arterial network takes little account of the functional tests which, on the contrary, patently prove that the *sclerosed* coronary system can allow of a considerable increase in coronary flow by vasodilation.

From the therapeutic angle, there is thus every advantage in trying to increase the coronary flow in the anginal subject since a reduction in myocardial hypoxia is thereby brought about. It would therefore seem desirable to have available medications which, in addition to their other pharmacological effects, clearly and selectively decrease coronary arterial resistance.

Recent clinical investigations have cast some light on the physiological mechanisms of anginal pain, in that fresh facts have been brought forward regarding the haemodynamic conditions under which anginal pain occurs. ROBINSON [1544] has shown that, in a given patient, the anginal pain always starts with a combination of cardiovascular disturbances which is remarkably constant during each attack. These haemodynamic conditions are represented by the product of the heart rate by systolic arterial pressure which both rise. In a given patient, each anginal attack always corresponds to a given level of this heart rate x blood pressure index, whether the painful attack is brought on by physical exercise or by a mental arithmetic calculation, or whether it occurs spontaneously. These observations suggest then that the development of the anginal episode can be related to the attainment of a critical level in this index, the latter being remarkably *constant* for each patient although varying considerably from patient to patient. Furthermore, it is interesting to note that this relation persists even when, with a given patient, there are wide variations in the characteristics of the angina-inducing stress: type, intensity and duration.

A further important fact has been demonstrated by ROBINSON, namely that a variation in tolerance to effort does not have any repercussion on the critical level of the pressure x heart rate index at which the pain starts.

If we examine the physiopathological significance of these data provided by ROBINSON, it is necessary to anticipate the notions of physiology which will be developped in Chapter II, namely that the heart rate and systolic blood pressure are amongst the essential determining factors in myocardial oxygen consumption [644, 979, 1316, 1355, 1644]. It follows that the product of these two factors is in strict correlation with the amount of oxygen consumed by the myocardium and that it can be considered as the expression of the internal, metabolic, working of the myocardium.

The constant nature of the heart rate x pressure index which is attained by a given anginal subject at the moment he develops his pain, means therefore that each painful attack occurs at an *identical level of myocardial oxygen consumption*. ROBINSON's findings also show that the normal cause of the anginal attack lies in an increase in the oxygen requirements of the myocardium to a critical level, which is fixed for each patient.

A further consideration arises from these clinical observations, namely that the anginal attack is conditioned by the extent of the work of *the myocardium* and not by that of the physical work done by the patient. The relationship between these two types of work is not necessarily constant. Indeed, the levels of heart rate and blood pressure reached during physical exercise of a given nature are not fixed: they may vary widely because of the interplay, to a varying degree, of different factors such as emotion, ambient temperature, etc. It follows that the *same physical work* carried out at different times can correspond to very *different levels of cardiac work*. It is not then surprising that the triggering of the anginal pain can often seem very capricious to the clinician [165c] if he refers solely to the extent of the *external stress* to which the patient is subjected.

In the same context, a further item of information is deserving of note. We know that nitroglycerin has the property of increasing physical performance in the angina patient: after taking nitroglycerin, he is able to accomplish much greater effort before the heart attack occurs. ROBINSON has shown that this improvement in physical effort is associated with a *lower level* of the heart rate x pressure index for a given work, whatever the amount of work done. These findings, which have been confirmed by MACALPIN and colleagues [1244], indicate that the increase in angina-inducing effort which reflects the beneficial effect of nitroglycerin can be related to a reduction in the heart rate x pressure index. It goes without saying that, under these conditions, the patient can produce more work before the combined rise in his blood pressure and heart rate reaches the critical level at which the painful attack occurs.

The proof that a clinically improved angina subject, whatever the method used to achieve this, does not experience angina pain even at higher effort heart rate because the *critical* level of oxygen consumption by his myocardium is not reached has been provided by FRICK et al. [592] who show that, during the speed-up in heart rate produced by atrial pacing bringing the normal rate up to almost double, the angina subject on nitroglycerin, whilst not suffering any heart attack, does not reach the myocardial oxygen consumption level (measured by the SARNOFF tension-time index) at which, in the absence of nitroglycerin, the angina pain occurs.

2. Cardiac Dynamics During the Anginal Attack

In 1970, CROSS [68c] rightly pointed out that until recently, little was known about the haemodynamic and physiologic events which are associated with angina [1568]. In recent years, however, far-reaching pathophysiological investigations have been devoted to this important question and they have demonstrated that the functioning of the heart is depressed during the anginal attack.

According to PARKER et al. [1415, 1418], angina-inducing exercise causes a marked rise in the left end-diastolic ventricular pressure (confirmed by MCCALLISTER et al., [1245], and by O'BRIEN et al., [1384]) and in the pulmonary arterial pressure. These findings corroborate others [431, 1213, 1328] but run counter to those of COHEN et al. [346]. PARKER believes that the divergences between his findings and those of COHEN are perhaps explained by the fact that his patients were at a more advanced stage of their heart disease. In any event, he shares COHEN's opinion in the sense that, during the attack of effort angina pectoris, the left ventricular function is lowered[9], as witness the subnormal rise in the cardiac index, the increase in left end-diastolic ventricular pressure, and the increase in pulmonary arterial pressure. This left functional deficiency is best reflected in the relationship between the stroke work and the end-diastolic ventricular pressure,

---

9 From the experimental angle, this tallies with the findings of certain authors [1338] who report a marked lowering of myocardial contractility at the ischaemic cardiac region drawing its supplies from the coronary artery previously occluded with an Ameroid type device in a dog kept alive. Similar findings are reported by ENRIGHT et al. [91c] who evaluated the immediate functional deficit resulting from acute regional myocardial ischaemia in 40 anaesthetised dogs. Ventricular function curves, maximum dp/dt, isovolumetric force-velocity curves, and peak systolic and resting diastolic length-tension curves were assessed at fixed heart rate and constant aortic pressure before and during occlusion of the anterior descending coronary artery 2—3 cm distal to its origin. Mild, moderate, or marked depression of the ventricular function resulted from occlusion of the anterior descending artery, depending upon the anatomy of the intercoronary collateral vessels. Maximum loss of function was apparent 2 min after occlusion, and was quantitatively reproducible by reocclusion after an intervening period of unobstructed flow. Resting diastolic length-tension relations were not significantly altered by occlusion of the anterior descending artery. In 12 dogs, force-velocity relations were determined during the inscription of ventricular function curves and in every instance when depressed function was evident from the ventricular function curve, the simultaneously determined force-velocity curve also demonstrated impaired performance.

since this work does not increase significantly in spite of a markedly increased left ventricular filling pressure.

In a subsequent publication [1414] PARKER points out that stroke work of the left ventricle decreases, which would indicate, in the light of the fact that the end-diastolic pressure does not decrease in the same proportions, that the ischaemic ventricle of the angina subject works to a depressed functional curve as compared with that of a normal ventricle. PARKER has also demonstrated that similar haemodynamic changes occur in the coronary patient in whom an attack of angina has been induced by atrial pacing of the heart rate [1416]: the left ventricle contracts along a depressed functional curve, and this ventricular depression can be reversed by stopping the stimulation and returning the heart rate to its normal level.

In a further very recent study [179c], PARKER and his colleagues compared and specified the haemodynamic response to exercise and atrial pacing in the same patients. There were 20 patients with coronary artery disease and 7 normal subjects. Angina developed in 13 patients during pacing and exercise, but was absent in 7 patients during both tests. During exertional angina, the average left ventricular end-diastolic pressure rose from 8 to 32 mm Hg and the stroke work fell. This signifies that the ischaemic left ventricle was operating on a depressed ventricular function curve. The elevated left ventricular end-diastolic pressure may have been due in part to decreased compliance during myocardial ischaemia but was probably related more to an augmentation in left ventricular volume. Such a change would increase myocardial fiber length which, by the LAPLACE relation, would raise oxygen consumption. This rise would be in addition to the normal heightening in left ventricular oxygen requirements during exercise related to the catecholamine release, increase in heart rate, systemic pressure and rate of fiber shortening [1116, 1789].

There was also clear evidence of depressed left ventricular function during myocardial ischaemia induced by pacing. Since there was no change in cardiac index and only minor changes in systemic pressure, there was an associated decline in stroke index and left ventricular stroke work inversely related to the change in heart rate. In the normal subjects and in those without angina, the decrease in left ventricular stroke work with pacing was accompanied by a fall in left ventricular end-diastolic pressure according to the STARLING relation. In contrast, however, the patients with angina during pacing showed no fall in left ventricular end-diastolic pressure in the face of similar reductions in stroke work. This abnormal pressure could be in part due to decreased compliance of the ischaemic ventricle, but it is more reasonable to consider that it is operating on a depressed functional curve. With interruption of pacing, the heart rate returned abruptly to normal and, assuming no change in cardiac index, there was an increase in left ventricular stroke work [1416]. In the groups with and without angina the left ventricular end-diastolic pressure returned to normal, but in the presence of myocardial ischaemia this post-pacing pressure rose to grossly abnormal levels. This is further evidence that the ischaemic ventricle is operating on a depressed ventricular function curve.

The performance characteristics of the left ventricle during pacing and exercise for the three groups are shown in Fig. 2. The normal group and the group without angina reacted similarly during pacing and in the immediate post-pacing period. However, during exercise there was a distinct separation of these two groups because in the normal group there was a shift to an augmented ventricular function curve, but in the group without angina there was an upward movement on the original curve: the increase in stroke work during exercise was thus accompanied by increased fiber length implying abnormal left ventricular function. Furthermore, it is also clear from this study that in coronary patients in whom angina was not precipitated by exercise or pacing, that is, the group without angina, functional abnormality of the left ventricle was demonstrated only during

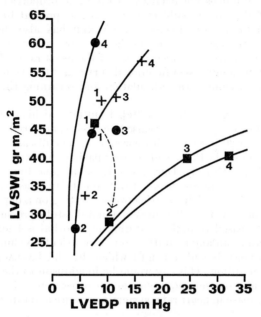

Fig. 2. Relation between the left ventricular end-diastolic pressure (LVEDP) and the left ventricular stroke work index (LVSWI) in three groups of patients (PARKER et al., [1416] and [179c]). Circles: normal group. Squares: angina group. Crosses: non-angina group. In the three groups: 1: during control period. 2: during atrial pacing. 3: during immediate post-pacing period. 4: during exercise. *During atrial pacing:* a) In the normal group, the decrease in LVSWI accompanying the increase in heart rate during pacing is associated with a reduction in LVEDP according with the Starling relationship. b) The group without angina reacts in the same way as the normal group. c) The patients in the angina group, in spite of a similar decrease in LVSWI during pacing, show no change in LVEDP and thus change from a normal to an abnormal ventricular function curve when ischaemia develops. The abnormal relationship between LVEDP and LVSWI in these conditions is illustrated by the dotted line showing the movement to a depressed ventricular function curve. This concept is supported by the marked elevation of LVEDP that occurs as LVSWI is suddenly increased by the abrupt fall in heart rate at the cessation of pacing, and this second point outlines the upper portion of the depressed ventricular function curve. Depression of ventricular function persists for a variable time during the post-pacing period, but the gradual return of LVEDP to normal indicates that depressed left ventricular function is a reversible phenomenon accompanying myocardial ischaemia. *During exercise:* the normal group moves to an augmented ventricular function curve, the patients without angina move upwards on the original curve, and the group with angina moves to a more depressed ventricular function curve than during pacing

exercise. The patients with angina during the pacing and post-pacing periods had a depressed ventricular function curve, but with exercise there was even further depression of ventricular performance, probably due to the volume load.

Tension-time index, which has been shown to be representative of myocardial oxygen consumption (see p. 93), and the importance of which in determining the threshold of pacing-induced angina has been stressed (see p. 100), increased to similar degree during pacing and exercise in the patients in whom angina developed. A closer analysis of individual factors responsible for myocardial oxygen consumption such as fiber length and rate of pressure development led PARKER to put forward the following considerations. Left ventricular end-diastolic dimensions decrease during pacing-induced tachycardia in patients presumably free of coronary artery disease [1789]. However, an increase in the end-diastolic heart size has been reported during pacing-induced angina in patients with coronary artery disease [1798]. Since changes in left ventricular end-diastolic pressure can be used as an index of changes in the end-diastolic fiber length [43c], it appears that fiber length was greater during exercise than during pacing in the group with angina. This increase would be associated with increased myocardial oxygen requirements during exercise. Consideration of tension-time index, which does not take the fiber length into account, fails to demonstrate this disparity. The small increase in dp/dt during both exercise and pacing which was noted by PARKER in the group with angina in comparison to the normal subjects, despite the increase in volume, suggests impaired myocardial contractility during ischaemia [215c].

From the above clinical observations, PARKER et al. conclude that in evaluating the haemodynamic function of the left ventricle in patients with coronary artery disease, pacing is of value only when ischaemic symptoms develop. This is in keeping with their previous observations that pacing in patients with coronary artery disease seldom induces lactate production in the absence of pain and that there is close correlation between the development of pain and electrocardiographic, metabolic and haemodynamic abnormalities [1417][10]. However, exercise is a superior stress, usually demonstrating functional abnormalities even in the absence of pain.

By studying left ventricular function, pressure-volume relationships and ventricular wall motion during acute myocardial ischaemia induced in ten coronary patients by atrial pacing and resulting in angina, DWYER [3e] also found that there was a deterioration in ventricular function — expressed in terms of the relationship between stroke work and end-diastolic volume — as manifested by a rightward shift of the ventricular function curve.

Other investigators also demonstrated that there is significant myocardial dysfunction during exercise in patients with occlusive coronary artery disease [29c].

WIENER et al. [1994] have on the whole confirmed these observations whilst at the same time pointing out:

— that the sudden rise in left end-diastolic ventricular pressure occurs, as had already been shown by ROUGHGARDEN et al. [1568], *before* the pain and the electrocardiographic signs of ischaemia;

— that the rise in pulmonary arterial pressure is quite abnormal;

— that certain determining parameters in myocardial oxygen consumption rise to a marked degree, heart rate by 43%, left systolic ventricular pressure by 20% and left ventricular dp/dt by 38%;

— that cardiac output would increase in proportion to the degree of exercise. This latter point is however at odds with the findings of COHEN et al. [346] and of NAJMI et al. [1335] who note a *subnormal* increase in cardiac output.

Whilst certain authors [1328] have interpreted the sudden rise in the left end-diastolic ventricular and pulmonary arterial pressures as obvious symptoms of acute failure of the left ventricle during the exercise-induced anginal attack, WIENER et al. [1994] consider that the combination of haemodynamic disturb-

---

10 In a study involving 41 subjects with coronary heart disease in whom right atrial pacing was performed, which resulted in anginal pain in 50% of cases, HELFANT et al. demonstrated however that, although development of angina pectoris appears to be related statistically to subnormal left ventricular function and abnormal lactate metabolism, there is considerable significant individual variation [144c].

ances arising points in favour of a different physiopathological mechanism than typical cardiac decompensation, because cardiac output and the velocity of ventricular contraction increase simultaneously. FRICK et al. [592] also believe that it is not a question of ventricular failure because the rise in left end-diastolic ventricular pressure seems to them to be due to a ventricle which does not adapt itself to the increase in return blood flow resulting from muscular exercise. An identical view is held by O'BRIEN et al. [1384] and by LINHART et al. [82a] who consider it to be a question of a lessening of myocardial compliance.

A more shaded opinion is put forward by GLANCY et al. [51a] who studied the effect of digitalis on left ventricular response to exercise in patients with angina. After ouabain, left ventricular end-diastolic pressure increased abnormally with exercise in only half of all the patients in whom it rose before administering the drug. Furthermore, ouabain improved the left ventricular function in several patients as assessed by the relationship of the stroke work index to ventricular end-diastolic pressure. Such results suggest that in some angina patients, the abnormal rise in left ventricular end-diastolic pressure during exercise is to a large extent caused by left ventricular failure, whilst in others, decreased left ventricular compliance appears to be a more important causal factor.

The same view is held by DWYER [3e] who studied left ventricular function, pressure-volume relationships, and ventricular wall motion by sequential cineventriculography during acute myocardial ischaemia induced in ten coronary patients by atrial pacing and resulting in angina. The observations made by this author suggest that both interpretations (reduction in ventricular compliance or ventricular failure) are valid, since both a change in end-diastolic compliance and a shift of the ventricular function curve to the right were observed: an abnormal pressure-volume relationship in the left ventricle was found during angina in five of the patients, while an increasing or stable filling pressure was associated with a declining end-diastolic volume in four other patients. Caution should be exercised not to extrapolate these data to explain changes occurring during exertional angina. Increased venous return occurring during exercise as well as increased sympathetic tone may induce different alterations in wall motion and volume.

As has been stressed by DWYER [3e], many experimental studies lay emphasis on the multifaceted picture of angina pectoris. A single view of this disorder will not provide an adequate explanation of all the observed clinical and physiologic alterations. The degree of ischaemia, the number of diseased vessels and the reserve capacity of nondiseased myocardium are a few of the many factors which determine the overall response of the heart to stress.

As pointed out by CROSS [68c] the riddle that remains to be answered is how are depressed contractility and angina related now that it is known they are associated. From simultaneous metabolic and haemodynamic studies carried out in angiographically proven coronary heart disease cases in whom atrial pacing resulted in angina, WIENER considers that the acute myocardial ischaemia thus induced, and depicted by abnormal lactate and pyruvate metabolism, is not directly responsible for angina; it is rather a sudden impairment of ventricular compliance which is thought to constitute the mechanical basis for the anginal syndrome [338c].

It is interesting to note that, *at rest*, without the stress of exercise or artificially induced tachycardia, patients with coronary disease without definite left ventricular dilatation often have abnormalities of ventricular performance. This was shown by BRISTOW et al. [46c], by calculating left ventricular volume and circumference from cineangiocardiograms in 15 patients with arteriographically proven coronary artery disease and five control subjects. The average end-diastolic pressure was found to be often abnormally high despite absence of significant left ventricular dilatation (lack of increase in end-diastolic volume). They concluded that significant abnormalities of diastolic compliance and of contractile performance of the myocardium were often present because they demonstrated a depression of ejection fraction and of the extent and rate of circumferential fiber shortening, i. e. variables which are considered as reasonable indicators of the competence of the contractile elements [96 c, 154 c]. Similarly, in patients with refractory angina pectoris due to severe coronary artery disease, measurements of left ventricular chamber volume and mass indicated the presence of left ventricle dilatation and a proportional hypertrophy, which are interpreted as manifestations of reduced left ventricular performance [264 c].

To complete the discussion on the cardiovascular disorders characteristic of angina pectoris, mention may be made of the pulmonary and cutaneous circulatory systems.

Regional distribution of pulmonary blood flow and ventilation was determined with the ^{133}Xe technic in the erect position at the bedside in 15 patients an average of 6 days after uncomplicated myocardial infarction and in five patients with severe angina. Follow-up studies were repeated within 3—25 weeks on six of the patients with myocardial infarction [172 c]. There was marked reduction in perfusion to the lung base after myocardial infarction. Patients with severe angina showed some underperfusion of the lower lung zones, but to a much less degree than those with acute myocardial infarction. The pattern of pulmonary perfusion reverted toward that seen in angina in the follow-up studies of patients with infarction. Distribution of ventilation was normal in all patients. The results of the study suggest therefore that there are probably chronic changes in the pulmonary vasculature of patients with arteriosclerotic heart disease which lead to redistribution of pulmonary blood flow toward the apex, and that the marked underperfusion of the lung base demonstrated following acute myocardial infarction reflects an acute increase in the pulmonary venous and interstitial pressures most likely due to occult left ventricular failure.

As far as the cutaneous circulation is concerned, liquid crystals, encapsulated onto black Mylar tapes, were used as cutaneous temperature sensors in 50 male patients, who had thermographic examinations while they were being exercised on the treadmill, in an attempt to induce angina pectoris [255 c]. Twenty-eight of the group remained free of pain and the exercise thoracic thermogram was essentially unchanged from the control or resting state. Twenty-two patients developed angina pectoris during exercise, of whom 21 had associated S—T depression in the electrocardiogram, and 17 thermographic abnormalities. When the pain was unilateral (9 patients), skin coolness was invariable and was within the distribution of the pain. When the pain was central (13 patients), skin coolness was present in 8 patients and was not always within the area of pain. When present, the skin coolness was transient and settled within minutes of relief of pain. This study therefore demonstrated that the majority of patients with exertional angina develop transient areas of skin coolness within or adjacent to the area of pain. In patients with lateral pain, skin coolness was invariable, while with central pain, about two thirds of the patients had regional cutaneous hypothermia.

3. Part Played by Hypersympathicotony in the Anginal Attack

The incidence of hypersympathicotony in the anginal pain is a further major aspect of physiopathology which deserves to be widely covered because of the essential place which it occupies in the modern concept of the angina syndrome.

It is obvious that the triggering factors in angina pain (effort, emotion, cold, stress, digestion, rarefaction in oxygen of the atmosphere) increase myocardial oxygen requirements through interplays of a nervous and/or biochemical nature.

Although no full explanation has yet been given on this point, the fascinating theory had been put forward as early as 1940 by RAAB [1478] that angina attacks are due to the hypoxia-inducing metabolic effect of sudden discharges of adrenaline onto a cardiac muscle whose sclerosed arteries are incapable of dilating sufficiently to meet the increase in myocardial oxygen consumption. RAAB shows the following year that exercise causes in the angina subject an acute and intense rise in the adrenaline level in the blood [1479][11]. This observation was subsequently confirmed [631, 1820]. Both adrenaline and noradrenaline increase [1523, 225c][12], a fact which has all the more clinical value in that it does not appear in the normal subject undergoing identical muscular exercise [1523]. It thus provides the proof that hyperactivity of the sympathetic system would appear to be a clinical feature of angina pectoris.

These facts led RAAB to suggest that the triggering factors in angina set up a condition of hypersympathicotony leading to the release of catecholamines from the surrenal glands and the sympathetic nerve endings in the myocardium. These catecholamines exert on the cardiac muscle a specific metabolic effect which is likely to cause hypoxia in those muscular zones whose irrigation has become marginal. Indeed, the increase in myocardial oxygen consumption which they cause is excessive and partly superfluous, in the sense that only a fraction of the oxydative energy is transformed into mechanical energy[13]. As a result of these observations, both RAAB [1485, 1491] and RICHARDSON [1523] advocate anti-adrenergic measures as a rational treatment for anginal coronary diseases.

The hypothesis by RAAB is supported by recent physiopathological data indicating that a condition of hyperactivity of the orthosympathetic nervous system does in fact appear to be one of the features of angina pectoris. Thus ELLIOTT and GORLIN [488] note that the anginal attack is very often associated with an abrupt rise in blood pressure by generalised vasoconstriction, and a rise in heart rate, the two phenomena being due to a sympathetic discharge. These haemodynamic disturbances have also been pointed out by PARKER et al. [1415]. ELLIOTT and GORLIN further point out that, during certain attacks, the coronary vascular system takes part in this constriction, since the arterial supply of oxygen to the cardiac muscle is reduced whereas its oxygen requirements are greater. Incidentally, these phenomena are identical to those observed during an intravenous perfusion of noradrenaline in man [2037], because the resulting increase in myocardial oxygen consumption is not accompanied by a lowering of coronary resistance but by a rise in the oxygen extraction coefficient, which indicates that the oxygen requirements are not covered by an adequate increase in coronary flow.

---

11 This observation is all the more remarkable in that it was made by means of a colorimeter, considered a posteriori as being insensitive as compared with current fluorometric methods.

12 Adrenaline is much more active in its effect on inducing myocardial hypoxia than is noradrenaline [1523].

13 It is interesting to note that with a conscious dog, various natural stimuli (food, sexual stimulation, cold, audible stimulus, spontaneous excitement) cause similar hypertension and tachycardia to those induced in the same animals by injecting intravenously adrenaline or noradrenaline. For this reason, these natural stresses probably cause considerable activation of the sympathetic system, leading to the discharge of catecholamines into the blood circulation [1217]. GRANATA [706] and PITT [1448] have also shown that excitement causes sympathetic stimulation of the conscious dog, leading amongst other things to an increase in coronary flow. According to GREGG [724] there is no longer any doubt that the sympathetic system is involved in the response to different stresses by the coronary circulation.

Thus, during the angina attack, myocardial ischaemia is in fact produced by the existence of arteriolar constriction which occurs when there is a considerable increase in myocardial oxygen requirements. These two phenomena aggravate the prejudicial effects of the reduction in coronary perfusion pressure (due to anatomical vascular stenosis) which may be found in particularly advanced cases of obstruction where it is not unusual to find complete occlusion of two of the three major coronary arteries [696].

In point of fact, the hypersympathicotony factor would come into play to a different degree depending on the various clinical forms of angina pectoris. In a treatise based on both clinical and physiological data at present available, GORLIN [696] has attempted to identify the factors which may come into play in the development of the different clinical forms of angina pectoris. To start with, he recalls that angina is not an inevitable consequence of cardiac ischaemia and that it is not known whether certain factors recognised as capable of promoting angina are likely *in themselves*, i.e. in the absence of morphological impairment of the coronary arteries, to bring on the anginal pain: it is a case of a chronic reduction in the oxygen content of the arterial blood as with severe anaemia, thyrotoxicosis, and polycythaemia.

As far as the physiopathology of the different forms of angina pectoris is concerned, we can summarise GORLIN's opinion in the form of a table (see Table 1).

A further clinical proof, this time indirect, of the part played by the sympathetic system in angina is that electrical stimulation of the carotid sinus nerve brings to the sufferer immediate relief from the attack [501] and prevents it occurring during exercise [215][14]: it involves a reflex reduction of the sympathetic tonicity in the heart and arterial vessels which leads to an immediate lessening in the heart rate, mean blood pressure and global vascular resistance [500].

If we consider the therapeutic implications which arise from the abundantly supported role of hypersympathicotony in the origin of the anginal attack, it will be understood why the supporters of this nervous effect — and they are becoming more and more numerous — advocate the use of therapeutic methods capable of moderating sympathetic activity [1148]. With this in mind, the fact that a medication which can reduce the work of the heart and increase its blood irrigation (see p. 27) possesses in addition anti-adrenergic properties of a global nature can only increase its therapeutic potential.

If by way of a synthesis we bring together all the notions on physiopathology which have just been expounded, we can accept the aggregate pathogenic ideas put forward by CONDORELLI [352] which can be summed up as follows. The anginal syndrome acknowledges two types of causes. The first is a *predisposing* cause, consisting of the latent permanent ischaemic condition resulting from atherosclerotic damage, stenotic and/or obstructive, to the coronary arteries. The *triggering* cause of angina attacks, whether these be due to effort, emotion, cold, digestion or lying in a prone position, consists of a stimulation of the orthosympathetic system which is objectified under clinical conditions by the appearance, *before* the painful attack, of a marked rise in blood pressure (systolic and diastolic) and heart rate [352, 1245]. Hypertension and tachycardia unduly increase the oxygen needs of the ischaemic cardiac muscle, with the result that the latent chronic myocardial hypoxia turns to acute hypoxia, the cause of the angina attack. These modern pathogenic concepts of the angina syndrome, which are based on widely documented pathophysiological observations remarkable for their con-

---

14 This observation has encouraged certain surgeons [501] to implant a pacemaker on the carotid sinus nerves, which the patient can bring into play whenever the need is felt (for details, see p. 315).

Table 1. *Pathophysiology of cardiac pain (see ref. [696])*

Angina of effort	Cardiac work increased. Coronary blood flow slightly increased. Inadequate elevation in cardiac output during exercise[a]. Inadequate elevation in mean ejection rate during exercise. Occasional abnormal increase in left ventricular end-diastolic pressure. Lactate production.
Angina with tachycardia	Reduction of coronary artery filling time in diastole, and augmentation of cardiac oxygen requirements, combining to produce selective myocardial ischaemia beyond a stenotic coronary artery.
Spontaneous angina	Cardiovascular hypersympathicotony leading to: — Increase in blood pressure. — Accelerated heart rate. — Increased vigor of contraction. — Elevation of cardiac work. — Reduction in myocardial blood flow by coronary vasoconstriction.
Angina of emotion	Dual origin (generalized sympathetic stimulation and coronary constriction) similar to that of spontaneous angina.
Angina of deglutition	Poorly understood. Most often: sign of advanced coronary disease or of the pre-infarction state. Occasionally: may serve as a clue to the presence of an associated disease in the gastrointestinal tract (unrecognized visceral coronary reflexes?).
Angina with cold wind	Characteristic for angina related to coronary heart disease. Mechanism unclear: perhaps hypertension and concurrent coronary vasoconstriction[b].
Nocturnal angina	Mechanism unclear. Three possibilities: 1. May point to early heart failure. 2. Fall in blood pressure with inadequate perfusion of the myocardium beyond a stenosed coronary artery. 3. Sympathetic discharge, as in spontaneous angina, brought about as a reaction to a dream[c].
Angina in aortic stenosis (20% incidence)[d]	Little or no reserve for increased coronary flow. Increased myocardial oxygen extraction during stress. *With coronary artery disease:* During stress: — increase in coronary flow (adequate overall coronary reserve). — abnormal lactate metabolism (evidence of regional ischaemia)

[a] GORLIN [696] believes that many patients with coronary heart disease have subliminal cardiac failure, as evidenced by measurable deficiencies in the response of cardiac output [346] and of velocity of cardiac contraction [1287] to stress and, in some cases, by an abnormal elevation of left ventricular end-diastolic pressure [696]. PARKER et al. [94a] think also that mild deficiency in left ventricular function is present in patients with coronary artery disease because the administration of digitalis during an imposed exercise reduces significantly the abnormal elevation of left ventricular end-diastolic pressure.

[b] See references [351] and [1816].

[c] Others admit tachycardia as possible cause [597].

[d] See reference [521].

sistency and coming from different research teams, enable a definition to be drawn up of the "ideal" pharmacological characteristics to which a medication intended for the long-term treatment of coronary insufficiency should measure up.

Such a medication must firstly be able to neutralise the latent myocardial ischaemia by correcting the imbalance which exists between the supply and demand of oxygen at the myocardium, the supply being handicapped by the fact that the coronary vaso-dilation potential, though real, is limited by vascular damage (see p. 25). This imbalance could therefore be resolved by a substance which reduces myocardial oxygen requirements by lightening its work, and at the same time increases coronary blood irrigation. This is also the opinion of MASON et al. [87a]. ROWE [1570] in fact suggests to those attempting to develop anti-anginal medications to get down to the job of finding substances which temporarily reduce the work of the heart. As for the increasing of coronary flow by specific coronaro-dilatory effect, this is theoretically ideal in the eyes of MODELL [1307, p. 363] because the cardiac work does not increase, whereas the rise in coronary flow which can be expected from a rise in cardiac output, for example, must be rejected because it can only be the consequence of myocardial stimulation and thus the work of the heart increases. It must not however be overlooked, as stressed by ROWE [1572] that in those cases where the increase in coronary flow remains an *isolated* phenomenon, clinical experience has shown, in the case of various medications of different chemical structure, that it was not of any advantage to the angina patient.

The onset of hypersympathicotony which is the triggering cause of the heart attack requires of such a medication that it also be endowed with antiadrenergic properties affecting both adrenergic α- and β-receptors. Indeed, if the activity of these receptors is lowered by the medication, it can be hoped to reduce the intensity of all the haemodynamic disturbances provoked by the hypersympathicotony, namely high blood pressure, tachycardia, increase in cardiac contraction power and acceleration of the rate of this contraction. In this way there will also be lessening of the excessive increase in myocardial oxygen consumption which, as we have seen earlier, characterises angina pectoris patients subjected to angina-inducing muscular effort or to angina-inducing artificial tachycardia (see p. 24).

4. Trends in Pharmacological Research for the Development of Antianginal Medications

If we review rapidly the various criteria on which pharmacologists have successively based themselves to find long term antianginal medications, we can reconstitute the major stages in their development. By so doing, we find that the tendency to connect together present-day pathogenic concepts has developed progressively [306].

4.1 Coronary Vaso-Dilation

First it was the concept of coronary vaso-dilation which prevailed. This was the case, in particular, with the derivatives of papaverine, the xanthines, khellin and even with the long-acting nitrates, of which it was thought at the time that the coronary dilating effect alone, and a real one at that, could provide a certain degree of clinical benefit.

Although for a long time there had been doubts as to the therapeutic role of the coronary-dilator effect of the nitrites, and that it is likewise known that the clinical benefit obtained by the use of *exclusive* vaso-dilators is usually no greater than that of placebo-therapy, the concept of coronary vaso-dilation has dominated pharmacological research for over thirty years during which period a veritable escalade towards the most powerful and longest-acting coronaro-dilator has taken place. This tendency is seen especially in the successive developments of prenylamine (see p. 165) and of benziodarone (p. 168), dipyridamole (p. 181), carbochromen (p. 188) and hexobendine (p. 192). Certainly, some of these medications are endowed with special action mechanisms likely to cause favourable changes in the metabolism of an ischaemic myocardium. The fact still remains that the goal originally pursued was to set up considerable and very prolonged hyperirrigation at the cardiac muscle, since the first pharmacological exploration took as a yardstick the effect on coronary flow. This tendency still remains today, as witness the recent development of lidoflazine, described as a coronary-dilating substance with a very lasting effect, which at certain doses succeeds in increasing coronary flow to as great an extent as respiratory anoxia [1660] (see p. 199). Witnesses also to this concept are new derivatives of dipyridamole, more powerful [927], and in 1969, amoproxan (p. 292) which, whilst remaining largely outside the field of certain existing drugs as regards the intensity and duration of its vaso-dilator effect, is purely and simply a coronary-dilating medication, being for instance without effect on cardiac work and on the adrenergic system.

Nevertheless the concept of *exclusive* coronary vaso-dilation seems nowadays to be largely outmoded, and, in the light of what we know of the pathophysiology of the angina syndrome, would not seem able *by itself* to exert any transcendent therapeutic effect. This opinion also finds its arguments in the fact that drugs with a powerful coronary-dilating effect have proved to be of doubtful clinical efficacy, and also that drugs which are really effective for the angina patient probably do not act by coronary vaso-dilation or that this mechanism is of secondary importance. There are good reasons for believing that the ability to increase total coronary flow in anaesthetised animals alone is largely irrelevant to the problem of increasing oxygen availability in the anginal patient [245c]. It follows that the fact of increasing the myocardial blood flow cannot, in itself, automatically lead to the assumption that the medication producing such an effect will be effective in man [1251].

4.2 Reduction in Cardiac Work

The efforts of pharmacologists were next concentrated on the type of drug which would be capable of reducing the work of the cardiac muscle so as to reduce its oxygen requirements. This aspect was dictated mainly by the results of clinical experimentation with the nitro-derivatives, especially nitroglycerin. In point of fact it was shown first that coronary flow *does not increase in the angina patient* at the moment the therapeutic effect shows itself[15], and then that the work of the heart decreases at that moment as a result of a lightening in the peripheral loads and of various changes in the cardiac dynamics which lead to a reduction in myocardial oxygen requirements (see details p. 128).

It was still necessary to achieve lightening of the cardiac work, not to the detriment of the normal processes of cellular respiration, but by reducing the haemodynamic loads imposed on the cardiac muscle, for instance by peripheral vaso-dilation which lowers overall vascular resistance (this, by the way, is, in order of priority, the type of activity by nitroglycerin in the anginal attack), and also for instance by lowering the heart rate.

Such a rational approach to the long term treatment of angina by using drugs which aim at reducing the work of the heart, and consequently its oxygen needs,

---

15 It may well be that this notion in turn must be revised and that it must be considered that nitroglycerin does in fact increase coronary flow in the coronary atherosclerotic subject. This is what COWAN et al. have just demonstrated by using a measuring technique enabling them to quantify the *very early* effects of nitroglycerin, i.e. during the 45—90 sec following its sublingual administration (see p. 126).

has later found solid experimental and clinical support. It has been demonstrated that when a coronary occlusion is performed in animals or occurs in a patient, there is always an ischaemic zone (where the oxygen supply is marginal) surrounding the necrotic area of that part of the myocardium which draws its supplies from the occluded artery [29a]. It is reasonable to suggest that since the blood supply to this ischaemic segment of myocardium is markedly reduced, its survival may depend on its oxygen consumption. Clearly, if the oxygen consumption of the myocardium is stimulated by factors such as increased intraventricular tension and/or augmented myocardial contractility, the viability of the ischaemic area may be reduced and the extent of the infarct increased by occlusion of a coronary artery at any given spot. Moreover, such an unfavourable change in the relationship between myocardial oxygen supply and demand may impair the contractile function of the myocardium at the margin of the infarct [15a].

When an occlusion occurs in a coronary artery, then it is likely that the quantity of infarcted myocardium and the area of the malfunctioning ischaemic zone will be increased. Conversely, reduction of myocardial oxygen demands (produced, for example, by slowing the heart rate and/or counteracting the augmentation of sympathetic influences) may reduce oxygen demands and thereby the size of the infarction and of the segment of ischaemic, inadequately functioning myocardium. Thus any augmentation of myocardial oxygen needs in the presence of coronary occlusion may be expected to increase the size of the necrotic zone and to impair the function of the ischaemic zone, while a reduction of oxygen consumption may be expected to exert the opposite effect [15a].

4.3 Inhibition of Monoamineoxydase

About the same period, it was thought for a time that the inhibitors of monoamineoxidase were about to constitute a major therapeutic advance. It was in 1957 that CESARMAN [287], whilst treating depressed patients with iproniazide, noticed by chance that one of his patients suffering at the same time from angina pectoris found his heart condition considerably improved. Subsequently, he treated a large number of angina subjects with this medication, and he obtained confirmation of its beneficial effect on the painful cardiac symptomatology. These unexpected results were confirmed a year later. They encouraged organicists to direct their efforts to the synthesis of other MAOI substances, and during the next few years there was a veritable crop of increasingly active MAOI medications which were tested by cardiologists with encouraging results. It was, however, found that the favourable effect on cardiac pain was only achieved at the cost of highly unpleasant side effects, effects which were even hasardous for the patient. Amongst these were three grave complications, namely: acute and unforeseeable hypotension, particularly dangerous for the coronary subject since it can lead to the incidence of myocardial infarct, toxic hepatitis or sexual impotence. It was thus seen in no uncertain fashion that the therapeutic effect was merely symptomatic, in the sense that the conditions governing myocardial nutrition were in no way improved, the imbalance between the supply and demand of oxygen remaining unchanged since cardiac work was not reduced and probably also that myocardial irrigation is not augmented, for in experiments on animals high doses of MAOI are needed to raise to a very moderate degree the coronary blood flow (see p. 161).

The favourable clinical effect of the MAOI's was ascribed to a genuine euphoric effect and to a probable action on pain perception, which might explain why the angina subject, improved by this type of medication, is not longer put on guard by the feeling of pain and thereby allows himself to indulge in excessive physical activity which may precipitate the incidence of infarction.

Despite their very real therapeutic effect on cardiac pain, the MAOI's are no longer used nowadays except in a few cardiological centres which reserve for them a role as a contributory form of therapy in particularly severe cases of angina pectoris (see p. 164).

4.4 Blockade of Hypersympathicotony

As regards the anti-adrenergic properties of such a type of medication, these were originally discovered incidentally and only in respect of the adrenergic α-receptors. Pharmacologists who have demonstrated α-anti-adrenergic properties in the case of substances otherwise possessing a coronary vaso-dilator effect have, with good reason, held that inhibition of this part of the adrenergic system should contribute to anti-anginal therapy. This is notably the case with prenylamine. This agent does not however provide particularly transcendent clinical results (see p. 168). Moreover, the therapeutic advantages of pure α-blocking agents in angina pectoris are practically non-existent [301]. Fundamentally, the precarious character of this transposition of pharmacology to the clinic may be explained by the fact that agents opposing the α-receptors only induce very partial neutralisation of the adrenergic system, the activity of the β-receptors remaining untouched. Although they inhibit the vaso-constricting effects of the circulating catecholamines, they neither modify their cardiac actions [1482] nor reduce their level in the cardiac muscle [1488]. For this reason they are unable to help in treating angina pectoris [1483] since the most harmful haemodynamic disturbances occurring in the angina subject during his pain attacks are primarily of a cardiac character and thus are ascribable to the β-receptors. This is why, in the anti-adrenergic sphere, pharmacologists have tended over the past years to develop medications able to block the activity of the β-receptors.

4.5 Blockade of the Adrenergic ß-Receptors

This concept by BLACK [180] has made possible the synthesising of various types of chemical structures whose essential biological feature is to antagonise the adrenergic β-receptors. These medications however modify certain haemodynamic parameters in such a way that, fundamentally, they provide a set-off which is unfavourable to the angina subject in particular and to the cardiac patient in general.

It must be stressed at the outset that they only partly meet the therapeutic implications of current concepts of the anginal syndrome, the reason for this being twofold:

a) Although they can in fact act on the latent ischaemia of the myocardium by lessening the oxygen demands of the heart, they reduce coronary irrigation (see p. 208) and thus the oxygen supply to the cardiac muscle. It follows that the imbalance between oxygen supply and consumption is liable to persist, since the decrease in oxygen supply seems to be parallel to the reduction in cardiac work [394, 1241]. In addition, β-blocking medications can increase the oxygen extraction coefficient of the myocardium [1258, 2032] whereas, as we have seen earlier (p. 24), what basically distinguishes the angina pectoris patient from the healthy subject during muscular effort is in fact because his myocardium extracts an additional amount of oxygen from the arterial blood, which is not the case with the subject who has no coronary disease.

b) If we consider the anti-adrenergic aspect of the β-blocking medications, it is evident that the adrenergic haemodynamic disturbances bringing on angina attacks can only be partly jugulated since only tachycardia and an increase in power and velocity of cardiac contraction are likely to be neutralised, hypertension arising from stimulation of the α-receptors on which the β-antagonists have no effect. Now although the cardiovascular disturbances arising from stimulation of the β-receptors mainly contribute to the excessive increase in myocardial oxygen requirements as a result of sympathetic hypertonicity, the fact remains that hypertension also plays a not inconsiderable part [352, 488, 1415, 1544].

The β-blocking medications have a further disadvantage from the clinical angle, namely a certain cardiac risk. It is currently accepted that their anti-anginal effect calls for the administration of comparatively large doses and that, this being so, decompensation symptoms may occur in subjects whose cardiac function has not remained intact (see p. 215). This potential cardiac risk inherent in β-blocking agents arises, pharmacologically speaking, from the depressive effect which they exert on the myocardium and which has been demonstrated under varied experimental conditions (see p. 215).

Other factors must however be taken into account, since they have major therapeutic consequences. It would appear that it is not so much the direct and non-specific cardio-depressor effect of the β-blocking agents which gives rise to the cardiac risk, but essentially the fact that the activity of the adrenergic β-receptors is suppressed by these drugs. Now adrenergic control of the cardiac function is an important factor in the normal response of the heart to exercise [1361]. It has been proved that β-blockade deprives the heart insufficiency patient (whether potential or declared) of a physiological mechanism which he normally brings into play in order to limit his circulatory deficiency[16]. This was demonstrated by GAFFNEY and BRAUNWALD [620]: the patient with cardiac insufficiency partly offsets this failure by a reflex mechanism whose efferent component follows the path of the β-adrenergic system and, amongst other things, leads to an increase in the power and velocity of myocardial contraction. It follows that if this sytem is put out of action by pharmacological β-blockade, the condition of cardiac insufficiency is thereby precipitated or aggravated. It is therefore logical to consider that the use of a β-blocking agent always entails a cardiac risk, whatever its chemical structure may otherwise be (see also p. 229).

4.6. Overall Inhibition of Hypersympathicotony

From the viewpoint of the anti-adrenergic properties which should be present in any medication intended for the fundamental treatment of angina pectoris, it would therefore appear desirable not to look for *complete* α-or β-antagonist properties, seeing the side effects which they can entail under clinical conditions. It would seem more logical to aim at damping down rather than suppressing the cardiovascular disturbances which characterise over-stimulation of the adrenergic system in its entirety. In so doing, we partly preserve amongst other things the major functions of the β-adrenergic system, and it can thus be hoped to maintain the physiological compensation which the cardiac patient brings into play to limit his functional deficiency. From the clinical angle, the cardiac risk should thereby be reduced accordingly.

---

16 In this context, it has been reported that propranolol induces deterioration of ventricular performance in calves with experimental heart failure [127a], and it is suggested that adrenergic support is necessary to maintain the ventricular function, this support being derived mainly from circulating catecholamines produced in the adrenal medulla.

This progressive advance of ideation, based on lessons drawn from animal and clinical experimentation, has led to the belief that progress could be achieved in the fundamental treatment of coronary insufficiency by developing a type of medication which, whilst reducing the work of the heart and increasing its blood irrigation, would be able — thanks to *incomplete* but *overall* antiadrenergic properties — to damp down all the adrenergic reactions of the cardiovascular system which end up by producing excessive and undesirable increase in myocardial oxygen requirements. It will be seen that a first attempt in this direction was materialised by the synthesis of a medication partly opposing the sympathetic system, which represents a new pharmacological type which we have called "adrenomoderator" [307, 314] and for which several years of multi-centre clinical research have confirmed the high hopes it had raised, thus proving the validity of the experimental concepts on which the working assumption was based (see p. 255).

To conclude this chapter, mention must be made of some very recent individual opinions which draw attention to the fact that pharmacological research should take more complex directions taking into account the vascular and metabolic state existing in the myocardium of the coronary atherosclerotic subject.

4.7. Dilatation of the Coronary Conductance Vessels

McGREGOR [1251] emphasises the fact that the experimental pattern generally used by pharmacologists, namely the normal coronary system formed by resistances *in parallel* (arterial, capillary and venous segments), obviously does not meet the conditions of human pathology, where account must be taken at least of the existence of intercoronary communications and also of the fact that the arterial segment could be made up of resistances *in series* [1251], the former consisting of the large *conductance* arteries (particularly when they are the seat of stricture) which are located on the heart surface, the latter of the small pre-capillary *resistance* vessels which are in close contact with the cells of the myocardium. It may well be that these two types of arterial segment have a distinct functional role and react differently to pharmacological agents. Although this structural pattern of coronary circulation in the atherosclerotic subject is only a supposition, yet one which finds certain bases in the opposite reaction to the catecholamines of the large and small coronary vessels [2053], McGREGOR considers, as a consequence of his hypothesis, that in the search for better vaso-dilators able to provide more blood for the ischaemic zone of the myocardium downstream of a complete obliteration of a large trunk, the tendency must not be towards substances which increase very considerably, and above all for a very lengthy period, the global myocardial irrigation and thereby increase appreciably the oxygen content of the coronary venous blood, but rather towards those which limit their vaso-dilatory effect selectively to the large *conductance* arterial vessels or to the collateral vessels, whilst at the same time respecting the normal function of auto-regulation of the small *resistance* vessels. In his opinion, only the nitrites act in this manner of the drugs he has used.

The pharmacological models to use in the study of vaso-dilators must therefore, according to McGREGOR [1251], comprise not only the setting up of zones of chronic arterial occlusion, but also the measurement, not of the *total* coronary flow, but of the blood flow *in the ischaemic zone*. It would thus appear that an interesting approach to the conditions of human pathology might consist in using animals in whom a gradual chronic coronary occlusion has caused collateral vessels to develop and in whom the *retrograde* coronary flow is measured, providing a good pointer to the collateral flow downstream of the occlusion [1240, 126 c].

In experimental coronary arterial constriction, the peripheral coronary arterial pressure (pressure distal to the point of constriction) appears also to be a good index of collateral vessel development [26 c].

4.8. Improvement of Functional Coronary Microcirculation

In the opinion of WINBURY, it is the concept of the nutritional microcirculation which should guide the quest for anti-anginal medicinal substances. Nutritional circulation is that portion of the regional blood flow which supplies the tissues with oxygen and substrates. In view of the fact that a certain part of the blood can pass via arterio-venous by-passes or via non-functional capillaries (low diffusion capacity), the total blood flow of a given region does not necessarily represent the nutritional circulation. RENKIN [1518] has shown that the trans-capillary exchange of the nutritional substrates and oxygen by diffusion and ultrafiltration is controlled by the vaso-motor adjustments in the capillary system. The main adapting mechanisms are the variations in *total* blood flow caused by the muscular cells of the arterioles, and the variations in the number of open capillaries which are conditioned by the pre-capillary sphincters.

It can thus be imagined that drugs can directly modify this circulation in such a manner that the measurement of *total flow* cannot provide any forecast of it. WINBURY, for instance, has demonstrated that as regards the skeletal muscle and the heart, the changes in regional vascular resistance caused by pharmacological agents are not necessarily accompanied by similar directional changes in the nutritive circulation, measured for example by the extraction of Rb^{86} [617, 2014]. He draws from this the conclusion that the pre-capillary sphincters, whose role is important for regulating the distribution of the nutritive circulation, can respond to drugs in a different way than the resistance arterioles, so that control of the myocardial nutritional circulation seems to him to be independent of the control of the arteriolar circulation [2008]. WINBURY considers that, under normal conditions, 75% of the functional myocardial capillaries are open. The remaining 25% may be open, either by direct action on the pre-capillary sphincters without total coronary flow necessarily changing (which is the case with some nitro derivatives), or by increase in total flow as a result of arterial dilation (such is the case, for instance, with Persantine). He assumes that the ideal anti-anginal agent is the one which would produce little arteriolar dilation, would have a specific action on the nutritional circulation thus diverting the available blood to the nutritional circulation by relaxing the pre-capillary sphincters, whilst at the same time lessening the work of the heart [2008].

4.9. Development of a Collateral Coronary Circulation

The advantage of developing a collateral circulation is also advocated by others, but under very different exploration conditions. Various German authors, for instance MEESMANN [1262] and SCHMIDT [1679], consider as a favourable indication for an anti-anginal substance the fact that it develops, after chronic oral administration, a collateral anastomotic circulation in dogs which is disclosed by X-raying the heart removed after sacrificing the animal and whose coronary system has previously been injected with material opaque to X-rays.

The development of such vessels is especially convincing in the case of certain substances, but no-one has yet proved the validity of the extrapolation to humans of such an effect demonstrated on the *healthy* heart of a dog, for it so happens that the few medicaments which effectively set up such a collateral system in animals only develop this effect at very high doses, considerably in excess of the posology advocated for the angina patient (refer, for instance, to p. 183). Moreover, clinical experiments with such medications have not given particularly outstanding therapeutic results since they have failed by a long chalk to win the unanimous verdict of clinicians.

The question of collateral coronary circulation has just been approached from a different angle by SCHAPER [1657]. On the basis of anatomo-pathological investigations, he considers that anastomoses, which constitute a potential collateral circulation which can be mobilised in the event of coronary insufficiency, form part of a functional arteriolar network. The transformation, in the case of an ischaemic heart, of normally non-functional anastomoses into an effective collateral circulation would appear to be based on a process of cellular growth leading to a veritable neo-formation of the vascular wall [1658]. SCHAPER suggests the following mechanism, for example from the heart of an animal which has been subjected to chronic constriction, by means of an Ameroid ring, of a large coronary trunk. Stenosis produces a pressure gradient between the poorly irrigated areas depending for their supply on the constricted artery and normal areas. The hypoxia in the ischaemic zone causes an extreme rise in the parietal pressure in arteriolar anastomoses, and this is the mechanical factor which speeds up cellular multiplication. After a certain time, the vascular wall thickens, which entails a drop in parietal pressure. Thus by a morphological process of cell multiplication, the anastomoses and arterioles are transformed into small functional arteries. This hypoxia must, however, be sufficiently extensive and relatively constant: if too little, it would be incapable of triggering off the mechanism of cell proliferation since it is offset by the physiological vasodilation, whilst it produces irreversible lesions of the myocardium if it is too severe and too sudden.

According to SCHAPER, the development of collateral coronary circulation following artificial stenosis of a large coronary artery could be followed up experimentally in time by working out what he calls the "coronary quotient", i.e. the ratio which exists between retrograde coronary arterial pressure and aortic pressure. The level of the retrograde coronary pressure downstream of the occlusion would depend on the number and diameter of the anastomoses which become functional. Where these are adequate, vascular resistance to the flow of blood decreases progressively to the point where the retrograde pressure tends to come up to the aortic pressure level. By working out the coronary quotient therefore, it would be possible to measure the quality of the collateral circulation development. According to SCHAPER, this coronary quotient would provide the most sensitive indication of the development and nutritional efficacy of a collateral coronary circulation.

By extending these concepts to practical application, he shows that in the case of lidoflazine (see p. 203), dogs in a state of chronic coronary deficiency which are treated daily with this medication show a statistically higher coronary quotient than untreated animals, this quotient tending towards unity.

Although the process is a neat one, attention must be drawn to a major source of possible error which the author [1659] appears to have overlooked (see also p. 203). The comparison of the mean coronary quotients is only made between two different groups of animals, some treated, the others untreated. Since the ischaemia induced in the two groups by chronic obstruction of the coronary artery would seem to be the cause of normal development of collateral circulation, and since the drug being investigated can only speed up that development, the validity of the comparison strictly depends on the identity between several factors within the two groups, namely the rapidity and extent of the setting up of ischaemia, and the degree of *final* ischaemia achieved. These factors have not been checked, nor is it seen how they could be with the technical means at present available to us.

This being so, it would seem risky to compare two mean coronary quotients when there are so many variables which cannot be checked.

To this must be added the fact that the animals are allowed to move within enclosures of very different capacities, to the extent that physical exercise (whose accelerating action on the collateral circulation is admitted by the author) is very different from one animal to another.

It might also be wondered to what extent these experimental and very interesting findings can be extrapolated for humans. Can we in fact liken the disturbances in myocardial irrigation caused in man by atherosclerosis to the reduction in coronary flow artificially induced in animals by fitting a constrictor ring? This latter is clearly an acute process by comparison to the atherosclerotic process. Hypertrophy of coronary anastomoses of the order commonly found in coronary heart disease appears to require a long time in human pathology [105c]. Furthermore, in the specific case of lidoflazine, even if the favourable effect on the coronary quotient were really due to the transformation of non-functional anastomoses into neo-formed arterioles, it is difficult to understand why, as in fact it does happen [39c], angina patients successfully treated with this medication suffer a relapse in their clinical condition when the treatment is halted or a placebo substituted (see p. 204). In this case it must be admitted that, as a result of suppressing the medication, the neo-formed arterioles degenerate and so lose their function. Although such degeneration has in fact been observed in animals [1658], it has not been evidenced in man [614], so that the objection remains valid.

Furthermore, the existence of secondary degeneration of the neo-formed collaterals in an animal would appear to indicate that the neo-formation of arterioles from pre-existing intercoronary anastomoses calls for the presence of a continual stimulus. It could well be imagined in this case that this stimulus consists in the hyperirrigation achieved by the medication, which is, in fact, the functional mechanism suggested by SCHAPER [1659]. But then this favourable effect on the collateral coronary circulation would have nothing specific about it and could be the attribute of any so-called vaso-dilator substance with a powerful and prolonged action. Another fact which further complicates the problem is that lidoflazine would not seem to increase coronary flow in man [248, 282c] despite its powerful effect on dogs. The neo-formation of collaterals which the drug is supposed to achieve in the angina subject, and which is alleged to be at the root of its therapeutic effect, cannot therefore be attributed to myocardial hyperirrigation. Should it therefore be admitted that the chemical structure itself of the drug is the stimulating factor in arterial neo-formation, a fact which remains in the realm of hypothesis as regards man?

It is clear that the interesting concepts advanced by SCHAPER deserve more intensive investigation, but in our present state of knowledge they are not without contradictions and do not provide an entirely satisfactory explanation of certain facts. It seems premature, therefore, to take such observations as a basis for arriving at a concept applicable to the perfecting of antianginal drugs.

4.10. Potentiation of the Endogenous Mediators of the Coronary Autoregulation

To conclude with the criteria which pharmacologists have adopted to try to perfect antianginal medications, mention must be made of attempts to modify favourably the autoregulating system of coronary circulation.

Attitudes to this concept still seem purely hypothetical and thus in complete contradiction. For instance, special interest has been shown for some considerable time in certain vaso-dilator drugs because, preserving the enzymatic degradation of adenosine, they considerably potentialise its coronaro-dilator effect (see for example p. 183). This property was considered as being very favourable because it provided an explanation of the potency and lasting nature of their increasing effect on coronary irrigation. Conversely, McGREGOR [1252] considers that the quest for medications which considerably increase coronary flow must definitely be avoided, since such an effect can only be achieved at the expense of disturbing the mechanisms of autoregulation (see also p. 44).

Before proceeding to the development of antianginal medications on the basis of currently held notions as to the autoregulation of coronary irrigation, it would thus seem desirable to await additional information regarding this fundamental aspect of myocardial physiology which has not yet been fully resolved (see Ch. II).

4.11. Prophylaxis of Cardiac Necrosis

A specific experimental approach to the development of medications intended to combat angina pectoris will be briefly considered. Truth to tell, it is aimed at reducing the incidence of those myocardial disorders which can lead to infarct and/or cardiac necrosis rather than at making a favourable change in the biological consequences of coronary heart disease which are responsible for the actual angina attack.

It is based on facts which demonstrate that if, as is universally admitted, atherosclerosis of the coronary vessels constitutes the largely preponderant substratum of angina pectoris, the possibility cannot be excluded of the existence of the angina syndrome which does not acknowledge any pathologically recognisable atherosclerotic cause. Indeed, post-mortem examinations [84, 1137] and coronaro-arteriographic explorations [697, 967, 1139, 1470] have disclosed the fact that 15—38%, depending on the authors, of patients suffering from angina pectoris are free from any perceptible deterioration of the coronary vessels.

If we add that clinical manifestations of infarction are frequently diagnosed as coronary thrombosis or coronary occlusion, whereas the autopsy reveals that one or other of these conditions is absent in half the cases [481, 1802], it is not surprising that RAAB [1486, 1487] considers that we overestimate the role of coronary *vascular* disorders in the history of the ischaemic heart diseases and that sufficient attention is not paid to myocardial metabolic disturbances as a possible cause of the common forms of heart diseases, including angina pectoris. In RAAB's view, the so-called "coronary" heart disease is in fact often a "myocardial" heart disease in whose pathogenesis three intricate factors play a combined predisposing and causal role, namely: coronary atherosclerosis which is the predisposing factor, whilst the causal factor consists of a disproportionate increase in myocardial oxygen needs due to the catecholamines, these latter making a fundamental contribution to the vulnerability of the cardiac muscle [1484].

By acting on an atherosclerotic terrain which limits the possibilities of coronary vaso-dilation and, consequently, the amount of myocardial hyperirrigation required to meet the excess demands for oxygen, these catecholamines set up myocardial hypoxia. To this is added the over-production of cortico-surrenal hormones (cortisol in particular) which potentialise the cardio-toxic effect of the catecholamines. These pathogenic concepts held by RAAB are remarkably in line with those of SELYE, based on animal experimentation. SELYE supports his view on the results of observations he was able to make on an experimental heart disease pattern, necrotic electrolyte-steroid cardiopathy. He believes [1716] that this type of experimental necrotic cardiopathy (which is induced by the administration to a rat of steroid — possessing both gluco- and mineralocorticoid properties — and electrolytes, to which may be added catecholamines and stress procedures in an alternative to this pattern) is a good test for investigating a medicinal medium which could prevent, or at least reduce, the incidence of myocardial infarction in man.

SELYE stresses the fact that the agents used in producing experimental heart disorders in an animal are not necessarily those which are responsible for myocardial infarction in man. He adds, however, that these factors are precisely the ones which are most frequently blamed by clinicians as probably being at the origin of the infarct, namely the overproduction of catecholamines and of 17-hydroxy-corticosteroids (especially cortisol) acting on a coronary atherosclerosis terrain. The disastrous action of these three factors on the myocardium upsets electrolytic balance, entailing the loss of cellular potassium and magnesium and overloading in sodium. This creates a favourable ground for critical disturbances of myocardial fibre which are probably the cause of impairment of myocardial contractility and of derangements in the source and conduction of the nerve-impulse in the specific system of the heart.

SELYE adds that the ease with which experimental infarctoid necrosis is induced depends on the extra sodium administered, and that agents which prevent the excretion of potassium protect the animal against these lesions.

He recalls that in his time he had suggested that the considerable number of myocardial infarct cases discovered in hospital and in which no coronary thrombus could be proved, might be due to a biochemical mechanism similar to that which is found in necrotic electrolyte-steroid cardiopathy.

A further important item provided by SELYE is the fact that potassium and magnesium have an anti-necrotic action [1716]. The same goes for certain anti-kaliuretic medicaments such as amiloride [1715] which, when administered as a prophylactic, is able to prevent this infarctoid necrosis in rats, whereas hydrochlorothiazide and ethacrynic acid prove inactive. This clearly shows that this type of experimental infarctoid necrosis is sensitive to various medicinal agents of the diuretic non-kaliuric type (amiloride) and recalcitrant to the diuretics which are both natriuric and kaliuric (chlorothiazide derivatives).

4.12. Inhibition of Platelet Aggregation or Adhesiveness

Over the past few years it has been found that certain antianginal medications have the property of inhibiting the behaviour of the platelets in the process of intravascular thrombosis. This property probably offers certain *additional* prospects for a future approach to the treatment of the clinical manifestations of coronary atherosclerosis and its possible thrombo-embolic consequences.

The part played by the platelets in the origin of thrombosis seems to be well established. We know little however of the origin and determinism of platelet anomalies in the pathogenesis of thrombo-embolic disease. Platelet adhesiveness is increased in patients with coronary sclerosis [158c], and substances which affect this activity (such as clofibrate and dipyridamole) are now being investigated. Although platelet adhesiveness is increased in patients with ischaemic heart disease, HAMPTON et al. [140c] consider that measurements of platelet adhesiveness are of little clinical value because such an increase is seen in a wide variety of illnesses. Therefore, measurements of the changes in platelet electrophoretic mobility induced by ADP provide more information, as it seems to exist a correlation between ischaemic heart disease and an abnormally increased sensitivity of platelets to ADP but not to noradrenaline. On the contrary KARPPINEN [170c] reported that in coronary patients, no significant differences in the surface charges of platelets and erythrocytes (electrophoretic mobility measured by means of the cell electrophoresis technique) were found when compared to healthy subjects, but differences are more likely to be found in plasma and serum factors. The view that the platelets of ischaemic heart disease patients are structurally and metabolically different (increased phospholipid/protein ratios) from those of normal subjects, in such a way that they favour thrombosis, is supported by NORDOY et al. [236c].

Investigation of human platelets is virtually limited to artificial laboratory situations. Several tests are currently used without any of them being specific to the thromboembolic diathesis. The most they can do in certain cases is to provide an element of diagnosis or provide a means for finding new anti-thrombotic agents. The problem is rendered even more complicated by the fact that, for instance, in both the rat and man (patients who had suffered a myocardial infarction or presented signs of coronary heart disease), a high thrombotic tendency may be associated with a platelet hypersusceptibility to thrombin-induced aggregation, which, in turn, is related to changes in fatty-acid composition (ratio of saturated + monounsaturated to polyunsaturated fatty acids) of platelets [268c].

From the experimental angle, the main laboratory tests [138c] relate to platelet adhesiveness and aggregation (see also ref. [229c]).

Platelet adhesiveness is determined by the counting of platelets after passing the total blood through a glass ball column. The agglutinant agent is the ADP freed by the erythrocytes.

Platelet aggregation in platelet-rich plasma goes hand in hand with the reduction in optical density of this plasma. It is increased by ADP, ATP, adrenaline, noradrenaline, 5-HT, and by thrombine and collagene.

The electrophoretic mobility of the platelets in diluted platelet-rich plasma expresses the changes in their surface charge. Agglutinant agents increase mobility at low concentrations and decrease it at higher concentrations. Dissociation of sensitiveness to ADP and to noradrenaline would appear to be characteristic of arteriopathy and hyperlipaemia (138c).

Various antianginal medications have been investigated for their effect on the behaviour of platelets and on experimental thrombosis.

a) Laboratory research into human platelets

Persantine is by far the most extensively investigated antianginal medication in platelet behaviour tests, but the results are not always in concordance with each other. Aggregation by ADP is inhibited at a concentration of $10^{-4}M$, but not at lower concentrations [90c], Persantine being less active than Intensaine [139c]. Spontaneous aggregation and that which is induced by noradrenaline are not changed. When administered intravenously, Persantine reduces spontaneous aggregation but does not modify the effects of ADP or of noradrenaline. For other investigators, Persantine inhibits the ADP- and noradrenaline-induced changes in human platelet aggregation and adhesiveness [87c]. Adhesiveness is not altered in normal men [90c] but it is reduced in post-operative states [51c]. The effects on changes in electrokinetic mobility are complex: Persantine is inactive in the case of diluted platelet-rich plasma, but it inhibits increase in the mobility due to noradrenaline following incubation in the total blood or after systemic administration [139c]. There is a paradoxical potentiation of ADP-induced platelet aggregation in the rat by adenosine and Persantine, which remains unexplained [247c].

From the clinical viewpoint, the activity of Persantine has proved to be the same as that of a placebo in three double-blind experiments, whether involving post-operatory incidence of thrombosis in the deep veins in 650 cases [51c], myocardial infarct complications in 103 cases [109c], or cerebral ischaemic incidents during long-term treatment in 169 cases [2c]. On the other hand, long-term treatment seems to reduce the frequency of thrombo-embolisms after replacing heart valvules in a group of 100 cases [306c, 307c]. When combined with anti-coagulants, Persantine has a favourable influence on the development of renal transplants by reducing the incidence of acute thrombosis and of progressive stenosis of the arterioles of the renal cortex [180c].

Intensaine is a powerful and lasting inhibitor of aggregation by ADP and noradrenaline. When administered intravenously, Intensaine suppresses the changes in mobility induced by the agglutinants [139c].

Nitroglycerin inhibits the aggregation induced by ADP but does not alter that caused by noradrenaline.

Papaverine inhibits aggregation by ADP and by noradrenaline.

Ronicol inhibits aggregation by noradrenaline, but is inactive as regards ADP.

Ustimon and nicotinic acid do not change aggregation.

The following adrenergic blocking agents are active against aggregation by noradrenaline: phentolamine, tolazoline, propranolol, isoxsuprine (Duvadilan) and iproveratril (Isoptin). Only propranolol and phentolamine are active against ADP. Changes in mobility induced by ADP and noradrenaline are eliminated following intravenous and oral administration of propranolol [139c].

b) Investigation into experimental thrombosis

Persantine prevents the formation of platelet masses in the cortical arteries of rabbits, induced by traumatising the vascular wall combined with the local application of ADP or 5-HT [107c, 223c]. It has a temporary protective effect against thrombosis caused by laser beams in rabbits ([10c]. It reduces the extent and duration of mesenteric occlusions induced by an electric current in rats [82c].

Intensaine and propranolol are inhibitors of platelet masses in rabbits, but just as with Persantine there is no parallel between the intensity of effect on human platelet aggregation and the prevention of experimental thrombosis [139c, 88c].

As things stand at the moment, it is difficult to see — and even more so to prove clinically — what possible therapeutic advantage might be offered for an antianginal medication by the fact that it inhibits platelet adhesiveness and aggregation. For the time being, the development of research of this nature would only appear to be a subsidiary but indecisive line.

Chapter II

Haemodynamic Basis
for Coronary Pharmacology

It would appear expedient, in opening this chapter, to anticipate the objection in a very general sense that drugs which increase coronary blood flow in animals are unsuited, for morphological reasons, to exerting their action on a sclerosed coronary system in a human being.

Certain clinicians are often heard to say that the extent of vascular impairment found in autopsies on angina patients excludes the possibility of a beneficial effect from a long term medicinal form of treatment. The least that can be said is that, for physiologists, this objection is not based on sufficient evidence [217] since it is important not to lose sight of some fundamental notions.

1. Certainly it would appear impossible to modify the vaso-motor function of a large coronary trunk which is atherosclerosed. It is nevertheless evident that it is not at the large trunk level that a pharmacological agent works on a normal coronary system, but rather at arteriolar and pre-capillary level. Indeed, the resistance of the large arterial trunks only plays a minor part in variations in the vaso-motricity, whereas this latter is maximal at arteriolar and minor vessel level [488]. Arteriolar resistance is so high that it is necessary to reduce to one third the diameter of the large vessels to see a significant drop in irrigation pressure take place [488]. Now anatomical impairment affects the large epicardial branches whereas the small intramyocardial branches are very rarely affected. In other words, the atheromatous process is segmentary and only affects the first few centimetres of the main arteries [1674], all authors being agreed on the fact that the small arteries, and especially the arterioles, are never affected [279].

It has further been shown that in pathological situations, the normal regulating mechanisms of the coronary circulation are not always able to ensure, within the limits of anatomical and physical possibilities, optimum adaptation of coronary irrigation to myocardial requirements [217, 225, 226]. However, certain anatomo-pathological and clinical findings show that a sclerotic coronary system may still react from the functional angle at the small vessels located in the myocardium which, since they are not affected by the degenerative process, represent a "coronary reserve" [656, 1690]. In the central zone of an anoxaemic area, local regulation causes what is probably a maximum vaso-dilation, whereas in the peripheral zones there are still unused coronary "reserves". It is therefore permissible to assume that appropriate substances capable of reducing coronary arterial resistance can improve the blood irrigation of the peripheral zones of a previously stenotic area [218].

2. Blood flow in a large coronary trunk whose diameter is considerably reduced by the atherosclerotic process obeys, as in the case of a normal vessel, the laws of fluid dynamics, i.e. it directly depends both on the velocity of blood flow and on the section of the arterial trunk, to the formula:

flow = velocity $\times$ section

viz: $$\frac{(\text{Perfusion pressure} - \text{capillary pressure}) \times R^2 \times \pi R^2}{4 \ln},$$

or yet again:

$$\text{Flow} = \frac{(\text{Perfusion pressure} - \text{capillary pressure}) \times R^4 \pi}{4 \ln},$$

where l is the length of the arterial segment considered, and n = blood viscosity. It is obvious that if arteriolo-capillary resistance decreases with the intervention of a pharmacological agent or of a natural biological mediator, arteriolo-capillary pressure reduces and thereby the flow must of necessity increase. Now, as stated by BRETSCHNEIDER [217], there is nothing to prove that a medicament is unable to reduce, in the angina subject, the resistance of that part of the coronary vascular system which is still intact, which has retained its capacity to react and which is still subjected to nervous and humoral regulation.

We have pointed out in Chapter 1 that the myocardial blood flow of a coronary patient with advanced arterial sclerosis which is clinically proved does in fact increase during effort or atrial pacing, and subsequent to the sublingual intake or intracoronary injection of nitroglycerin, or following an intravenous infusion of small doses of adrenaline (see p. 28).

3. We know that the reduction by the stenotic process in the functional reserve of the coronary vessels is partly offset by the development of a collateral circulation. It has been proved that this development may be speeded up in animals by means of pharmacological substances [523, 1261, 1659].

4. In the zones adjacent to a stenotic area, such physiological vascular dilation as has developed by hypoxia probably does not reach its maximum level, and there is nothing to prevent us thinking that we can further increase it by means of substances which reduce coronary arterial resistance.

5. It has also been shown that there are many anastomoses in the heart of a healthy subject. These are of two types: *intracoronary*, i.e. connecting two branches of one and the same coronary artery, and *intercoronary*, i.e. connecting branches of different major coronary arteries [89, 892, 1539]. These latter have an average diameter of up to 40—200 microns [191]. In patients who have suffered from coronary insufficiency, an autopsy reveals that the number and size of these anastomoses are considerably increased [89, 191, 892] reaching as much as 2 mm in diameter [89], and that their histological structure is in no way incompatible with normal vasomotor function since they are free from atherosclerosis. Evidence was put forward by stereoarteriography in support of the existence of coronary arterial anastomoses as normal structures in man [105c]. In the subendocardial layers of the left ventricle, the anastomoses are commonly 100—200 μ or more in lumen diameter in normal hearts and they are capable of great enlargement in ischaemic heart disease. In the latter case, the anastomotic vessels are more numerous but chiefly of larger size [105c]. The anastomotic reserve seems to be able to compensate for the progressive evolution of the atherosclerotic coronary disease, as demonstrated by the high incidence of cases with one or more occlusions and stenoses with normal myocardium or with only minimal myocardial damage [16c].

6. It is possible that under the effect of certain pharmacological substances, some redistribution of intramyocardial blood flow may occur at capillary level, from non-functional vascular zones to functional zones, thus increasing the *nutritive* blood flow without it following that the *total* coronary flow necessarily increases. According to WINBURY [2014], who is at present working on this problem, such redistribution would arise from a dilator action exerted preferentially on the pre-capillary sphincters (see p. 45).

7. The possibility of an improvement in angina pectoris by pharmacological media which increase coronary flow is still accepted by GORLIN [694], although

as far back as 1960 he disclosed the paradoxical fact that nitroglycerin does not increase coronary flow in the subject suffering from angina pectoris.

In the light of all these facts, we are entitled to ask whether the increasingly unfavourable attitude of clinicians as regards the use of vaso-dilator medications in angina is based rather on arguments of a post-mortem character than on the somewhat disappointing experience they have had with the use of older types of medications, insufficiently investigated from the pharmacological angle and where it was only necessary to demonstrate the existence of vaso-dilator properties for them to be submitted for their medical assessment.

It is permissible to think that this attitude can change, since pharmacologists are suggesting substances which are more and more active and with increasingly lengthy activity, certain of which act by new mechanisms and which are even better studied from the experimental angle in that technological methods are rapidly improving, not to mention the fact that advances in clinical pharmacology are constantly providing fresh information regarding the patho-physiological aspect of coronary insufficiency. Medical disaffection to the vaso-dilators also has a local character depending on the school of thought: for instance German clinicians still believe in them.

Fashion also plays a part in the doctor's opinion. The therapeutist does not turn up his nose at innovations. Once it was a question of the "coronaro-dilators". A little later it was the inhibitors of mono-aminoxydase. Today it is abstention, the doctor too often restricting himself to nitroglycerin, sedatives, tranquillisers, anticoagulants and an invitation to lead a quiet life, away from the stresses of present-day living, ideally in a secluded spot, advice which is certainly wise but which the majority of patients cannot put into practice.

Since therapeutic fashions are in a constant state of change, tomorrow will perhaps see a return to new vaso-dilators, but on the strict understanding that this is not their only activity and that they also meet certain criteria as regards their other effects on the cardiovascular system. It is these criteria which we propose to examine.

Any substance which increases coronary irrigation in animals does not ipso facto offer a potential advantage for human treatment (see p. 40). From the pharmacological angle, it should have certain haemodynamic features for it to have any chance of being effective for man as a preventive medication for anginal attacks[1]. Although they might not have gained unanimity of opinion, these characteristics have attracted a sufficiently wide audience for them to be considered as essential, at least from the experimental viewpoint, and in the light of our existing knowledge.

These essential criteria are as follows:

— Not to lower too much general blood pressure

— Not to increase myocardial oxygen consumption, in other words, not to increase either the work of the heart, nor its output, nor its rate.

— Not to cause myocardial oxygen shortage by an uncoupling effect on the oxidative phosphorylations (of the dinitrophenol type) or inhibition of cellular respiration (of the cyanide type).

---

1 It goes without saying that such a substance must first meet other fundamental requirements, viz: its resorption as regards the methods of administration adopted under clinical conditions, good tolerance, low toxicity and rareness of side effects. Specifically as regards gastro-intestinal resorption, LENKE [199c] has demonstrated that in the case of several substances which are endowed with important coronary dilating properties following intravenous administration in dogs, some of them had only a weak or no effect at all when they were administered into the duodenum. He considers therefore that an early test of activity by enteral administration is suitable.

— Not to disturb the metabolic mechanisms alleged to be at the basis of auto-regulation of the coronary circulation [1252].

These characteristics find their justification in the multiple aspects of the physiology of coronary circulation.

Blood pressure may not drop too steeply under penalty of seeing this hypotension have a harmful effect on myocardial irrigation. This factor is too well known to need further emphasising: it has for a long time been shown that, all other haemodynamic factors remaining constant, any variation in blood pressure, in either direction, entails a *like* change in coronary arterial flow [36, 44, 470, 715, 718, 791, 950, 954, 1222, 1398, 1682]. It is therefore obvious that any marked hypotensive property in a substance which lowers coronary arterial resistance is liable to harm myocardial irrigation.

The second haemodynamic characteristic required of a coronarotropic substance is that it should not increase myocardial oxygen consumption. This is vital: it has, in effect, been shown that it is the myocardial oxygen consumption which determines *pari passu* the level of coronary flow.

This fundamental concept is comparatively recent since it was in 1950 that FOLTZ [570] demonstrated the key-role played in coronary flow regulation by the myocardial oxygen requirements. Obtained with an anaesthetised dog, this notion was subjected to criticism until 1965, when GREGG [979] demonstrated the validity of the phenomenon on a non-anaesthetised dog.

The ingenious technique adopted by GREGG consists in implanting, by an acute operation, a flow transducer onto the coronary artery, a second flow transducer onto the aorta root, a catheter into the arch of the aorta, and a catheter into the coronary sinus, all these devices making possible the simultaneous measurement of the coronary arterial flow, cardiac output, work done by the heart and myocardial oxygen consumption. The animal is treated as a thorax operation case, and after several weeks of patient training it is able to comply with all the requirements of the experimenter; amongst other things, the myocardial oxygen consumption can be modified at will be subjecting the animal to muscular effort of variable and measurable intensity, consisting in making it run on an endless belt. With this type of preparation, GREGG shows that there is a linear relationship between the work done by the heart and its oxygen consumption.

SARNOFF [1644] and NEILL [1355] have clarified this concept by showing that it is not the cardiac work as defined conventionally (i.e. the product of cardiac output x mean blood pressure) which governs the oxygen consumption, but rather what they refer to as the tension-time-index, viz: the product of three haemodynamic parameters: — mean systolic blood pressure, duration of the ventricular ejection and heart rate. It is interesting to note that this index can be estimated clinically, the heart volume, measured by X-ray, being a valid expression of the duration of the ventricular systole [280].

GREGG [979] has disclosed a second very important phenomenon, namely that there is an equally satisfying linear relationship between myocardial oxygen consumption and coronary arterial flow.

Thus there is no doubt that under physiological conditions it is the extent of the myocardial oxygen needs which precisely conditions the level of coronary arterial flow.

Thanks to the application of bloodless methods for measuring the various parameters required, it has been possible to demonstrate that in man also the coronary flow is directly dependent on myocardial oxygen demands [694, 1569] and that, during exercise, it increases as a function of the myocardial oxygen consumption [1171].

It therefore follows that if we attempt to administer to the angina pectoris subject a medication which is liable to increase his myocardial oxygen requirements, there is the risk of setting up myocardial hypoxia since his coronary reserve is considerably lowered.

It is easy to understand why any increase in the oxygen requirements of the cardiac muscle urgently calls for an increase in blood flow, unlike what happens, for instance, in the case of the skeletal muscle (Table 2). Here the amount of oxygen extracted from the arterial blood only represents 25% of the amount available. It follows that the oxygen content of the venous blood remains high, viz. 75% of the saturation, and that any increase in work is covered by higher oxygen extraction and not by a rise in blood flow.

Table 2

| | Rest | | Effort | |
	Arterial oxygen extraction (%)	Oxygen content in venous blood (%)	Arterial oxygen extraction	Blood flow
Skeletal muscle	25	75	↗	→
Cardiac muscle	75	25	→ (exhausting work) ↗ 95%	↗ ↑ max (5 times)

In contrast to what takes place at the skeletal muscle, oxygen extraction by the cardiac muscle is, under normal conditions, exceptionally high. It is 75% [471] which explains why the coronary venous blood is very poor in oxygen, the level of the latter only reaching 25% of the saturation. It therefore follows that *the coronary oxygen reserve is very low*. If the subject is given considerable muscular effort to do, it is found, as stated in Chapter I, that the oxygen extraction rate by the myocardium does not change, which means that the increase in myocardial oxygen demands is fully covered by an increase in blood flow. It is only when this reaches its maximum — it can be increased up to fivefold [1706, 35a] — that the oxygen extraction rate from the blood becomes more marked, reaching as high as 95% under very severe work conditions [1706]. This is the reason why the myocardium depends to such a critical extent on its temporary blood irrigation.

To return once more to the pharmacological criteria, it is therefore obvious that in order not to raise the oxygen demands of the cardiac muscle, a given substance must not increase the work of the heart since any excess work can only be accomplished at the cost of increased oxygen consumption [979].

This concept also implies that cardiac output must be only slightly altered. The work of the heart is, in effect, directly dependent on cardiac output and mean blood pressure. It follows that in order not to increase the work of the heart, a substance, even with minor hypotensive properties, may only very moderately increase cardiac output, barely in an identical proportion to the drop in pressure, under penalty of increasing the work load.

The repercussion of changes in heart rate on coronary flow can only be clearly seen if account is taken of the coronary flow distribution in relation to the two phases of cardiac contraction, systole and diastole.

In 1940, GREGG [727] showed as a result of observations on anaesthetised dogs that the coronary blood flow was always very low during the systole, even to the extent of being retrograde, and that in fact what really counted for the regulation of coronary flow was what happens during the diastole. Taking these observations as a basis, the conclusion was reached that there was an advantage for an anti-anginal medication to slow up the heart rate, since by so doing it extended the diastolic period which could only improve coronary flow.

Back in 1963, GREGG used a more accurate technique for measuring the phasic coronary flow enabling him to work with an unanaesthetised dog, as a result of which he completely revised his opinion and showed that in fact the coronary flow during the systole amounted to 25—60% of the flow during the diastole [722], that it could increase by from 300 to 400% during intensive exercise, at which time it would be equal to the diastolic flow [723, 724, 728]. These later facts show that it is illusory to want to lower the heart rate of the angina subject in the hope of increasing his coronary flow. The fact still remains that a lowering of the heart rate can be an advantage since it contributes to a lowering of myocardial oxygen needs [118a][2].

The above physiological considerations thus stress the need, when making a pharmacological study of a substance which reduces coronary resistance, to take a close look also at its effect on myocardial oxygen consumption. It should be added that an analysis of the elements thus gathered provides highly informative *additional* information, because the direct quantification of oxygen consumption calls for the measuring of three factors, viz. coronary arterial flow, the oxygen content of the arterial blood and the oxygen content of the coronary venous blood (see p. 93).

A comparison of the variations occurring in these four parameters will provide five interesting additional indications.

1. The first of these concepts is the determination of the type of effect in the case of a substance which increases coronary irrigation. If this substance does not increase the oxygen needs of the cardiac muscle, its "benign" character is demonstrated at the same time along the lines of GREGG's definition [732]. The substance with a benign character is, in fact, the one in which the increase in coronary flow which it causes is not conditioned by an increase in oxygen requirements. Conversely, the substance which increases flow by an inevitable increase in oxygen consumption is of a "malignant" character.

2. The second concept gathered is the behaviour of the oxygen content of the coronary venous blood. Its interest lies in the fact that it enables a relationship to be established with variation in flow. For instance, where we find ourselves faced with a substance of the benign type (i.e. one which increases flow without changing the oxygen consumption), it is found that the oxygen content of the coronary venous blood increases. This phenomenon is logical since the excess oxygen supplied to the myocardium by the speeding up of the blood flow is not used by the muscle.

3. The third notion, which derives directly from the foregoing, is the behaviour of the oxygen coronary arterio-venous difference. Let us take the case of a benign type substance which thereby increases the oxygen content of the coronary venous blood. If the oxygen content of the arterial blood does not alter, which is usually the case, it follows that the oxygen coronary arterio-venous difference drops correspondingly. If during the investigation of a substance it is shown that, at different doses, there is good correlation between the increase in blood flow and

---

2 In normal human subjects, myocardial blood flow increased with cardio-acceleration by atrial pacing to an average rate of 130 beats/min. With average rate of 150 beats/min, myocardial flow fell significantly after the initial rise at 130 beats/min [182c]. In man with abnormally low heart rates (idioventricular rate), myocardial blood flow was found to be positively related to the increase in heart rate induced by pacing [141c].

the reduction in the oxygen coronary arterio-venous difference, a second element is introduced, as GREGG points out [732], which provides an experimental check on the benign nature of the coronary dilator effect.

4. A fourth item of information provided by this type of investigation lies in the fact that it is possible not only to exclude the malignant character of a substance which improves coronary irrigation, but also to make it clear why it does not act in the same way as substances of a malignant nature, whether they be inhibitors of tissue respiration like cyanide or uncoupling agents of the oxidative phosphorylations such as dinitrophenol.

Cyanide causes a very sharp rise in the oxygen content of the coronary venous blood (it becomes almost on a level with the arterial blood), which is the direct consequence of inhibition of tissue oxidation which leads to a marked drop in oxygen consumption by the myocardium [1086, 1165, 1284]. Furthermore, there is a simultaneous production of lactic acid by the myocardium (which reflects the transition from the normal phase of aerobic metabolism to that of anaerobic metabolism) in such a quantity that there is found an inversion of the lactate arterio-venous difference.

Dinitrophenol increases very considerably the myocardial oxygen consumption, and this increase in needs is only partly covered by the increase in coronary flow. For this reason, the myocardium increases its coefficient of extraction of oxygen from the arterial blood, which entails oxygen desaturation of the coronary venous blood [222, 223, 1168].

5. If we establish the relationship which exists between the variation in blood flow and the variation in myocardial oxygen consumption, we define the *coronary efficiency*, a concept which corresponds to what GOLLWITZER-MEIER [686] calls the "quality of coronary irrigation". It goes without saying that this efficiency increases in the case of a substance which increases coronary irrigation whilst not at the same time increasing myocardial oxygen needs, whereas it does not alter or decrease in the case of a malignant type substance.

A final aspect of the physiology of coronary circulation deserves some enlargement: this is the automatic regulation of coronary irrigation.

We have seen that there are very close correlations between cardiac work, oxygen consumption, and coronary arterial flow. This dependence proves that the level of the blood flow is strictly conditioned by the myocardial oxygen requirements, and that there exists an intramyocardial system of regulation for coronary vasomotor functions. This regulating system must obviously be very sensitive, instantaneous and of a permanent nature [1252], as witness more especially the extraordinary constancy of the oxygen content of the coronary venous blood and the considerable reactive hyperaemia which occurs immediately on the restoration of a coronary arterial circulation which has been temporarily arrested.

As far back as 1880, the question arose as to whether there was not an intermediary of a metabolic nature which might play a predominant role in this automatic regulating system. Although a large number of physiologists have bent their efforts to this important question, it has still proved impossible to find a completely satisfactory answer as regards the nature of the metabolites or of the transmitters involved. On the other hand, there is no doubt whatsoever that local myocardial factors play a vital part in changing the tonicity of the coronary vessels which is very high — and which is directly subordinated to the orthosympathetic nervous system [488] — and thereby adjusting the blood flow to allow it to meet the myocardial oxygen demands. A study of these intramyocardial mediators has involved particularly interesting investigation work. Several lines have been suggested.

Let us first take a look at hypoxaemia. It has long been accepted that hypoxia is the most powerful physiological stimulus in relaxing the coronary vessels, a fact which has also been demonstrated in man [805]. But although the effect of hypoxaemia is disputed by no-one, there is no general agreement as to the mechanisms involved in this effect. It would seem, however, that unlike the conclusions of HILTON and EICHHOLTZ [833] it is not the oxygen content of the *arterial blood* which is the critical factor, but rather the oxygen content at the *myocardial cell*. Indeed, BERNE [143] has shown that whatever the amount of oxygen supplied to the myocardium by the arterial blood, coronary flow does not alter as long as the oxygen content of the coronary *venous* blood remains *in excess of 5.5 volumes*%. He proceeds as follows. A heart is first perfused at a pressure of 160 mm Hg with arterial blood containing 18.5 volumes % of oxygen. During a second phase, pressure is maintained but use is made of blood with a low oxygen content, 12.5 volumes %: it is seen that coronary flow increases by 60%, the oxygen content of the venous blood then being 2.5 volumes %. If for a second experimental sequence the same conditions of arterial oxygen concentration are adopted, viz. 18.5 and 12.5 volumes %, but at a higher perfusion pressure to ensure an oxygen content of more than 6 volumes % in the coronary venous blood, it is found that coronary flow no longer alters on transition from normoxaemia to hypoxaemia. BERNE pointed out these facts by showing that the coronary flow increases from the moment when the oxygen content of the coronary venous blood drops below 5.5 volumes %, and also that the increase in flow is proportional to the reduction in the oxygen content of the venous blood.

This observation by BERNE was likewise confirmed by KATZ [950] who, during the hypoxaemia phase, finds a satisfactory correlation between the oxygen concentration in the coronary venous blood and coronary arterial resistance, this relationship being completely independent of the oxygen content of the arterial blood [143]. These experimental data do not therefore bear out the idea that coronary dilatation caused by hypoxaemia is due to the diminution of oxygen in the arterial blood as such. It suggests on the contrary that arterial hypoxaemia sets up tissue hypoxaemia which triggers the release mechanism of vaso-dilator metabolites from the under-oxygenated myocardium. A similar argument lies in the fact that the increase in blood flow caused by hypoxia persits for some time after the reestablishment of a partial oxygen pressure exceeding that available prior to the setting up of the hypoxia. CRONIN et al. demonstrated that the coronary arterioles are directly insensitive to hypoxaemia or acidaemia *of the blood* within the lumen of these vessels but respond to factors which affect the aerobic metabolic state of the contracting myocardial *fibers*, notably reduction in the rate of oxygen delivery or reduction in intracellular pH [71 c].

The nature of these metabolites has formed the subject of considerable research in the field of fundamental physiology.

Although CO_2 and lactic acid are products of cardiac metabolism, aerobic or anaerobic, and that they possess vaso-dilator properties, their role appears to be a minor one in the automatic regulating system in view of the fact that concentrations exceeding those found in the coronary venous blood during hypoxia only result in very much less coronary vaso-dilatation than that caused by hypoxia [833].

Recent works have shown [1035] that the level of blood pH appears to play a critical role, since several drugs known for their property of increasing coronary flow have only seen their activity displayed in a restricted pH zone of 7.0—7.8, to disappear at 7.9. Within the same context, the hypothesis has recently been advanced that, although the pH level does in fact play a major part, it is not a question of the extra-cellular pH, viz. the blood pH, but rather of the intra-cellular pH at the myocardial cell level [467].

In 1935, ANREP [42] suggested histamine as a regulating substance, but various researchers including CODE [338] were unable to repeat his results, so that the hypothesis was abandoned.

Although DAWES [395] had suggested that the potassium freed by the cardiac muscle during its working could contribute to the local regulation of coronary circulation, DRISCOL and BERNE [450] demolished this hypothesis by showing that intra-coronary infusion of KCl causes mediocre vaso-dilatation which is not related to the dose, and also that various experimental manipulations which lead to a considerable increase in coronary flow do not trigger the release of potassium by the cardiac muscle.

The nucleotides of adenine, which have long been known as powerful vaso-dilators, have attracted attention as possible regulators of coronary circulation. This hypothesis is of special interest because of the important role played by these substances in the energy-producing metabolism of the myocardium. Now despite their powerful coronarodilator action, there is no evidence that the phosphorylated derivatives of adenine, viz. ATP, ADP and AMP, are capable of passing through the membrane of the myocardial cell to reach the resistance vessels. But it is quite the reverse with adenosine, which easily passes through this membrane [883]. If we add that this substance is a powerful vasodilator [2028], that it is quickly rendered inactive by deamination in inosine, and that it has a great potential source in the form of the adenine nucleotides, we see that *adenosine would seem to be a serious challenger for the role of biochemical mediator.*

BERNE [141] has added suggestive arguments in favour of this theory by showing that, during experimental myocardial anoxia, there is observed in the coronary venous blood a considerable freeing of inosine and hypoxanthine, products of the degradation of adenosine caused by the splitting up of the intra-myocardial adenine nucleotides in the presence of hypoxia.

If we take it as agreed, with BERNE, that the adenosine formed in the myocardium during hypoxaemia passes *in its entirety* through the cellular membrane, we can accept the regulating pattern which he suggests [142] and which is seen as follows. Any reduction in oxygen pressure in the myocardial cell, caused either by a drop in coronary arterial flow or by hypoxia or by an increase in myocardial oxygen consumption, leads to the degradation of the adenine nucleotides into adenosine. This spreads through the cell membrane and brings about arteriolar dilatation, which in turn increases the blood flow. The increase in flow has two consequences: firstly it speeds up the elimination of the freed adenosine, and secondly it reduces any additional intracellular formation of adenosine by raising the intratissular oxygen pressure. Thus a new steady-state is reached, which is maintained for such time as fresh changes in the initial factors do not take place.

This attractive assumption can only be valid if it is shown that the adenosine is not de-aminated *prior to leaving the myocardial cell*, since its two breakdown products, inosine and hypoxanthine, do not possess any vasodilator properties.

Quite recently, BERNE [945] has provided experimental proof of the last link in his hypothesis: by operating with an inhibitor of adenosine deaminase, 8-aza-guanine, he detects the presence of adenosine in the coronary venous blood of hearts which are given a perfusion extremely low in oxygen.

These experimental facts are therefore compatible with the idea that adenosine is formed during myocardial hypoxia and that it spreads from the myocardial cell into the blood before being broken up there.

This concept finds a further argument in the fact that, in 1967, BERNE found adenosine in the coronary venous blood during the phase of reactive hyperaemia which follows removal of occlusion of a coronary artery which has previously been occluded in an animal [1581].

Finally, in 1969, BERNE [109a] recalls that before being able to accept the hypothesis of the role of adenosine in the physiological regulation of coronary irrigation, three things must be shown: 1. that there is a continual release of adenosine from the normal myocardial cells into the interstitial fluid; 2. that the substance released is in fact adenosine and not one of its precursors; 3. that there is a precise quantitative cause and effect relationship between the adenosine content in the interstitial fluid and the diameter of the coronary resistance vessels. He provides at the same time a positive answer to the first of these three requirements by showing that the normal myocardium releases adenosine into the pericardial fluid and that this releasing action is speeded up by asphyxia. BERNE stresses the fact that the assumption as to the regulating role of adenosine does not imply that adenosine is the sole determining factor in vascular resistance, and he suggests that adenosine modulates the effects of the other known or accepted factors, thus adjusting the coronary flow in such a way as to maintain a correct supply of oxygen to the cardiac muscle. It still remains to be shown, however, that the basal concentration of intramyocardial adenosine is in fact reduced where there is excess coronary irrigation.

Consonant with this hypothesis, the adenosine content of the left ventricular muscle has been shown to rise sharply during acute occlusion of the left coronary artery in anaesthetised dogs [28b]. The increase is the more important as the duration of occlusion is long (from 5—15 sec), but it appeared to be more closely related to the number of beats occurring during occlusion than to its duration. This evidence suggests that adenosine production is somehow linked to the metabolism of the heart, as heart rate is an important determinant of myocardial oxygen consumption. The myocardial content of the sum of inosine and hypoxanthine also rose, though at a slower rate; the limited data on individual nucleoside content would suggest that the increase in the sum of the two compounds was largely due to an increase in inosine content, as the hypoxanthine content did not appear to change during coronary occlusion.

Among the several chemical changes initiated by myocardial ischaemia and capable of producing arteriolar dilatation, only adenosine can account for the entire coronary dilatation observed. However, other factors, such as reduction in pO_2, increase in pCO_2, increases in the concentrations of lactic acid and potassium in the interstitial fluid of the myocardium probably contribute to the relaxation of the vascular smooth muscle [26c and 27c]. A further step has been recently made by SNOW and OLSSON [295c] who demonstrated that in dogs, adenosine is readily extracted by the myocardium and they have given evidence in support of an hypothesis that adenosine is actively transported by the heart. It has also been suggested by RABERGER et al. [263c] that a primary step in the coronary dilator action of adenosine could be concerned with the myocardial uptake of adenosine and the production of 3'—5' AMP leading to an increase in myocardial glycolysis and lipolysis.

Other indirect arguments in favour of the key-role played, according to BERNE, by adenosine in the regulation of coronary circulation are to be found. These are supplied by BRETSCHNEIDER [221, 224] who shares BERNE's notions. To start with, the dilator effect of adenosine on the coronary vessels is specific, since it takes effect at very low dosage, and it is vaso-constrictive as regards other areas, the kidney for instance [220, 790]. Next, certain coronaro-dilator drugs —

with particular reference to Persantine—would seem to owe their coronarotropic action to the fact that they considerably potentialise the dilating effect of adenosine at this level [220, 790], one of the possible mechanisms being the inhibition by Persantine of adenosine deaminase [256]. Persantine does in fact exert a competitive inhibition effect *in vitro* on adenosine deaminase [422], a fact which in the view of those responsible for such findings bears out the idea that the coronaro-dilator effect of Persantine results from the action of endogenous adenosine accumulated in the myocardium. These results (see p. 185) would therefore suggest that adenosine plays the part of mediator in coronary dilation due to hypoxia.

The fact that intracoronary injection of Persantine potentialises both the coronaro-dilator effect of adenosine (but not that of bradykinine and acetylcholine) and the intensity of the reactive hyperaemia following arterial occlusion [1302] is likewise in favour of the mediator role of adenosine.

Certain facts however argue against the hypothesis as to the mediator role of adenosine:

a) potentialisation of the coronaro-dilator effect of adenosine by Persantine is not found *in toto* with animals when adenosine is injected into the coronaries [1694]; it is also non-existent on the isolated heart of dogs and guinea-pigs [1694] although it is found in the case of cats [1813];

b) the said potentialisation would seem to rest, to a considerable extent, on a process, having the blood as its seat, of inhibition by Persantine of the permeation of the erythrocyte membrane as regards adenosine [256, 1049, 1050];

c) Intensaine, a coronary vaso-dilator with powerful and prolonged action, does not intensify the coronaro-dilator effect of adenosine [226, 1694];

d) the findings of BERNE are not proof against criticisms of an experimental character, in view of the fact that prolonged anoxia leads to membrane lesions and increased cellular permeability, and that the discharge into the coronary venous blood from the myocardium of products of adenosine breakdown has only been demonstrated under conditions of anoxia and not during hypoxia of a physiological nature.

These facts lead SCHOLTHOLT et al. [1694] to dispute the regulator role of adenosine in myocardial blood circulation, and favour instead bradykinine (see p. 63).

Another mediator has been advanced, in the context of the adenosine hypothesis. BRETSCHNEIDER [226] offered the suggestion that in the action mechanism of certain vaso-dilator substances there comes into play a specific "sympathine" for the coronary vessels which is discharged by adenosine at the myocardium and which stimulates the adrenergic β-receptors. This could be isopropylnoradrenaline (isoprenaline) which, in a very small quantity, causes a considerable increase in coronary flow [837, 1087] which is merely ascribable to a reduction in vascular resistance without there being any increase in myocardial oxygen needs [837]. The validity of this hypothesis has been examined by KRAUPP using a dog previously treated with reserpine, and by HIRCHE with a dog previously treated with a β-blocking agent. KRAUPP found that, in the case of various long-acting coronarodilators (Persantine, Ustimon, Isoptin), there is no significant shift in the dose/activity relation after reserpine; the action of Intensaine is however suppressed at therapeutic doses, but reinforced at higher doses. HIRCHE [837], for his part, found that prior treatment by a β-blocking agent suppresses the coronaro-dilator action of isoprenaline but leaves that of adenosine practically unchanged. These facts would therefore appear to contradict the sympathine hypothesis, although the individual behaviour of Intensaine is remarkable.

However, according to BRETSCHNEIDER [225], the known fact that the functionally important fractions of the cardiac catecholamines are not rendered inactive by reserpine, and also that the β-receptors of the myocardium and of the coronary vessels probably do not react functionally in the same manner, would seem to lessen the significance of these results arguing against the sympathine hypothesis.

BRETSCHNEIDER's arguments do not seem to have carried the day, and it can be taken as valid that metabolic regulation of the coronary circulation functions independently of the sympathetic innervation, of a β nature, of the coronary vessels, an intrinsic innervation whose reality has been amply demonstrated [999, 1280], which is independent of the adrenergic receptors of the cardiac muscle [1449], and which would seem to be exclusive to the small arteries [197, 1894], whereas it is of a mixed nature, a and β, in the case of the large trunks [197][3]

A third transmitter has been suggested as a biochemical regulator of coronary circulation. This is bradykinine, which is one of the most powerful endogenous vaso-dilator substances known for humans and animals [1133]. It is the natural biochemical mediator for functional vaso-dilatation in the case of certain glands [834, 835], and it could play a preponderant role in the regulating of blood pressure at the periphery [575]. Moreover bradykinine is the most powerful reducer of coronary vascular resistance [47, 1169, 1419, 1423]. It exerts its effect by direct action on the smooth muscle of the vessel itself and not by increasing myocardial metabolic requirements, since at the active doses it does not change the heart rate, intraventricular pressure, or myocardial contractility in dogs [1169], and it leaves practically unchanged the frequency and amplitude of the cardiac contractions of an isolated heart [47].

These harmonious findings led PARRATT [1419] along with LOCHNER [1169] to suggest that bradykinine could be implicated in functional vaso-dilatation in the myocardium and play a preponderant part in the local automatic regulation of the coronary arterial flow, not only because of the very high reactivity of the coronary system to bradykinine, but also because the latter is considerably more active than adenosine as regards its coronaro-dilator effect, in the region of 50 to a 100 times greater [1694].

In support of the hypothesis as to the role played by bradykinine in coronary irrigation, recent observations by PITT et al. [98a] must be mentioned. Having recalled that it is from the kallikrein in the plasma that bradykinine is

---

3 No evidence has been found by KABELA and co-workers [67a] indicating the presence of a-receptors in the coronary circulation of the isolated dog heart, since a-receptor blocking agents did not antagonise the effects of adrenaline, noradrenaline and phenylephrine upon the a-receptors in isolated heart preparations, although they were effective in the whole animal. The fact that butoxamine, a β-blocking drug with vascular specificity (see p. 237) reduces myocardial blood flow and increases myocardial vascular resistance can be taken as evidence for the existence of myocardial vascular β_2-adrenoceptors [246c]. Furthermore, histochemical studies on the binding of perfused catecholamines by vascular smooth muscle suggest a predominance of β-adrenergic receptors in small coronary arteries [8c]. However, LUCCHESI and HODGEMAN [7e] suggest that the β-adrenergic receptors in the coronary vascular bed represent β_1-receptors and not β_2-receptors because practolol, which is a cardioselective β-blocking agent, produced, along with a significant reduction in the cardiac positive inotropic and chronotropic response to adrenergic stimulation, a marked decrease in the coronary vasodilator response to intracoronary injections of isoprenaline while it did not affect the isoprenaline-induced vasodilator response in the hind-limb (see p. 235). The hypothesis has been recently raised that there is only one type of adrenergic receptor, a-receptor, which could be transformed in β-receptor when cardiac activity is increased, by the release of a modulator substance which, it is said, has been extracted from the plasma of the coronary sinus blood while cardiac sympathetics were stimulated and was also found in high concentration in myocardial tissue homogenate [310c].

formed in man, these authors take venous blood samples from the coronary sinus of 7 angina patients in whom myocardial ischaemia (marked by cardiac pain or the appearance of electrocardiographic symptoms of ischaemia) occurs spontaneously or by atrial pacing of their heart rate. They find that there occurs in five of these patients considerable activation of the kallikrein system which is manifested by an abnormal increase in arginine esterase activity, a lowering of the kallikreinogen level and the absence of kallikrein inhibitor. The interest of these findings lies in the fact that activation of the kallikrein system does not appear in two patients who do not develop cardiac ischaemia. Since myocardial ischaemia is associated with activation of the kallikrein system, the authors suggest that plasma kallikrein could play a major role in the response to ischaemia and could be the mediator in the coronary vaso-dilatation which is triggered off by myocardial ischaemia.

A new substance has recently been proposed, hyperemine, which is said to condition the response of reactive hyperaemia to the temporary interruption of coronary irrigation [1869, 1870]. Its structure has not yet been defined, and no confirmation of its mediator role has been provided by other authors.

If we take a close look at the notions regarding the mechanisms which govern the regulation of coronary circulation, it is clear that a complete picture will only be obtained by an investigation, of both a physiological and biochemical nature, on a non-anaesthetised animal. Recent advances in technology give room to believe that this question could find a satisfactory answer in the fairly near future. The importance of these methodological advances will emerge in the following chapter where it will be seen that the point has been reached where research can be carried out, both on animals and humans, into many aspects of coronary circulation under fundamentally physiological conditions which exclude, for instance, having recourse to general anaesthesia and to damaging surgical operations.

Chapter III

Pharmacological Methodology for Testing Antianginal Drugs

In this chapter will be described the experimental methods which are now available for measuring the various haemodynamic parameters which are necessary to determine the profile of the pharmacological properties of a given compound which may be recommended for clinical use as an antianginal drug.

The nature of such biological parameters is of course closely related to the haemodynamic properties which such a substance should possess if it is to be considered of therapeutic interest. It follows, therefore, that such methodology applies chiefly to the quantitative measurement of coronary blood flow, of cardiac output, of heart work and of oxygen consumption by the myocardium. Other special methods will also be described namely the techniques which are advocated to study the nutritional myocardial microcirculation and the collateral coronary circulation. The procedures used to create chronic coronary insufficiency in animals will also be given some attention.

Coronary Blood Flow

The correct quantitative evaluation of coronary blood flow is hindered by certain anatomical factors. This accounts for the fact that a good many of the techniques which were initially proposed reflect the ingeniousness of the investigators concerned in getting round obstacles.

Because progress in methodology has been very rapid during this last decade, certain of the older procedures with only historical interest will be briefly commented so that greater attention can be paid to the more elaborate methods evolved in recent times.

To begin with a few words about the procedures which operate with isolated heart.

In 1895, LANGENDORFF [1074] published a method for perfusion of the isolated mammalian heart, which he used on dogs, cats and rabbits to study changes in the rate and amplitude of the cardiac contractions produced by various means. By reason of the principle on which the perfusion was based, which was the introduction of an irrigation cannula into the aorta in such a manner that it did not pass the aortic valve, the nutrient fluid (normal saline) entering the coronary vessels, this technique also implied the possibility of collecting the fluid leaving the venous system and measuring the changes in the coronary flow. In 1898, PORTER [1463] used an arrangement closely resembling that of LANGENDORFF to record changes in the flow from the coronary veins occurring in response to experimental modification of the cardiac contraction, particularly in force and rate.

The original apparatus of LANGENDORFF rapidly became the object of diverse and numerous technical improvements, the most outstanding of which were the work of HEUBNER and MANCKE [825] whose object was to obtain constant perfusion conditions (pressure, rate and temperature) and to be able to use continuous perfusion, the duration of which could be controlled, with drug solutions of known concentrations for pharmacological investigation, instead of simple injections. The satisfactory settlement of this method is due to UHLMANN and NOBILE [1910] who were apparently the first to use it for measurement of the coronary flow. These authors advanced the technical features of the perfusion apparatus to a high degree of precision, endeavouring above all, by means of arrangements which were sometimes complicated but effective, to obtain stable experimental conditions, particularly in regard to the physical constants of the perfusion and the chemical characteristics of the perfusates. The apparatus of UHLMANN and NOBILE is still currently used, as initially intended, by pharmacologists concerned with coronary circulation problems [1899, 1900].

Another variant of the LANGENDORFF technique, which has been used extensively on the cat and dog by KATZ and his co-workers [958], is perfusion of the coronary system by means of a pump, under a constant pressure of 100 mm Hg with defibrinated heparinized blood. The animal whose heart is to be perfused is first heparinized, after which all the mediastinal vessels are ligatured with the exception of two: the aorta, into the root of which the irrigation cannula is inserted, and the left pulmonary artery, which is used for the introduction of the drainage cannula into the right ventricle. All the coronary venous blood that discharges into the two right cavities is thus collected and measured in a graduated vessel, and is then returned to the pump after oxygenation. The heart is kept in permanent fibrillation by means of a faradic current so that coronary flow changes brought about by injected drugs are solely the result of their direct action on the musculature of the coronary vessels.

The system proposed by BAKER [72] improves the stabilization of temperature. Finally, the apparatus produced by ANDERSON and CRAVER [32] and subsequently improved [31, 1096] is merely a commercial form of Langendorff's arrangement, rendered practical, constructed in Pyrex and suitable for use with small hearts (guinea-pig) or large (dog). The fact that substances are administered by injection and not by perfusion necessitates a complicated rinsing system which may give rise to errors. Considering that the injection principle is unsatisfactory, particularly as the effects produced by test substances vary with the rapidity of their injection, which is difficult to control, TRUITT [1901] has modified this apparatus to make it suitable also for the perfusion of drug solutions.

Believing that the normal coronary flow of the perfused heart was, in most cases, too large — and this would made comparative tests difficult — some authors introduced a vasoconstrictor substance into the perfusate: polyvinylpyrrolidone [777] or privine, which, in strengths of 1—2 mg per litre, reduces the coronary outflow by almost 50% without altering the rate or amplitude of the cardiac contractions [272].

Equally open to criticism, in our opinion, is the idea expressed by these authors that the dilator effects of pharmacological substances, when recorded by the Langendorff technique with a perfusion fluid to which a vasoconstrictor has not previously been added, are of short duration and difficult to measure, and that this tends to limit the importance of the method; this is probably due to the fact that these experimenters injected the test substances into the aortic cannula; if the substances are administered as perfusions, dilator effects, significant both in size and duration and easily measurable, are obtained even with very low concentrations [301].

Whereas the original Langendorff technique measures the flow of perfusion fluid entering or leaving the coronary vascular bed under *constant perfusion pressure*, some authors, supporting the conceptions of KATZ [951] recommended that, instead of measurement of changes in coronary flow under constant perfusion pressure, changes in perfusion pressure under *constant rate of perfusion* should be recorded, as these would reflect the changes in tone of the coronary vessels. According to LUDUENA et al. [1191], the importance of this procedure lies in the fact that pressure changes are much more sensitive than changes in flow, so that very slight reductions in vessel tone, incapable of causing any technically appreciable increase of flow, are registered by significant falls in the perfusion pressure.

RYSER and WILBRANDT [1621] have applied a variant of Luduena's method to the guinea-pig. LARSEN [1075] suggested another variant, the beating isolated heart of the cat or rabbit being perfused with defibrinated blood, the volume of perfusing fluid per unit of time being constant. While the author's intention was to study the direct activity of different substances on the musculature of the coronary vessels, he was working with the beating heart and was therefore making a summated assessment, without recording, of the effects on the vessels of concomitant changes in the extravascular support. It becomes difficult under these circumstances to dissociate direct and indirect effects.

The principle of recording variations in perfusion pressure, on which the preceding systems are based, has no major advantage over measurement of the flow of fluid. Therefore, it is in this latter form, whatever technical variants are favoured, that the Langendorff technique has been most widely employed on various animal species — the rabbit, guinea-pig, cat, dog, and even the resuscitated human heart [1023].

One may reasonably question the value of the results derived from pharmacological investigations carried out by the Langendorff technique and the validity of the extrapolation of these results to the whole organism.

Although one certainly cannot claim that the values, relative or absolute, furnished by this method can be extrapolated to the coronary circulation of the intact animal, the figures obtained on the isolated heart do, however, give relatively exact indications as to the activity relations existing at the level of the coronary system in the intact animal. Comparing the coronary vasodilator activity of khellin with that of aminophylline, ANREP et al. [45] found an activity ratio of 4—1 in favour of khellin by the Langendorff method, and they obtained the same coefficient in the whole dog by the heart-lung preparation method. HANNA and SHUTT [779], comparing the coronary vasodilator effect of 65 analogues of papaverine, found that the respective activities were the same, whether they worked by the Langendorff method or on the whole dog, the coronary arterial flow being measured by means of a rotameter. WINBURY et al. [2015] also reported good correlation, in respect of 25 compounds belonging to the same chemical series, between the figures furnished by the Langendorff procedure and those obtained by a technique applied to the heart in situ in the dog, the coronary inflow being measured with a sensitive rotameter. We ourselves have found, in respect of various substances, coefficients of coronary vasodilator activity close to those we established by employing the much more complex method of GREGG on the heart in situ in the dog [301].

All these facts indicate that the investigation of the coronary circulation on the isolated heart, perfused by techniques derived from Langendorff method, has made an extensive contribution to our present knowledge of the pharmacology of the coronary circulation. The data they furnish acquire particular significance when one works under experimental conditions which, whatever they may be (for example with permanent ventricular fibrillation [956, 958]), ensure constancy of the extravascular support during the tests, as the effects recorded can then be regarded as the expression of a pharmacological activity exerted exclusively on the intrinsic resistance of this vascular bed.

Needless to say, the quantitative results which have been obtained *in vitro* must be carefully analysed since the physiological conditions have been in many ways altered. According to some investigators, some correlation could however exist between the quantitative data recorded *in vitro* and those which result from intracoronary injection in the whole dog [925]. Nevertheless, it stands to reason that this route of administration is only experimental and far removed from the usual therapeutic modes of administration.

Although perfusion techniques on isolated heart fall in particularly well with investigations on cardiac metabolism because the nature and the concentration of the substrates may be modified at will, they are at the present time largely superseded by the in vivo procedures for measuring coronary irrigation, which enable experiments to be carried out in conditions where all the determinants of the coronary flow play their normal role.

Methods working on the anaesthetized entire animal, with the heart in situ, may be grouped into two general categories: some measure the quantity of blood issuing from the venous territory, or the coronary outflow; the others measure the coronary inflow, that is, the quantity of blood that enters the coronary system.

1. Measurement of Coronary Outflow

It is chiefly for reasons of anatomical disposition that many workers have chosen to measure the *venous* coronary flow since the coronary sinus can be reached more easily than the coronary arteries, and very often without opening the thorax, which is not the case when measuring the *arterial* coronary flow, except when indirect procedures are employed, involving radioisotopes for example. Unfortunately, the flow from the coronary sinus cannot be in any way compared with the arterial blood flow.

The procedures which collect the venous coronary blood flow admit of serious sources of error which throw doubt on their validity. The main objection that can be made is that they only measure the sinus outflow, which is a fraction of the total coronary outflow as only a part of the coronary venous blood returns to the general venous circulation by the coronary sinus, the remainder discharging into the cardiac cavities by the anterior cardiac veins and the thebesian vessels. According to physiologists who have given serious attention to this problem, only 60% of the coronary venous blood drains off through the sinus [43, 1067]. If this proportion remained fixed under all haemodynamic conditions, then measurement of variations in coronary flow by cannulization of the sinus, although only partial, would naturally be valuable. While, unfortunately, as a result of early investigations the most recent of which dates back to 1929 [43, 512, 1222], the ratio of the coronary venous outflow through the sinus to the total coronary venous outflow has long been considered constant, even when wide variations in cardiac output, in heart rate and in intra-aortic pressure are present, it becomes more and more apparent in the light of subsequent investigations by the more exact methods which have been made possible by certain technical advances, that there is no fixity in this relationship [705, 954, 955, 959, 1308, 1965].

The method is based on the assumption that every change in the total coronary venous outflow finds constant proportional reflexion in the outflow from the coronary sinus. JOHNSON and WIGGERS [902] have shown that the relative outflows from the sinus and from the thebesian veins exhibit considerable variations in the cat and the dog, the ratios going from 1:1·3 to 1:4·8 in favour of the thebesian outflow; these facts confirm both WEARN's conclusions [1965] for the human heart and the observations of KATZ et al. that the proportion of venous blood passing through the coronary sinus varied greatly in different animals of the same species [955] and still more in the same animal under different haemodynamic conditions [954], particularly when the strength of the cardiac contraction was modified, which is a very frequent occurrence in connexion with substances acting on the coronary circulation. According to JOHNSON and WIGGERS' experiments, the distribution of the venous return between the sinus and the thebesian system is determined not only by the respective anatomical vascular resistances of these two systems, but also by the height of the pressure in the right ventricle in each systole, rise of this pressure alone (produced experimentally by mechanical compression of the pulmonary artery) being capable of increasing the sinus outflow. They attributed this phenomenon to the fact that the increased resistance against which the thebesian vessels drained into the right ventricle caused diversion of the blood from these vessels towards the coronary sinus so that a fraction of the blood in the cavity of the right ventricle came to be added to the coronary sinus blood, after passing in the reverse direction through the thebesian vessels. It is true that this opinion of JOHNSON and WIGGERS on the suggested action mechanism has not been confirmed experimentally in the course of subsequent investigations by WIGGERS himself [634, 1995]: the increase in the sinus flow is not a mechanical phenomenon because it is delayed, is preceded by reduction of outflow, and because the outflow remains increased after the intraventricular pressure has returned to normal, regaining its control values only slowly. Whatever may be the mechanism or mechanisms involved in these conditions, it nevertheless remains a fact that a slight increase of systolic pressure in the right ventricle causes the sinus blood flow to increase to an extent very close to that very frequently reported in the literature as resulting from administration of various substances when the coronary flow is measured by collection of the venous blood from the sinus only [902]. These changes in the outflow from the coronary sinus cannot therefore be regarded as reflecting vasomotor effects upon coronary vessels unless it is proved that the systolic pressure in the right ventricle remains unchanged. This, however, is never taken into consideration by the pharmacologists who use such a procedure. Sharing the opinion of the authors quoted on the absence of any constant relationship between sinus outflow and thebesian outflow, GRAHAM [705] has shown that the ratio may vary from 40 to 80%, which likewise proves that the outflow of the coronary sinus cannot be taken as an index of total coronary flow, and that changes in the sinus outflow may well represent changes in the distribution between coronary drainage by the sinus and coronary drainage by the thebesian vessels, rather than changes in the total coronary flow [957].

In an attempt to reconcile these divergent opinions, GREGG and SHIPLEY [720, 734] made simultaneous determinations of the coronary inflow and outflow in the entire animal and showed that, under a variety of experimental conditions, the relationship between inflow in the left coronary artery and the sinus outflow was constant in a given animal as long as reasonably normal haemodynamic conditions prevail; it follows that, for GREGG, the changes in the outflow from the coronary sinus in a given experiment can probably serve as purely directional but not quantitative indications of changes in the flow in the left coronary artery and presumably also in the total coronary arterial flow. GELLER et al. [634] and WIGGERS [1995] do not, however, agree with this reconciliatory view, as their experiments indicated that the right coronary artery is concerned in the venous flow from the coronary sinus to a much greater extent than is stated by GREGG, because the flow from the coronary sinus increased when the right ventricle increased its activity as well as when the left ventricle increased its activity. The fact is that considerable areas of the myocardial musculature supplied by the right coronary artery drain into the coronary sinus in the same way as those receiving their blood from the left coronary artery.

It would appear, then, to be well established that the magnitude of changes in venous flow from the coronary sinus cannot be taken as a measure of changes in the coronary arterial flow. Until a satisfactory answer to this very important question of the fixity of the ratio between coronary sinus venous outflow and total coronary venous flow is obtained, it must be considered that any technique for measurement of the coronary blood flow based solely on cannulization or catheterization of the coronary sinus is vitiated by a serious source of error and that *quantitative* results arrived at by this method must be accepted with the greatest reserve, the main reason for this being that the distribution of the venous coronary blood between the coronary sinus and the other vessels is extremely *variable*, a fact which has been once again confirmed recently [97].

1.1. Morawitz Technique

MORAWITZ and ZAHN [1321] suggested cannulization of the venous coronary system. They drained the coronary sinus by means of a special type of cannula which they inserted into the large venous trunk through an opening made in the right atrial appendage, the cannula passing through the right atrium. This method was much favoured because of its relative simplicity [667, 912, 913, 914, 915, 1390]. A recently proposed modification [22c] which measures coronary venous flow by means of an electromagnetic sensor does not seem to offer any advantage.

1.2. Heart-Lung Preparation

Very commonly employed, especially on the dog, this classical method, which we owe to Starling, allows of measurement of the coronary sinus outflow by means of a special cannula introduced into the sinus through the right atrium. This is a denervated preparation. This technique has made a powerful contribution to our knowledge of many aspects of the coronary circulation and it is still extremely useful for studies on cardiovascular physiology by reason of the possibilities it offers for control, in the investigation of a variety of circulatory problems, of all the haemodynamic elements affecting the coronary flow, and consequently for demonstration of the effects of one determinant factor, all others being maintained constant. In the sphere of pharmacology, it thus allows assessment of the contribution to a given overall effect upon the coronary outflow made by each of the factors influencing this outflow. It also facilitates approach to the investigation of intimate mechanisms in the activity of a substance on the coronary circulation.

1.3. Rodbard Technique

With a view to overcoming the inaccuracies of techniques which collect the venous blood from the coronary sinus only, RODBARD et al. [1548] have suggested an ingenious method whereby, in the anaesthetized dog, the *total* coronary venous outflow can be continuously measured at the same time as the cardiac output. The procedure is to divert all the venous blood returning by the two venae cavae into a reservoir, whence it is pumped out through a flowmeter into the right pulmonary artery and then to the lungs. The coronary venous blood entering the right atrium and ventricle, that is, 95% of the total coronary venous outflow, is driven by the right ventricle into the pulmonary trunk and then into the left pulmonary artery, where it is measured by a second flowmeter before reaching the lungs. The sum of the flows measured simultaneously by these two flowmeters gives the value of the cardiac output. Although the heart is functioning under conditions which are relatively different from normal conditions (the right ventricle particularly is only contracting on a reduced mass of blood represented by the coronary flow), this technique has the advantage, from the coronary point of view, that it maintains the general arterial circulation intact while measuring almost the total venous outflow.

1.4. Busch Technique

BUSCH [263] reported on a method which can be applied only in the rabbit and does not require cannulation of the coronary vessels as it takes advantage of a special anatomical arrangement of the venous system in this animal species namely that, as a result of peculiar embryological growth, there is a direct communication between the left external jugular vein and the coronary sinus. Thus, avoiding the opening of the thorax, it makes use of a specially designed cannula introduced in the jugular vein in order to collect only the coronary venous blood from the sinus without draining any blood from the two venae cavae. The method is difficult to apply and causes considerable loss amongst the experimental animals. It has since been abandoned.

1.5. Catheterization of the Coronary Sinus without Thoracotomy

From the moment the radioopaque intracardiac catheter was developed, it became easy to enter the coronary sinus without thoracotomy, the catheter being introduced into the right external jugular vein and inserted into the coronary sinus under fluoroscopy. This technique was applied more particularly by WEST et al. [1978, 1980], who designed, for this purpose, a special catheter, the intracoronary end being provided with two additional side holes. Coronary venous blood flowed through the catheter, was measured by different devices, and then generally reinfused into the general venous circulation.

It was soon realized that this procedure was capable of providing very inaccurate values for sinusal flow because the existence of additional resistance to venous flow, created by both the catheter and the flowmeter, altered the normal distribution of flow between the coronary sinus and the thebesian vessels to the advantage of the latter and thus to the disadvantage of the sinus.

In order to reduce to the minimum the undesirable variations of sinus flow due to artificially increased resistances, BRETSCHNEIDER [219] proposed in 1960 a special catheter of original design which allows the blood issuing from the coronary sinus to be measured and thereafter to flow into the right atrium as in normal conditions. The catheter is bent 20 mm from its intracoronary tip. It is passed along the external jugular vein, the bent portion being guided into the sinus. An inflatable small balloon permits firm fixation. Blood coming from the sinus enters the catheter, is then measured by a sensitive device located in the tip, goes out by a large hole located at the external curve of the bend, and finally returns via the right atrium.

A slight variation to this catheter has been constructed by LOCHNER [1162] who uses an electromagnetic sensing element, supplied by a square wave current, instead of the measuring device adopted by BRETSCHNEIDER.

GANZ and FRONEK [624] elaborated a method for measuring blood flow in the coronary sinus by local thermodilution method [608], which makes measurement of blood flow possible by injecting and mixing an indicator (glucose or physiological saline at a temperature of $\pm 20°C$) with the coronary venous blood and then detecting the resulting change in the immediate neighbourhood of the site of mixing. The injecting orifice and the detector (thermistor) are located near the tip of a specially designed catheter which is introduced by the way of the jugular vein into the coronary sinus.

The validity of the method has been checked in animal experiments by comparison with the volumetric values. The method has been recently applied in man [152c].

2. Measurement of Coronary Inflow[1]

There are many procedures for measuring the coronary arterial blood flow. They may be classified in three main groups according to whether they are based on extra-arterial cannulation or intra-arterial cannulation, or do not involve any arterial cannulation at all.

2.1. Techniques With Extra-Arterial Cannulation

As they require the partial or total section of a coronary artery, they are being progressively abandoned. Only two of them are described.

2.1.1. Melville Technique

Utilizing the principles enunciated by STEHLE [1827], MELVILLE and his co-workers [1184, 1276] have devised an ingenious variant of the perfusion technique and recording devices in the Langendorff method which enabled them to observe the coronary inflow and the characteristics of the cardiac contractions simultaneously.

It has been used on the heart *in situ* in the dog [1182], the animal being heparinized, the blood perfusing the heart from the apparatus coming from one of the animal's carotid arteries and entering the coronary system by the anterior interventricular artery, which is previously dissected out and cannulized. One disadvantage of this technique seems to be a certain inertia in the recording system which entails some asynchronism between the development of pharmacological phenomena and their graphic recording.

2.1.2. Schofield Technique

With the object of rendering the coronary flow independent of arterial pressure so that fluctuations in the latter would not alter it in a manner which could not be controlled and measured, SCHOFIELD and WALKER [1692] proposed a technique for artificial perfusion of the coronary arteries whereby they were able to measure, in the dog, changes in flow due purely to pharmacological effects produced upon the vascular system of the heart beating *in situ*.

The method, conceived by DAWES, MOTT and VANE [396, 1917], is itself an improved version of the procedures of GADDUM et al. [619] and of BINET and BURSTEIN [163] which, despite their simplicity and the advantage of using a relatively small quantity of extracorporeal blood, present, in the opinion of DAWES et al., certain disadvantages, mainly deriving from the fact that the perfusion pressure is not independent of the animal's systemic arterial pressure.

---

1 Much technical information about arterial flowmetry can be found in a recent monograph published by Chr. CAPPELEN Jr.: "New findings in blood flowmetry" Universitetsforlaget, AAS and Wahls Boktrykkeri, Oslo, 1968.

SCHOFIELD and WALKER's procedure is to perfuse the anterior interventricular coronary artery by means of a Dale-Schuster pump, which ejects into a rotameter, and then into the coronary artery, arterial blood from a femoral artery, kept at 37°C. In this way the coronary flow is independent of the level of the animals' general arterial pressure, and changes in the flow reflect changes in resistance developing in the coronary vascular system following the intracoronary injection of drugs. With the heart beating normally, the method does not, however, permit detection of those among the cardiac factors which are responsible for the changes in coronary flow recorded or differentiation of active changes in the calibre of the vessels from changes due to variation in the compression exercised on these vessels by the cardiac extravascular support. Although it offers the advantage that the pharmacological reactions of the coronary system can be examined without interference from concomitant changes in the arterial pressure, the method is open to one major criticism, namely, that the pulsatile rhythm of the pump differs from the rhythm of the heart perfused; the artery cannulized is irrigated artificially at the arbitrary rate of the pump while the rest of the coronary arterial system (circumflex and right coronary arteries) is subject to a different rate (that of the heart) as well as a different pressure (that of the animal), particularly when the systemic arterial pressure is altered by the substances injected. In addition to this major disadvantage it may be mentioned that the preparation of the artery for perfusion necessitates section of nerve fibres in the arterial wall, which may modify vasomotor control.

2.2. Techniques With Intra-Arterial Cannulation

Three of them are described.

2.2.1. Gregg Technique

The technique employed by GREGG and his co-workers [731, 733] allows of correct measurement of the coronary arterial blood flow in conditions which approximate closely to the physiological state, apart from the general anaesthesia and artificial respiration. It provides for normal irrigation of the left coronary artery in the dog from the animal's own carotid artery, the blood passing through a measuring apparatus interposed between the carotid and the coronary.

The thorax is opened at the level of the fourth left intercostal space. The left subclavian artery is dissected out from its origin in the arch of the aorta for the insertion of a cannula of special type which, travelling in a retrograde direction, is brought into the ascending part of the aorta so that its tip enters the left coronary artery, where it is maintained in position by a ligature. The blood from a common carotid artery is diverted to the inlet of a flowmeter from which it emerges to perfuse the territory of the left coronary artery, travelling by way of the cannula. The drug injections can be made as desired, either into a peripheral vein or into the stream above the arterial cannula in intracoronary administration.

The apparatus used originally by GREGG et al. [735] for measurement of the flow was a SHIPLEY and WILSON type rotameter [1747]. It consists essentially of a vertical tube tapering towards the base and containing a small float moving freely in the vertical direction, the position of which varies with the rate of flow and is picked up by an induction mechanism connected to a recording system. The GREGG's procedure requires heparinization of the animal and allows the measurement of the *mean* blood flow only. Any of the following three flowmeters can be used as measuring apparatus in place of the rotameter:

a) the bubble-flowmeter as finally designed by SOSKIN et al. [1796], which was used by ECKENHOFF et al. [470] and improved by DUMKE and SCHMIDT [461], is based on the principle of the displacement of a bubble of air injected into the blood stream which travels through a glass tube of known volume and special shape inserted into the circulation under study; the mean blood flow is measured by timing the speed of the air bubble. This instrument has been only occasionally used because it cannot provide continuous measurement;

b) the electromagnetic flowmeter of DENISON et al. [414], applicable to intact vessels, which is an improved and modified version of the flowmeter of RICHARDSON et al. [1522] which could be used only on cannulized vessels;

c) the drop-meter of VERA et al. [1936], which consists of a transit chamber for insertion into the continuity of a coronary artery; a photoelectric cell counts the drops at the entrance into the chamber and recording is effected electronically.

2.2.2. Pieper Technique

This method, which was proposed in 1964, has undeniable advantages compared to the preceding one. PIEPER [1441] has designed a particularly ingenious catheter-tip flowmeter for measuring coronary arterial flow in closed-chest dogs.

It is a rigid catheter which is inserted through the right carotid artery and pushed into the aorta till the intracardiac tip enters the orifice of the left coronary artery. When the tip is wedged in place, it is kept from slipping out by an outer oversized rim which provides also a positive seal preventing any blood flow past the rim. Three side holes, near the proximal end of inflow cannula, and spaced 120 degrees apart, provide for the entrance of blood. Blood flow is measured by a miniaturized flowmeter which is attached to the tip of the catheter, and the signal is then amplified. The flowmeter is placed in the ascending aorta where it measures the inflow into the left coronary artery. A brass sleeve is attached to the main tube. By sliding the main tube, one may occlude the inflow openings during a few seconds; this allows the establishment of zero flow whenever desired during an experiment. Performance tests showed the reliability of the instrument for the measurement of pulsatile flow: the relationship between actual flow velocity and flow signal gives a curve which is slightly parabolic. This may be made linear by passing the flow signal through a function generator.

Use of this catheter offers two important advantages: it does not require thoracotomy and phasic as well as mean flow may be measured.

2.2.3. Berne Technique

BERNE [139] employed an elegant and rather complex technique whereby, in the dog, simultaneous recordings could be made of inflow in the circumflex coronary artery, outflow from the coronary sinus, the oxygen tension in the coronary venous blood, the intramyocardial pressure, the whole being completed by measurements of the oxygen consumption of the myocardium from determinations of the oxygen content of the arterial and venous coronary blood. The technique was to introduce an ECKSTEIN cannula [475] by the endo-aortic route into the left coronary artery and to perfuse the vascular area with the blood of a dog donor, distributed by means of a perfusion pump [143], the pressure of which could be regulated very exactly in relation to the arterial pressure of the recipient dog. The coronary flow was measured with a SHIPLEY and WILSON rotameter [1747] and the oxygen tension in the coronary venous blood was recorded continuously by the polarographic method of CLARK et al. [331], while a GREGG and ECKSTEIN apparatus gave the intramuscular pressure in the myocardium [725].

This method is applied by its author to both the beating heart and the fibrillating heart.

The experiments on the fibrillating heart appear to be particularly interesting: as the cardiac extravascular support is constant and pharmacological changes in the systemic arterial pressure do not affect the coronary flow, the flow is determined solely by changes in the intrinsic resistance of the vascular bed. In the case of the beating heart, the simultaneous recording of the various functions mentioned above allows of rational analysis of the respective roles of the factors concerned in a change of flow, namely, the tone of the smooth muscle fibres in the coronary vessels, the intramyocardial pressure (extracoronary cardiac support) and the metabolism of the cardiac muscle.

BERNE's technique has constituted an advanced experimental attempt to measure the changes occurring simultaneously in the coronary flow and myocardial metabolism; thus, the combination of data collected in the case of administration of a substance which increases the blood flow makes it possible to follow the evolution of the coronary efficiency and to assess the importance or unimportance of a coronary vasodilator activity in accordance with whether the metabolism of the myocardium shows very little change or increases in parallel manner.

One criticism can unfortunately be formulated, not against the measurement of the coronary inflow, but in relation to the estimation of cardiac metabolism. This is, in effect, regarded as being the metabolism of the left ventricle, which presupposes that the coronary sinus blood is necessarily that returning from the left ventricle and can thus be used for venous oxygen determinations and consequently for metabolic determinations in respect of the left ventricle. According to GELLER et al. [634], there is here an erroneous interpretation of the opinion of GREGG [720], who considers that the venous outflow from the coronary sinus can reasonably be used to estimate directional (not quantitative) changes in the arterial flow in the left coronary artery, on the assumption that the latter, which supplies the left ventricle, contributes 80—90% of the venous outflow from the coronary sinus. Now, the right coronary artery, which supplies the right ventricle, also contributes to the venous outflow of the sinus and, as a result of the findings of WIGGERS and his co-workers [634, 1995], it is even very probable that this contribution of the right coronary artery is considerably in excess of the 10—20% accepted by GREGG. It would follow, therefore, that the coronary sinus drains a not inconsiderable fraction of blood from the area of the right ventricle, so that the arterio-venous oxygen difference, as calculated by use of venous blood from the coronary sinus, does not express the quantity of oxygen taken up solely by the left ventricle. The values for cardiac metabolism calculated from this arterio-venous difference are not, then, exclusively those of the left ventricle as the arterial circulation of the left ventricle and that of the right both contribute to the venous flow in the coronary sinus, and do so in an irregular manner, impossible to foresee.

Moreover, it must be stressed that according to more recent investigations [1067], the oxygen content of the blood in the coronary sinus could not be representative of the *mixed* coronary venous drainage.

2.3. Techniques Without Arterial Cannulation

They can be gathered into direct methods and indirect methods.

2.3.1. Direct Methods

Four of them will be considered.

2.3.1.1. The Thermostromuhr

The first thermostromuhr was constructed by REIN [1517] in 1928. The apparatus comprises a small diathermy unit (which supplies a small and constant amount of heat) and two thermocouples. When the instrument is applied firmly around an intact blood vessel, part of the heat supplied by the diathermy unit is removed by the blood stream and this produces a difference of temperature between the two thermocouples which is a function of the speed of the blood flow and is recorded by a highly sensitive galvanometer. REIN's thermostromuhr was modified slightly in 1934 by BALDES and HERRICK [81], who used direct current instead of high frequency current.

This method has inestimable advantages; while allowing continuous recording of the mean coronary flow, it is applied to the normal, unanaesthetized animal for, although the fitting of the device around a coronary artery requires a major surgical operation under anaesthesia, the procedure can be performed under conditions of asepsis and the animal can be permitted to recover, the leads connecting the thermostromuhr to the galvanometer emerging from the thorax through the operation wound. The animal can naturally be used over a number of weeks.

The thermostromuhr offers the great advantage of experimentation under conditions exactly similar to those existing in normal man, that is, experimentation on a coronary circulation which is still an integral part of the whole circulatory system and is subject to the influences of the various physiological factors which can modify it. It thus furnishes information on the overall pharmacological effect at this level. Unfortunately some very exact investigations by GREGG and his co-workers [730, 1746] ended in the conclusion that this procedure could not be used for quantitative estimations under most experimental conditions. The physical proof of this produced by these authors has no place here. Briefly, the flow values established in chronic experimentation from preliminary calibration, carried out either in vivo or in vitro, can be grossly incorrect as the relationship between the blood flow and the galvanometer deflection varies with a number of variables which cannot be estimated and the existence and magnitude of which cannot be anticipated; these are the degree of stretching of the artery, the position and degree of angulation of the instrument in relation to the artery on which it is applied, the presence of backflow in the flow measured, the nature of the tissues in the immediate neighbourhood, the movements of extravascular and intravascular fluids in the tissues, the viscosity of the blood flow measured and changes in the temperature of the blood.

2.3.1.2. The Calorimetric Method

This method for measurement of the intramyocardial blood flow in animals, which we owe to KIESE and LANGE [980] is based on the technique employed by HENSEL et al. [815] to effect continuous measurement, by means of a calorimetric probe, of the blood flow in the skin and the muscles in man.

The method employs a differential thermo-element, which is introduced into the cardiac muscle, consisting of two metal needle points, one of which measures the temperature of the muscle, the other being heated, and its temperature will vary with the blood flow as the heat transmitted to it is carried away by the blood. The difference between the two thermal currents is recorded continuously by means of a highly sensitive mirror galvanometer. After thoracotomy, the thermo-element is fixed through an opening in the pericardium in the cardiac muscle so that the tips of the probes penetrate the muscle 3 mm under the epicardium. The flow values obtained by this method would appear to correspond to those afforded by the nitrous oxide and the heart-lung preparation techniques. The calorimetric method has the advantage that it leaves the vessels undamaged as it does not require any vascular cannulization; moreover, the estimation of the coronary blood flow in an experimentally infarcted area of the heart is made possible.

One drawback inherent in the method is that the calibration of the measuring device is critical, the results being therefore more or less quantitative. Some technical progress has been recently made in this field [1421].

The calorimetry method has been slightly modified so as to record myocardial metabolic heat production at the same time as blood flow [1421, 245c].

2.3.1.3. Method Using the Electromagnetic Flow Transducer

The third method for getting a direct reading of coronary arterial flow without resorting to vascular cannulation is due to GREGG and dates from 1963. It uses small electromagnetic flow transducers which are implanted around the artery. The method has several advantages:

— precision of measurement, since the blood flow is measured to within 5%;
— the possibility of measuring simultaneously the mean flow and phasic flow, the electromagnetic sensor providing the best method for phasic flow [1248];
— the possibility of measuring, at the same time as the coronary flow, the flow at several other arteries, including the aorta, whatever their diameter may be providing they are anatomically accessible;
— the possibility of working out simultaneously the cardiac output;
— its applicability to chronic, non-anaesthetised animals.

The principle behind this method was described by KOLIN in 1936 [1012, 1013, 1016]. When a blood vessel is located in a magnetic field whose lines of force are at right angles to the blood flow axis, the latter develops a difference in potential whose amplitude is a direct function of the velocity of the blood flow and thus a direct function also of the flow (FARADAY's law). From the technical viewpoint, therefore, all that was needed was to produce solenoids which were small enough to fit the usual arterial diameter, to find a method for implanting which would not injure the vessel, and to design amplifiers capable of continuously picking up the electromagnetic signal both for phasic flow and mean flow. Although the principle is simple, the technical manufacture of miniature flow transducers proved highly complex. In point of fact it needed 25 years, since it was only in 1963 that GREGG and KHOURI [977] managed to perfect them.

The miniature flow transducer is in the shape of a horseshoe. It consists of a solenoid contained in a plexiglass sheath and powered by a sine-wave type current. The artery is inserted through the slot, then the flow transducer is closed by fitting a small plexiglass plug. The measuring and amplifying apparatus also enables the *datum zero* to be determined, which must of necessity be a mechanical zero. It is arrived at experimentally for each artery by placing around the latter, downstream of the transducer, a plastic slip-knot (snare) which is fully closed when it is wished to check the flow zero [728][2]. Only one vessel does not lend itself to occlusion: the aorta, whose flow zero is taken as coinciding with the diastolic moment of the phasic flow.

---

2 In chronic experiments, on conscious dogs, it is advisable to use a pneumatic occlusive cuff which is placed around the blood vessel. Air injection causes inflation and closure of the lumen [979].

Once the test is finished, readings are taken of the flows recorded by referring to the calibration curve previously established *in vitro* for the transducer used, such calibration enabling the construction of a scale of flows which is linear in character[3].

In order to implant a flow transducer on the left coronary artery, it only requires a left thoracotomy after which the artery is freed at its source over a few millimetres to provide sufficient space for fitting a sensor and the "snare". If the aortic flow and mean systemic arterial blood pressure are measured simultaneously, a set of recordings is obtained which makes it possible, by means of a single type of experiment on one and the same animal, to establish a very wide picture of the essential haemodynamic changes which have occurred, since in addition to the three parameters measured it is possible, by combining them in various ways, to arrive at four more: cardiac output (see p. 92), the work of the left ventricle (see p. 92), coronary arterial resistance by dividing the arterial pressure by the coronary flow, and total arterial resistance by dividing the arterial pressure by the cardiac output.

Electromagnetic transducers are currently applied in reconstructive arterial surgery during intervention [53 c].

Recently [1017], an electromagnetic transducer of this type has been fitted at the end of a catheter (intravascular flow sensor). This new device has the advantage, amongst other things, of not requiring the isolation of the artery, but its end shape makes it more likely to damage the arterial endothelium than would the usual type of catheter, so a technical improvement is still being sought [1015]. Physiological intravascular flow sensors emerged from three types of physical intraluminal velocity meters developed two decades ago, one of which consists of a large magnet which is external to the conduit, and only miniature electrodes are introduced. Devices of this type offer the most effective means for probe miniaturisation because the magnet is eliminated from the artery lumen and placed outside the experimental subject. Flow probes as small as 0.5 mm in diameter passing through a small intravascular catheter have been designed [186 c]. In an external magnetic field, they permit measurement of total rate of volume flow and offer the possibility of percutaneous introduction into the vascular tree [222 c].

2.3.1.4. Method Using the Ultrasonic Flowmeter

The ultrasonic flowmetry based upon the Doppler effect has been designed very recently. The ultrasonic flowmeters are true volume flow instruments in that they measure flow velocity integrated over the circular area involved. The Doppler flowmeters are very sensitive and they possess good zero stability. Because of the small size and light weight of most ultrasonic flow transducers, they lend themselves well to chronic implantation and are potentially superior to the electromagnetic type for this kind of application. Clinical applications of the directional Doppler flowmeter are twofold: transcutaneous and intravascular or intracardiac [168 c]. By transcutaneous application, the Doppler flowmeter makes it possible to record the flow velocity curves of the superficial arteries (especially femoral, brachial, subclavian, carotid) and to determine the normal pattern of peripheral flow. It can contribute to assess the flow velocity variations under the influence of physiological factors [234 c] and of drugs. The flowmeter can also record the peripheral

---

3 Whereas the blood flowmeter suggested by GREGG powers the transducer by means of a current of the sine wave type, the supply by square wave current has recently been perfected. Its principles are exactly the same. Under certain application conditions, measurement of the flow could be done without it being necessary to prepare calibration curves *in vitro* for each transducer.

venous flow. By intravascular and intracardiac application, the catheter tip flowmeter can record in man the flow velocity curves in both venae cavae as well as in the right atrium and right ventricle.

2.3.2. Indirect Methods

One method uses nitrous oxide, whilst the others use radio-isotopes. *These are the only methods applicable to humans*, and in fact are being used on an increasing scale, especially the isotope techniques which have now reached, as will be seen on p. 81, a high degree of accuracy.

2.3.2.1. The Nitrous Oxide Technique

Recommended by KETY and SCHMIDT [973] and originally used for measurement of the cerebral blood flow, this technique was applied by ECKENHOFF et al. [469] for calculation of the coronary blood flow through the left ventricular muscle. It is based on Fick's principle that the blood flow through an organ per unit of time is equal to the amount of a substance (oxygen or foreign gas administered) extracted from the blood by this organ in a unit of time divided by the difference between the concentrations of the substance in the arterial blood and in the total venous blood leaving the organ at the same moment.

In the method as applied to measurement of the coronary flow, the concentration of nitrous oxide in the arterial blood is estimated on blood drawn from any artery, and the venous blood concentration is determined for blood taken from the coronary sinus, preferably by catheterization [690, 691].

The quantity of coronary blood passing through the part of the myocardium, venous drainage of which is effected by way of the coronary sinus, is equal to the amount of nitrous oxide taken up by the cardiac muscle divided by the arterio-venous nitrous oxide difference.

The numerator in this fraction is calculated from the weight of the heart (determined after the experiment in the anesthetized sacrificed dog, or derived according to the usual standards for the conscious dog or man) and the concentration of nitrous oxide in the myocardium, the latter being assumed to be identical with the concentration of the gas in the venous blood after equilibrium has been established between the blood and the myocardial tissue; a coefficient for the partition of nitrous oxide between the blood and the myocardial tissue enters into the calculation. The denominator of the fraction is obtained by graphic integration of the clearance from the myocardium and of the coronary arterio-venous difference for nitrous oxide [1707][4] during the period of equilibration, a period during which the subject inhales a mixture of 15% nitrous oxide, 21% oxygen and 64% nitrogen under uniform standard conditions. From the formula it is easy to obtain the value of the coronary flow per minute and per 100 g of myocardium, or more exactly, according to the advocates of the method, of left ventricle. The dangers of contamination of the venous blood taken from the coronary sinus with atrial blood and of mechanical occlusion of the coronary sinus would appear to have been eliminated by the technical conditions under which GOODALE et al. [690, 691] perform the catheterization of the coronary sinus.

This procedure has the advantage that it can be used in lightly anaesthetized or even unanaesthetized animals which are therefore in states approximating closely to the normal condition. Another important advantage of the method is that

---

4 An improved technique for measuring blood N_2O levels by gas chromatography allowed myocardial concentration/time clearance curves to be plotted more precisely [59a].

it determines myocardial metabolism and left ventricular efficiency as well as the coronary flow; an idea of the coronary efficiency can be derived from it.

While it is suitable for employment when it is desired to determine the value of a *steady* coronary flow, the limitations of the nitrous oxide method become at once obvious when an attempt is made to measure even relative changes in terms of a reference value, as is always done in pharmacological work. In effect, it can only be used in conditions in which the flow remains constant for at least the 10 min required for the carrying out of the procedure; it cannot, therefore, be applied in circumstances in which *rapid* fluctuations occur in the coronary blood flow. Another disadvantage, inherent in the procedure itself, is that measurement is periodic and not continuous; the various determinations required to demonstrate a pharmacological effect and the repetition of which is limited by the time required by each of them can only be carried out at moments chosen empirically by the experimenter.

In 1953, GOODALE and HACKEL [688] modified their technique and measured the coronary blood flow from the rate of *desaturation* and not in the phase of saturation of the myocardium with nitrous oxide, that is to say, on the basis of the elimination of nitrous oxide from the myocardium from the moment the animal or subject, who had first been saturated, was returned to breathing room air. The authors showed that the desaturation procedure affords definitive technical advantages as it avoided the real danger of leakage from the respiratory apparatus during the phase of saturation. Moreover, desaturation technique reduced the source of error in the saturation procedure noted by GREGG et al. [729], and on the existence of which GOODALE and HACKEL expressed their agreement; this was that nitrous oxide could diffuse outward through the pericardium into the thoracic cavity at a rate which increased the closer the myocardium came to saturation. Furthermore, as the nitrous oxide levels in the arterial blood and in the venous blood often approximate to one another more quickly during desaturation than during saturation (a fact which supports the occurrence of external gas loss noted by GREGG), the period of observation required to obtain arterio-venous nitrous oxide equilibration is so reduced that the determination actually requires only 5 min instead of 10.

Making on several occasions two successive determinations on the same subject (animal or man), first by the saturation method and then by the desaturation method, GOODALE and HACKEL obtained values which were in perfect agreement, the indication thus being that the desaturation procedure was valid in comparison with the saturation technique.

A criticism has been formulated by WIGGERS and his co-workers [634, 1995]. The nitrous oxide method is claimed to measure the coronary arterial flow and the oxygen consumption of the myocardium for the left ventricle, on the basis of GREGG's observations [734] that 90—95% of the venous flow in the coronary sinus comes from the left ventricle. Now, WIGGERS et al. have shown that the right coronary artery, which is the main supply of the right ventricle, contributes much more to the venous flow in the coronary sinus than was found by GREGG. According to WIGGERS, the nitrous oxide method cannot, therefore, claim to measure the coronary flow and the oxygen consumption of the left ventricle as the arterio-venous difference in nitrous oxide is calculated on the basis of the nitrous oxide content of venous blood taken from the coronary sinus which also drains, and probably to quite a considerable extent, myocardial areas belonging to the right ventricle.

On the whole, however, it can be assumed that the nitrous oxide method constitutes an important approach to determination of the coronary flow under conditions which are peculiarly physiological as it necessitates no surgical intervention or anaesthesia.

The accuracy of the data it affords is, however, conditioned by the number of tests made for a single study, and it is greater in the anaesthetized animal because the method requires a steady state which is sometimes difficult to obtain in the waking animal, even when it is trained to remain still [570]. In spite of the major disadvantage of necessitating a steady state during the *entire period* of collecting blood samples, the method has nevertheless some outstanding advantages: neither thoracotomy nor general anaesthesia (at least in man) is required, the haemodynamic state is not altered [1574] and the results obtained in man and dogs concord [1571]. Owing to its relative simplicity, the procedure has been very often applied in man. It is in the course of being superseded by the more recent isotopic methods, although these require far more expensive equipment.

2.3.2.2. Methods Based on the Employment of Radioactive Substances

During recent years, advantage has been taken of the development of equipment for detecting radioactivity in the blood and the tissues to elaborate many methods which are based on the use of radioactive tracers. Several isotopes have been proposed: non-diffusible substances, diffusible substances, and finally diffusible inert gases.

2.3.2.2.1. Non-Diffusible Substances

The chief isotopic method which is based on the principles of the dilution of a non diffusible tracer makes use of radioactive iodine [1723]. Radioactive iodinated human serumalbumin is injected into an antecubital vein in dosage of 0.2—0.4 ml (0.05—0.1 ml for dogs). The passage of the radioactive tracer through the heart is rated by a gamma-ray detector placed on the precordium and measuring the chronological change in counting rate. The curve produced during the first circulation of the radioactivity is known to consist of two well-defined peaks representing the passage of the radioactivity through the right and left sides of the heart. SEVELIUS and JOHNSON have recognized that the typical curve is composed of three peaks, the second classical main peak being closely followed by a third peak, the onset of which coincides with the appearance of the radioactivity in the periphery (detected and recorded by a second detector placed over a carotid artery). That this third peak is, for JOHNSON and SEVELIUS, related to myocardial blood flow and that the area beneath the peak may be taken as a measure of the coronary blood flow is demonstrated by the fact that, in dog experiments, the third peak of the curve which may be seen in normal conditions disappeared completely when both main coronary arteries were occluded. The third peak thus appears at a time which could represent myocardial blood flow. Unfortunately, because of an insufficient time lag, it is difficult to differentiate the peak of precordial radioactivity related to myocardial flow from other rapid changes in precordial activity, such as that resulting from the preceding passage of blood through the left side of the heart, or that due to subsequent recirculation from the most rapid noncoronary circuits [213c]. Until the true coronary precordial peak in radioactivity can be more sharply defined, it is difficult to place reliance on data obtained with this method as representing coronary flow [726].

2.3.2.2.2. Diffusible Substances

Amongst the most widely used diffusible tracers are potassium (K^{42}) and rubidium (Rb^{86}). The principle behind the method is as follows. The isotope administered into the arm vein as a slug injection has a large volume of distribution within the myocardium. Over a period of at least 1 minute, coronary venous drainage of the isotope is negligible as compared with its initial deposition. In view of the fact that the isotope extraction rates by the heart and by the body are identical, it is possible to calculate the coronary flow since the uptake or the clearance by an organ of a rapidly diffusible substance depends on the flow of blood through that organ.

At the outset, the limitations of such methods were very real. For instance, in 1966, MOIR [1309] considered that the method using the rubidium then available only gave a very inaccurate quantitative measurement and only gave a guide as to variations in coronary flow. Later on, the technical procedure was improved to such a degree that at least two teams of research workers [167, 1008] were able to demonstrate the reliability of the method (see further).

Rubidium quickly took preference over potassium since, whilst metabolically behaving in the same way as the latter because its turnover rate is identical, it has an advantage over it in that it has a longer half-life. Rubidium has been used in two forms, Rb^{86} and Rb^{84}. LOVE and BURCH [1179] used Rb^{86} on animals, which calls for continuous intravenous infusion so as to keep constant the concentration of the isotope in the arterial blood; it does not enable measurement to be made of any changes in coronary flow in the same subject. A few years later, DONATO et al. [438] adapted the method for use in man, but the use of Rb^{86} has two drawbacks: firstly, because of the low percentage of gamma rays emitted, that of requiring comparatively heavy doses, which limits to two the number of assessments which can be made for a given patient [437]; secondly, it presents the difficulty of differentiating between the specific activity of the cardiac muscle alone and that of the surrounding tissues and of the blood contained in the cardiac cavities [438, 1203], with the result that the relationship between coronary flow and extraction of the isotope by the myocardium is not close. It was to mitigate this drawback that DONATO [438] used two isotopes at different times, adding to the diffusible Rb^{86} a non-diffusible substance, I^{131}, which enabled him to dissociate the radioactivity of the cardiac muscle from that of the intracardiac blood.

Other authors then chose Rb^{84}, which emits positons (i.e. free positive electrons). BING [165] was the first to use it in 1964. With his colleagues, he perfected a technique known as the "coincidence counting technique" which measures the disappearance of the Rb^{84} as a function of the coronary flow in man. This method was not strictly quantitative, but it did provide information as to changes in the clearance of the Rb^{84} by the myocardium. Its main advantage lies in the fact that, by monitoring the right hemi-thorax by a second counting system, it makes it possible to arrive at a distinction between the radioactivity of the cardiac muscle and that of the surrounding tissues and of the blood in the heart cavities. It still had the drawback of not being able to detect *rapid* changes in flow, because statistical error is too great when periods under 5 minutes are considered.

In 1968, i.e. after 4 years of experimenting, BING provided a clear definition of the technical conditions and improved the method [167]. There are two methods of injecting Rb^{84} and determining coronary blood flow using this technique. The first is by constant intravenous infusion of Rb^{84} chloride over a 30 min period. A distinct drawback in constant infusion is that a long steady state is required, rapid changes in coronary blood flow being obscured. Moreover, the accuracy of flow measured is difficult to ascertain because the long steady state period is not compatible with simultaneous direct Fick principle determinations. The second variant of the method is rapid intravenous injection of Rb^{84} given as a bolus; its theory and principle are described in a very recent paper by BING and colleagues [27a]. The development of coincidence counting and *rapid* bolus injections of $Rb^{84}Cl$ has the advantage of allowing determination of myocardial blood flow over short periods following administration of a drug. The calculation of coronary blood flow from rapid injections is much simpler than in the case of constant infusion, and it does not require a computer. In addition, the accuracy of the figures can easily be ascertained by direct Fick principle measurements. It must be stressed that as this method determines clearance of the radio-isotope by the myocardium, nutritional blood flow concerned with active myocardial uptake is measured, rather than total flow. The reproducibility of the values for coronary blood flow in man is excellent since two determinations, five minutes apart in resting individuals, revealed no significant difference, values being reproducible within 2.1% [27a].

Using the same method, KNOEBEL et al. [1008] obtain with a dog normal coronary flow values comparable to those given by the Fick method [1254]. Like BING, they show the reproducibility of two measurements made consecutively on 10 normal subjects at rest, which are respectively 243 ± 64 and 236 ± 62 ml/min.

2.3.2.2.3. Diffusible Inert Gases

Two diffusible inert gases have been used: krypton[85] and xenon[133]. The flow measuring techniques using them would appear to be more deserving of confidence in that these two indicators freely diffuse through the cell membranes [1078]. They can be administered either by inhalation or (in saline solution form) by injection into the left ventricle or directly into the coronary artery. Inhalation and intraventricular injection call for catheterisation of the coronary sinus but dispense with external counting. Selective injection into the myocardium via the coronary artery calls for catheterisation of the latter and precordial count.

The intracoronary selective administration of krypton has been used by HANSEN et al. [780] and by HERD et al. [816] on dogs. Left intraventricular injection following left catheterisation has been used by GORLIN [344] on man and dogs: the normal coronary flow values obtained are comparable to those provided by the nitrous oxide method.

As regards Xe^{133}, this has been used for intracoronary injection in humans by Ross et al. [1562] and by BERNSTEIN et al. [146]. Xe^{133} was used in preference to krypton because its gamma emission is greater [1562] and its lower emission energy means less irradiation hasard for the patient. The advantages of this technique over the foregoing method are:

a) delivering the isotope selectively to the myocardium so that all immediate precordial radioactivity comes from the myocardium and the speed of its disappearance from the precordium is a dependent variable of the coronary blood flow: 90% of what returns to the right side of the heart disappears from the blood during a single pulmonary passage, and it has also been shown that coronary venous drainage into the right auricle plays no part in the precordial radioactivity curve [493]. It follows that recirculation presents no significant problem. Moreover, the method allows repeated measurements to be taken since these do not require more than 2—3 min.

b) enabling separate investigation of right and left coronary circulation, depending on which artery is catheterised. It has thus been possible to demonstrate that, in relation to the weight of cardiac muscle, left coronary flow is considerably greater than right coronary flow, the respective values being, per minute and per 100 g of muscle, 86 and 40 ml for dogs and 76 and 48 ml for men [1447]. The accuracy of the method can be considered as satisfactory since the values for total coronary flow obtained in the case of dogs are in agreement with those provided by direct rotameter measurement [1504], and furthermore [146], with

12 dogs where two measurements were taken at 3 min interval, the mean difference between the two measurements amounts to 17% of the actual mean value for the coronary flow, this mean difference being 14.5% in 22 human subjects.

By way of concluding this survey of the methodology used for measuring coronary flow, it would seem pertinent to round off by summarising the methods which can be adopted under conditions which do not call for general anaesthesia, that is to say on conscious dogs and humans.

1. *For the non-anaesthetised dog.* Two methods can be recommended. The first uses miniature electromagnetic flow transducers (see 2.3.1.3.). Under an anaesthetic, a transducer is fitted to the coronary artery and the cable connector is attached to the skin. The thoracic opening is closed up and the animal is treated as a thorax operation case. After 4—6 weeks, one animal is available for measuring variations in coronary flow under the influence of a wide variety of agents. This method allows the simultaneous chronic implantation of other transducers, particularly on the aorta, and various catheters — for instance in the aorta and in the coronary sinus — with the result that the same animal can be used for a whole set of measurements of a fundamental nature making it possible to assess coronary flow, cardiac output, the work done by the heart and myocardial oxygen consumption. It is difficult to see how physiological conditions could be more closely approximated for simultaneous measurement of the major haemodynamic parameters.

The second method enabling coronary flow to be measured in a non-anaesthetised dog is the most recent one. Perfected by FRANKLIN [582], it uses ultrasonic waves and measures the flow by telemetry on a dog in freedom. The potential advantages of this method are considerable [1916], but for the moment results present some interpretation difficulties which can only be solved by experts.

2. *For use on man.* The nitrous oxide method which has long prevailed is likely to give place to the isotope methods for two essential reasons: it calls for catheterisation of the coronary sinus and requires a steady state of several minutes, a fact which excludes the possibility of detecting rapid variations in coronary flow.

As far as the isotope methods are concerned, a choice may be made between:

— the use of Rb^{86} according to the DONATO method, limited by the need to apply high radioactive doses;

— the use of Kr^{85} by the GORLIN method [344] which calls for the catheterisation of the left ventricle;

— the use of Xe^{133} with the ROSS technique [1562] which requires catheterisation of the coronary artery;

— the use of Rb^{84} by the BING technique [167] which dispenses with any cardiac catheterisation. This seems especially promising, particularly as regards its method of rapid isotope injection, since it has proved itself on over 1000 patients, it provides a coronary flow measurement in 30 sec, it supplies excellently reproducible values, and enables very early variations in blood flow to be detected.

It is also necessary to point out the special interest offered by selective coronarography (whose data make it possible to establish an excellent relationship between clinical symptomatology and coronary arterial lesions [1470, 1471]), associated with the measurement of coronary flow by the Ross method [1561], thus enabling investigations which correlate physiological results and anatomical pictures. It can therefore be expected that it might provide the answer to several pressing questions which have not been solved as to the efficacy of the therapeutics advocated in the fight against coronary atherosclerosis, and also provide a sound basis for a rational evaluation of antianginal medications under these pathological conditions.

3. Nutritional Myocardial Micro-Circulation

The nutritional myocardial circulation is studied by means of Rb^{86} since its extraction by the tissues from the arterial blood is in relation to the flow of the blood-stream through the capillaries and to the total capillary surface available for the diffusion of this isotope [1518], this latter depending on the number of open capillaries whilst the former depends on arteriolar resistance. For this reason, Rb^{86} can be used as a quantitative indicator of the capillary blood flow [601].

It was WINBURY [2008] in particular who developed this type of method on animals. It calls for the injection of the isotope into the coronary artery and the determining of its concentration in the blood of the coronary venous sinus [2014]. The difference between the radioactivity injected and the radioactivity recovered in the venous blood represents what has been picked up by the tissues, and the percentage of Rb^{86} extraction is an index of the distribution of blood as between the nutritional vessels and non-nutritional passages. The uptake of Rb^{86} is a direct function of the blood flow.

Despite all the interest of this type of research, WINBURY's investigations probably only constitute an initial attempt to meet the vital need, stressed by ROWE [1572], for methods enabling the nutritional circulation to be investigated which in fact is the only circulation which is of any account as regards the metabolic needs of the cardiac muscle.

4. Collateral Coronary Circulation

The effect of a drug on collateral coronary circulation can be examined either in acute or in chronic experimentation.

4.1. Acute Experiment

There are at least three ways of tackling the problem.

4.1.1. Linder Technique [1142]

An acute coronary arterial occlusion is carried out on a dog, and a measurement is taken of the collateral blood flow intended for the ischaemic zone thus created by using inert radioactive gases such as Xe^{133} or Kr^{85}. The substances being investigated may be administered as required by general or local route.

4.1.2. Rees Technique [1505, 267 c]

Myocardial infarction is induced in a dog by acute ligaturing of the anterior descending coronary artery. Then a fine catheter made of nylon is inserted into the artery distal to the ligature. The thorax is closed up again. Small quantities of Xe^{133} are injected down the catheter as required during the recovery period. The disappearance of the isotope, which is a dependent variable of the anastomotic blood flow, is measured by an external precordial scintillation counter. This method thus provides a means of measuring the immediate effect of drugs on the anastomotic blood flow.

4.1.3. McGregor Technique

The foregoing technique can be used for acute pharmacological tests. This in fact is the procedure recommended by McGREGOR for research into anti-anginal substances (see p. 44) because it enables the collateral intramyocardial blood flow to be assessed at the opposite end to the occlusion by measuring either the retrograde coronary flow [1240], or the elimination of an inert indicator injected into the ischaemic zone [972], or the thermal conductivity in that zone [683], or finally the partial oxygen pressure by means of a micro-electrode fitted into the ischaemic zone [524].

4.2. Chronic Experiment

Here again several methods have been suggested.

4.2.1. Meesmann Technique [1262]

The substance under investigation as to its effect on collateral coronary circulation is administered to conscious dogs over a lengthy period of daily treatment. At the end of the chosen period, the animal is killed. The heart is removed and then chilled for 24 hours. For preparing the visualisation of the coronary arterial tree, the organ is warmed up again and the three coronary arteries are fitted with cannulae. The arterial system is first carefully rinsed out with Ringer fluid at 37°, then a contrast substance is injected under constant pressure. Finally the organ is X-rayed.

With this method, it is possible to assess the extension of the retrograde refilling of the adjacent coronary vessels, which is an index of the collateral coronary circulation. Amongst other things, MEESMANN demonstrated by this technique the need which exists, in the case of Persantine, for administering high doses for several weeks to develop a considerable collateral circulation, the usual doses being unable to set up an anastomotic system (see p. 181).

4.2.2. Schmidt Technique

SCHMIDT and SCHMIER [1679, 285 c] follow a different course than MEESMANN after sacrificing the animal. After closing the aortic valves, they inject into the coronary arterial tree a plastic material, Araldit, which produces a moulding of the entire myocardial vascular system after intravascular polymerisation. The heart is then treated with a 35% soda solution. Once the myocardial tissue has been destroyed, the vascular cast can be examined. It shows the density of the arterial network and the presence of intercoronary anastomoses whose number and size can provide an indication as to the favourable effect of medications administered during chronic treatment. In addition, when use is made of animals which have been subjected to ligature of a large coronary trunk and which, on recovery, are given repeated doses of a medicament, the cast of the heart of the control specimens is cut off from all the vascular area depending for its supply on the previously occluded artery, whereas in the case of animals pre-treated with certain medicaments to which is attributed the property of encouraging the development of collateral coronary circulation, the destruction of this part of the arterial cast may be less marked, or even non-existent, the filling up of the distal portion of the ligatured artery taking place from the arteries left intact and via the newly-formed collateral anastomotic system or one which has been boosted by the effect of the drug.

4.2.3. Schaper Technique [1657, 283 c]

We have mentioned on page 46 that, in SCHAPER's view, the most sensitive indicator of the development and nutritional efficacy of a collateral coronary circulation is the coronary quotient which is arrived at by dividing the retrograde coronary arterial pressure measured downstream of a chronic coronary occlusion by the aortic pressure. The technique therefore consists in incompletely occluding the circumflex coronary artery of a dog by means of an Ameroid type ring (see p. 90). This operation is used at the same time to insert two catheters, one in the aorta root and the other in the distal portion of the coronary artery downstream of the ring. The animal is treated as a thorax operation patient. After it has recovered, measurements are taken at different times of the two pressures. The development of an effective collateral coronary circulation is reflected in a progressive increase in retrograde coronary pressure, so that the coronary quotient rises, and at its optimum approaches the value of one. The quotients are compared at given times of animals treated with a medicament and those of untreated animals. This method has been used to demonstrate the favourable effect of lidoflazine on the development of collateral coronary circulation (p. 199). The limitations of this method and the sources of error to which it exposes the investigator in assessing the effect of a drug on the development of collateral circulation have been outlined already in Chapter 1 (see p. 46).

5. Experimental Chronic Coronary Insufficiency

The demonstration of any new antianginal drug capable of being used clinically demands an extremely searching and laborious experimental investigation, which is rendered particularly difficult by the complexity of factors concerned in regulation of coronary flow and metabolism of the myocardium. Nevertheless, experimental pharmacological investigations aimed to find out powerful and long-acting antianginal medications were and remain intensive. Several compounds have been shown periodically to exhibit on animals some properties related to the coronary circulation and the metabolism of the myocardium which answer best to the pharmacological requirements at present accepted for an antianginal compound and which therefore raised the hope of using them for the effective prophylactic management of the anginal syndrome (see p. 39). But search for a medication which will effectively prevent or reduce in man the frequency and severity of the anginal attacks has been up to now rather disappointing.

There are many reasons which could partially explain why pharmacological properties cannot often be extrapolated to clinical medicine. Some of them relate to the experimental conditions inherent in pharmacological investigation while others, which will be considered in chapter IV, are to be found in the difficulties which necessarily arise when correct clinical assessment is undertaken.

The majority of the many drugs in use at the present time were recommended as antianginal medications on the basis of animal experiments, and though preliminary clinical trials of some have been encouraging, subsequent controlled trials have in almost every case failed to confirm the initial claims. Thus, there is the fact that pharmacologic properties demonstrated in the laboratory animal may not be reproduced in the human patient. Possibly one of the main factors responsible for failure in this transposition from pharmacology to clinical trial is the fact that the pharmacological experimental work is carried out mainly on normal coronary circulations whereas the medication has to deal with coronary arteries which are generally very much altered by pathological processes.

It can therefore be taken as probable that any important advance in this field will be effected by the creation in animals of coronary and cardiac lesions of chronic type, comparable to those occurring in man, and capable of causing the development of anastomoses between coronary arteries, similar to those seen very frequently in human subjects with obliterating coronary arterial sclerosis. Experimental pathology of this kind would provide us with "coronary animals" in which the haemodynamic disturbances produced by operative technique or by sclerogenic agents could be investigated and correlated with the pathological lesions produced. It would also enable the study of the pharmacological effects of compounds on hearts already provided with vicarious anastomotic circulation. Thus, in order to complete this methodological survey, it seems worthwhile to review briefly the various attempts aimed to elaborate an experimental model that could realize a chronic coronary insufficiency in animals. There are many various procedures which have been advocated. Only the most interesting which are also the most recent will be described.

MARCUS, KATZ, PICK and STAMLER [1219] have succeeded in producing chronic coronary insufficiency and a chronic cardiopathy of coronary origin in the dog by the intracoronary injection of spherules of divinylbenzine, of average diameter 500 μ, in a dose of 2—3 mg/kg. Electrocardiograms recorded more than 15 months after the operation show frank signs of myocardial infarct, in agreement with the pathological findings in those of the animals which were purposely killed; they showed the presence of old infarcts involving the right ventricle, the anterior and posterior walls of the left ventricle and, almost always, the interventricular septum.

The facts described by these authors in 1958 indicate that the procedure is worthy of the attention of experimenters as it provides dogs with chronic cardiac lesions corresponding exactly, from the pathological standpoint, with those seen in man with cardiac involvement of coronary origin and which are expressed by comparable electrocardiographic signs. It is therefore astonishing that the powerful interest which these observations must have aroused has not led to the extensive employment of this method. Its protagonists themselves do not appear to have extended their study of the basic technique by physiological or pharmacological investigations.

The same comment can be made for the method used by KURIJAMA [1059]. The anterior descending coronary artery having been dissected near its origin in dogs, the vessel is then surrounded with a gelatin sponge containing dicetylphosphate which is finally held in place with a wire. Chemical irritation induces the formation of granulomatous tissue leading, in all cases after 3—4 weeks, to vascular stenosis by external compression, which is severe in 63% of cases and provokes histological deterioration, characteristic of acute myocardial infarction, in that portion of the muscle whose irrigation is dependent upon the stenosed artery.

The lack of continuity in the utilization of such procedures is sufficient comment on the difficulty of experimental physiopathological approaches to the problem of coronary affections in man. The concern to produce in animals cardiovascular disturbances which are as like to those deemed to occur in the subject suffering from coronary heart disease continues nevertheless to stimulate research workers, since it is a truism that this method of approach in pharmacological work should provide the vital link between investigations into normal animals and clinical research on angina pectoris subjects. Proof of this is provided by the fact that at the 1st World Pharmacological Congress in Stockholm (August 1961), where the pharmacology of coronary circulation was tackled albeit in a very limited manner, two new experimental methods were suggested.

According to BUSCH [264, 265], cardiovascular disturbances very similar to those found in coronary subjects could be produced by rendering rabbits sensitive to various proteins (notably egg white or sheep serum). Their coronary vessels and cardiac muscle are considerably impaired and present, under histological examination, a picture of tissue changes similar to those found in a man suffering from coronary sclerosis; the haemodynamic consequences of this experimental "coronary disease" would seem to be those which occur in humans during an angina attack or during the development of infarction, with particular reference to a marked reduction in coronary blood flow [265]. As a result of these observations, Busch considered that myocardial ischaemia of an anaphylactic type in rabbits would provide a particularly apt experimental procedure for investigation into coronaro-dilator substances. It was abandoned, probably because it is still to be proved that there is a close correlation between the capacity of various substances to antagonise anaphylactic ischaemia and their effectiveness in the case of angina pectoris subjects.

Another method was proposed by VARMA and colleagues [1921]. They found that with a rabbit anaesthetised with pentobarbitone, subjected to vagotomy, given curare followed by artificial respiration, the injection of 0.1 mg of picro-toxine into the lateral cerebral ventricle induces, after a temporary period of cardiac irregularity, profound depression of the S-T segment of the electrocardio-gram which lasts for 30—120 min and which would appear to indicate the exist-ence of serious myocardial ischaemia. This effect seems to admit of a stimulation of the central sympathetic mechanisms leading to hypersympathicotony. Despite all the interest offered by this method, which can be adopted, for the same reason as the injection of vasopressine and experimental hypoxia, for the purpose of inducing myocardial hypoxia objectified by electrocardiographic indications of ischaemia (and which has the additional merit of revealing the possible role of certain central sympathetic nervous mechanisms in the origin of ischaemic dis-orders of the cardiac muscle), it is clear that it only produces ischaemia of a functional nature (coronary spasm with a pharmacological character). It therefore seems farther removed from experimental coronary pathology than the BUSCH technique where the anaphylatic type ischaemia produced would appear, accord-ing to details at present available, to be of an essentially organic nature.

Comparatively simple, the SALAZAR technique [1630] applied to a dog under light general anaesthesia consists in inserting a catheter into the carotid artery and guiding it towards the left coronary artery until its extremity fits into one of the two large branches. A steel wire, acting as an electrode, is inserted into the catheter lumen and adjusted in such a way that it extends 3 mm beyond the end of the catheter tube. With a negative electrode placed on the thorax, a 3-volt d/c current is applied to the intracardiac electrode, initially at a low intensity then gradually increased to between 100 and 900 micro-amps. After a period ranging from 20—90 min, depending on the animal, the continuously recorded electro-cardiogram shows the emergence of undoubted myocardial ischaemia, and a coronary arteriogram provides proof of the fact that there is coronary thrombosis. Catheter and electrode are withdrawn, and the precarotid incision is stitched up. This method, which has the advantage of avoiding any surgical operation properly so called, did not entail any fatal results: it proved effective with the 23 animals used. Anatomopathological examinations carried out on sacrificed animals disclosed the existence of ventricular infarction and coronary arterial thrombosis.

WEST et al. [1979] use a catheter inserted into the coronary artery of a dog to inject a suspension of lycopod spores measuring from 20 to 40 μ in diameter.

NAKHJAVAN et al. [1337] describe a closed thorax technique used on dogs which briefly consists in sliding along from the carotid artery a small metal cylinder on a guide wire and fixing it permanently either in the anterior inter-ventricular artery or in the circumflex artery. The diameter of the cylinder used to reduce the vascular lumen can be selected in accordance with the size of the vessel whose lumen it is desired to restrict.

Over the past few years, other improved methods have been suggested.

Firstly, the method proposed by Vineberg [1943] and Litvak et al. [1161]. This is of special interest because it permits of slow coronary arterial occlusion, gradually progressive and permanent, in a dog which is kept alive. By means of an acute operation, a constrictor ring of the Ameroid type is fitted around a coronary artery, usually the left circumflex. This ring consists basically of an outer steel sleeve lined on the inside with a layer of ameroid (a plastic substance with a casein base) and which has a central aperture in which the artery is housed. Once the ring is in position, the plastic layer gradually swells by absorbing water from the tissues. Since he has a range of rings whose centre aperture is of different sizes, the experimenter selects the ring whose aperture is best suited to the size of the artery, and he fits it around the latter during an aseptic operation. The thorax is closed up, and the animal is treated as a patient recovering from a thorax operation. The Ameroid slowly swells by water absorption and causes a gradual arterial constriction: after 4—6 weeks, the diameter of the artery is reduced by 80—90%. Unfortunately, operational wastage is enormous, only 10% of the animals surviving the operation.

It is possible to use this method to examine the surviving percentage of animals treated with an antianginal medication and compare them with a batch of untreated controls [1196]. The retrograde coronary flow in the distal portion of the occluded vessel can also be measured. In addition, the coronary arterial tree can be injected with plastic moulding material to show the extent of any collateral circulation which has developed. This method also lends itself to pharmacological research on artificially reduced blood circulation [137]. A large number of applications of this technique have been reported (see p. 86).

A further method of coronary restriction was perfected in 1966 by Khouri and Gregg [978, 127 c]. As compared with that of Vineberg, it has the dual advantage of being adjustable at will, and operating on a "determinable" basis. The technique consists of fitting around the circumflex coronary artery a rigid ring with an inflatable lining into which air can be pumped. At the same time, an electro-magnetic transducer is fitted upstream of this pneumatic cuff. The transducer supply wires and the tube leading to the occlusion device are sunk into and secured to the skin. Once the animal has recovered, it is possible to inflate the constrictor ring and adjust compression in such a way as to reduce the blood flow to the desired level, the reduction being measured by means of the flow transducer fitted upstream of the occlusion. Anatomical examination of the hearts injected, after death, by the Schlesinger method [1673] and which have been subjected to partial coronary occlusion over a period of some forty days reveals that compensating and collateral flow vessels have developed. Similarly, the blood flow in the non-occluded arterial trunk increases considerably and appears to perfuse more myocardial tissue than prior to the occlusion. This very promising method is still at the moment limited to laboratories highly specialised in fundamental research.

The above enumeration shows that there is no lack of techniques. They make it possible to foresee that progress can be expected of pharmacological research carried out along these experimental lines.

Measuring Cardiac Output

Several methods are available for obtaining direct measurement of cardiac output, and these have formed the subject of a recent critical survey by Lequime et al. [1103]. Basically they are:

— the original Fick method which calls for the insertion of a catheter as far as the pulmonary artery. The method is too conventional to be given in detail.

Mention need only be made of the fact that the accuracy and reproducible nature of the values which it provides are highly satisfactory [1717].

— the calorimetric method which also calls for the insertion of a probe, of the DELAUNOIS thermistor type for instance [402], into the pulmonary artery.

— the indicator dilution method which uses radioactive iodinated human serum albumin: cardiac output is calculated from the radioactivity decline curve [99], usually the portion relating to the passage through the right ventricle, taking into account the circulating blood volume and several biological constants, as per the HAMILTON formula [772]:

cardiac output $= \text{VS} \times \dfrac{\text{S}}{\text{H}}$, where VS is the circulating blood volume (in ml),

H = the height of the equilibrium plateau obtained ten to fifteen minutes after injecting the tracer (in cm), and

S = the surface defined by the curve and worked out by planimetry (in cm^2).

— the so-called dilution method, whether it entails a dye injected into a peripheral vein (e.g. Cardio-green), or physiological fluid either cold or at room temperature (method by thermodilution). This method is simple and quick; it enables very frequent measurements to be made, particularly in the case of thermodilution, and it provides cardiac output values which are in excellent agreement with those provided by the FICK method, especially if use is made of the procedure recommended by GOODYER et al. [693], namely, if the injection of saline is done in the right auricle and the cooling off of the blood stream is read off in the aorta root[5]. As regards the dilution method (whether using dye or saline), planimetric measurement can be avoided by using a computer, which offers the advantage of providing an immediate reading whose accuracy is greater than the planimetric calculation since the computer automatically cancels out any error due to possible recirculation. The validity of certain types of computer has been the subject of intensive technical research by TAYLOR et al. [1876] who find that they are of great practical interest.

— the fiberoptic hemoreflection method [92c, 93c, 106c] incorporating in-stantaneous as well as continuous measurement of oxygen saturation without withdrawal of blood samples and using special intracardiac catheter (intracardiac oxymetry) has also been used to record dye-dilution curves for determination of cardiac output [92c, 155c]. The results were in good agreement with those obtained by a conventional densitometer method [155c] or by the direct FICK method [331c], or by thermal dilution method [294c].[6]

— a very recent method, but one whose validity has not been checked other than on primates, uses 50 μ microspheres marked either at ^{125}I, or ^{51}Cr or ^{85}Sr. Some 5000—10000 microspheres in 7—10 ml of saline solution are infused over a period of 15—20 sec through a catheter inserted into the left ventricle. Under these conditions, there is excellent correlation between the measurements taken by this method and the values obtained with the same animals and under the same conditions by the FICK method [61a].

---

5 Our own fairly extensive experience in this technique with anaesthetised dogs enables us to give it an error limit which does not exceed 12%, worked out over two hours of observation at a rate of 12—20 readings an hour.

6 The technique is sufficiently accurate for acute studies but until the long-term risk of clot formation on the catheter tip is thoroughly evaluated, the use of this method in chronic studies of patients under intensive care is questionable, while the thermal dilution method is uniquely attractive for use in the long-term monitoring of cardiac output necessary to the management of the critically ill patient [294c].

Besides these direct methods, there is one which enables the cardiac output to be calculated from certain parameters. This is the electromagnetic flow-measuring technique by means of which the flow of the left coronary artery and aorta flow can be measured simultaneously. The sum of the two flows gives the cardiac output. The value thus obtained is obviously incorrect by default since it only takes into account the left coronary flow and not the total coronary flow, the flow of the right coronary artery not being measured. When they wish to work out cardiac output by this method, physiologists do not measure the right coronary flow because the anatomical position of the right coronary artery is such that access to it entails major surgical impairment. The omission of the right coronary flow, however, is negligible since it amounts to only one sixth of that of the left coronary artery [726], and furthermore the total coronary arterial flow only represents between 4 and 5% of cardiac output [726, 1008, 1571].

Measuring Cardiac Work

For physiologists and pharmacologists, the concept of cardiac work covers merely the work of the ventricles, the auricles being only of limited interest from the haemodynamic viewpoint. Of the two ventricles, it is more especially the left one which engages the attention of researchers.

The work done by the left ventricle is expressed by the following equation:

$$\text{C.W.} = \underbrace{\text{C.O.} \times \text{M.B.P.} \times 13.6}_{(1)} + \underbrace{\frac{pV^2}{2g}}_{(2)}$$

where:

C.O.   = Cardiac output
M.B.P.   = Mean systemic blood pressure
13.6   = Specific weight of mercury
p   = weight of volume of blood ejected
V   = velocity of the blood flow
g   = gravity acceleration

The term (1) represents that part of the cardiac work which ensures the ejection of a certain quantity of blood at a given pressure into the general arterial circulatory system, whose resistance it must overcome.

The term (2) expresses that portion of cardiac work which ensures the velocity of the blood flow in the aorta and its branches.

Under physiological conditions, term (2) is a negligible fraction of ventricular work since it represents only one hundredth part [511]. It follows that when researchers want to measure cardiac work, they ignore term (2) and keep merely to term (1). Measurement of the left heart work consists therefore in quantifying the cardiac output and the mean systemic blood pressure.

Measuring Myocardial Oxygen Consumption

Physiologically speaking, oxygen consumption by the left ventricle is governed by several factors [1790]:

(1) the contractile state of the myocardium [1790];

(2) the tension developed in the ventricular wall throughout the systolic phase [1116, 1644], this tension itself depending on the systolic ventricular pressure and the volume of the ventricular chamber [611, 1116];

(3) the velocity of ventricular contraction [1791];

(4) the external work of the ventricle [700], itself depending on the heart and the total vascular resistance (see p. 92).

Although the measuring of myocardial oxygen consumption encounters special difficulties from the technical angle, it can now no longer be accepted that experimental research on a substance intended for the treatment of angina pectoris does not supply accurate details as to its effects on the oxygen requirements of the cardiac muscle (see Chapter II).

Two methods may be used, one direct and the other indirect.

1. *Direct method.* This is based on the FICK principle according to which the amount of oxygen consumed by the left ventricle is obtained by multiplying the left coronary arterial flow (in ml/min) by the arterio-venous difference which is found between the oxygen content of the coronary arterial blood and the oxygen content of the coronary venous blood. It follows that, from the technical viewpoint, a calculation of the myocardial oxygen consumption calls for the simultaneous measuring of the following three parameters: coronary arterial flow, oxygen content of the coronary arterial blood and oxygen content of the coronary venous blood.

We will not again be going over the measuring of coronary arterial flow.

All that is needed to measure the oxygen content of the coronary arterial blood is to take a sample of the blood in any peripheral artery, since the oxygen content of arterial blood is identical at all points of the arterial system.

Measuring the oxygen content of the coronary venous blood is technically more complex. Numerous reports have shown that only the venous blood of the coronary sinus is representative of myocardial drainage circulation. Technically speaking, it is therefore necessary to sample the coronary venous blood from the sinus [1392]. The latter is catheterised by means of a SONES catheter with three eyes (one terminal and two lateral) at its endocardiac extremity, inserted in the right external jugular vein and introduced under radiological control into the coronary sinus.

Arterial and venous blood sampling, and measurement of coronary flow, must of necessity be simultaneous. The blood samples are analysed for oxygen content either with the Van Slyke gasometric apparatus or by means of an analyser of the Beckman type for instance.

It should be recalled that measurement of myocardial oxygen consumption also provides additional vital notions which are arrived at by comparing such variations as occur simultaneously in the four terms of the formula. These details have been outlined in Chapter II (see p. 57).

2. *Indirect method.* Its advantages lie in the fact that it is technically very simple and that it calls for no surgical damage.

It involves the measuring of the tension-time-index [1644, 1355] which is an accurate haemodynamic index of myocardial oxygen needs (see Chapter II). Since it is the product of three haemodynamic parameters, the mean systolic blood pressure, heart rate and duration of the ventricular ejection, it is easy to measure since it only requires a recording of the central arterial pressure (in the aortic arch) and heart rate, and eventually of an electrocardiogram, the latter giving also the heart rate and the duration of ventricular systole by working out the Q-T space. The procedure can be easily applied in conscious dog and in man [249 c].

The value of the tension-time-index as an accurate pointer to myocardial oxygen consumption has been confirmed by various authors [167, 592, 984, 1543, 1798].

A new complex haemodynamic parameter for the evaluation of oxygen consumption of the left heart in dog and man has been recently proposed by STRAUER et al. [302c]. According to these investigators, the best correlation was found between left ventricular oxygen consumption and the product of the square root of left ventricular work by the sum of dp/dt max + dp/dt min.

The ultimate aim set itself by pharmacology is to build up, for the benefit of the clinician called to study the therapeutic effects of an antianginal drug, a dossier in which the key piece is the overall effect of this substance on the general and coronary circulations of an intact organism, animal or human subject, the conditions in which, as in the patient, all the factors influencing the myocardial metabolism operate. Only when made on the whole organism can determinations of the effect of a substance on the coronary efficiency have true values. The pharmacodynamic investigation of substances liable to be used in the clinical treatment of man must of necessity, therefore, be carried out on intact laboratory animals in conditions as close as possible to those existing in the case of the human patient. These methods, however, have their place only in the final, preclinical stage of experimental investigation. The information they supply is, of course, essential for any inference of therapeutic value, but it is not enough as it does not throw very much light on the intimate mechanisms involved in an overall effect and these procedures do not enable the total phenomenon to be broken down into all its components. It is only recourse to simpler, partial preparations that allows of analysis of the mechanisms operating. The experimental investigation of an antianginal drug thus implies the employment of a batch of different techniques, adapted for certain well-defined ends, each of which has its usefulness provided its possibilities and limitations are known.

The simple methods, and particularly the techniques on isolated heart, have the additional advantage of permitting the screening of large series of compounds. The current investigation of chemical series requires more elementary methods, which nevertheless enable the nature of some pharmacological properties to be determined, for example a direct dilator effect upon the coronary vessels when fibrillating hearts are used, and the possible intervention, in a given increased blood flow, of some modifications of strength and rate of cardiac contractions when the investigations are carried out on normally beating hearts.

Chapter IV

Clinical Methods for Assessment of the Therapeutic Value of Antianginal Medications

The multiplicity of methods which have been recommended for appraisal of the clinical effectiveness of antianginal medications indicates that none of them is entirely satisfactory and that such appraisal still leaves something to be desired.

It is naturally not a question of evaluating whether a particular drug has an effect or not on the developed anginal attack. As BATTERMAN [105] has stated, the clinical problem that presents itself is that of assessing change produced by prolonged administration of a drug in the frequency and severity of the attacks of pain.

However logical the point may appear, it is fitting to recall that exactitude in the diagnosis of angina pectoris constitutes the indispensable premise to every experimental therapeutic investigation. And while, since the time of Heberden's classical description of this syndrome, numerous medical contributions, both clinical and instrumental, have facilitated its diagnosis to a singular degree, even at the present time the correct diagnosis may eventually prove especially difficult. In the course of a symposium devoted to the differential diagnosis of thoracic pains [1860], seventy-eight different conditions, other than coronary insufficiency, were enumerated as capable of occasionally simulating the anginal syndrome[1]. As the several types of specialized knowledge required for the exact diagnosis of most of these pathological states are lacking in a good number of doctors, even if they are cardiologists, it can be taken as very probable that some patients without any heart disease must have been included in series of patients selected for experimental investigations on the anginal syndrome [320].

Diagnosis of Angina Pectoris

Various types of clinical examination are used to assist the physician in his diagnosis, particularly electrocardiography, ballistocardiography and vectocardiography. As for the electrocardiogram, the type of tracing termed "coronary" is far from being constant as 40% of patients with clinically well-established coronary involvement have, in addition to negative general and *objective* cardiological examinations, a normal resting electrocardiogram [1233]. Furthermore the electrocardiogram is in poor correlation with the data collected in patients in whom selective cinecoronarography has demonstrated the presence of obstructive atherosclerotic coronary lesions to various extent [1141]. In the case of the ballistogram, the abnormalities described for the anginal syndrome, although characteristic [240] and present in 90% cases [418, 419, 1651], are not specific [1650, 1824]. As regards the vectocardiogram, its morphological alterations are not related with the data derived from the visualization of the atherosclerotic

---

1 According to RICHARDSON [1521], the cartilaginous joints of the thorax seem particularly liable to acute or chronic trauma and they are probably the source of a number of painful anterior chest-wall syndromes.

coronary damages appearing by selective cinecoronarography [1141]. The diagnostic accuracy of combined electrocardiogram, vectocardiogram, and exercise-electrocardiogram was found greater than that of any one taken singly [316 c].

The inconstancy of the electrocardiographic changes and the lack of specificity in the ballistocardiogram and in the vectocardiogram as well have led to the elaboration of laboratory tests based on the fact that, the anginal syndrome being the reflection of distress of the coronary circulation, a coronary insufficiency, superimposed by the operation of an experimental stress that increases the work of the heart and its oxygen requirements, is reflected either in the reproduction of an attack of pain or in typical electrocardiographic changes, identical with those recorded in the course of a spontaneous crisis [1664] namely, depression of more than 2 mm of the S-T segment in at least one lead [1664] and complete reversal of the T wave in a left precordial lead [990].

Such experimental standard tests are the two-step exercise of MASTER et al. [1233] and the generalized hypoxia test of LEVY et al. [1129]. While very useful in most cases, these tests do not have the value of unquestionable diagnostic elements as many patients with undeniable coronary disease give negative responses. This is particularly true in relation to the effort electrocardiogram. For example, MASTER test (see p. 103) was negative in 18% of proved cases of angina [1593] and, according to the recent statistics of MASTER himself [1230], there was still a negative response in 3.2% of cases even when MASTER double test was applied or the variant of the simple test suggested by LITTMAN [1160]. However, the value of this test should be more doubtful for FRIEDBERG et al. [598] because they found, as the result of a double blind study, that the proportion of the false negative tests was 12% instead of 3.2% according to MASTER, while the number of the false positive tests averaged 39%. Following further studies, especially by MASTER, the diagnostic significance of this test could be improved if, instead of considering exclusively *the magnitude* of S-T depression, more attention were paid to *the duration* of the depression [1236, 1556], adding a careful examination of a specific configuration of the segment [1235] to which BRODY drew particular attention [231]. As the MASTER test is always negative in the normal subject [1593], only a positive test is of real value and affords a considerable degree of support to a suspected diagnosis of coronary involvement.

While it seems to be well established that LEVY's hypoxia test (see p. 106) is always negative in the normal subject and that a considerable number of anginal subjects exhibit typical electrocardiographic abnormalities, points indicating quite close correlation between these electrical signs and angina [168, 169, 259, 1474, 1839], it is less frequently positive in the coronary patient than the exercise test of MASTER [510, 1380, 1839].

An important modification of the LEVY's test has been proposed by MALM-STROM [1214]: by use of a gaseous mixture containing only 6.5% oxygen and 4.5% carbonic anhydride (the concentration of CO_2 has been lowered to 3% by KATZ and MESSIN, 949), MALMSTROM showed that his technique furnished 90% of positive results in anginous patients with atherosclerotic coronary disorders, a fact that gives answer to the objection commonly raised against the hypoxia test of LEVY which, by use of a 10% oxygen and 90% nitrogen mixture, afforded positive results in only 50% of cases with undoubted coronary insufficiency. In the hands of COULSHED [372], the MALMSTROM's procedure should even provide a positive response in 95% of patients suffering from myocardial ischaemia.

All these considerations led DRY [452], ELLIS et al. [489], BATTERMAN [105], ANDRUS [33], FRIEDBERG [597] and SOMMERVILLE [1787] to state that the diagnosis of angina pectoris should in fact be established primarily by extremely careful interrogation of the patient and that instrumental examinations as well as induced coronary insufficiency tests merely provide additional elements, the value of which is important but not decisive [366, 520, 860].

We should, however, take a look at the diagnostic value of the methods which have been proposed over the past few years and which for the most part are based on recent concepts of human physiology. One of these, advocated by SHEFFIELD since 1966, would appear to make an interesting contribution to the problem of diagnosing angina pectoris.

In the view of SHEFFIELD et al. [1736, 1737], it is not a standard *skeletal muscle* load which should be imposed on the patient, but a specific and reproducible degree of *cardiac* stress, independent of age and work capacity. Working from this assumption, they suggest a type of test known as GXT (graded exercise test) which should, in the case of a given patient, increase in a standard manner the myocardial oxygen demands. Taking as a basis the physiological notion that any increase in myocardial oxygen requirements calls for a parallel increase in coronary flow (see p. 55), and that this oxygen consumption tends in fact to vary in proportion to the heart rate [195], they deem it reasonable to assimilate the functional potentials of coronary circulation with the heart rate measured during the exercise.

They select a level of tachycardia which is 85% of the *maximum* possible rate for each patient in the light of his age. They take as the criterion for ischaemic depression of the S-T segment the critical value of 1 mm in any derivation where this segment is isoelectric prior to the exercise, and not 0.5 mm as in the MASTER test, because from their own experience any depression of 0.5 mm appears difficult to them to reproduce accurately.

Working on a total of 216 subjects, of whom 112 were deemed to be normal and 104 suspected cases of angina pectoris on the basis of purely clinical criteria, they find that, as compared with the MASTER test, their method has greater sensitivity and greater specificity since it provides less responses which are falsely negative and falsely positive respectively. They add that their method does not increase the potential risk of the test for the patient, and perhaps even lessens it.

Applying the technique suggested by SHEFFIELD, SOLVAY and VAN SCHEPDAEL [1774, 1775] go even further in the application of this method, because they believe that it is capable of providing a fairly accurate assessment of the coronary reserve of an angina subject. They make simultaneous measurements of the extent of ischaemic phase shift in the S-T segment of the ECG and the heart rate, corresponding to the emergence of the electrocardiographic anomaly (known as *dynamic*) *at the moment of the triggering of the cardiac pain induced by the Sheffield effort test*. In their view, the coronary reserve is defined by the *maximum* heart rate level which a given individual can tolerate without the appearance of pathological manifestations (angina attack, dynamic electrocardiographic anomaly, etc). Amongst other things, they base their opinion on the fact that a dynamic ischaemic S-T always worsens with effort or appears only on such an occasion, unlike rest condition ischaemic S-T which does not necessarily vary. They also consider that the call made on the patient's coronary reserve is directly linked to the increase in heart rate. The view of SOLVAY and VAN SCHEPDAEL is based on their personal findings with 145 obvious coronary cases (i.e. who had had a myocardial infarct and/or who were subject to unquestionable angina attacks brought on by effort), followed up over a period of from 1 to 7 years and subjected at different stages in the development of their illness to a strictly standardised effort test. They find that the extent of the call on the coronary reserve during effort can vary considerably from subject to subject and also in a given subject from one moment to another, but that it is *the same for a given level of heart rate in relation to the maximum possible level*, this latter being essentially related to the age of the subject.

The efforts to which the patients are subjected are achieved by the use of the ergometric bicycle, using the technique prescribed by MESSIN et al. [1290] by increasing muscular load by 300 kgm/min every 3 min without interruption until such time as there is fatigue, dyspnoea or chest pains. The E.C.G., monitored throughout the duration of the test, allows the heart rate to be calculated and the extent of the shift in the dynamic ischaemic S-T segment to be measured. All anomalies showing up on the effort electrocardiogram are systematically noted, although giving first priority to the ischaemic S-T criterion which is considered as the most valid criterion for diagnosing with any degree of certainty electrical myocardial ischaemia during or following an effort test, a very large majority of authors pronouncing in favour of the ischaemic configuration of the S-T segment for which they measure the depression which should reach a certain figure, usually 0.5 mm but sometimes as much as 1 mm. This measurement makes it possible to assess the coronary reserve of a subject but with the strict proviso that the effort applied represents a sufficiently heavy load for the coronary system, the best way to assess this load being to note the heart rate obtained *at the end of the test* and to compare it with the maximum possible rate for the age, corresponding to an intact coronary reserve. The essential facts observed by SOLVAY and VAN SCHEPDAEL are as follows:

a) In the case of 70 patients they study the behaviour of the coronary reserve as a function of the clinical condition of the patient. In 42 clinically stabilised cases, the extent of dynamic S-T segment shift increases in parallel with heart rate, but does not change, as between one test and another, with an identical effort-induced heart rate. Of 12 clinically improved cases, 9 no longer show any signs of S-T shift at an effort heart rate level identical to that found prior to the clinical improvement, whilst in the remaining 3 cases the S-T shift is fifty per cent less with an identical heart rate during the effort. Finally, in the 16 cases where the clinical symptomatology becomes worse as time goes on, the shift in dynamic ischaemic S-T becomes considerably more marked at identical heart rate levels.

It is thus clear that with these 70 patients, there is a marked correlation between the development of their clinical condition ,whichever direction this may take, and the extent of the dynamic ischaemic S-T shift with identical effort-induced heart rate.

b) With an eye to the correlation which could exist between the cardiac pain occurring during the effort test and the dynamic E.C.G. in the case of 145 patients, SOLVAY and VAN SCHEPDAEL arrive at the conclusion that the effort-induced pain attack seems to occur in the stabilised coronary subject as soon as a certain level of heart rate, which is always the same for a specific individual, is overstepped[2].

Effort-induced angina pectoris would thus appear to depend both on the degree of lessening of coronary reserve at rest and the extent of the call made on that reserve during exertion. The call made on the coronary reserve can be assessed roughly from the highest level of heart rate attained at the end of the angina-producing exertion with a standard muscle loading. Taking as a basis the level of effort-induced heart rate at which there occurs a 1 mm shift in the dynamic

---

2 This conclusion is very much like that of ROBINSON [1544], although he takes into account a more comprehensive parameter in that not only the heart rate is measured, but also the systolic blood pressure, so that in the case of ROBINSON, it is not the heart rate level but the level of the heart rate $\times$ pressure index which is fixed to a remarkable degree in any given individual (see Chap. I — p. 29).

ischaemic S-T, SOLVAY and VAN SCHEPDAEL classify all their coronary subjects into 14 arbitrary groups according to their effort-induced heart rate which ranges between extremes of 50 and 180 beats per minute, each group differing from its adjacent groups by a total of 10 beats per minute. In this way, each group represents a different level of coronary reserve integrity which increases from the 50 group to the 180 group.

In this way, the three groups in which effort-induced heart rate amounts to 160, 170 and 180 beats per minute respectively constitute the category of patients who possess an intact coronary reserve and therefore are not subject to angina pectoris during the effort test.

At the other end of the scale there is a category made up of the four groups of patients for whom effort causes angina to occur at a heart rate of from 50—90 beats per minute: these subjects retain only about one fifth of their coronary reserve.

All the remaining groups form three intermediate categories whose effort-induced heart rate ranges from 90—160 beats per minute and whose coronary reserve is estimated approximately and respectively at $^2/_5$, $^3/_5$ and $^4/_5$.

These authors therefore find that there is good correlation between the extent of the anginal pains as emerging from interrogation and the degree of *dynamic* S-T ischaemic shift, but subject to taking into account the heart rate level present at the same moment, the latter reflecting the degree of coronary reserve and also the degree of its use under effort conditions.

SOLVAY and VAN SCHEPDAEL finish by showing that, in the case of their patients, there is a good degree of relationship between the extent of mortality of cardiac origin and the level of coronary reserve, since it is in the group of patients where there is the most pronounced decrease in this reserve that the mortality rate is highest.

A further application of the SOLVAY and VAN SCHEPDAEL method consists in the objective quantitative assessment of the efficacy of medicines intended for the long term treatment of coronary insufficiency. Amongst other things, it makes it possible to investigate subjectively effective drugs which enable the angina subject to carry out the standard test with less speeding up of the heart rate. This being so, the reduced call which the patient makes on his coronary reserve, whatever the original level of this reserve, enables those angina patients who have benefited from the treatment to be "de-classified" and placed into categories with a *lower* level of effort-induced tachycardia, at the same time specifying by how many groups they have been down-graded in the light of the number of tens of beats by which their effort-induced heart rate has been reduced as a result of the functional benefit bestowed by the treatment. An example of therapeutic application of their method is given on p. 281.

ROOKMAKER [1552] also suggested in 1969 an effort test for diagnosing angina pectoris which offers the additional possibility of assessing the efficacy of long term antianginal medications. Basically it consists in applying a physiological exercise which eliminates the interplay of psychological stresses. The ECG is taken by remote control reading, and the diagnosis based on two morphological criteria provides many more positive answers than the MASTER test.

A very recent technique, which probably offers genuine future prospects, has been suggested by BALCON et al. [80]. This is based on the temporary inducement of artificial supraventricular tachycardia brought on by atrial pacing of a resting patient. Since it only imposes effort on the heart and not on the body, there is no increase in the return venous flow and consequently in cardiac output, nor are there any changes in general oxygen consumption or in the rate of circulating catecholamines. A bipolar conductor is inserted percutaneously into an antecubital vein as far as the right auricle, the positioning being done without fluoroscopy but with electrocardiographic monitoring [1798]. The heart rate, controlled by an external pacemaker, is increased by stages until the appearance of the first feeling of substernal pain reported by the patient. The heart rate need only be reduced to halt the pain and stimulation to be discontinued to restore the control condition. The method can be applied to hospital out-patients.

This method presents no hasard, is reproducible and easy to check [1080]. Its diagnostic value and its validity lie in the fact that this supraventricular tachycardia does not cause either pain or electrocardiographic impairment with healthy subjects [1450], that each heart attack thus induced is triggered, for a given patient, at an identical level of myocardial oxygen consumption worked out from the tension-time index [1215] — this index being a highly reproducible parameter of the "angina level" [592, 1798] — and that finally, with a given patient, this "angina level" is the same for any pain induced by atrial pacing or by physical exercise [80, 1082]. According to O'BRIEN et al. [1384], a correction should be made to this latter concept, since they find in each of their 7 patients examined that the tension-time index level at which the angina attack occurs during physical exercise is significantly higher than during the cardiac pain induced by atrial pacing. Furthermore, O'BRIEN et al. consider that this method has certain limitations because two other patients suffering from severe coronary disease did not develop an angina attack with atrial pacing whereas physical exercise triggered off cardiac pain.

Electrical pacing of the heart is also readily achieved with the catheter electrode positioned in the coronary sinus ("coronary sinus pacing") [254c]. It is easily controlled, reproducible and can be terminated abruptly. It simplifies myocardial metabolic studies by allowing simultaneous pacing and withdrawal of coronary venous blood through a single catheter.

The use of the coronaro-arteriographic method has also been advocated for discovering the myocardial origin of a thoracic pain. By revealing the undoubted presence of any coronary atherosclerosis, it is a very good method for proving that the angina pectoris is associated with and probably due to impairment of the myocardial vessels [1470]. It is, however, ineffective for relating a thoracic pain to angina pectoris where clinical diagnosis is doubtful, because the arteriogram may be normal in cases of classic angina and even fatal angina [765]. Its chances of success as regards clinical diagnosis are difficult to assess. In view of the anxiety state which a coronaroarteriographic examination induces in the patient, the amount of time and skill which it requires on the part of radiologists, and the morbidity risks which it entails, SOMERVILLE [1787] feels that its routine application for diagnosing a thoracic pain is a retrograde use for what is otherwise a very useful test in other applications.

Another trend in connexion with the physiopathological diagnosis of coronary insufficiency should be noted. Apart from the data furnished by the electrocardiogram which, as we have just pointed out, are far from having absolute value, there has hitherto been no procedure whereby functional coronary insufficiency could be objectively assessed in man. It is for this reason that the observations of GORLIN et al. [698] acquire particular importance; they have shown that in angina pectoris the coronary flow, otherwise normal in the resting state, does not increase after the absorption of nitroglycerin as it does in the healthy subject. As they attribute this fixity of the coronary flow to the fact that in these subjects the potential of vascular dilatation is exhausted as a result of the existence of maximum dilatation directed to correction of the troublesome effects of the arteriosclerotic disorders, these authors think that, in any subject suspected of angina, the nitroglycerin test should have a diagnostic value not possessed by either anamnesis, electrocardiogram or effort test: invariability of the coronary flow under these conditions they regard as indicating coronary insufficiency.

This opinion has been recently confirmed by BING. As this author considers that SONES' coronaroarteriographic method [1788] represents probably the most objective procedure of which the regular use is restricted by the fact that it can only be carried out in specialized centers by an experienced team of physicians [164], he relies on another diagnostic procedure [165, 2042]. According to the latter, the coronary blood flow is measured, after sublingual administration of nitroglycerin, in every patient who is suspected of suffering from angina. In BING's opinion, the value of this test lies in the fact that coronary blood flow increases in normal subjects while it does not change or may even decrease in coronary patients. It should, however, be pointed out that this test may well no longer present today the value that BING assigned to it in 1965 because by using, in 1969, a method which is capable of measuring the effects of nitroglycerin on coronary blood flow as early as within 45 sec after administration, he found that both the normal subject and the coronary patient reacted by a significant increase in myocardial irrigation (see p. 126).

ISAACS et al. [879] have proposed an objective method for measuring standardized treadmill exercise tolerance in the anginal patient, which combines ECG and vectocardiogram, while SPECKMANN et al. [1804] prefer to rely on a group of eight tests which are considered to enable the cardiac origin to be excluded in cases presenting precordial pain due to extra-cardiac causes.

An observation of importance, reported by GAZES et al. [631], may open up new possibilities in the differential diagnosis of angina pectoris in that it offers laboratory evidence of a biochemical nature in support of the clinical features of diagnosis. These authors found that, in twelve cases of angina, the performance of a double MASTER type test produced definite increase in the blood plasma content of noradrenaline in eight cases and of adrenaline in five[3].

This phenomenon does not appear either in the normal subjects or in those suffering from extracardiac pains when they are subjected to exercise of this type. According to GAZES et al., the biochemical mechanism involved in this phenomenon is the following. These catecholamines are liberated to some extent from the myocardium and the coronary vessels, altered by the pathological process, as well as from the adrenal medulla. As lactic acid is a powerful stimulant of the chromaffin tissue of the adrenal medulla [2036], it can reasonably be assumed that the anoxia induced by the exercise in the patient with angina pectoris will result in accumulation of lactic acid in the myocardium, this lactic acid stimulating the chromaffin tissue of the heart and thus liberating the catecholamines.

Such a diagnostic procedure requires a careful titration of the plasmatic catecholamines, a laboratory test which is not yet available in every cardiological center.

Let us finally recall the use, for diagnostic purpose, of measuring the lactates levels in the coronary venous blood, a subject which we dealt with largely on p. 25.

Clinical Assessment of Antianginal Drugs

The need for an exact diagnosis and the reliability of the various experimental tests which have been proposed for helping in an accurate diagnosis having been

---

3 Identical phenomena are seen in the dog 24—36 hours after experimental occlusion of a coronary artery [1524].

recalled, the methods which are currently favoured by clinicians with the object of assessing the therapeutic value of drugs in angina pectoris may now be approached.

If there is no clinical method for the evaluation of antianginal drugs which has received, if not unanimous, at any rate majority support, the main reason is that there are at the outset profound differences of opinion as to what should be the aim. Two opposed general trends declare themselves: some clinicians focus their attention more on the anginal pain factor and, in consequence, prefer to adopt an essentially subjective method. Others seek to be able to calculate the effect of drugs and, to that end, ignore the immensurable pain factor and turn to measurement of an indirect objective element which, rightly or wrongly, they consider to be the expression, if not of the pain, at any rate of the degree of coronary insufficiency. Within each of these two general conceptions there are many different methods.

It would, in fact, hardly be an exaggeration to say that each group of clinicians who have specialized in the study of this problem has its own method which it justifies by apparently sound arguments, even if some aspects of the problem are overlooked.

The following are the main methods:

1. Assessment of the ability of a drug to produce favourable changes, to the point possibly of complete prevention, in the electrocardiographic signs of ischaemia developing during the performance of a standardized exercise.

2. Measurement of the resistance to experimental hypoxia, carried to the point when an attack develops, with and without medication.

3. Measurement of the quantity of standardized work that can be performed by the patient, with and without medication, before pain develops.

4. Assessment of changes in the incidence and severity of the anginal attacks.

For convenience, we shall group these methods as objective and subjective; this distinction is arbitrary in view of the fact that some experimenters, and this is particularly true of those who hold by the objective method, employ procedures of the other type along with their basic method.

1. Objective Methods

1.1 Russek Method

RUSSEK [1591] rightly emphasizes that there is no field in human therapeutics in which there are so many discordant opinions on the effectiveness of drugs as in that of angina pectoris. The difficulties which clinical experimenters encounter arise from three facts: a) the anginal syndrome is not linked with any well-defined anatomopathological entity; b) the subjective changes produced by a particular treatment are difficult to classify or standardize and an unconscious element of preconception, on the part of doctor or patient, may enter into such appraisal; c) the methods applicable to man for determination of coronary flow, metabolism, the work and the efficiency of the heart are extremely complicated.

The subjective sensation of anginal pain might, conceivably, constitute an acceptable index of assessment if it were the exact reflection of the disparity existing between the coronary blood supply and the demands of the myocardium. This is not the case as there is no simple and direct relationship between the degree of coronary insufficiency and the intensity of the pain experienced, a minute ischaemic area being capable of causing as severe discomfort as that produced by a massive ischaemia involving a wide extent of the ventricular mass

[434]. Moreover, in the same patient, a strictly standardized pain-producing test exercise will sometimes cause a barely perceptible sense of discomfort and at other times a very distinct pain. Again, it would be essential that the pain should be a well-defined entity and that it should be capable of quantitative measurement in man, which is obviously not the case.

Furthermore, the anginal sensation is more than a simple reflexion of the cardiac hypoxia as it is also determined by the psychic reactions to its perception. It is important, therefore, in the assessment of the effects produced by a given drug, to neutralize or to be able to estimate the psychic component, the strength of which varies considerably and unpredictably from day to day and even from attack to attack. The utilization of a placebo, especially in the "double-blind" method (see p. 110), is intended to minimize or even neutralize psychic and other factors which might falsify assessment of the true effects of a drug.

RUSSEK considers that pain as a criterion is misleading as it also fails to differentiate powerful analgesics like morphine, which abolish the pain by action on its anatomical support and on the psychical reaction, from true antianginal drugs like nitroglycerin, for example, which act on the physiopathological cause of the pain — the myocardial hypoxia.

RUSSEK holds also the view that the keeping of a daily record by the patient, in which all aspects of the pain are entered (see p. 111), cannot provide any elements of value for an appraisal, no matter what the system of annotation, as the patient's impression may be influenced, without his being aware of it, in either direction by normal, exceptionally bad or particularly good periods, themselves determined by unfortunate or pleasing events.

All these considerations led RUSSEK to choose an objective element, the "morphology" of the electrocardiogram, in preference to pain as criterion. He therefore investigated the power of drugs to prevent, wholly or in part, the development of ischaemic changes in the electrocardiogram after the performance of a standard exercise by anginal patients. The exact conditions in which these investigations were conducted are of paramount importance. RUSSEK selected his subjects carefully, retaining only those coronary patients whose resting electrocardiograms were normal and who, every time they performed the standard exercise, which was always carried out under exactly the same conditions, exhibited a practically constant, positive ischaemic electrocardiographic response. The experience of the doctors in the RUSSEK group, extending over more than 20 years, has shown them that only one coronary subject in fifty could be considered suitable for this type of investigation [1591, 1616]; in such patients the performance of a standard exercise reproduced virtually identical electrocardiographic changes, even after intervals of months.

The experimental effort chosen was the "two-step" exercise of MASTER. It is a standardized test, imposing a load on the cardiovascular system. Initially regarded as a simple examination test for the functional capacity of the circulatory system as a whole and consequently applied only in connexion with blood pressure and pulse estimations [1234], the effort test was subsequently extended by its author to the diagnosis of angina pectoris [1233] and was then used, particularly by RUSSEK, for evaluation of the effectiveness of antianginal drugs. The principle of the test is that it imposes a definite, strictly standardized effort demand on the patient [1229]. An electrocardiogram is recorded before the exercise, which is to ascend and descend two steps of a stair repetitively for a period of exactly 90 sec. Each step is 9 in. (22.86 cm) high. The number of ascents that the patient has to make varies with age, weight and sex, and is shown in tables drawn up by MASTER et al. [1233]. Immediately after the test another electrocardiogram is recorded, with the patient seated, the pathological changes in the tracings being generally of short duration. Additional ECG are taken, preferably every two minutes, until the tracing again becomes normal.

The following changes in the electrocardiogram are considered to be abnormal and typical of coronary insufficiency:

1. Depression of the RS-T segment more than 0.5 mm below the mean iso-electric level, established from the P-R segment.

2. Flattening or inversion of an originally positive T wave.

3. Flattening or inversion of an originally negative T wave.

These electrocardiographic changes are similar to the abnormalities seen in the electrocardiograms of the same patients recorded during spontaneous anginal attacks, and they are widely accepted as reflecting myocardial hypoxia; they can, in fact, be reproduced exactly in the same subjects when they inhale an atmosphere containing 10% oxygen [1233].

Control tests on 2000 healthy subjects of both sexes and all ages have shown that these changes in the configuration of the electrocardiogram never appear in subjects who have no coronary involvement. A positive result is thus patho-gnomonic [1231]. Abnormal electrocardiograms of this type can therefore be taken as proof of functional coronary insufficiency.

RUSSEK et al. [1612, 1614] were struck by the fact that, among anginal patients and particularly those whose resting electrocardiograms were normal, there were some who, having performed the "two-step" exercise, exhibited these electrocardiographic changes in a qualitatively and quantitatively constant manner every time the standardized effort was imposed on them. These changes regressed after ten minutes or so, and the electrocardiogram became normal. Some patients came to be submitted to more than 200 identical tests in the course of several years, and these furnished a tracing of myocardial ischaemia which was reproduced with remarkable constancy [1591]. The method thus made it possible to determine which substances, administered before the exercise, act like nitro-glycerin in preventing development of the abnormal electrocardiographic changes produced by pain-causing effort. By way of example, RUSSEK et al. [1591] show that, in the same patient, an induced anginal attack could be countered as effec-tively by alcohol as by nitroglycerin; but, whereas the former drug did not modify the ischaemia-producing effect of the exercise performed on the myo-cardium, the exercise failed to produce any change in the electrocardiogram when it was preceded by the administration of nitroglycerin. It is obvious that in this particular case only nitroglycerin, and not alcohol, can be described as an anti-anginal drug [1612].

Convinced that the evaluation of antianginal medications, based on electro-cardiographic effort tests, although difficult to carry out and necessitating careful and patient investigation, represented the most reliable clinical method available today for the identification and assay of agents which would be useful in the prevention and treatment of myocardial hypoxia underlying the anginal syn-drome, RUSSEK and his co-workers have investigated a large number of medi-cations on a group of almost 200 patients who have been under observation for more than ten years [1589, 1590, 1591, 1612, 1613, 1614, 1615, 1616, 1619, 1620]. We shall have occasion to state their opinion on each of the drugs they have considered.

Although the electrocardiogram does not reflect the effects of a substance on metabolism, the work and efficiency of the myocardium or the coronary flow, the changes in the ECG do indicate whether the effects are favourable or not for the myocardium. Moreover, this method eliminates the problem of the placebo.

The main charge that the supporters of the pain factor make against RUSSEK's method is that an exact parallelism between neutralization of the electrical signs of effort ischaemia and the prevention of anginal pain has not been established. This is particularly evident in the case of Peritrate, which RUSSEK [1620] classifies as a powerful long-acting coronary vasodilator but does not state that it influences the pain syndrome as favourably as the effort electrocardiogram.

Other authors criticize the actual technical conditions of RUSSEK's method. For example, on the basis of his very thorough personal experience, FRIEDBERG [596] thinks that the response to RUSSEK's test is never constant in a given subject, and that the results obtained are difficult to assess. For his part, he has been unable to assemble a sufficiently large number of patients presenting reproducible reactions whenever examinations are repeated fairly frequently and also when the conditions in which the test is performed are slightly modified by the unavoidable intervention of emotional factors, which vary from one test to another and which escape medical control. For FREEDBERG [583], the effort tests are without significance when they are conducted at 23—24°C or when they are imposed more than once a day. In his opinion, these tests must be performed in a temperature of 10°C (see p. 107), and in each instance at the same time of day, i.e. in the morning, and the patient fasting, the last meal having been taken on each occasion at the same time the previous day.

In our view, there are other objections that can be advanced.

As a matter of fact, the RUSSEK technique has the validity of an acute experiment and, even if it does actually permit of differentiation between substances which improve the metabolic state of the myocardium from substances which might simply be termed antalgics (that is, capable of abolishing the pain without improving the coronary circulation), it still only evaluates their *immediate* and transient effect, whereas any drug to be used in coronary disease is destined to be administered over prolonged periods. As FREIS recently stated [13b], even the prevention or diminution of ST-T changes in the electrocardiogram during exercise by a coronary vasodilator drug provides no assurance that the drug will be effective in the long-term prophylactic treatment of angina. Although the exercise electrocardiogram test may provide an additional index of effectiveness in a well-designed clinical trial, it cannot be regarded as a substitute for such a trial.

It is of course undeniable that the ability of a given substance to prevent the development of electrical abnormalities due to effort is an indication of its beneficial effects on myocardial blood supply and coronary efficiency. When, however, RUSSEK thinks that a substance which counters development of the ECG changes of induced ischaemia can be classified as a coronary vasodilator, his opinion is going beyond the facts for, as no measurement of the state of the myocardial irrigation has been made, he can only state that the substance corrects the disequilibrium existing between the supply of the myocardium and its oxygen requirements; he is not entitled to assume a coronary vasodilator action (which is, however, likely) or to prejudge the manifold effects which can be brought into action at the level of the heart muscle.

RUSSEK's technique (for the same reason as other clinical objective methods) does not furnish any element which affords information on mode of action and it is impossible to say whether a drug is effective because it increases the amount of blood delivered to the myocardium or diminishes the work of the heart, or because it increases the coronary efficiency or combines different effects.

RUSSEK's technique affords thus the possibility to select substances which reduce the relative myocardial hypoxia induced by effort, and which, by virtue of this fact, are beneficial to the patient; it does not establish that a specific coronary vasodilator effect is concerned[4].

1.2 Levy Method

LEVY et al. [1128, 2003] employ a generalized "anoxaemia test" and take as criteria of the possible anti-anginal activity of a drug two phenomena produced by the test: one is objective — changes in the ECG, and the other, subjective, is the anginal pain. They use an apparatus designed in 1938 [1126] by means of which an atmosphere consisting of 10% oxygen and 90% nitrogen is administered to the subject in the rhythm of normal respiration. There is then development in the ECG of characteristic and definable changes, which can be used as an index of coronary insufficiency [1127, 1129]; these are changes in the S-T segment and in the T wave. As the displacements of the S-T segment are measurable and the changes in the T wave do not lend themselves to any correct comparative quantitative measurement, only the former are considered. These concepts of clinical physiopathology have been given an experimental basis in the animal as LESLIE, SCOTT and MULINOS [1108, 1711], working with the cat, have shown that the breathing of oxygen-deficient air produced in every instance electrocardiographical changes identical with those that followed ligation of a coronary artery in the same animals.

In a majority of patients the anoxaemia test also induces development of an attack of pain comparable to those developing spontaneously in the same patients [1126].

The procedure is as follows. The experiment itself is preceded in the case of each patient by several control experiments intended to familiarize him with the apparatus and to establish a standard, reproducible response. This response is calculated on the basis of: a) the deviations in millimetres of the S-T segment of the electrocardiograms recorded in four leads (three standard and a precordial) every 5 min from the commencement of the inhalation and during the painful crisis; the sum of the four deviations is determined; b) the duration of the inhalation required to produce the anginal pain. A treatment phase is then started (the patient is ignorant of the type of drug administered) and the effect is checked every week by the anoxaemia test. The activity of a drug is assessed by comparison of the responses obtained during medication with the control responses. The effect is estimated as a percentage. Every drug used is tested in relation to a placebo.

1.3 Riseman Method

According to RISEMAN and his co-workers [1531], the fact that a substance prevents or reduces, probably by a coronary vasodilator action, the electrocardiographic signs of myocardial ischaemia induced by an exercise (RUSSEK's method) or by hypoxia (LEVY's method) constitutes an indication of true pharmacological activity but cannot be accepted as evidence of therapeutic effectiveness for the following reasons. a) There is no constant relationship between the electrocardiographic signs of induced ischaemia and the development of cardiac pain. b) A very limited proportion of patients are suitable for these tests [584, 1536, 1616]; consequently, although the hypoxic electrocardiograms recorded

---

4 In the opinion of REDWOOD et al. [266c], workloads causing angina in less than 3 min cannot reliably be used for studying the effects of therapy. However, if progressive workloads are chosen that cause angina to occur in the control studies in more than 3 min, exercise capacity and tension-time index at angina provide important information relating to the efficacy and mechanism of action of a therapeutic intervention.

after these tests reveal a pharmacological effect, they do not supply any information of the incidence of the beneficial clinical effect, so far as the considerable proportion of patients excluded from the tests are concerned. c) Certain technical difficulties may render it impossible to reproduce identical results in the course of repeated tests as, in the anginal patient, the resting electrocardiogram may spontaneously show varying degrees of depression of the S-T segment on different days.

RISEMAN therefore suggests another method, based on an experience of twenty-five years acquired in a special clinic for the management of angina pectoris. The experimental work was carried out on a group of patients who were chosen for their intelligent cooperation and whose clinical state was stable in that their affections did not involve any spontaneous remissions. This mode of selection retained an average of 20% of the patients. The therapeutic efficiency of a drug was determined on the basis of three elements:

a) a purely clinical evaluation of the subjective effects of the medication;

b) assessment of the exercise tolerance, that is, the quantity of work (performed under standard conditions) that could be effected by the patient before development of an anginal attack; and

c) the characteristics of the effort electrocardiogram recorded at the end of a period of treatment, comparison being made with a tracing taken under the same conditions but after a period of placebo treatment.

The patients were examined every week. At the time of the first visit a complete clinical examination, and particularly a record of all the features of the anginal syndrome, was established by three doctors, first independently and then together. After the patient had rested for 20 min a fourth doctor who, throughout the investigation, would not know the nature of the medication received by the patient, calculated his exercise tolerance.

This exercise, which was strictly standardized [1535], involved ascent and descent of MASTER type steps, which the patient effected at a fixed rate until the development of anginous pain, but never (in subsequent examinations) beyond the point when the work performed was 50% more (after effective treatment) than he could do before receiving the medication.

This exercise took place in a special room at 10°C as the vasomotor changes in the size of the coronary arteries due to cold, which are probably of reflex origin, contribute to the precipitation of anginal attacks, so that the amount of work necessary to induce an attack was less than at ordinary temperatures of 23—24°C [586].

At each weekly visit the patient was questioned, always by the same doctor, as to his opinion on the effectiveness of the medication received in the preceding week, the number of attacks occurring (a daily record was kept), and any unusual circumstances which might have influenced the attacks; his exercise tolerance was also measured.

After the first visit the patient was left without treatment or was given a placebo for several weeks or months so that the subject's usual clinical record and his average exercise tolerance could be established over a period of some length; the tolerance was regarded as adequately stable as the quantity of work a patient could perform before the advent of pain is comparatively constant [584]. It was only then that the substance to be tested was administered; the total period over which this drug was taken included terms of placebos during which the clinical picture and the exercise tolerance were redetermined. At the end of each weekly visit the patient received his week's supply of medicine from a doctor who did not know its nature. The patient himself did not know what he was taking. The conditions of a "double-blind" were thus operative. Between two periods of true different medications, effective or ineffective, there was a long period of placebo treatment.

When a substance had shown itself to be active, effort electrocardiograms were recorded for the patients who had been improved to determine if the benefit achieved (subjective and objective) was evident in the tracings: improvement in the coronary circulation was indicated by the absence of S-T segment depression in the ECG recorded after exercise identical with that which caused significant depression, coupled with an anginal attack, when the patient was taking a placebo.

The final evaluation of the results was formulated by combination of the conclusions afforded by the three methods of examination, namely, the patient's opinion, the clinical medical assessment and the exercise tolerance. These results are divided arbitrarily into four categories:

1. Good response: cases in which the exercise tolerance, when tested repeatedly, was found to have increased by 50%; these patients reported disappearance or definite reduction of their attacks.

2. Moderate response: cases whose exercise tolerance had increased by 20 to 49%; there was concomitant reduction in the number of attacks.

3. Poor response: cases in which exercise tolerance had risen by 10—19%; the clinical condition showed no change.

4. No response: the subject experienced anginal pain after an exercise similar to that producing pain when he was taking a placebo.

The patients who participated in an experiment of this nature were divided into three groups according to the magnitude of the increase in exercise tolerance they showed when the exercise was performed two minutes after sublingual administration of 0.3 mg nitroglycerin: group 1 consisted of patients who showed a clearly defined response, group 2 of those whose response was moderate and group 3 was that of patients responding little or not at all to nitroglycerin. Thus the total activity of a drug under investigation could be classified as good, moderate, poor or nil and could also be compared with the activity of nitroglycerin administered as a test, and this in the three groups of patients, those who reacted well, those who reacted moderately and those who reacted poorly to nitroglycerin.

The importance of exercise tolerance measurement, which is for RISEMAN the most useful part of his method, is underlined by the following facts. First of all, there is close correlation between increase of exercise tolerance and the subjective response in ordinary life in the sense that definite or moderate improvement in tolerance is always associated with disappearance of or reduction in the number of anginal attacks [584]. Further, many patients consider themselves improved by the treatment given, whatever it may be, although the disappearance or reduction of their attacks is not regularly accompanied by increase of exercise tolerance; expressed differently, apparent clinical improvement develops more frequently than the objective evidence of such improvement [1301]. This is in agreement with the opinion of other authors that many patients are incapable of deciding between the effect of a drug and the effect of a placebo [677, 1752].

The value of the method employed by RISEMAN is supported by the fact that the placebo always produced negative results [584, 1534].

1.4. Solvay Method (1774, 1775)

As has already been said on p. 97, SOLVAY estimates coronary reserve of the anginous patient from two parameters: heart rate which is attained at the end of a standardized exercise and degree of S-T depression at the same moment. When administering long-term effective treatment, he noted some reduction of these parameters, which enabled him to determine the degree of improvement of coronary reserve in each patient treated with the medication of which he was attempting to evaluate the efficacy. An example of the use of this method is given on p. 281.

In view of the fact that SOLVAY employs a cycloergometric exercise, it should be mentioned that the possibility has been contemplated of progressive habituation on the part of the patient on whom such an effort has been imposed on several occasions. If such should be the case, the validity of this method would be unreliable. A recent clinical statistic analysis [262] has shown that there existed between the haemodynamic changes (heart rate, aortic pressure, pulmonary blood pressure, cardiac output, stroke volume, work of the left ventricle, tension-time index, peripheral vascular resistance) which were observed during two identical cycloergometric tests imposed at different moments on a fairly large number of patients, some clearly discernible differences, but which were in most cases without physiological significance. Thus, any important change in the results of the effort-test, due, for example, to the administration of a medicament, is of real value and cannot be attributed to any habituation on the part of the patient to the exercise so performed.

1.5. Rookmaker Method

ROOKMAKER applied his diagnostic method (see p. 99) to assess the efficacy of antianginal drugs [1552]. The test is based upon the disappearance or the reduction by at least 0,1 millivolt of the S-T segment depression present during the effort-test.

1.6. Frick Method

FRICK et al. [592] demonstrated that their technique of producing angina in the coronary patient by artificially increasing heart rate by atrial pacing, is suitable for use in assessing the therapeutic potential of antianginal drugs. For example, the efficacy of nitroglycerin has been expressed in terms of tension-time index level, in other words in terms of myocardial oxygen consumption level (see p. 30).

2. Subjective Methods

Methods of this type are used by clinical experimenters who consider that the evaluation of medication for angina is the measurement of a completely subjective sensation.

As in clinical work on man pain cannot be expressed numerically, such measurement must necessarily be based on a verbal and/or written report by the patient on his reactions, it being understood, of course, that the patient must be cooperative [121].

Those who favour this type of method rely on the widely held view — it is held, for example, by KATZ [952] and by BATTERMAN [104] — that the pain is a variable subjective manifestation, with only a negligible quantitative relationship to the underlying coronary disease and showing little correlation with the changes in the effort electrocardiogram.

The view of SILBER and KATZ [1752] is that angina is a pain which must be analysed and assessed from the standpoint of the physiopathology of sensation, without regard to factors which determine coronary flow as, according to these authors, it cannot be proved that there is any strict correspondence between the power of a substance to counteract the ischaemia-producing effort effects in the electrocardiogram and the power of the same drug to prevent anginal pain.

As the anginal pain is not only a matter of physical perception but is also a psychological reaction [2027], the magnitude of which depends on a host of factors which are beyond human control and are not subject to scientific measurement, it is of the highest importance that the effects of these psychological reactions on the patient's assessment of the evolution of his pain syndrome under treatment should be neutralized. This is the reason for the employment of the placebo. It is a reactor the response to which is an all or nothing response. In any patient an inactive placebo cannot be made active by simple suggestion. This explains the fact that the percentage effectiveness of a placebo is found to be very noticeably the same by all authors.

Without probably being as great as some would have it [1076], the effectiveness of the placebo is appreciable, as EVANS and HOYLE [514], GREINER et al. [738] and BEECHER [122] estimate it at 35—38% of cases in a series of patients exceeding a thousand. This is important as, if the effectiveness of a substance exceeds 40%, this fact becomes highly significant because it is impossible to exceed this figure with a placebo [105].

In effect, the total subjective effectiveness of a drug is equal to its true effectiveness augmented by that of its placebo which represents the alleged beneficial effect which the a priori favourable anticipation associated with the trial of a new treatment can have and actually does have. Not only has the placebo been repeatedly shown to be effective in reducing episodes of angina pectoris [56, 349, 514, 1232] but, quite unexpectedly, ARONOW and CHESLUK [11 c] have demonstrated, in a double-blind crossover study, that the placebo can exert a favourable effect on such an objective criterion as capacity for effort since 6 of 17 patients, i.e. 35%, had significantly improved exercise tolerance while taking the placebo compared to no medication and only 2 of 17 patients, i.e. 12%, had significantly improved exercise tolerance while on no medication compared to placebo.

Each medication studied must have its own placebo, identical with the drug itself in form, size, appearance, colour and taste, so that it cannot be distinguished from the actual drug[5].

The introduction of a placebo into investigations of this nature does not go far enough. It is advisable to use the double-blind system in carrying out the investigations, the direct examiners as well as the patient not being aware of the nature of the medication (real or placebo) administered. The need for this procedure, which is intended to eliminate the psychological factors (enthusiasm or scepticism) which might interfere in one direction or the other, on the part of both the doctor and the patient, is generally admitted as a result of the investigations of GOLD [676] and SILBER and KATZ [1752], who have shown in an attempt to assess the therapeutic value of khellin in angina that this substance was considered to be active when the doctor knew the manner in which the experimental work had been carried out, but was subsequently judged to be exactly equal to its placebo when the investigation was repeated on the same group of patients and by the same experimenters, ignorant this time of the nature of the drugs supplied to the patients.

Another essential experimental condition is the institution of a period of control prior to the investigation. Like the double-blind administration of the placebo, this condition is intended to neutralize the importance of psychic factors by protecting the examiners from the danger of false assessments based on the natural instability of the anginal state in which spontaneous remissions, some-

---

5 Interesting and original considerations concerning placebos have been reviewed by WOLF [2026].

times complete, are known to occur and which, in some patients, may last for several weeks [206]. COLE et al. [349] have demonstrated the importance of these psychological factors experimentally by showing that 50% of the patients selected for such investigations reported definite reduction in the frequency of their attacks during the first three months of observation, irrespective of the nature of the drugs administered (active drug, placebo or no medication). These phenomena are probably due to the special attention given these subjects and to the exceptional psychological climate such an investigation automatically creates between the patients and the doctors [1232]. A drug study of this kind should include a preliminary period of clinical observation lasting three months, termed the "rapport period" by COLE [348, 350], after which the experimental investigation proper is initiated, first by a period of control during which the placebo is administered. COLE also insists that the treatment periods (both real and with the placebo) should be relatively long so that the evaluation may gain in accuracy. A revealing feature of COLE's study was that half of the placebo-treated patients reported a decrease in the frequency of attacks continuing over the first 2—4 months of treatment. This illustrates the potent effects of the placebo and of the doctor-patient relationship on the manifestations of an illness such as angina pectoris.

Some of the practical problems that occur even in a well-designed therapeutic trial have also been described by COLE. Only about one fourth of the patients referred for angina were judged acceptable for the trial. Some of those rejected had chest pain from other causes or had such conditions in addition to angina which made analysis of results impossible. Others were suffering primarily from anxiety and were unable to differentiate minor chest discomforts from true anginal attacks. Some patients were unable or unwilling to keep records of the daily incidence of attacks or number of nitroglycerin tablets used. Still others had attacks too infrequently to permit valid comparison of active drugs with placebo.

The three requirements essential to every subjective method having been stressed, it only remains to consider the manner in which the effect of a drug on the anginal syndrome should be assessed. The procedures employed are extremely varied and their analysis is not of any practical importance. One method alone which, since its publication, has been adopted by other authors on a number of occasions, will be described because of the progress it represents in comparison with preceding methods.

Greiner Method

GREINER's purely subjective method [738] is based essentially on the employment of a daily report card which the patient keeps day by day. The card, which covers a week, is in this form

Day of the week	Same heart pain as usual	Less heart pain than usual (good day)	More heart pain than usual (bad day)	No heart pain at all
Monday				
Tuesday . . .				
Wednesday . .				
Thursday . . .				
Friday				
Saturday . . .				
Sunday				

The question to which the patient has to reply is very simple as he has only to decide whether, from the standpoint of cardiac pain, the day which is ending at the time he marks his card has been, when compared with the usual state, the same, definitely better, definitely worse or one with no pain at all. The answer was made daily at bedtime; the patient put a cross in the appropriate space on the card. The questionnaire thus calls for a minimum of intelligence, judgment and memory on the part of the subject.

The periods of true treatment and the periods of placebo administration are alternated randomly. The length of these courses varies considerably, ranging from two to a number of weeks in different cases.

When the investigation of a drug (with its placebo) is considered to be completed, the days of treatment are totalled for each patient and then for all the patients together in respect of the drug and the placebo separately. The separate results under each of the four types of day are established by simple addition of the crosses marked on the daily report cards. The result for each type of day is calculated as a percentage of the total number of days of treatment and figures which can be compared are finally obtained for the drug and for the placebo. In the case of an active drug, the comparative examination reveals definite disparity in the figures yielded by the medication and those relating to the placebo under the four types of day.

This method of quotation makes it possible to group the observations in a great variety of ways, particularly in relation to each patient, details of the calculations being supplied by the authors (see the original work). The true pharmacological effect of the drug under investigation is represented by the difference between its established activity and that of the placebo.

GREINER's original method has subsequently been amplified by GABRIELSEN and MYHRE [618] who attach the arbitrary values 0, 1, 2 and 3 to excellent, better, usual and worse days respectively. This enables them to express the results numerically and to proceed to statistical evaluation, with calculation of the possible errors, although this tabulation is of decisive value only if the clinical investigation has been very prolonged and has included a sufficient number of cases.

Assessment of the therapeutic value of the substances employed for the control of cardiac pain in patients with angina constitutes a problem of unusual difficulty as experiments pointing to favourable effects cannot be completely dissociated from the force of suggestion and as the methods employed may very well not be sufficiently free from faults to carry complete conviction.

Although convinced of the need to find an objective experimental equivalent for the pain symptom, which would provide a scientific basis for this problem, GREINER et al. [738] consider that their subjective method is of very considerable importance. The objections they make to certain objective methods appear justified. LEVY's technique particularly can only furnish a presumptive assessment as there is no close correlation between the ECG changes and the anginal pain. RISEMAN's technique appears to them to be scientific as they have re-examined it themselves [75] and were able to confirm his conclusions on the effects of a given drug (aminophylline) in fixed dosage by using, like RISEMAN, the pain factor as criterion. In view, however, of the special conditions under which the exercise test applied by RISEMAN is carried out (see p. 107), they think that data collected in this manner cannot necessarily be applied to the effort pain developing in the ordinary circumstances of daily life. WOLFF, HARDY and GOODELL [2027] have, in fact, shown that the natural pain is not a simple perception but a mixture of perception and reaction. The total distress that the patient expresses by the term "pain" does not depend solely on the intensity of the pain, but also on the feeling states that may exist or may be aroused by factors associated with the pain perception, such as anxiety, frustration, fear and panic which are contributing to the anginal syndrome [597]. There is interaction between pain perception and such feeling states, each of these factors being capable of intensifying or diminishing the total experience expressed as pain. Now, at the time of the performance of exercise tests, the particular conditions in which the exertion is carried out practically neutralize the feeling states, so that the perception of pain alone limits and measures the capacity for exercise. It does not necessarily follow, therefore, that the favourable effect of a drug, as revealed by an effort test, will manifest itself in relation to efforts made in the course of ordinary life. The results of standardized effort tests can, therefore, only be generalized with circumspection.

Other experimenters [485, 514] who, like GREINER et al., prefer the purely subjective method, recommend a quotation system in which are entered so many details relative to the anginal syndrome and to incidents, favourable and unfavourable, in the daily life that the investigator finds himself confronted with an insurmountable tangle of material on which it is difficult for him to express an accurate judgment. They select well-established cases of anginal syndrome which have already been under treatment for six months at least. A complete history, including social and family background, is made. The clinical physical examination is complemented by a very detailed biological schedule. The patients are submitted to a control period of two to four weeks during which they receive no medication (with the exception of nitroglycerin) or are given a placebo. Particular emphasis was placed on the following cardinal features during this period: the number of attacks in each 24 hours, the duration of each attack, the severity of each pain, the degree of activity indulged in during an attack, the average distance the patient could walk before an attack develops, the number of tablets of nitroglycerin required in 24 hours to alleviate severe pain. All this information is entered by the patient on a special card which is examined on each visit to the clinic. At these times the patient is questioned as to his subjective condition, his reactions to medication, the weather conditions that have prevailed, any unforeseen changes in his mode of life (daily activities and occasions of stress). All these elements are collected in the same manner for the period during which the drug under test is administered. When the investigation ends, all the documents are carefully examined, classified, analysed and compared, after which they are subjected to criticism and the experimenters express their verdict.

In our opinion, GREINER's method has many advantages.

— The keeping of the daily report card is simple because it involves a minimum of judgment, intelligence and memory.

— It provides for investigation of the placebo over identical periods, which does not eliminate the effect of suggestion in an investigation of this kind but neutralizes it.

— It involves use of the double-blind system.

— Applied to patients who do not modify their ordinary life in any way, it respects the conditions in which a drug prescribed by the medical practitioner would exercise its effect.

— It does not have the disadvantages of the weekly or fortnightly assessment ("interval evaluation") so commonly employed; the latter does not permit of uniformity of the criteria on which judgment is based and cannot avoid the risk of the patient's impression for the entire period (week or fortnight) being coloured by one or two particularly good or bad days; nor does it take account of days without pains, a notion which can prove very useful.

— The method supplies the maximum of subjective information and the data are entered in such a manner that they can be referred to easily for statistical

8*

analysis. Furthermore, the system of annotation is such that the facts secured can be re-examined at any time, their primary meaning can be reconsidered, and they can be re-interpreted from various angles on the basis of any new concept which may subsequently be introduced.

— It records only facts and offers the greatest freedom from distortion by innumerable factors affecting patient's statements on the evolution of his cardiac pains.

— It has the advantage of assessment of the remote effect of a drug administered daily over long periods.

AMSTERDAM et al. [30] have recently suggested a change in the procedure usually adopted for double-blind experimentation. It aims at minimising the placebo effect which is associated with the use of a new medicament, but above all, that which, according to SHAPIRO [1732], may be the true expression of the most important factor of all, namely the favourable rapport established between the patient and the doctor carrying out the experiment. It is with this in mind that AMSTERDAM et al. introduce into this type of investigation the two following points. Firstly, they administer the new medication openly for one to two months. In addition to the fact that this preliminary stage enables the level of effective dosage to be determined, it partially obviates the placebo effect linked to the adoption of a new form of treatment. As for the double-blind stage proper, it consists in returning the patients to their medical practitioner, asking them to keep a daily chart of the development of their condition, and above all only collecting the results by correspondence. This form of procedure ("remote" double-blind test) avoids any direct contact between the experimenter and the patient, so that there is little chance of any rapport building up between them which may cause any significant change in the patient's response to the course of treatment adopted.

Mention must be made at this point of the development of a new type of procedure covering the investigation of antianginal drugs under double-blind conditions which makes a definite break with the procedures hitherto adopted. It should be made clear that, for the moment, it has only been put into practice in a few clinical investigations and then only in the case of a specific drug, lidoflazine (see p. 199).

The method consists in drawing a distinction between two stages [39c]: a first so-called open stage lasting for at least 6 months, during which the drug is administered openly to a given batch of angina patients. This is followed by the second stage, double-blind, *in which only those patients showing marked improvement during the initial stage take part.* The patients thus involved are split into two groups of equal size from a list of participants drawn by lot, one group being treated with the placebo and the other continuing on the drug under investigation. The experimenter only breaks the code prematurely in the event of the patient's condition deteriorating, and in any case after a certain length of time in the case of patients whose clinical condition, improved by the drug during the open phase, does not deteriorate.

In the view of the originators of this procedure, the overall investigation which results makes it possible to objectify the therapeutic effect under double-blind conditions, since any deterioration occurring under placebo in a patient originally improved with the active product would demonstrate that the therapeutic benefit was in fact due to the drug.

The clinician is thus required to give his opinion, before the code is made known, as to the nature of the treatment administered, taking it that he assumes that this was the placebo if the patient's condition deteriorates and that it was the drug under investigation if the clinical condition continues to be favourably affected. To give only one example [1938], one clinician's guesses were all accurate in the case of lidoflazine, a fact which according to the law of probability and in the light of the number of patients has only one chance in 32,768 of being due to luck.

This original type of procedure is at first sight highly attractive. It may however be wondered whether it is not likely to distort the results of the investigation and whether it represents a genuine advance over the methods normally used, since if this were so it would deserve to be generally adopted for this type of research work.

The following comments may be made.

1. When, in the course of the double-blind phase, the clinician assumes that the deterioration in the patient is due to the placebo, and also that the continuance of the initial improvement can be ascribed to the drug, he cannot definitely eliminate two major factors which are likely to upset his prediction. Firstly, both the deterioration and the continuance of clinical improvement can be due, in a manner which it is impossible to check, to a spontaneous aggravation of the angina condition or to a similarly spontaneous abatement in the disease, whose essentially cyclic course need not be gone into again. The argument is still valid even if account is taken of the severity of the selection criteria, which include amongst other things a stabilised symptomatology and sustained clinical observation over a period of at least a year by the same cardiologist. It must further be admitted that clinicians who adopt this procedure strictly apply these criteria and can keep continuous observation on their walking patients throughout the entire investigation period. The second factor lacking from the clinician's assessment, during the double-blind phase, is the therapeutic effect of the placebo, generally accepted as being in the region of 40% of the patients taking part in a given experiment (see p. 110). It is difficult to accept the view of the originators of this procedure that the placebo effect can no longer enter into it since the selection criteria were very strict and the duration of the double-blind phase sufficiently long to eliminate the placebo effect. In this connection, there only remains to recall the conclusions put forward by BERNSTEIN [145] on the basis of a survey of various investigational reports. This author draws attention to the fact that patients who are given a placebo for 3 months find their clinical condition improved by 50%, a concept which answers to the generally accepted view (see p. 111).

2. If we analyse the five clinical reports on lidoflazine which are at present available [400, 412, 1670, 1925 and 1938], and if we take the predictions which mistakenly attributed to the placebo a relapse in the clinical condition, we find these covered 3 out of 76 patients where the test was deemed to be complete. Since the patients were split up into two equal groups of 38, this means that the placebo effect only appeared in 3 out of 38 cases, i.e. in only 8% of the cases, a figure far below the generally accepted percentage (see p. 110). In other words, it must be admitted either that the application of this type of procedure leads practically to the disappearance of placebo-prone subjects or that lidoflazine improves the clinical condition of the patient to the point of rendering him insensitive to placebotherapy. Both these eventualities are hard to accept.

It would thus appear that this type of procedure solves none of the difficulties met with in the investigation of the actual therapeutic effect of antianginal drugs, and that its application to the investigation into an isolated drug leads to results which can invalidate any comparison which one may be called upon to make with the effects of other medicaments investigated double-blind in accordance with the usual methods.

3. Conclusions on Methods of Clinical Assessment

Because of its many advantages, the method of GREINER and his co-workers would appear to be of greatest importance as it represents the best attempt at estimation of the subjective effect of drugs on the anginal syndrome. Its limitation is that it provides no element of information on the mode of action of antianginal drugs which prove to be effective. Substances which improve conditions for the work of the heart cannot therefore be distinguished from those acting in other ways such as, for example, analgesics and central depressants. Now, therapeutically speaking, the only drugs of importance are those that can, by action upon the myocardium, re-establish equilibrium between the oxygen supply and the oxygen demands. It seems therefore necessary to employ in the same time another method of examination which will provide objective proof of improvement in the circulatory conditions. Measurement of the exercise tolerance, as carried out by RISEMAN, will allow the effect of a drug, given continuously, to be translated into figures. This method seems preferable to the RUSSEK technique, which gives expression only to the immediate effect and not to the result of a prolonged treatment, and which is only applied to patients subjected to very severe selection for reproducibility of the electrocardiographic changes, involving an enormous number of patients.

It is obvious that even if one employs the objective test of RISEMAN, together with subjective clinical assessment based on use of the card recommended by GREINER, the accuracy of the data provided by such investigations will still be a function of the number of patients treated and of the duration of the experiment; a hundred patients under observation for a year would appear to represent minimum conditions [1752]. This is an important requirement to be met, as particularly stressed by RUSSEK [1601], who rightly emphazises that a double-blind clinical study could hardly be found which has been conducted as it should be made, i.e. involving at least one hundred patients which should be followed up during one year. It must effectively be admitted that too many double-blind clinical studies which are concerned with the therapeutic evaluation of some antianginal drugs are currently published involving the participation of too few patients. In chapter V, it will be repeatedly seen in the case of different drugs that only ten or a dozen anginal patients which were drugged during one fortnight or one month took part to many clinical studies. Numbers were evidently too small to yield a statistically significant result. Under such conditions, anybody can obtain any result as RUSSEK has so rightly pointed out [1601], and it is not surprising that some clinical investigations which have been conducted by separate teams on a given drug led to conflicting reports as to the estimation of its therapeutic effectiveness. As has been emphasized by LASAGNA [1076], the most satisfactory situation is for a drug to be carefully investigated by independent observers in a number of clinics on different groups of patients and under different conditions. If such investigations are in general agreement on the effectiveness of the drug, there is then little room for doubt.

It is now generally recognized that in the case of many medications which have been proposed as long acting antianginal drugs, many claims of therapeutic effectiveness rested on flimsy evidence. Well-designed, controlled clinical trials were nonexistent. The supporting clinical data often consisted of nothing more than a few reports in which no attempt was made to control observer bias or the placebo effect. Therapeutic claims often were only based on a few clinical studies, none of which bore any semblance of a controlled therapeutic trial.

In an editorial headed "Cardiovascular drugs: Experience of the drug efficacy study", a study in which panels of specialists evaluated the cardiovascular drugs used in their various disciplines, FREIS [13b] expressed very recently the following views: "Many cardiovascular drugs need restudy using the technics of controlled clinical trials. Knowledge gained from a review of past deficiencies can be used in designing future, more definitive studies. In the case of the antianginal agents, for example, because of the limited numbers of acceptable patients the trial should be organized on a multiclinic basis. Precautions must be taken to provide a foolproof double-blind study, and the active agents should be given for a sufficient time to determine long-term effectiveness. The use of a pre-randomization trial period of several months' duration would allow a sufficient interval to establish a reasonably stable base line for the frequency of anginal attacks and also would serve to eliminate additional unreliable, uncooperative, or otherwise unsuitable patients. During this period the patients would continue to take nitroglycerin as needed but would also receive a placebo of a long-acting preparation. The post-randomization period could be interspersed with additional control periods as check points on the long-term fluctuations in the frequency and severity of anginal attacks."

To close this chapter, it is fitting to mention the particularly well informed opinion of some outstanding cardiologists. FISCH and DE GRAFF [553, 547] think that the subjective techniques are indispensable in spite of the difficulties inherent in appraising all subjective reactions. But elimination of bias by double-blind studies is essential and one must select patients with significant unequivocal angina, namely those experiencing an average of at least seven attacks of angina per week. This selection is justifiable because, clinically, these are the patients that require continuous treatment and also because, on an experimental basis, it assures collection of significant numbers for statistical validation. Moreover, they state that in spite of its limitations, the quantitative exercise tolerance test designed by RISEMAN approaches the ideal assay technique.

Severity in selecting all the criteria which must form the basis of a well conducted clinical investigation is justified by the fact that it is essential to avoid drawing over-hasty conclusions from the results of badly conceived clinical trials, not only with regard to the efficacy of drugs which are in reality ineffective but also with regard to the inefficacy of drugs which are in fact effective. As RUSSEK [1608] points out, much emphasis has, in fact, been placed on the fact that uncontrolled clinical observation has often falsely endowed inert agents with powers that they do not possess, but it should be equally recognized that improperly designed double-blind studies could divest potent agents of actions clearly and consistently evident to patient and physician alike. The problem of treating the anginal patient is of such social importance that failure to utilize available benefits may deprive the patient with angina pectoris of considerable comfort, assurance and productivity [1608].

Chapter V

Pharmacological and
Clinical Features of Antianginal Drugs

The pharmacological effects on the myocardium and the coronary circulation, as well as the antianginal properties are not specific to one or even several well-defined chemical functions, as such properties have been found in a great variety of chemically quite unrelated substances. There is thus no structural specificity for such a type of medication. Moreover, very dissimilar chemical structures are endowed with pharmacological effects on the coronary circulation and cardiovascular system which are essentially the same, and also with a comparable level of antianginal properties.

In this chapter are set forth the pharmacological properties and the therapeutic antianginal effects of a very large number of medications which have been used or are still employed by clinicians for the treatment of angina. With the exception of nitrites which are assembled in the same group and discussed in respect of the oldest of them, namely nitroglycerin, the drugs considered are filed according to a sequence which corresponds more or less with their chronological presentation to the medical profession.

However, for the purpose of rational classification, the antianginal medications have been arranged in different groups. The first group has been given special attention because it includes those drugs which have been experimentally studied on a large scale and which constitute the back-bone of present day antianginal medication. They are listed in the contents and discussed between pages 150 and 288.

The other drugs which are placed together under the heading "Miscellaneous drugs" are divided into three secondary groups (see p. 288) according to the progress so far achieved in the pharmacological and clinical studies which have been and are being carried out, and also according to the nature of their pharmacological properties. The criteria upon which such classification is based are outlined on pages 288, 299 and 307.

Nitrites

The term "nitrites" is applied both to nitrites and to nitrates; it has been sanctioned both by long usage and by the similarity of their actions on the smooth muscles of the body.

The nitrites which were or are still most used in clinical medicine are: sodium nitrite, amyl nitrite, octyl nitrite, glyceryl trinitrate or nitroglycerin, erythrityl tetranitrate or erythrol, pentaerythritol tetranitrate, mannitol hexanitrate, triethanolamine trinitrate and isosorbide dinitrate. Their structural formulae are given in Table 3.

Although it has long been accepted that nitrates act after having been reduced to nitrites in the body, it is certain that, for reasons developed mainly by GOOD-MAN and GILMAN [692] and by DRILL [449] and which cannot be detailed here, this conception requires re-examination before it can be given the validity of fact. Recently, DiCarlo and Melgar [33a] studied the biochemical events which follow the absorption of nitroglycerin. C^{14} labeled nitroglycerin was incubated with fresh rat blood serum under a variety of experimental conditions. The data

Table 3

Nitrites:

Sodium nitrite: $NaNO_2$
Amyl nitrite: $CH_3—CH(CH_3)—CH_2—CH_2—NO_2$
Octyl nitrite: $CH_3—CH_2—CH_2—CH_2—CH(C_2H_5)—CH_2—NO_2$

Nitrates:

Nitroglycerin (Glyceryl trinitrate)

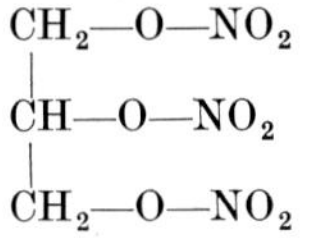

$CH_2—O—NO_2$
$CH—O—NO_2$
$CH_2—O—NO_2$

Erythrityl tetranitrate

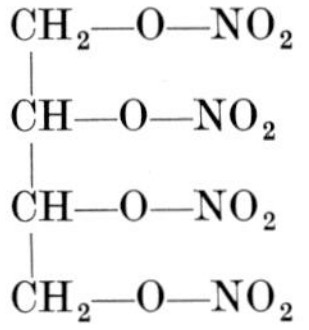

$CH_2—O—NO_2$
$CH—O—NO_2$
$CH—O—NO_2$
$CH_2—O—NO_2$

Pentaerythritol tetranitrate

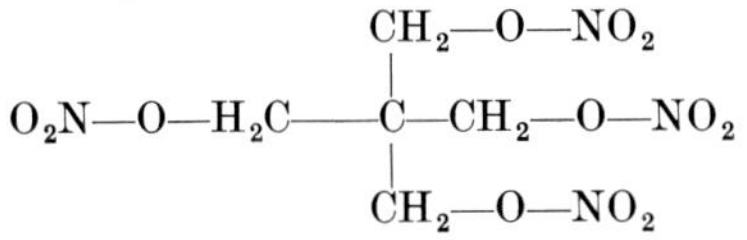

$CH_2—O—NO_2$
$O_2N—O—H_2C—C—CH_2—O—NO_2$
$CH_2—O—NO_2$

Mannitol hexanitrate

$CH_2—O—NO_2$
$O_2N—O—CH$
$O_2N—O—CH$
$C—O—NO_2$
$C—O—NO_2$
$CH_2—O—NO_2$

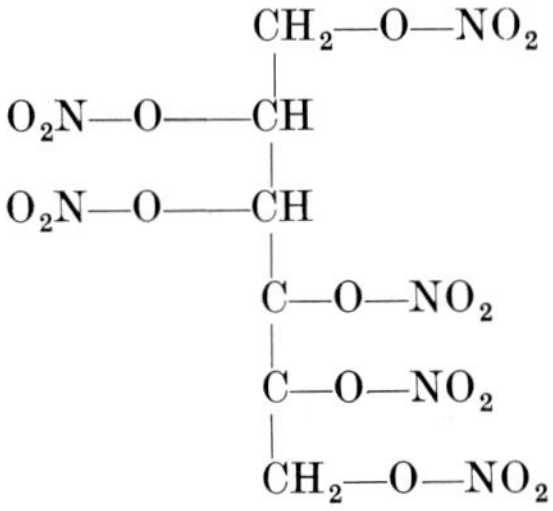

Triethanolamine trinitrate
(biphosphate)

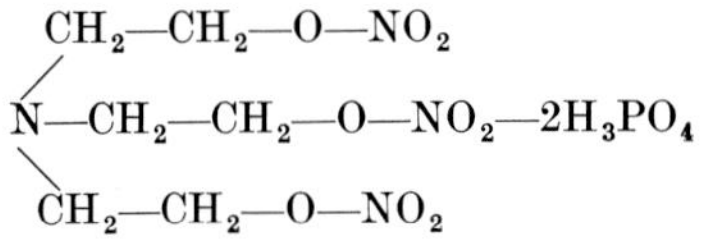

$CH_2—CH_2—O—NO_2$
$N—CH_2—CH_2—O—NO_2—2H_3PO_4$
$CH_2—CH_2—O—NO_2$

Isosorbide dinitrate

$H_2—C$
$H—C—O—NO_2$
$C—H$
$H—C$
$O_2N—O—C—H$
$C—H_2$

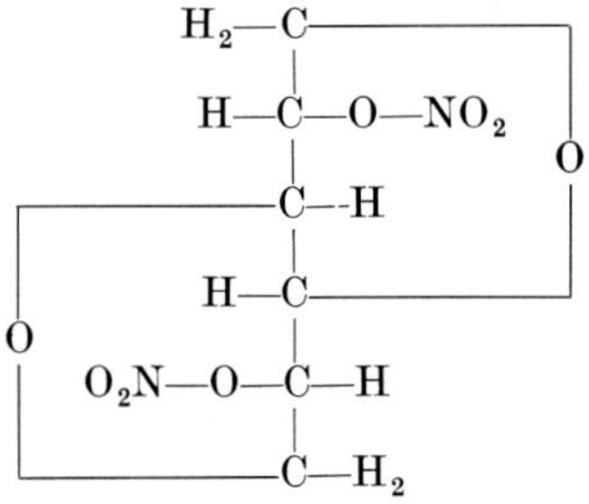

indicated that the degradation of the drug proceeded by a 2-step mechanism involving the reduction of nitrate to nitrite *in situ*, followed by hydrolysis to release inorganic nitrite. The serum enzyme differs from the previously described liver organic nitrate reductase since addition of reduced glutathione to the preparations was unnecessary to the enzymatic activity. The speed of the bio-transformation of nitroglycerin by serum correlates with the short duration of action of the drug.

The basic effect of nitrites is relaxation of all smooth muscles, particularly those of the small blood vessels, arterioles, capillaries and venules, but this vasodilatation is specially marked in the post-arteriolar section of the vascular bed. The spasmolytic effect of nitrites is direct, and independent of the nerve supply. There is, however, considerable variation in the sensitivity of the different vascular areas in the body to the action of nitrites; the intensity of their vaso-dilator effect depends largely on dosage employed; the rapidity and duration of their action vary considerably for the different compounds. The coronary vaso-dilator activity of nitrites is very much reduced in the case of the isolated rabbit heart when the nutritive fluid used for perfusion is poor in potassium [1273]. It is accompanied by a definite increase in the potassium content of the cardiac muscle. These observations suggest that nitrites have an effect on muscle nutrition or on the metabolism of the myocardium but their exact significance has not yet been clearly defined.

By measuring the oxygen uptake of isolated rabbit left atria, LEVY [24b] studied the direct effects of various organic nitrates on basal myocardial oxygen uptake, in order to provide further information on the basic actions of nitrates on cardiac metabolism. A significant decrease in oxygen uptake was observed with a 442 μM concentration of nitroglycerin. In a similar concentration, isosorbide dinitrate and erythrityl tetranitrate had no significant effect while mannitol hexanitrate, iditol hexanitrate and sorbitan tetranitrate produced significant increases. No simple relation was found between the lipoid solubility or per cent nitration of the compounds under study and their effects on oxygen uptake.

Of the nitrite compounds, nitroglycerin has been the subject of by far the greatest number of experimental and clinical investigations and is the one most used in human therapeutics. If we omit sodium nitrite, use of which has been very much restricted in favour of other nitrites, nitroglycerin, amyl nitrite and octyl nitrite can be regarded as substances of rapid but transient action particularly in respect of their therapeutic effect, while the five other compounds in the series have a more prolonged action.

1. Nitroglycerin
(Trinitrin, Anginine)

Since the middle of the nineteenth century, the time when MURRELL [1334] recommended the use of nitroglycerin in angina pectoris on purely empirical grounds, an impressive number of investigators have rightly interested themselves in the pharmacological properties of nitroglycerin, especially the effects on the cardiovascular system and the coronary circulation.

First of all, the outstanding data derived from the experimental work which has been done before 1960 will be summed up. Then, will be considered in more detail the investigations which were carried out from 1960 in animals and also in man by means of some very elaborated methods and also in such clinical situations that the haemodynamic changes induced by the drug as soon as it is swallowed could be followed up step by step during its therapeutic effect.

Given to the unanaesthetized dog in an average dosage of 0.04—0.06 mg/kg, nitroglycerin increases coronary flow, the effect being extremely transient with intravenous administration, and 5—15 times longer with oral administration [508, 509]. In the anaesthetized dog, intracoronary or intravenous injection yields similar results, which are attributed to reduction of resistance in the coronary vascular bed (by direct vasodilator action) as the systemic arterial pressure falls in the same time [205].

Under the same conditions, WEGRIA et al. [1968] observed tachycardia additionally. The minimum active dose which, given by intracoronary injection, increased the coronary flow was from 0.02 to 0.002 mg [468]; the flow only increased as long as the arterial pressure did not fall (this was particularly true for the stronger doses), and it fell as soon as systemic hypotension developed, whatever the route of administration (sublingual, intravenous, intramuscular, subcutaneous). This is in accordance with the observations of DÖRNER and WICK [443] showing that it is common to record in anaesthetized and in conscious dogs as well a decrease in coronary blood flow which is either primary or secondary to the general haemodynamic effects.

The coronary vasodilator effect of nitroglycerin is the result of direct action on the muscle of the vessel. Indirect and direct proofs demonstrate effectively that this is the case. Nitroglycerin produces a generalized arterial vasodilation, particularly at arteriolar level, as well as considerable dilatation of the capillaries and venules [1972, 2000]; these phenomena result in accumulation of blood in the venous territories with reduction in the quantity of blood returning to the right heart, whence develops a fall in the systolic output with, by reason of the tachycardia present, an unchanged cardiac output [211]. As otherwise the work of the heart is hardly changed [211, 1969], the increase in the coronary blood flow must arise from a direct coronary vasodilator effect by a reduction in the intrinsic component of the coronary vascular resistance. The experimental proof of this was provided by work on the perfused fibrillating isolated heart of the dog [957, 958], on the fibrillating isolated heart of the rabbit [301] and on the heart in situ [606]. The employment of a coronary arteriographic method has also shown that nitroglycerin injected through a catheter into the root of the aorta increased the arterial calibre by more than 50%, the heart rate and arterial pressure being unchanged [764].

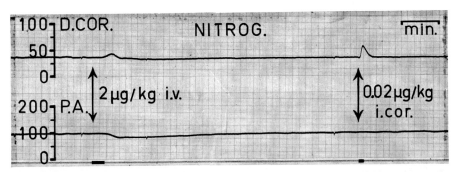

Fig. 3. Effect of nitroglycerin on coronary arterial blood flow and systemic blood pressure in the anaesthetized dog. From top to bottom: D.Cor.: Mean blood flow in the left circumflex coronary artery, measured with an electromagnetic probe (ml/min). P.A.: Mean blood pressure in the femoral artery (mm Hg). At first signal mark: intravenous injection of nitroglycerin, 0.002 mg/kg. At second signal mark: intracoronary injection of nitroglycerin, 0.00002 mg/kg

Actually, the effect of nitroglycerin on coronary blood flow in the animal varies according to the routes of administration. Fig. 3 gives a good example which illustrates the present current opinion. When nitroglycerin is injected into the coronary artery, myocardial blood flow increases sharply. This rise is very short, lasting only 10—15 sec, and is not followed by any reduction. When a dose which is 100 times larger (corresponding on a weight basis to the recommended dose in man by i.v. injection in case of emergency, for example Veinitrine) is injected into a peripheral vein in the same animal, the increase in coronary blood flow is much smaller and this primary rise is followed by a moderate and progressive sustained fall, which is probably a direct consequence of the decrease in systemic blood pressure[1].

What is the effect of nitroglycerin on the work of the heart and the coronary efficiency ? According to BOYER and GREEN [205], the work of the heart is reduced. With very small doses, the coronary vasodilatation is not accompanied by any concomitant changes in the rate or amplitude of the cardiac contractions, although these two functions are definitely depressed with large doses [1274]. ECKSTEIN et al. [476] consider that a minute increase in the consumption of oxygen by the myocardium accompanies increase of coronary flow, but the hyper-irrigation is more than enough to supply the heart with several times the additional quantity of oxygen required. SARNOFF et al. [1645] also concluded that the oxygen consumption was unchanged. Despite a multiplicity of observations indicating that the gaseous metabolism of the myocardium is unaltered, GORLIN and his co-workers [208, 1761] report that it increases appreciably in healthy man (by 63%) and that, as the coronary flow raises in parallel, the hyper-irrigation is probably secondary to the elevation in the consumption of oxygen by the heart. This discordant result should be accepted with caution in view of the objections that can be made in relation to the nitrous oxide method which they employed (see p. 79). As long as the facts cited by GORLIN have not been confirmed by others, it can be taken that the effect of nitroglycerin on the coronary efficiency is positive; SCHIMERT [1669] considers that, in dilating the coronary arteries, the drug has a favourable effect on what he calls the "coronary reserve" by reducing the overload on the heart. The amount of oxygen available per work unit of the left ventricle is significantly increased [609], as a consequence of the strong decrease in the ventricle work that accompagnies the coronary vasodilation [625][2].

Nitroglycerin enhances the backflow developing in the distal end of the circumflex coronary artery, ligated at its origin, by 20% [1095] but, according to KATTUS and GREGG [947], the drug does not modify this retrograde blood flow, under the same experimental conditions.

Nitroglycerin was unable to improve in rabbits the functional conditions of coronary circulation impeded by ligation of the left coronary artery performed 3—4 days previously [1295]. On the other hand, nitroglycerin antagonized the electrocardiographic S-T depression due to injection of picrotoxine into the lateral cerebral ventricle in the rabbit [1921].

In the anaesthetized dog, nitroglycerin reduced blood flow in the inferior vena cava, inducing thereby peripheral venous stasis [857]. This finding concords with the fact that for doses ranging from 5 to 80 γ/kg i.v., nitroglycerin diminishes blood pressure, coronary vascular resistance, cardiac output, heart work and myocardial oxygen consumption, coronary blood flow remaining unaltered. All these effects occur immediately but do not last more than 5 minutes. The reduction of total peripheral resistance reflects the peripheral vasodilator action of the drug, an effect which is considered by these investigators as being the essential primum movens for the haemodynamic cardiac modifications, and

---

1 The same findings have been very recently reported by COWAN et al. [28a] in anaesthetized open chest dogs, left circumflex coronary artery flow being also measured with an electromagnetic device.

2 RAFF et al. [105a, 265c] have recently demonstrated that the fall in the pressure rise velocity of the left ventricle which occurs in anaesthetized dogs after i.v. injection of nitroglycerin is due to the reduction in general blood pressure since an acceleration of the pressure rise velocity was seen when blood pressure was artificially stabilized. Furthermore, a similar increase in pressure rise velocity occurred when nitroglycerin was infused directly into the left coronary artery, a mode of administration which did not alter the systemic blood pressure.

consequently also for the antianginal effect, the coronary action being subordinate in their opinion [1712].

The biochemical mechanism involved in the action of nitroglycerin has been investigated. RAAB et al. [1489, 1490] consider that favourable effects in angina are due to metabolic neutralization of the anoxiant properties possessed by sympathicomimetic amines for the myocardium. Their opinion is based on the fact that, in the atropinized cat, tachycardia and T wave depression in the electrocardiogram induced by adrenaline or noradrenaline failed to develop when nitroglycerin was administered before or at the same time as the catecholamines. Neither ECKSTEIN et al. [476] nor POPOVICH et al. [1461] have been able to confirm these findings, however, although the latter repeated RAAB's experiments very exactly (the same dosages, particularly) with, additionally, measurement of cardiac metabolism, which is definitely increased after administration of both amines; in their opinion, nitroglycerin produced no change in any of the three phenomena. Nitroglycerin is not, therefore, an anti-adrenergic metabolic agent at myocardial level, and it can be taken as probable that it does not act by chemical blocking of the effects of sympathicomimetic amines formed in the heart or liberated in the blood during anginal attacks. The biochemical mechanism concerned in the favourable effect of nitroglycerin in angina pectoris has not, in fact, been identified yet (see p. 128).

Such were the essential principles established some 10 years ago regarding the pharmacological and biological general effects of nitroglycerin. Since that time, the properties which nitroglycerin brings to bear on haemodynamics have formed the subject of numerous investigations which have provided explicit information regarding these effects. Certain of these investigations have the special advantage of having been carried out with angina pectoris patients during the period when the heart attack was wearing off after sublingual absorption of the medicament. For this reason they are of exceptional interest.

Effect on the Coronary Flow in Dogs

In the case of a conscious dog, nitroglycerin administered in food at a daily dose of 0.1—0.5 mg/kg moderately increases the coronary flow measured by means of an electromagnetic flow transducer [887].

Applying the Xe^{133} technique [1562], REES et al. [1510] show that an intravenous injection of 0.01 mg/kg of nitroglycerin over a period of 1 min (which corresponds to human practice) increases coronary flow for 3 min, then subsequently lowers it. The effect is therefore of a dual phase nature, coronary resistance being considerably reduced during the initial phase with peripheral resistance following this same pattern. Myocardial oxygen consumption drops throughout the entire action period, probably because of the drop in blood pressure.

As far as REES is concerned, these findings in dogs would appear to cast doubts on the validity of the reducing effect on coronary flow which certain clinicians have observed in coronary subjects [698], arguing that the method used (nitrous oxide) is unable to register rapid variations in blood flow. However, the data provided by BERNSTEIN [146] and obtained by the Xe^{133} radio-isotopic method provide a partial answer to REES' objection, since they indicate a marked drop in flow in the angina subject 3 min after *sublingual* intake. BING [167] also shows that when taken by the sublingual route nitroglycerin does not alter coronary flow in the angina subject at the end of 2—3 min, whereas it increases myocardial irrigation in the healthy subject. There is therefore only one explanation for these discrepancies: the effects of an intravenous injection are not necessarily the same as those for sublingual administration. Furthermore it is dangerous to extrapolate to the coronary subject facts observed in the case of a normal coronary system in an animal.

REES is of the opinion that nitroglycerin has on animals two effects which are potentially interesting for therapeutics: initial increase in coronary flow and prolonged reduction in the oxygen requirements of the heart. So REES asks himself what happens in the case of the angina sufferer (see p. 128).

Having found in the course of a previous investigation that nitroglycerin increases, in dogs, the *collateral* blood flow at the far end from a chronic coronary occlusion [523] without there being any change in *total* coronary flow, FAM and McGREGOR [522] show that the intravenous injection of nitroglycerin into a dog has the effect of dilating, above all, the conductance vessels (this observation is also consonant with the coronary dilatation visible in man and animals under X-ray, 635, 1093, 1788) without significantly affecting the small pre-capillary resistance arterioles. On the basis of this finding, they suggest that where there are conditions of myocardial ischaemia, the hypoxic zone (where there is already maximum physiological compensatory dilation of the resistance vessels) can find its irrigation increased by enlarging the diameter of the conductance vessels and of the collateral vessels. This would seem to be one of the action mechanisms of nitroglycerin in an anginal attack.

WINBURY [2011] shows that nitroglycerin increases nutritional coronary circulation (see p. 45) and lowers coronary vascular resistance. Since there is little change in *total* flow, this means that the bloodstream supply is diverted to nutritional vessels, either the number of open capillaries increasing or the capillary blood flow increasing as a result of relaxation of the pre-capillary sphincters. These experimental findings suggest for WINBURY the idea that nitroglycerin could, in the case of the angina patient, redistribute the available blood flow through the myocardium in such a way that the ischaemic zones are given extra blood at the expense of the normal zones [2009]. In a very recent report published in 1971, WINBURY et al. [11c] demonstrated that nitroglycerin given intravenously (0.005—0.02 mg/kg) or directly into the coronary artery (0.002—0.004 mg) selectively increases oxygen tension of the subendocardium but not the subepicardium and that this change is not dependent upon an increase in coronary blood flow or a decline in aortic pressure (incidentally, it may be mentioned that dipyridamole does not produce a significant change in intramyocardial oxygen tension, in spite of a large increase in coronary flow). These results support the hypothesis that nitroglycerin causes redistribution of myocardial blood flow from the epicardium to the ischaemic subendocardium and an increase in the density of open capillaries in the epicardium to compensate for the loss of blood flow to that region. These overall modifications are presumed to be the result of dilatation of the intramural arteries in the left ventricle, which determines the distribution of blood flow between the superficial and deeper regions of the left ventricle.

A few authors have looked into the effect of nitroglycerin on a previously modified coronary circulation. For example, the drug slightly and temporarily increases the circumflex coronary flow in a dog whose anterior coronary artery has been occluded between 20 and 30 hours earlier [627]; it antagonises the reducing effect of norepinephrine on this flow. With a dog whose anterior coronary artery has been gradually occluded by an Ameroid ring over a period of 2 months, an intravenous injection of 0.5 mg/kg of nitroglycerin modifies the coronary flow of the infarcted myocardium and of the normal myocardium in a very changeable manner, even being able to reduce it in certain cases [928]. In case of acute severe ischaemia in dogs, nitroglycerin dilates the coronary arterioles further in spite of maximal ischaemic dilatation but, due to the accompanying hypotension, the coronary flow can no longer increase [211 c]. In trained conscious dog with experimental chronic obstruction of the left circumflex coronary artery, nitroglycerin causes sustained and large dilatation of a heavily stressed normal descending bed in the presence of left circumflex insufficiency, but dilates the ischaemic circumflex bed only when its collaterals are well-developed. No evidence was found that nitroglycerin could dilate coronary collaterals [128c]. Finally, nitroglycerin prevents the coronaro-constrictor effect of pituitrine in dogs [1272].

Effect on Coronary Flow in Humans

Using their technique for measuring coronary flow (see p. 83), KNOEBEL et al. [1007] show that nitroglycerin taken under the tongue does not cause any foreseeable changes in a *normal* man in the coronary flow over the next 3—10 min, 7 subjects showing an increase and 10 a reduction. There is however a highly significant correlation for the 17 subjects between the modification of the flow and that of the pressure/min (i.e. the product of the heart rate x mean systolic blood pressure and the duration of systolic ejection), which suggests that nitroglycerin has no incidence on the mechanisms which govern the automatic regulation of coronary flow, a conclusion which falls in line with that of McGREGOR and FAM [1252] outlined in p. 124.

By using the method for measuring myocardial irrigation by means of perfused Rb84 at a constant flow rate, BING [167] manages to test the effect of nitroglycerin with effect from the *3 min* following its sublingual administration. Under these conditions, he finds that the drug causes a marked increase in the coronary flow of the *healthy* subject, but does not change it in the case of the coronary atherosclerotic subject, thus confirming the opinion of BRACHFELD [208] and that of LICHTLEN [1136]. It must however be pointed out that with certain coronary patients, the effect of nitroglycerin on myocardial flow would appear to be of a dual phase nature, an initial moderate and short-lived increase (2 min) being followed by a similarly moderate reduction [278], which is exactly what REES [1510] found with dogs (see p. 123).

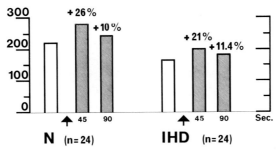

Fig. 4. Very early effect of nitroglycerin (0.8 mg by sublingual administration) on coronary blood flow in normal subjects (N) and in patients with ischaemic heart disease (IHD). For both groups of patients: Open column: Control coronary flow, in ml/min. First hatched column: Coronary flow 45 sec after nitroglycerin (at arrow). Second hatched column: Coronary flow 90 sec after nitroglycerin. There is an increase in blood flow in both groups of subjects. (COWAN et al., [27a])

The development of coincidence counting with *rapid* bolus injections of Rb84 (see p. 82) might give a new dimension to the action of nitroglycerin on coronary blood flow in man as compared with the effect when measured with the constant infusion of Rb[84]. According to very recent studies by BING and his team [27a] dealing specifically with the *very early* effects of nitroglycerin, tests performed on 24 normal subjects and 24 coronary heart disease patients revealed (Fig. 4) that there was a significant increase in myocardial blood flow 45 sec after sublingual administration of nitroglycerin in both normal subjects (26% increase) and patients with coronary heart disease (21% increase). Ninety seconds after administration, there were smaller increases in flow which were not significant in normal subjects (10% increase) but remained significant in coronary patients (11.4% increase). These data demonstrate an *early* increase in nutritional blood flow in both series of subjects, thus suggesting a redistribution of blood flow within the heart muscle. In the light of these findings, and also the observed prolonged peripheral haemodynamic effects of nitroglycerin, which will next be discussed, BING is of the opinion that early direct cardiac action, together with a reduction in myocardial oxygen needs, may well explain the beneficial action of the drug. It is also interesting to point out that when tested in patients undergoing internal mammary artery implantation for coronary artery disease, nitroglycerin given sublingually during the operation increased both rapid phase and slow phase coronary flows, thus improving perfusion in regions of ischaemic myocardium [150c].

Haemodynamic Effects in Humans

The special interest of the latest haemodynamic studies carried out on man lies in the fact that they examined the effects of nitroglycerin when *administered by the sublingual route*.

In the case of a normal man, nitroglycerin reduces the systolic, mean, and mean-systolic blood pressures, and also the work of the left ventricle [208, 845, 1543]. When administered during exercise, it lessens the increase in cardiac and systolic flows, but increases tachycardia [1376]. An identical response is found with the sufferer from coronary insufficiency. BING and his colleagues took simultaneous measurements of a large number of haemodynamic parameters under the effect of nitroglycerin, with the result that they are able to establish a consistent table of disturbances occurring. They show [167, 1543] that with the *coronary subject whether anginal or not*, the drug lessens after 5 min the shortening of the ventricular fibres, the speed at which this shortening takes place, the left ventricular systolic and end-diastolic pressures, the tension-time index, peripheral resistance and left ventricular work; the heart rate increases. In short, these effects — shown in schematic form in Fig. 5, lead to a reduction in myocardial oxygen needs and can be considered as being the result of the peripheral vasodilator effect and of the reduction in venous return which results therefrom [167].

As a matter of interest, the same authors point out that comparable cardiovascular changes occur in the *normal* man, so that the overall haemodynamic effects of sublingual administration of nitroglycerin do not differ as between the healthy subject and the coronary anginal patient other than in the effect on coronary flow, the latter increasing in the case of the former whereas it does not alter in the second instance. LINHART et al. [1153] arrive at similar general conclusions as regards the anginal subject, since in their view the peripheral actions of nitroglycerin result in a reduction in left ventricle work and in its oxygen needs.

This impact on ventricular dynamics also explains why nitroglycerin increases myocardial oxido-reduction potential. Negative in the case of the coronary subject, this becomes positive [1475] and so indicates an improvement in myocardial oxygenation, itself probably due in part to the reduction in muscular

fibre tension and the speed at which these fibres are tightened. SOMANI [66] takes
the view that the reduction in oxygen requirements could be independent of the
general haemodynamic changes and be due to an oxygen-saving effect at cell
level, since he observes the phenomenon on a specimen heart subjected to constant work and also on a dog's heart homogenate.

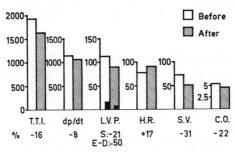

Fig. 5. General haemodynamic effects of nitroglycerin (0.8 mg by sublingual administration)
in patients with coronary heart disease. Open columns: before nitroglycerin. Hatched columns:
5 min after nitroglycerin. TTI: Tension-Time Index (mm Hg sec/min). dp/dt: rate of rise in
left ventricular pressure (mm Hg/sec). L.V.P.: left ventricular pressure (mm Hg), S: systolic
pressure, E-D: end-diastolic pressure (black columns). H.R.: heart rate (beats/min). S.V.:
stroke volume (ml). C.O.: cardiac output (1/min). (BING et al. [167])

The possibility of an MAOI effect has also been mooted [1475] to explain the
improvement in myocardial oxygenation due to nitroglycerin. In point of fact,
OGAWA et al. [1386] have recently demonstrated that nitroglycerin inhibits the
mono-amine oxydase of the mitochondriae of the heart of a rat both in vitro and
in vivo. In a later paper [1385], they confirm this effect on the same substrate,
showing at the same time that the same applies to three other organic nitrates,
erythrytol tetranitrate, mannitol hexanitrate and isosorbide dinitrate (Tables 4
and 5).

Table 4

Nitro derivatives	Molar concentration (mM)	MAO inhibition as a percentage
Nitroglycerin	0.66	26.1
Erythrol tetranitrate . . .	2.48	35.2
Mannitol hexanitrate . . .	3.58	23.5
Isosorbide dinitrate	50.	21.1

and, at a concentration of $5.4 \cdot 10^{-4} M$:

Table 5

Nitro derivatives	MAO inhibition as a percentage
Nitroglycerin	49.4
Mannitol hexanitrate	39.7
Erythrol tetranitrate	32.1
Pentaerythritol tetranitrate	15.

Measuring the level of the inhibition phenomenon at different concentrations,
they find that for these nitro derivatives there is a close relationship between
MAO inhibition and the dose usually administered under clinical conditions in the

treatment of angina pectoris. They do not draw the conclusion that the MAOI effect is responsible for the anti-anginal effect, but they do emphasise that the close relationship between the MAOI effect and the therapeutic effect could be more than a coincidence and that this study deserves to be gone into further. We should point out in this connection that the biochemical effects of nitroglycerin are still not properly known. It inhibits ATPase activity in rats [1027], which would explain its vaso-dilator action, and at very high doses it is an uncoupling agent of oxydative phosphorylations [873].

Haemodynamic Effects in the Case of the Angina Patient Suffering an Attack

Because angina-inducing exercise causes haemodynamic disturbances in the coronary subject which differ from those which appear in a healthy subject with an effort of equal intensity (see p. 24), haemodynamic investigations carried out on an angina subject suffering an attack, during the palliative effect of nitroglycerin administered by the sublingual route, stand out to a remarkable extent in that they enable certain mechanisms of the antianginal effect to be defined.

By means of the atrial pacing method [1798], FRICK et al. [592] show that nitroglycerin, administered to the angina subject in whom an attack has been induced by controlled artificial acceleration of his heart rate, reduces the aortic, right auricular, and arterial and venous pulmonary pressures, cardiac and systolic outputs (with compensatory tachycardia), the tension-time index and the end-diastolic cardiac volume. These facts indicate that nitroglycerin reduces the oxygen needs of the heart by two mechanisms: peripheral vaso-dilatation and reduction of the ventricular volume (and thus reduction in the ventricular wall tension according to LAPLACE's law), this latter mechanism being in line with what has been demonstrated by other techniques on humans [211, 2002].

In the case of a coronary subject who has suffered an infarction and who is free from effort-induced anginal pain [1418], nitroglycerin administered during an exercise decreases the left ventricular volume (as witness a drop in left ventricular end-diastolic pressure), and consequently, in the light of LAPLACE's law [1116], also reduces the tension of the left ventricular muscle and thereby its oxygen needs. Ventricular performance is therefore improved during the exercise (in the same way as with the coronary subject suffering from angina pectoris) and once more becomes comparable to what it is in the normal subject.

With the coronary subject suffering from effort-induced angina pectoris [1415], the same authors examine under particularly conclusive conditions (namely, exercise applied in the absence of nitroglycerin and after its administration) the effect of the drug on the cardiovascular disturbances caused by an angina-inducing exercise. They find that after taking nitroglycerin the majority of the patients are able to accomplish the same external physical effort *without displaying the haemodynamic disturbances* appearing in the absence of nitroglycerin, namely: rise in end-diastolic left ventricular pressure, pulmonary hypertension and *subnormal* rise in the cardiac index, all these symptoms bearing witness to the ventricular depression during the effort-induced anginal attack (see p. 30). Furthermore, after taking nitroglycerin, the exercise is accompanied by a significant increase in systolic volume and work, phenomena not found in the absence of the drug. These facts indicate that nitroglycerin increases myocardial performance during the angina-inducing exertion. The mechanism of this effect seems to the authors to be the reduction in heart oxygen needs as a result of a reduction in left ventricular volume.

The results of all these haemodynamic studies carried out on angina subjects make it possible to start discussing the probable mechanisms of the antianginal effect of nitroglycerin.

Mechanisms of the Antianginal Effect

The haemodynamic mechanism by which nitroglycerin exerts its beneficial effect on the coronary subject was very generally considered as being coronary vaso-dilatation before GORLIN and coll. [698], taking as a basis original patho-physiological observations on haemodynamics, suggested a concept which was the opposite of conventional notions. They had found that whereas nitroglycerin considerably increases the coronary flow in a healthy man [208, 903], this flow did not increase in the case of the angina subject; in fact it dropped by an average of 16% in 7 patients. This absence of rise in coronary flow in the angina subject was put down as the result of prior exhaustion of the dilation capacity of the coronary arterioles, a dilation which had progressively developed to offset the consequences of atherosclerotic vascular obstruction. The favourable subjective effect which the administration of nitroglycerin had on the patients could not therefore be explained by any generalised coronary vaso-dilatation. Since myo-cardial oxygen consumption increased as compared with the cardiac work accom-plished, the authors likewise rejected the possibility of an improvement in cardiac efficiency. They therefore advanced an old theory by suggesting that the remark-able clinical effect of nitroglycerin on an angina pectoris subject could be due to a decrease in the contractility of the heart. This concept, which was in direct opposi-tion to hitherto accepted theories, upset the generally accepted notion that the beneficial effect of a coronaro-dilator drug on the patient, whatever this drug might be, is due to an improvement in his coronary arterial flow. It was not backed up by subsequent tests by JOHNSON and SEVELIUS [903] who, in the case of patients suffering from coronary disease, found that the sublingual administra-tion of nitroglycerin at therapeutic dosages caused a marked increase in intra-myocardial blood flow. SKINNER et al. [1756] also thought that, as regards nitro-glycerin, the fact of lessening or suppressing the kinetocardiogram anomalies found in the angina subject provided indirect evidence of an increase in coronary flow.

GORLIN and his colleagues [699] felt that the lessening of cardiac contractility caused by nitroglycerin was a haemodynamic consequence of its peripheral vascular action. Since this effect had in fact been observed during experimentation on dogs by DARBY and ALDINGER [390], these latter also considered that it is secondary to a reduction in the load which must be borne by the heart. Thus they suggested that the mechanism of the favourable effect of nitroglycerin on the angina subject might be of a dual nature: the drug increased coronary flow whilst at the same time reducing the work imposed on the myocardium by the peri-pheral load. FERRERO and coll. [538] wanted to see proof of the lessening by nitroglycerin of the work of the left ventricle in a coronary subject in the fact that the U wave of the electrocardiogram dropped more often and to a more marked degree in the case of such a patient than for a healthy subject. The opinion as to the dual mechanism is not shared however by HONIG et al. [857]: experimental research on humans and animals having shown them that the amount of oxygen supplied to the myocardium increases under the influence of nitroglycerin, and that the work done by the heart does not decrease, these authors conclude that nitroglycerin combats ischaemia in the coronary subject merely by the mechanism of vaso-dilatation.

The mechanisms of the therapeutic effect of nitroglycerin are not easy to elucidate, particularly in view of the fact that under clearly defined experimental conditions, on a normal man for instance, changes in coronary arterial flow caused by nitroglycerin reported in published works vary according to the measuring method used: some find that flow increases [165, 208, 339, 1192, 27a] whilst others find that it drops slightly [146, 851, 1562]; when measured by a given method, further authors [1007] find that it increases for half the patients and decreases for the other half. Furthermore, the effect of nitroglycerin varies according to the method of administration and the experimental pattern. This fact emerges very clearly from the study made by BERNSTEIN into the haemodynamic effects of nitroglycerin on three groups of subjects: normal animals, healthy humans and patients suffering from coronary atherosclerosis [146].

When injected into the *coronary artery* via a catheter, nitroglycerin considerably increases coronary flow in all three groups. Even 30 sec after injection, the blood flow increases by 59% in the case of dogs, 64% in the case of the normal human and 38.5% in the case of the sufferer from coronary insufficiency. One of the interesting features is the demonstration of the fact that the impaired coronary system of the angina subject is capable of dilating under the effect of nitroglycerin.

The most attractive portion of BERNSTEIN's work is that in which he studied the haemodynamic changes brought about in man by *sublingual* administration of nitroglycerin. In both groups (normal and anginal), the work of the ventricle, myocardial oxygen consumption, blood pressure and coronary flow show a marked decrease and in a comparable manner from one group to the other.

LUEBS et al. [1192], however, find the coronary flow increases in the healthy subject and decreases in the angina patient, whereas BING [167] finds also that it increases in the normal subject but does not alter in the anginal patient. Despite these differences as to coronary flow behaviour (it should still be noted that all these authors are unanimous in accepting that this flow does not increase in the case of the angina subject), BERNSTEIN's research thus confirms in the coronary patient the phenomena which had been partly reported back in 1960 by GORLIN [698], namely that nitroglycerin has general haemodynamic effects which may well explain, at least in part, its antianginal effect: the work of the heart is considerably reduced, as a result of the combined action of a reduction in blood pressure and a lowering of cardiac output, the latter phenomenon having been confirmed by CHRISTENSSON [328]. Taking all these observations as a basis, BERNSTEIN suggests that the beneficial effect of nitroglycerin in angina pectoris seems to follow two phases: during the first, it is the coronaro-dilator effect which comes into play, being immediately replaced by the systemic effect leading to a reduction in the work done by the heart. It is this reduction in work, leading to a decrease in oxygen requirements, which constitutes the vital factor in the view of FRICK [592, 1415], BING [167, 1543] and PARKER [1418], who base their opinion on the phenomena which they see take place during sublingual resorption of nitroglycerin in the case of the angina victim suffering an attack (see p. 128).

Although additional information is still required before all the mechanisms which contribute to the therapeutic effect of nitroglycerin for the angina pectoris subject are known, the predominating mechanism of its antianginal effect does indeed seem to be the reduction in myocardial work and its oxygen requirements following lightening of the peripheral vascular loads by arterial and venous vasodilatation [716]. The part played by the vein network is far from being negligible, since nitroglycerin increases venous compliance in man and thereby causes peripheral venous stasis [86a], the latter bringing about a drop in end-diastolic ventricular pressure and forming the basis of the reduction in cardiac loading [20a, 87a]. LINHART et al. [82a] stress the fact that following the administration of nitroglycerin to an angina patient suffering an attack (in this case triggered off by atrial pacing), the cardiac pain only recedes after the appearance of the drop in heart work load and in the end-diastolic ventricular pressure, which does in fact prove that it is these haemodynamic changes which condition the therapeutic effect.

These haemodynamic effects probably play the vital role in increasing the oxydo-reducing potential of the myocardial cell observed by ROBIN in the angina subject [1543] and which testifies to an improvement in myocardial oxygenation (see p. 126).

Thus after having tried for a century to demonstrate on animals and on healthy and coronary human subjects that nitroglycerin improves the irrigation of the cardiac muscle, and having taken it as probable that it owes its antianginal effect to this action on myocardial vascularisation, we find ourselves back, on the basis of the concordant results of numerous haemodynamic studies carried out on the anginal subject, with the concept advanced in 1867 by BRUNTON [250], and afterwards discarded, that the sedation of anginal pain ensured by nitroglycerin is due to a reduction in cardiac work which finds its basic justification in a decrease in peripheral vascular resistance.

A slightly different opinion is detected in certain authors [51] who, working on the angina subject required to undergo angina-inducing exercise on the ergometric bicycle, report that nitroglycerin administered during the attack caused a highly significant drop in the systemic blood pressure, the pulmonary blood pressure and the pulmonary venous capillary pressure, *without altering cardiac output and work*. They therefore consider that nitroglycerin neutralises the pain without reducing cardiac work. They think in terms of a reduction in heart oxygen requirements through a lessening in ventricular volume, itself due to peripheral dilatation which lowers the blood return flow and the pressure of ventricular filling.

The same view is held by PARKER et al. [242c] whose recent findings deserve particular consideration by reason of the fact that, at the present time, it is not yet clear whether nitroglycerin acts by increasing myocardial oxygen supply or by reducing myocardial oxygen requirements through haemodynamic alterations or by affecting metabolic processes in a manner yet unknown.

One of the actions of nitroglycerin appears to be the reduction in left ventricular volume, probably by venous pooling. Support for this is present in the observation that left ventricular filling pressure decreases sharply after nitroglycerin [208, 1415, 1335], and in left ventricular volume measurements made in man following nitroglycerin [211, 2002]. A reduced myocardial oxygen consumption associated with the decreased left ventricular volume would contribute to the beneficial action of the drug.

In view of the complex interaction of the effects of nitroglycerin, an effort was made by PARKER et al. [242c] to simulate the peripheral pooling action of nitroglycerin unassociated with any effects on the coronary vasculature. This was accomplished by observing the effects of phlebotomy during angina produced by right atrial pacing. Anginal pain was precipitated by this technic in 15 patients with coronary artery disease. This was accompanied by haemodynamic evidence of impaired left ventricular function (see p. 30). In a first group of eight patients, while pacing was continued, a phlebotomy averaging 276 ml was carried out and in all but one patient angina was relieved and ventricular function returned to normal. Phlebotomy was accompanied by a decline in cardiac index (9.6%) and left ventricular filling pressure, but no change in brachial artery mean pressure, tension-time index, or dp/dt. With reinfusion of blood, angina returned in all but one patient and there was a rise in left ventricular end-diastolic pressure but no change in cardiac index, brachial artery pressure, tension-time index, or dp/dt. In the second group of seven patients, alterations of blood volume were carried out by a larger venesection between three 9-min periods of atrial pacing and similar observations were obtained.

When discussing the results of their study, PARKER et al. begin with a reminder that a reduction in myocardial oxygen consumption as an important action of nitroglycerin has frequently been considered, but they stress the fact that the multiple and interrelated circulatory effects of nitroglycerin make an analysis of its action difficult. Recent literature has emphasized that myocardial wall tension is the most definitive determinant of myocardial oxygen consumption [42 c, 270 c]. The magnitude and frequency of systolic pressure generation, commonly expressed as the tension-time index [1644] are closely correlated with the rate of myocardial oxygen consumption. However, oxygen consumption will also vary with ventricular volume [271 c]. Ventricular volume and pressure are related through ventricular wall tension, which is a linear function of the two factors [42 c]. Thus, calculated ventricular wall tension and myocardial oxygen consumption are directly affected by changes in ventricular volume [270 c], even though ventricular systolic pressure, tension-time index, and the velocity of contraction [1791] remain unaltered. The regular occurrence of a fall in left ventricular end-diastolic pressure after nitroglycerin, assuming no change has taken place in ventricular compliance, implies a decrease in left ventricular volume, and this has been demonstrated in man [211, 2002]. Wall tension will be reduced by this smaller ventricular volume and oxygen consumption thereby decreased.

The dramatic clinical relief afforded by phlebotomy in seven patients with angina, who were paced continuously in PARKER's study, was also accompanied by haemodynamic alterations indicative of improved ventricular function. During pacing, normal patients and patients with coronary disease who remain free from angina show a decline in left ventricular end-diastolic pressure in association with the accompanying decrease in stroke work [1416]. With cessation of pacing, there is a return of left ventricular end-diastolic pressure and stroke work to control levels. In contrast, the patients with angina provoked by pacing show no change in left ventricular end-diastolic pressure in the face of a similar decrease in stroke work and thus are operating on a depressed ventricular function curve (for details, see p. 31). The upper portion of this depressed ventricular function curve is described by the grossly abnormal relationship between stroke work and left ventricular end-diastolic pressure at a lower heart rate during interruption of pacing (see Fig. 2). The symptomatic improvement with bleeding is accompanied by a shift to the normal ventricular function curve during both pacing and interruption. After reinfusion there is a return to the depressed ventricular function curve both with pacing and interruption.

In examining the reasons for the improvement in symptoms and in ventricular function following bleeding, PARKER considers that there is no reason to suggest an increase in coronary blood flow since there was no change in perfusion pressure or heart rate. Of the factors known to affect myocardial oxygen requirements, all were constant except left ventricular volume. It seems probable that ventricular volume was decreased with consequent reduction in myocardial oxygen requirements resulting in the relief of angina.

Amelioration of angina by phlebotomy did not alter dp/dt, and this finding may represent the opposing effects of reduction in ventricular volume and relief of ischaemia on myocardial contractility [215 c]. During reinfusion there was recurrence of angina without a change in the factors affecting oxygen requirements other than the increase in left ventricular end-diastolic pressure and presumably in left ventricular volume.

In the second group where patients were studied in three consecutive pacing periods, the clinical improvement appeared related to both a reduction in ventricular volume and tension-time index. This latter effect, which was not seen in the continuously paced group, appears to be a consequence of the larger phlebotomy with a greater fall in cardiac index. However, it is notable that angina returned or increased in severity in five of the six patients with reinfusion, and this was not associated with a change in tension-time index and would suggest that the ventricular volume change is paramount.

In conclusion of this study, PARKER et al. state that their observations indicate that phlebotomy exerted its beneficial effect in atrial pacing-induced angina presumably through a reduction in left ventricular volume. Thus, angina can be relieved or prevented solely through a reduction in blood volume, left ventricular end-diastolic pressure, and left ventricular volume. They also suggest that this reduction in ventricular volume may be the major mechanism through which the beneficial effects of nitroglycerin are achieved.

Some interesting comments to PARKER's work can be found in a leading article which appeared in Brit. Med. J. [235 c]. PARKER and his colleagues found no changes in either the tension-time index or the rate of change of pressure in their patients, and they argued that this was further evidence that nitroglycerin acts chiefly by its effect on cardiac volume. Phlebotomy had no effect on the vasoregulatory mechanisms, and the total peripheral resistance increased as expected with a reduction of circulating volume. In a very similar study [592] in which cardiac function was measured in patients with angina treated with nitroglycerin, the effect of the drug was to lower the systemic pressure and also to reduce the size of the heart, both actions diminishing the demands of the myocardium for oxygen. How much either of these effects plays a part when the drug is used to treat patients is not, however, clear. In common with many workers [698, 146, 1192], PARKER [242 c] pointed out that nitroglycerin was unlikely to have any beneficial effect on the already maximally dilated coronary circulation in patients with angina. This argument ignores the part played by the myocardium in coronary resistance. The diastolic intramyocardial pressure is dependent on the left ventricular end-diastolic pressure. In normal circumstances this component of coronary resistance is nil, but as the end-diastolic pressure rises there is considerable obstruction to coronary flow [225]. The development of angina may, therefore, lead to a reduced coronary flow, and nitroglycerin, which returns left ventricular end-diastolic pressure to normal, could counteract this effect.

So the mechanism of action of nitroglycerin is complex, and several factors, all of which tend to improve the relationship between myocardial oxygen supply and demand, are concerned. It seems certain that a reduction in left ventricular volume plays an important part, but so do reductions in peripheral resistance and changes in the myocardial component of coronary resistance. Finally, a direct beneficial effect on the myocardium cannot be excluded (see further). PARKER's study adds to the fund of information about its mechanism of action, but the complete answer is still to come, and the dramatic action of nitroglycerin in angina has yet to be fully explained.

There is no doubt, however, that one of the main mechanisms of the beneficial effect of nitroglycerin in angina lies in a decrease in myocardial oxygen consumption. But beside this major mechanism, and despite the many clinical testimonies that nitroglycerin does not increase coronary flow in the anginal patient (see p. 125

and 130), the fact cannot be ignored that the antianginal effect could in part be due, at least with certain patients, to moderate and short-lived increase in myocardial irrigation, since this phenomenon has in fact been demonstrated in certain cases by CARSON [278] (see p. 125), and also quite recently by COWAN et al. [27a] who report a significant increase over the 45 and 90 seconds following sublingual intake of a therapeutic dose (see p. 126). This latter observation provides arguments for those who consider that if the antianginal effect must be attributed above all to a reduction in cardiac work, it may well be that the increase in coronary irrigation also plays a part *during the initial seconds of the effect*, to be taken over in turn by the general haemodynamic action. The same opinion is held by VYDEN et al. [330c] because an intravenous injection of nitroglycerin in the anaesthetised dog briefly increased coronary flow, then markedly decreased cardiac work.

Finally, other effects may play a part in the angina subject, but these have only be demonstrated in animals, and there is nothing at present to give reason to believe that they could play a part in the coronary subject. They are:

a) preferential dilatation of the myocardial conductance vessels, bringing an improvement in the irrigation of ischaemic zones [522] without the coronary flow as a whole necessarily increasing. It ought to be mentioned that SOMANI et al. [1781] take the view that this effect is doubtful (and deserves going into more thoroughly) since, following intracoronary injection of nitroglycerin, they observe no phenomenon giving reason to conclude in favour of dilatation of the capacitance vessels on an isolated heart preparation from a dog which was supplied by a donor and whose myocardial circulation was perfused at a constant rate of flow;

b) a favourable action on the collateral vicariance circulation, since FAM [523] has shown that nitroglycerin increases collateral blood flow in a dog with chronic experimental coronary deficiency without thereby increasing the total coronary flow;

c) a redistribution of myocardial blood flow in favour of the functional capillaries, which also ensures improved irrigation of ischaemic zones [1571, 2007, 2011, 2013]. Details on this point have already been given (see p. 124). Doubt is once more cast on this effect by SOMANI et al. [1781] because, in the case of their special preparation (see above), they found no change in Rb^{86} clearance following the intracoronary injection of nitroglycerin;

d) an inhibiting effect on the central adrenergic mechanisms, since, according to KAVERINA [964], nitroglycerin reduces the noradrenaline content of the hypothalamus, bulb and upper medulla of a cat, and depresses the tonic activity of the sympathetic nerves and the intensity of pressor vasomotor reflexes, these actions being ascribed to changes in adrenergic processes in the central nervous system and effected through an increase in the content of functionally active forms of monoamines liberated from the labile reserves in granules [171c];

e) BECKER et al. [9a and 251c] produced ischaemia by ameroid constriction of the left circumflex coronary artery in conscious dogs. Three to eight weeks later, radioactive microspheres were injected into the left ventricle before and after 0.4 mg i.v. nitroglycerin. The hearts were removed and the ventricle cut into endocardial and epicardial halves. Results were expressed as the ratio of counts/g of endocardial to epicardial part. Compared to controls, the ischaemic dogs had reduced endocardial/epicardial ratio. The ratio increased 5 minutes after nitroglycerin. It is suggested by the investigators that chronic myocardial ischaemia results in endocardial underperfusion, which is relieved by nitroglycerin. In their opinion, this effect on regional myocardial blood flow may be important clinically.

f) Two hypotheses which have been advanced and which are still under investigation deserve mentioning: firstly, NEEDLEMAN [1353] suggests that the nitro-derivatives exert their therapeutic effect by reacting with the SH groups in the cardiac mitochondria, leading to the uncoupling of the phosphorylations; secondly, OGAWA [1386] puts forward the hypothesis that inhibition of mono-amine-oxydase could occur under the effect of nitroglycerin, which might explain, for instance, the reduction in the levels of vanillo-mandelic acid in the urine observed in man following the administration of nitroglycerin [273].

Therapeutic Effect of Nitroglycerin[3]

So far as the therapeutic value of nitroglycerin in angina pectoris is concerned, it would probably be impossible to find a single clinical work in the literature which is not in favour of its effectiveness. Nitroglycerin is probably at the moment the only antianginal substance to collect unanimously favourable reports from therapeutic trials.

For RUSSEK and his co-workers [1614] nitroglycerin is the classical anti-anginal drug, reliable, capable in an average dose of 0.4 mg by sublingual absorption of cutting short the attack of pain and also of preventing, in almost all cases, development of the pathognomonic ischaemic electrocardiographic changes that follow the performance of a standard exercise by the patient with an anginal syndrome of coronary origin. This activity, however, only lasts for 15—30 min. Taken by the oral route, nitroglycerin, even in a massive dose, has much less action, and then only after a latent period exceeding 30 min [1591, 1614, 1616, 1619].

Although considered the drug of choice for arrest of the anginal attack and for the prevention of an attack in the case of foreseeable exertion, provided it is absorbed just before the effort [1616, 1619], imperiously recommended for preventing the foreseeable attack and for relieving the cardiac pain [258], and although it is regarded by some [1410] as the only drug required by a number of angina pectoris patients, nitroglycerin does not afford prolonged protection to the patient because of the evanescent nature of its effect; it cannot therefore be regarded as a fundamental therapy.

According to FISCH [548] however, the effectiveness of nitroglycerin in the treatment of an established attack of angina of effort must be considered to be unproved because approximately 75% of all attacks of angina of *effort* end within two minutes of cessation of activity and that most patients overestimate the duration of the attack. In the course of his experimental work on angina, FISCH has been able to treat successfully several hundred episodes with sublingual lactose placebo. It can, in fact, be conceded that in some patients, the anginal pain of effort ceases so quickly when physical activity is stopped that it is doubtful that the use of nitroglycerin offers any advantage [451].

RISEMAN [584, 1531] likewise considers nitroglycerin to be the most active, particularly by the sublingual route, of all the nitrites; sublingual administration is the method which gives the highest percentage of patients reporting great beneficial subjective effect and the greatest tolerance of the patients for a standard exercise. This effect is brief. Investigating the influence of mode of administration on the effectiveness of nitroglycerin in proved coronary patients, RISEMAN and his co-workers [1531] concluded that there was comparable activity by the sublingual and subcutaneous routes (the latter is of little clinical importance),

---

3 A brief review concerning the clinical use of the nitrites in angina pectoris has been recently published [132a].

that the oral route was not very effective unless the dose was increased greatly, and that the percutaneous route was readily effective[4].

Nitroglycerin increases by 50% the time required for development of the pain induced by the anoxaemia test and it also reduces the intensity of the electrical signs typical of myocardial hypoxia [1128].

Nitroglycerin significantly increases the tolerance to effort in anginal patients [5, 1244]. Cardiac pain and ECG ischaemic signs appearing during effort are definitely delayed. PETZEL and MOLL [1435] reported a beneficial effect on both the pain and the ECG ischaemic signs consequent on exercise on the ergometric bicycle.

In order to find out to what extent the reduction of myocardial oxygen consumption induced by nitroglycerin could be offset by a decrease in myocardial irrigation due to the fall in general blood pressure, KLENSCH and JUZNIC [995] have shown on a group of 15 anginal patients that, in all cases, the saving in oxygen (evidenced by physical methods, [994]) distinctly outweighed the allegedly reduced supply.

Nitroglycerin can, however, be ineffective in angina and can even produce paradoxical reactions [514, 1232] — the development of an anginal attack [423] and electrocardiographic tracings characteristic of myocardial ischaemia, comparable with those engendered by exertion [1617]. Reasoning from data collected in animal experiments and from certain clinical features observed in 16 of their patients in whom nitroglycerin, in the usual or a larger dose, had a paradoxical effect, RUSSEK et al. [1617] take the view that, in these cases, the general effect of the drug overshadows the coronary vasodilator effect; the powerful vasodilator action of the drug at the level of the capillaries and venules [1972, 2000] causes a fall in the tone of the venous reservoir, diminishes the amount of venous blood returning to the right heart, reduces cardiac filling and, consequently the cardiac volume and the systolic output [211]; tachycardia and systemic hypotension are added. Little in evidence with the usual doses and in the great majority of subjects, in whom they are rapidly compensated by reflex mechanisms, these phenomena, which culminate in a reduction of coronary flow, are not sufficient in most instances to outweigh the powerful coronary vasodilator effect of nitroglycerin. Conversely, in particularly sensitive subjects or with relatively large doses, these general effects are more pronounced and the reduction in coronary flow which they engender overshadows the normal consequences of the coronary vasodilator action. These interrelations end in reduction of myocardial irrigation in subjects suffering from coronary insufficiency; hence there may be development of anginal pain, possibly accompanied by electrocardiographic signs of hypoxia, signs which are due neither to rotation of the heart as GOLDBERGER claimed [681] nor to increase of tone in the sympathetic nervous system as administration of the alkaloids of ergot do not prevent their development [1617].

In view of the possibility that nitroglycerin, even in the usual dosage, may produce opposite effects, one of the essentials in this treatment for patients with angina pectoris is the discovery of the optimal dose [1617] which varies greatly from patient to patient. The effect of nitroglycerin on the venous and general arterial systems, with all its consequences, forbids its use in acute myocardial

---

4 In the light of the results obtained by BOGAERT et al. [34c, 35c, 36c] from experimental studies in animals concerned with the effects of nitroglycerin on vascular smooth muscle and its metabolic fate in relation to its vascular effects, the ineffectiveness of nitroglycerin in the case of oral administration could mean that the increase in plasma levels is too slow to give a concentration gradient large enough to induce pharmacological effects.

infarct [1617], an opinion which is generally accepted. Nitroglycerin thus possesses a latent potential of unfavourable effects, and this is probably the reason for the development of acute infarct in patients who, to combat a severe attack of angina, have recourse without medical advice to excessive doses of nitroglycerin. RUSSEK's well-founded opinion is supported by various observations that over-dosage can be highly prejudicial; cases of collapse have been reported [1468, 1809] as well as instances of acute coronary occlusion which, by reason of their recent character, could undoubtedly be attributed to nitroglycerin [190].

Although the general view is that the efficacy of nitroglycerin diminishes with the age of the commercial preparation [1387], SAGALL et al. [1626] are of the opposite opinion as preparations more than 11 years old, provided they had not been stored in temperatures above normal, yielded results comparable with those of fresh preparations.

The reported lack of activity of nitroglycerin is due to inactivation by time, light, heat, air and moisture [258]. Therefore, it is recommended that nitroglycerin tablets should be purchased fresh and kept in a refrigerator in a tightly stoppered dark bottle or a plastic container [258], conditions which avoid deterioration [83].

Repeated use of nitroglycerin may give rise to some tolerance to its beneficial effects [451]. It has also been reported that the systemic haemodynamic actions of nitroglycerin in man are significantly reduced as early as after one week of daily treatment with Peritrate, which means that there is a crossed tolerance [1662].

Special Galenic Preparations

1. A special galenical preparation (nitroglycerin retard) has been introduced under the name Nitroglyn (Sustac, Nitropol), containing granules specially coated with nitroglycerin and capable theoretically of providing slow, continuous and uniform absorption after ingestion. Thus the theoretical possibility exists for the patient of being under the effect of nitroglycerin for several hours. The peripheral vasodilator effect of Nitroglyn in man is estimated to be twenty times longer than that of nitroglycerin administered sublingually [1216].

Nitroglyn has been found to be extremely useful in the anginal subject and to remain active much longer than nitroglycerin or Peritrate by some investigators [869, 882, 1064, 220 c]; it is reckoned to reduce the nitroglycerin requirements of 60% of subjects [874]. According to RUSSEK [1619, 1620], however, contrary to the hope engendered by the logical idea responsible for its conception, Nitroglyn in the recommended dosage of 2.4 mg produces no change in the adverse effect seen in the electrocardiogram of coronary patients after Master's exercise; a dose of 9.6 mg yielded but slight improvement in the ECG of only 65% of the patients, and in no case was there a normal response to the exercise. The absorption of the nitroglycerin is obviously, therefore, too slow, even with large dosage, to give a satisfactory clinical response, as understood by RUSSEK.

RISEMAN et al. [1531], who assess the effectiveness of a substance by combining subjective and objective methods, also consider that Nitroglyn is less active than nitroglycerin, even in the massive dose of 20—30 mg.

According to recent clinical controlled trials, the therapeutic importance of this medication is very limited [1427, 1444].

2. According to SÜTTINGER (1852), Nitrolingual-spray, a stable oily solution of nitroglycerin which can be vaporized and which is resorbed through the tongue and the mouth mucosa, is more quickly active than the usual tablet form, a fact which, together with the ease of its use, is considered to represent an advantage compared to the usual tablet presentation.

3. Nitrospan which contains 2 mg of nitroglycerin in a gelatin capsule should provide a permanent liberation of active nitroglycerin. At a dose of 1 capsule twice daily for 14 days, Nitrospan was reported to have an important prophylactic effect in angina [1806].

4. Depot-nitroglycerin (Nitro Mack Retard) which contains 2.5 mg nitroglycerin per capsule has been reported after a 4—6 weeks treatment at 2 capsules daily to relief anginal pains completely in 60% [931] to 80% [1138] of treated cases, and to promote rehabilitation of patients who had a myocardial infarction [495]. Nitro Mack Retard induced tachyphylaxis and for this reason a rest interval of 3 days is recommended after a 4 weeks treatment [931]. In conscious dogs, Nitro Mack Retard given by oral route with the food at the daily dose of 2 capsules for 10 weeks increased significantly myocardial blood flow [41 c].

Depot-nitroglycerin has been associated with phenobarbital in the form of Seda Nitro Mack Retard. In 50 patients with diagnostically verified angina pectoris due to coronary heart disease which were treated with this preparation twice daily for 5 months, a satisfactory to very good response was shown by 43 patients. Thus, addition of a sedative to nitroglycerin was thought to improve therapeutic results [50 a].

5. Another form of depot-nitroglycerin, which is presented in sustained release tablets (Nitro-bid Plateau) containing 2.5 mg nitroglycerin prevented at a dose of two tablets daily the anginal attacks in 21 patients out of 24 [1546], an appreciation which is in accordance with the excellent results previously reported in a double-blind study in 70 anginal patients [1207]. Accordingly, the use of this special form is advocated preferably to Peritrate for the long term treatment of angina.

6. As nitroglycerin is absorbed through the skin [1948], a fact which is responsible for the headaches found in workers engaged in the manufacture of dynamite, a commercial ointment preparation (Nitrol) containing 2% nitroglycerin has been produced, being intended primarily for treatment of peripheral vascular disorders. This galenical preparation has had some successes in angina pectoris [393, 797, 1531]. Nitrol is said to be particularly useful in nocturnal angina. Required amount can be measured on disposable "Appliruber" and is than applied to precordial skin area. As there is a slow and steady absorption of nitroglycerin, prolonged action may entail some side effects, and individual need must be adjusted to avoid headache which indicates overdosage.

7. According to SANDLER [1640], nitroglycerin is ineffective in angina when given in aerosols (Cardamist).

8. Nitroglycerin has been combined with a cardiotonic-sedative association under the trade name of Steno-Valocordin. This preparation was said to be an excellent antianginal drug [1046].

2. Triethanolamine Trinitrate

Triethanolamine trinitrate biphosphate (see p. 119 for chemical structure) or trolnitrate phosphate (Metamine, Nitretamin, Ortin, Aminal, Prenitron, Angitrit) was synthetized in the hope of obtaining a nitrite compound which did not have the two undesirable properties of nitroglycerin, namely, the transience of its coronary vasodilator action and the intensity of its peripheral vasodilator effect.

Its coronary vasodilator properties are approximately equal to those of nitroglycerin at doses from 5 to 100 mcg/kg i.v., but they develop more slowly and are much more lasting [203, 686, 922, 1436]; the considerable increase in the coronary flow is not accompanied by appreciable changes in the systemic pressure, even with the largest dose [686]. These observations were amplified by MELVILLE and LU [1275]: (i) on the isolated rabbit heart, Metamine and nitroglycerin had equal coronary vasodilator activities at all the used doses (0.008—0.04—0.2 and 1 mg), but that of Metamine was more prolonged; nitroglycerin caused greater reduction in the amplitude and frequency of the cardiac contraction; (ii) on the heart-lung preparation of the dog the two substances reduced cardiac output in identical manner at doses of 25 and 50 mg; (iii) in the anaesthetized dog, Metamine at the dose of 0.12 mg/kg i.v. produced a much smaller fall in arterial pressure, even in doses ten times stronger i.e. 1.2 mg/kg; and (iv) Metamine prevents the coronaroconstriction provoked by pituitrine [1272].

According to SCRIABINE [1712], Metamine when injected i.v. at a dose of 0.08 mg/kg induces in the anaesthetized dog haemodynamic effects which are similar to those seen after nitroglycerin, viz: a reduction of cardiac output, heart work, blood pressure, heart oxygen needs, and coronary and total vascular resistances. Coronary blood flow was maintained. On a weight basis, the effect of Metamine is less important, less rapid but more prolonged. Thus, the peripheral vascular effects could be responsible for the therapeutic effect of the drug.

On the basis of comparable experimental findings, BUJANOV [268] reported that Metamine only slightly increased venous coronary blood flow in cats, the chief pharmacological effect being a reduction of the myocardial oxygen consumption, as a consequence of diminished cardiac work.

The agreement presented by pharmacological observations encouraged clinicians to try the effects of Metamine in angina pectoris. As usual, the first studies, conducted with neither placebo nor double-blind system were particularly favourable [290, 381, 648, 806, 1286, 1409, 1436, 1811]. FULLER and KASSEL [613], who adopted a severe system of recording for the clinical effects observed and employed comparison with a placebo but not the double-blind procedure, concluded that the drug was truly effective in the prevention of anginal pains, 82% of their patients reporting considerable improvement. The clinicians whose observations were satisfactorily controlled by use of a placebo and the double-blind technique found that the beneficial subjective effects produced by Metamine were moderate [594, 602, 1427, 1752], and for COLE et al. [349] they were not superior to those given by the placebo. This unfavourable opinion on the clinical effects of Metamine has been corroborated by experimenters who concerned themselves with objective elements of assessment. The drug produced only a moderate increase in exercise tolerance (and it was still necessary to administer it by the sublingual or intramuscular route, as it was inactive by mouth [1531]) and it had no effect on the ischaemic electrocardiographic changes produced by exertion in two-thirds of the patients and only a very slight effect in the other third [1619, 1620]. Use of the effective administration routes was restricted by troublesome reactions — glossitis in the case of the sublingual and pain in the case of the intramuscular route [1531].

Accordingly, the majority of cardiologists who have investigated the effect of Metamine in angina pectoris on scientific lines are of the opinion that this substance does not measure up reliably to the claims of its manufacturer and that the slight improvements that it introduces are not sufficient to justify its employment as a long-acting antianginal agent. For example, it was found barely equal to placebo by FISCH [549].

It has been incidentally reported that Metamine succeeded in relieving anginal pain in two patients which were non-tolerant for nitroglycerin [806].

3. Erythrityl Tetranitrate

Erythrityl or erythrol tetranitrate (Cardilate, Cardiloid, Tetranitrol, Tetranitrin) is absorbed slowly from the intestine, which partly explains the delay in and duration of its effect. Theoretically, this nitrite should be an ideal drug as it differs from nitroglycerin only in the presence of an additional $COH-NO_2$ group, which produces a molecule a third heavier — a fact which could prolong the effect and yet maintain its strength. According to KRANTZ et al. [1030], erythrol tetranitrate has an equal but more prolonged effect on the arterial pressure than nitroglycerin.

Sublingual administration of 10 mg of Cardilate induces in both healthy and anginous subjects a drop in coronary resistance, but coronary blood flow remains unchanged because systemic blood pressure diminishes appreciably [1575]. Such findings suggest that the antianginal effect of the drug is not due to an increase in myocardial irrigation but rather to a decrease in cardiac work, as a consequence of a reduction in total vascular resistance.

In clinical work, although it has a certain prophylactic value in various patients, Cardilate is much less effective than nitroglycerin, both in respect of the number of patients who benefit in subjective effect and also in respect of the degree to which tolerance for a standard exercise [584] or for the anoxaemia test [1128] is increased. As this difference might be due partly to the fact that the two substances compared were administered by different routes, sublingual in the case of nitroglycerin and oral for Cardilate, RISEMAN, ALTMAN and KORETSKY [23, 1531] re-examined the question, using the three routes, oral, sublingual and parenteral. By the sublingual route and given in a dose fifty times larger, Cardilate proved as active as nitroglycerin, both subjectively in relation to the acute attack, and objectively in relation to the degree of increase in exercise tolerance; its effect was of slower development but was definitely more prolonged. By the oral route, Cardilate was, like nitroglycerin, much less effective than by the sublingual route, a fact which confirmed the previous experience of the same authors [1532, 1533]. This nitrite is also active by the subcutaneous and percutaneous routes, but these are of no clinical importance.

The therapeutic value of Cardilate would appear, therefore, to be somewhat limited, although RUSSEK [1592] has expressed the opinion that this drug by the sublingual route is very effective in prolonged prophylactic treatment and that it prevented the electrocardiographic signs of ischaemia due to the Master test in 72% of patients [1588]. In a recent trial [74c], DAGENAIS et al. found that Cardilate at the daily dose of 10 mg significantly decreased the frequency and severity of the ischaemic S—T depression induced by standard exercise in angina patients, and increased exercise duration by 80%.

The main drawback of Cardilate is the occurrence of severe pulsatile headaches which were present in 40% of cases [1602].

4. Pentaerythritol Tetranitrate

Pentaerythritol tetranitrate (Peritrate, Pentanitrine, Pentafin, Pentritol, Quintrate, Vasodiatol, Myocardol) is the oldest long-acting nitrite and also one of the best known to the physician. Much more stable than nitroglycerin and Cardilate, Peritrate is absorbed slowly from the intestine [1948]. Although the drug increased the coronary arterial flow in the dog when administered sublingually [2021] — its effect is less and develops more slowly than that of nitroglycerin — into the vein or in the duodenum [62], it seems that this observation should be considered as unusual because in the hands of most workers either the blood flow changed little [2008] or it decreased moderately as a consequence of a fall in blood pressure [1853], which is however weaker than in the case of nitroglycerin [2021].

Whereas for some investigators [268, 1853], the reduction in heart work seems to be the dominant haemodynamic effect of Peritrate, WINBURY [2008] expresses the view that the main action of the drug lies in a redistribution of the blood flow at the level of the myocardial microcirculation via the functional vessels, thereby improving the oxygenation of the heart muscle. He demonstrated that Peritrate increases the nutritional circulation while reducing coronary vascular resistance [2011]. Such an effect could be ascribed, probably as a result of elective relaxation of the precapillary sphincters, to an increase in the number of open capillaries. This process of selective orientation of blood flow should explain that the *total* coronary blood flow does not necessarily rise [2017]. Consequently, it was proposed by WINBURY that Peritrate, as nitroglycerin, does have a direct action on the capillary coronary circulation, and little if any effect on the arterioles [2008].

In the pig with chronic experimental coronary insufficiency, the daily administration of Peritrate has been reported to increase significantly the percentage survival rate [1196].

It has been noted that in patients with coronary insufficiency, Peritrate 80 (see p. 142) has not modified the cardiac output, nor has it changed the stroke volume, or the heart rate, or the blood pressure [1891]. As the work of the heart and its oxygen needs are determined by the above haemodynamic parameters, the therapeutic effect of the drug cannot be claimed to be due to a decrease in cardiac work and resultant oxygen myocardial consumption.

Therapeutically, pentaerythritol tetranitrate was considered excellent in angina by all clinicians who used purely subjective methods of assessment without employment of the double-blind system [78, 380, 1431, 1460]. ROSENBERG and MICHELSON [1553] expressed a more guarded opinion, however, as only 25% of their patients reported significant improvement and fifty-five others declared themselves satisfied, although their assessment was not statistically acceptable. COLE et al. [349], DEWAR et al. [424] as well as ORAM and SOWTON [1395], who used the double-blind procedure, did not consider Peritrate superior to the placebo, whereas ROBERTS [1541], using the same procedure for assessment found it much more active than the placebo, and considered it an effective preventive agent in a dose of 30 mg morning and evening.

For the authors who favour objective methods, the results were hardly favourable [594, 932, 1020, 1629, 1872], although exercise tolerance was increased in a large percentage of cases [1563, 1973, 2020, 2021]. On the other hand, RUSSEK, who assesses the power of a substance to prevent development of the electrocardiographic signs of ischaemia induced by Master's two-step exercise, found Peritrate, in a dose of 10—20 mg, to have an effect comparable in almost all his patients with that of nitroglycerin, with the additional advantage of more prolonged action, possibly exceeding 5 hours [1616, 1619, 1620]; this effect was, however, only evident when the drug was taken on an empty stomach. This all referred to an "acute" effect, observed for a matter of hours after a single administration of the drug. RUSSEK does not report, for example, that Peritrate modified the frequency or severity of the attacks, as his experimental work did not deal with the effect of prolonged treatment. While he considered nitroglycerin to be the drug of choice for the acute attack, RUSSEK thought that Peritrate would be unequalled for sustained protection; this was also the opinion of WINSOR and HUMPHREYS [2020]. RUSSEK believes that Peritrate alone merits at the present moment to be called long-acting coronary vasodilator.

RISEMAN et al. [1531] consider that Peritrate is less active than nitroglycerin but, when allowance is made for the fact that he did not rely on the same criterion as RUSSEK, RISEMAN admits that his assessment is very close to that of RUSSEK; RISEMAN thought the oral and sublingual routes about the same, an opinion shared by WINSOR and SCOTT [2021]. The employment of Peritrate will obviously be limited by its frequent irritant effect on the intestine [490, 1387]. In the opinion of RUSSEK [1602] the fact that the therapeutic effect is slow in occurring constitutes a disadvantage.

Peritrate has recently been made up in a stronger form, Peritrate 80 or Peritrate S.A., containing 80 mg per unit and with a recommended dosage of 2 per day. According to AMMERMANN [26], this form causes anginal pains to disappear in 91% of cases treated.

Much has been said about the effect of Peritrate at strong doses (80 mg twice a day) on the immediate sequels to myocardial infarction considered from the complications and fatality angles. Two double-blind experiments arrive at opposite conclusions: whereas OSCHAROFF [1396] reports that mortality is significantly reduced from 22 to 4%, MELLEN et al. [1266] find no difference as compared with the group of patients given the placebo. PALMER [1408] and MELLEN [1266] explain this apparently beneficial effect of Peritrate by the fact that in the two groups of the OSCHAROFF experiment the percentage of cardiovascular complications present at the time the patients were admitted was far higher in the control group than in the group treated with Peritrate, so that the difference in mortality rate found in the two groups reflects a difference in human material and not an effect of the drug.

There should also be caution in considering the interpretation put on his results by SCHWARTZ [1701]. Taking two groups of 25 patients, one group treated with 80 mg twice daily, and the other with 30 mg twice daily, the author concludes that his findings unquestionably militate in favour of the low posology because, over a period of 1 year, he only had one death at this dose whereas 4 patients died and two others developed acute infarction at the high dosage. The clinical material and observation period are obviously too limited to draw such a forthright conclusion. NEWELL and collaborators [231c] describe a multicentre trial of Peritrate (sustained action) given in a dose of 80 mg b.i.d. to 346 patients in the three months after they had suffered an acute myocardial infarction. The trial was double-blind, 181 patients being given Peritrate and 165 control patients receiving placebo. Treated and control patients were standardised for age and sex, blood pressure, heart rate, incidence of shock, number of infarctions, history of angina and diabetes, and for the different types of sedatives or anticoagulants that they were receiving. The overall mortality rates at 6 months were almost identical in both groups at 23%, but, within the treated group, the mortality was reduced in men under 50 years and increased in women over 70 years.

Peritrate has been made up in a special galenic form designed to prolong its therapeutic effect: Duotrate or Pentritol-tempules. This consists of a capsule containing a great many tiny granules coated with a semi-permeable plastic membrane, with a total of 45 mg of the active substance per capsule, and which disintegrate over a period of from 8 to 10 hours, thus providing, according to PLOTZ [1459], a better antianginal effect than that obtained with the Peritrate *tablets*. In his report on a double-blind experiment, SAPIENZA [1643] also concludes in favour of the undoubted superiority of this galenic form at a daily dose of 90 mg as compared with Peritrate tablets at a dosage of 80 mg per day, whose therapeutic effect is no greater than that of the placebo.

Another delayed action form, Tetrasule Timesule, has been investigated double-blind [347]; it reduces nitroglycerin needs and increases tolerance to exercise in 65% of patients examined.

Peritrate has been associated with other medicaments: nitroglycerin in a, preparation for sublingual administration, hydrochlorothiazide (Perithiazide) meprobamate (Equanitrate, Miltrate) and hydroxyzine (Cartrax).

Dilcoran (an association of 40 mg Peritrate and 20 mg phenobarbitone) ensures 78% favourable results, and Dilcoran 80 (80 mg Peritrate + 20 mg phenobarbitone) is very effective in over 90% of cases treated [1413].

Pentrium, which brings together Peritrate and Librium, has been the subject of clinical investigation covering 372 angina subjects treated for 3 years with very good results and without side effects [1718]. Peripheral arterial resistances are reduced.

Although Peritrate has had tremendous success, particularly in the United States, its efficacy is now increasingly questioned. According to FISCH [549], no clinical research provides any proof of a genuine beneficial effect from Peritrate, and its widespread medical use would seem to be due to the fact that the practitioner must prescribe something rather than to abstain from so doing, and also because the anginal syndrome is essentially elusive and sensitive to the effect of placebotherapy. With this in mind, we should point out that in the view of other authors [5], Peritrate does not increase the tolerance of the angina sufferer to effort, whereas it is increased significantly in the same patients following the administration of nitroglycerin. Similarly, DAGENAIS et al. recently found that at the daily doses of 20 or 40 mg in chronic administration, Peritrate did not decrease the frequency and severity of the ischaemic S—T depression induced by standardised exercise, and did not increase significantly the duration of effort [74c].

It is not without interest to note that long-term treatment with Peritrate significantly lessens the circulatory effects of nitroglycerin, which discloses the existence of a cross-tolerance [1662], and explains the diminished therapeutic effect of nitroglycerin.

5. Mannitol Hexanitrate

This nitrated derivative (see formula p. 119) which is known under the name of Nitranitol or Maxitate is absorbed slowly through the intestinal mucosa and its effect is consequently slow and prolonged. Used in a dosage 200 times as great as that of nitroglycerin, i.e. 65 mg (3 times daily) instead of 0.3 mg, mannitol hexanitrate is very effective by the sublingual route in angina pectoris, in respect of both the frequency of the attacks and the exercise tolerance. It ranks very close to nitroglycerin and Cardilate in its effectiveness by the sublingual route. Its action is less by the oral route [1531].

6. Amyl Nitrite

Introduced independently by RICHARDSON and by BRUNTON about 1860, at the same time as nitroglycerin, for the treatment of the attack of angina pectoris, amyl nitrite gave BRUNTON [250] the opportunity to describe the first positive antianginal effect in a coronary patient. A highly volatile liquid with coronary vasodilator properties [578], amyl nitrite, 3—5 minims over a period of 5 min, increased coronary flow in the anaesthetized dog but reduced it in the anaesthetized rabbit, although coronary vascular resistance decreased in both species [713].

Furthermore, a decrease in myocardial metabolic heat production has been noted, suggesting an increase in the efficiency of metabolic energy. GRAYSON et al.

think that such an effect might partially explain the therapeutic action of nitrites in angina [713]. The drop in arteriolar resistance provoked by amyl nitrite inhaled for 10 seconds has been decisively demonstrated by KOT et al. [1022], proving that there is relaxation of the smooth muscle in the resistance as well as in the capacitance vessels.

In normal man, amyl nitrite increased heart rate and cardiac output [642]. These phenomena lasted only 2 min and were not suppressed by β-blocking drugs.

MASON and BRAUNWALD [86a] have studied the effects of sublingual nitro-glycerin and inhaled amyl nitrite on the arteriolar and venous beds of the forearm in normal subjects. Both drugs reduced systemic arterial pressure, elevated fore-arm blood flow and decreased forearm vascular resistance. But, in contrast to nitroglycerin which decreased venous tone, amyl nitrite augmented venous tone strikingly. MASON and BRAUNWALD concluded that since amyl nitrite and nitro-glycerin have directionally opposite effects on the venous bed, the efficacy of both of these drugs in angina can obviously not be explained by their effects on veins alone. Inhaled amyl nitrite results in a marked and sudden arteriolar dilatation, and it is probable that the coronary vessels participate in this response. As a consequence, systemic pressure declines markedly, thus also reducing myocardial oxygen requirements. It seems likely that the beneficial clinical effects of amyl nitrite in angina result from a combination of these two actions.

Easily absorbed by the transpulmonary route, amyl nitrite is administered by inhalation from ampoules which the patient crushes in a handkerchief when it is to be used (Vaporol). It is therefore the most rapid of all the nitrites, acting within 30 sec. Its use is becoming increasingly unpopular because of the frequency of its disagreeable effects (marked facial congestion, pulsating intracranial sensations, nauseating tendencies sometimes causing vomiting), and also because of its unple-asant odour and its high price. Dosage is very difficult to control so that its admini-stration involves more risks than in the case of nitroglycerin. Its use should be restricted to hospital [1307, p. 365]. Amyl nitrite remains the form for extremely urgent states, particularly spontaneous anginal attacks of long duration, in which its effect may be spectacular. According to CONTRO et al. [356], it should be admini-stered with great caution in the individual with coronary arteriosclerosis as, in 50% of the cases examined in this connexion, the electrocardiogram revealed clear signs of coronary insufficiency, evidence of a myocardial ischaemia due mainly in all probability to a fall of arterial pressure, which deprived the coronary circulation of blood, and also to a slight increase in the work of the heart resulting from the tachycardia that developed.

A special galenic preparation of amyl nitrite in the form of a small pocket aeroliser, which is known under the name of Frenodosa, should permit a correct control of the dose; it should also avoid the unpleasant smell and should be very quickly active [1265].

7. Octyl Nitrite

This liquid, which can be administered by the respiratory route because of its high volatility, is presented in the form of an inhalant for clinical use. The inhala-tion of 0.3 ml of octyl nitrite induces an immediate arterial hypotension in the animal, the intensity of which is comparable to that produced by the same quantity of amyl nitrite, but its duration is six times longer [1028]. There is also a fall of pressure in normal man, with tachycardia, the maximum of which occurs 2 min after the strong dose of 0.2 ml inhaled in 1 min [1028]. The coronary flow of the perfused isolated rabbit heart and the coronary sinus flow of the dog heart *in situ* increase just as much as in the case of amyl nitrite, despite the intense peripheral vasodilatation. Unlike amyl nitrite, octyl nitrite has but little tendency to cause methaemoglobinaemia; its acute toxicity is less than a fourth of that of amyl nitrite.

Although such pharmacological results lead their authors to recommend octyl nitrite in the treatment of the acute anginal attack, only one experimental clinical investigation on the treatment of anginal patients with this nitrite seems to have been undertaken [585]: given when an attack was in progress, it cut down the duration of the usual attacks very considerably, definitely increased the tolerance for an anginogenic exercise and counteracted development of the electrocardiographic signs of effort ischaemia. The favourable effects did not appear to increase with increase of the dose inhaled but the unpleasant reactions were intensified. The optimum dose would appear to be one single deep inspiration.

Although its beneficial effects are hardly inferior to those of nitroglycerin or amyl nitrite, although its absorption, and consequently its activity, is much more rapid than that of nitroglycerin, octyl nitrite does not appear to have won general sanction, probably because its price is much higher than that of nitroglycerin (although less than that of amyl nitrite) and also because, by reason of the ease of its employment and the impossibility of getting an accurately adjusted dose, patients are more liable to troublesome, serious or even dangerous reactions inseparable from the powerful effect of nitrites.

8. Sodium Nitrite

Sodium nitrite (Erinitrit) appears to be absorbed better in the intestine than nitroglycerin; it acts in the same manner on the cardiovascular system but much higher dosage is required, doses of 3—30 mg in intracoronary injection and of 30—100 mg in intravenous administration being needed to enhance coronary blood flow in the anaesthetized dog [205].

On the heart-lung preparation of the dog, sodium nitrite increases the coronary flow in doses of 0.05—0.15 g, while the arterial pressure and cardiac output remain unchanged [193]. This substance can thus reduce coronary resistance by relaxation of vascular tone but, as the heart increases in volume, the change in the extracoronary myocardial support contributes to the fall of the vascular resistance.

The proof of direct coronary vasodilator action was supplied by, among others, KATZ [957, 958] who showed that the coronary flow increased in the heart brought to a state of ventricular fibrillation, and by FROHLICH and SCOTT on the dog heart in situ [606], for a dose of 8.7 mg, the same effect being attained in the case of nitroglycerin with a dose which was 70 times smaller. We have been able to establish an identical finding with the fibrillating isolated rabbit heart for a concentration which was 50—70 times higher than in the case of nitroglycerin, and this implies a reduction in the tone of the smooth muscle fibre of the coronary vessels [301].

SMITH [1759] has shown that in the anaesthetized dog sodium nitrite at the dose of 60 mg i.v. increases the blood flow measured in a distal branch of the left coronary artery after ligature of a neighbouring branch, which signifies dilatation of collateral vessels joining the two branches, but WIGGERS and GREEN [1996] think that this improvement in collateral circulation is not large enough to be functionally useful.

The lack of consistency between the powerful effects exercised by sodium nitrite in the animal following parenteral administration (when it stimulates development of the functional inter-coronary anastomoses occurring after incomplete occlusion of a coronary artery [2052]) and its low efficiency when given by the oral route in patients [1532] has led RISEMAN and his co-workers [1531] to re-examine its therapeutic value in the coronary subject when the dosage was increased and it was administered parenterally. Sodium nitrite in a dose of 300 mg (five times the usual clinical dose) is effective, although much less so than nitro-glycerin; it is as active by the oral as by the sublingual route, but acts better when given intramuscularly.

Undesirable reactions, particularly the hypotensive effects, are much more frequent than with other nitrites and must obviously limit its therapeutic employment. Sodium nitrite is no longer used in the treatment of angina pectoris.

9. Isosorbide Dinitrate

Suggested to clinicians for the long-term treatment of angina, Isordil or Carvasine or Sorbitrate (see formula p. 119) is isosorbide dinitrate or 1,4,3,6-dianhydro-sorbitol-2,5-dinitrate. It was investigated under experimental conditions by KRANTZ et al. [1029] who showed that the presence of the ether linkage in the nitrate sugar alcohols lessens the potency whilst increasing the duration of the vascular depressive effect[5].

Isordil increases the coronary blood flow and reduces the general blood pressure [679], whether it be administered intravenously or intraduodenally to anaesthetised dogs at doses ranging from 0.125 to 0.5 mg/kg [9, 251]; its depressive effect on coronary vascular resistance would appear to be greater than that of Peritrate [9, 251]. According to BUYANOV [268], Isordil only slightly increases coronary venous flow in cats, and in particular causes a reduction in myocardial oxygen requirements by lessening the work of the heart.

In closed-chest dogs, an intravenous infusion of Isordil over a period of one hour (0.013 mg/kg/min) resulted in significant falls in mean aortic and left ventricular end-diastolic pressures. Heart rate and systemic vascular resistances showed no significant change, nor did coronary blood flow and coronary arterio-venous oxygen difference. Myocardial oxygen consumption and left ventricular work fell, but cardiac efficiency did not change. Effects persisted for one hour post-infusion. It was concluded that sustained mild systemic hypotension caused by Isordil can reduce workload and oxygen requirements of the heart without adversely affecting the delivery of blood to the myocardium [131a].

Isordil quantity determinations effected in the blood of subjects to whom it is administered show that it is found in the lipid phase of the serum and does not change into a nitrite [68]; it appears to act as a whole molecule, a fact which seems to single it out from the nitro-compounds currently used in clinical treatment. Isordil is completely metabolised by the body [429] but its urinary mononitrates constitute only 1% of the quantity ingested, and it is probable that the major metabolite is completely denitrified.

Isordil does seem to be one of the most effective nitrated substances for the treatment of coronary insufficiency. This impression emerges from the following clinical investigations whose results show an amazing degree of agreement. Those carried out by SHERBER and GELB [1739, 1740] who, with 120 angina patients (108 of whom were unaffected by Peritrate), observe excellent effects in 75% of the cases and satisfactory effects in 20% at a daily oral dose of 4×10 mg; a survey by FISCH et al. [552] and a report by SHAPIRO [1734] who both conclude likewise in favour of the efficacy of the drug in over 75% of cases; an investigation by RUSSEK [1602] who confirms the excellent effect of the medication on the

---

5 Isomannide dinitrate, which has been found more potent than isosorbide dinitrate [1030] did not lend itself to medication.

frequency of attacks, while at the same time showing its favourable incidence on the ischaemia patterns of the Master effort test; the experiments of BAEDER [68] whose results can be superimposed on those of RUSSEK; the three clinical explorations by ALBERT [18], LESLIE [1109] and JOSEPH and MANCINI [910] whose results appear to have been excellent in 75% of cases and non-existent in only 5%: the benefits provided by the medication are reflected both in a very considerable subjective improvement, a lessening of needs for nitroglycerin, an increase in tolerance to exercise and certain favourable changes in electrocardiographic patterns. When used double-blind, Isordil has proved very much better than the placebo [147].

In an evaluation of the efficacy of nitrates in patients with angina, the effects of sublingual Isordil on capacity for upright bicycle exercise, blood pressure, heart rate and ejection time were determined in 23 subjects [54a, 55a and 118c]. The degree of clinical improvement following Isordil can be adequately explained by circulatory changes causing decreased myocardial oxygen demand. Tachyphylaxis does not develop at usual therapeutic doses (5—10 mg qid) and improvement after Isordil does not last appreciably longer than that following nitroglycerin.

The effect of a single oral dose (5—30 mg) appears within half an hour and lasts for over four hours [1602, 1740].

Isordil is similarly active in sublingual administration, proving as rapidly effective as nitroglycerin by this route but for a much longer time than with the latter [1740]. It is as effective as regards rapidity, intensity and duration as Cardilate [1602]. Because of these therapeutic characteristics, Isordil is considered by RUSSEK [1602] to be the only nitrated substance with a powerful antianginal effectiveness both in oral and sublingual administration. The major unpleasant reaction, headache, occurs in 20% of cases for RUSSEK [1602], 67% for LESLIE [1109].

Starting from the concept that the coronaro-dilator effect of Isordil could neutralise the coronaro-constrictor effect which is so undesirable in propranolol, and that the latter's heart-slowing effect might in turn counter the tachycardia induced by Isordil, RUSSEK [1607] carried out a clinical test as to the possibility of there being a synergy between these two drugs. He proves the existence of such synergy on twelve angina subjects by obtaining with the association considerably better therapeutic results than those arrived at by the separate administration of each of the two substances to the same patients. This advantage is reflected in a remarkable improvement as regards pain, effort capacity and electrocardiographic ischaemia patterns. However, other clinicians do not share RUSSEK's opinion as regards the synergy of this therapeutic association (for details see p. 213 and 214).

According to GIUSTI [114c], the combination of Isordil (5 mg) and prenylamine-theophylline acetate (40 mg) in treating angina patients would appear to be superior to either drug separately and to combined Isordil-propranolol therapy; such a combination also entails fewer side effects inherent to nitrates (headaches).

As far as the therapeutic effect of Isordil in angina is concerned, recent clinical trials throw some doubt on its efficacy. A double-blind crossover study comparing the effects of 5 mg of Isordil given sublingually four times daily for 4 weeks to those of a placebo also administered sublingually four times daily for 4 weeks was performed on 19 male patients with classical exertional angina pectoris due to coronary artery disease [11c]. Two of these patients were unable to tolerate the drug, because of severe throbbing headaches lasting for 2—3 hours after each dose. Isordil, compared to placebo, significantly reduced the number of anginal episodes requiring nitroglycerin in only one of 17 patients, did not significantly improve exercise tolerance in any of 17 patients, and did not improve the resting or exercise electrocardiograms in any of 17 patients. Isordil produced headaches in 12 of 19 patients. Isordil administered *sublingually* is therefore considered being no more effective than placebo in treating angina pectoris. GOLDBARG and his associates [53a] have also reported that isosorbide dinitrate given *orally* 10 mg four times daily to patients with angina pectoris due to coronary artery disease was no more effective than placebo therapy in reducing the number of anginal episodes or the number of nitroglycerin tablets consumed. Isosorbide dinitrate, in this study, also did not improve exercise tolerance or the ischaemic S-T segment changes following exercise. A similar opinion is put forward by others [31a, 52a] (see also p. 213 and 214).

The possibility having been contemplated that long-acting nitrites might reduce the beneficial peripheral vascular effects of nitroglycerin, calf blood flow and calf venous volume were measured plethysmographically in six subjects [140a]. After a six week administration of Isordil (120 mg/day), nitroglycerin still increased blood flow, but venous volume was no longer altered. It would therefore seem that Isordil in chronic administration does not modify the arteriolar action of nitroglycerin but does abolish the venodilator response, thus establishing a basis for vascular tolerance and possibly diminished salutary effect in relieving angina pectoris attacks. This action of isosorbide dinitrate may theoretically be responsible for diminished effectiveness of nitroglycerin during chronic administration of long-action nitrites. Furthermore, NICKERSON [232c] has pointed out that tolerance to the production of headache during chronic administration of long-acting nitrites develops readily and that the possibility of cross tolerance decreasing the effectiveness of nitroglycerin used for treating angina should be investigated. MODELL [226c] has also drawn attention to this possibility and has stated that an ineffective long-acting nitrite may possibly make nitroglycerin ineffective. As a consequence of these considerations, ARONOW and CHESLUK recently investigated the possibility of clinical ineffectiveness to nitroglycerin developing in patients receiving isosorbide dinitrate sublingually [12c]. Seventeen male patients with angina pectoris due to coronary artery disease who had not received long-acting nitrites for at least one month prior to this trial were evaluated in a double-blind crossover study to determine whether the presence of isosorbide dinitrate interfered with the effective response of exercise-induced angina to nitroglycerin administered sublingually. There was no significant difference in the duration of angina following nitroglycerin whether the patients were on no medication, sublingual placebo or sublingual isosorbide dinitrate. There was no significant difference in the blood pressure, heart rate, product of systolic blood pressure and heart rate, or electrocardiographic response after the complete relief of angina following sublingual nitroglycerin whether the patients were on no medication, sublingual placebo, or sublingual isosorbide dinitrate. These results indicate that long-acting nitrites do not cause any clinical impairment of the effectiveness of nitroglycerin given sublingually in relieving angina pectoris.

Sorbitrate and Isordil are proposed under two presentations: an oral form (5 or 10 mg) for chronic administration and a sublingual form (5 mg) to treat acute attacks. Isordil is also proposed in a third form, named Isordil Tembids (40 mg sustained action tablets) for oral basic prophylactic treatment.

10. Nilatil

Nilatil is p-toluolsulfonate or nitrolamine tosylate (or Itramin) which answers to the formula: $H_2N—CH_2—CH_2—O—NO_2$. It possesses general vasodilator properties which have been explicitly defined by BOVET and coll. [203]: following intravenous injection, the coronaro-dilator and hypotensive effects are less marked but are more prolonged than is the case with nitroglycerin. It is active when taken orally [985].

When used clinically, Nilatil at an average dose of 10 mg administered orally neutralised, in 18 out of 29 angina subjects, the ischaemia symptoms occurring during the Master test and brought about a considerable reduction in the number of painful attacks in 20 patients [1587]. These good antianginal effects have been confirmed by EHRENBERGER [480], by EJRUP and KUMLIN [483] and by BATTER-MAN and MOURATOFF [107]. According to FREMONT [587], Nilatil at the maximum tolerated dose (2—8 mg) taken half an hour before meals three times a day developed a very favourable effect in 90% of medium and severe cases of angina and in 67% of very severe cases. The effort electrocardiogram improves in half the cases.

11. Etrynit

Etrynit (Gina, Vasangor), is the trinitric ester of trimethylol propane (generic name: propatylnitrate):

$$H_3C - H_2C - \overset{\displaystyle CH_2ONO_2}{\underset{\displaystyle CH_2ONO_2}{\overset{\displaystyle |}{\underset{\displaystyle |}{C}}}} - CH_2ONO_2$$

On an isolated rabbit heart it has a coronaro-dilator effect which is exactly the same, in its different characteristics, as that of nitroglycerin [1801]. Compared with the latter, during a double-blind experiment, to determine its ability to abate the anginal attack in 35 established coronary patients, this nitro derivative proved equally active in sublingual administration [1801]. It must be made clear that Etrynit was used during this test at a dose twenty times stronger than nitro-glycerin.

Effective against an acute attack, and very useful in this respect for subjects who are especially sensitive to the undesirable actions of nitroglycerin [1639], Etrynit is ineffective as an antianginal medication with a lasting action [1395, 1639]. In an open clinical study in which 45 general practitioners were involved and which comprised 287 cases of angina pectoris, the therapeutic effect of Etrynit (average dose of 3 tablets a day) assessed by very simple subjective criteria was considered to be favourable in 75% of cases [4d].

12. Propanediol Dinitrates

a) Nitral, or 2-methyl-2n-propyl-1, 3 propanediol dinitrate, is stated to exert an excellent prophylactic effect in almost half the cases treated [1237].

b) Chloroglyceryl dinitrate or 1-chloro-2, 3-propanediol dinitrate is an oily liquid which is alleged to offer various advantages over nitroglycerin [261]: better coronaro-dilator effect on isolated rabbit heart, reduced systemic hypotensive effect on an anaesthetised dog, equal therapeutic effect on the angina pectoris subject whilst at the same time causing far less undesirable reactions.

A general comment must be made regarding all the nitro derivatives. This deals with their property of inducing methaemoglobinaemia. It is known that the uitrite ion oxidises haemoglobin to become methaemoglobin, both *in vitro* and *in vivo*. This is the case for example with amyl nitrite. On the other hand, the methaemoglobin-producing property of the nitrates is much less marked, for although its existence has been demonstrated *in vitro*, it has never been possible to prove the presence of methaemoglobin *in vivo*, even at large doses which induce complete vascular depression. It follows that, as things stand at the moment, it is considered that the formation of methaemoglobin by the administration of nitro derivatives, whatever they may be, for prolonged treatment of angina is no longer to be feared. The only danger there is lies in the possibility of poisoning by massive ingestion [692].

Papaverine

Papaverine (Pavabid), one of the main benzyl-iso-quinoline alkaloids found in opium, is a general inhibitor of the smooth muscle fibre and is considered to be one of the most powerful coronary vasodilators.

Administered intravenously, it increases the coronary flow considerably in the dog, whether anaesthetized or not, this increase being accompanied at any rate with the mean dose of 1 mg/kg, by systemic hypotension and tachycardia [468, 509, 1968].

It is not uncommon to record a reduction in blood flow which is secondary to the general haemodynamic modifications [443]. Papaverine increases strongly the oxygen content of the coronary venous blood in dog [1166], a phenomenon which is thought to result from an elevation in myocardial blood flow. Although the respective shares referable to direct action on the coronary vascular system and to other factors, and particularly to a marked increase in cardiac output [778] and to possible increase in the work and metabolism of the heart, have not yet been determined, there is true reduction of coronary vascular tone, as LINDNER and KATZ [1149] found increase of flow in the perfused isolated heart of the dog in fibrillation, an effect also observed in the isolated guinea-pig heart [799], in the resuscitated human heart [1023] and on the fibrillating isolated rabbit heart [301].

The direct action of papaverine on the coronary vessels has been confirmed on the dog's heart *in situ* [606]. The consequent fall in vascular resistance is accompanied by a distinct reduction in work of the left ventricle [610], the result of both phenomena being a large increase in the amount of oxygen which is delivered to the cardiac muscle [610].

By measuring the activity of phosphodiesterase in isolated bovine coronary strips, KUKOVETZ et al. [73 a] observed that the relaxing effect of papaverine on muscles which were previously contracted by barium chloride is accompanied by a 60% inhibition of phosphodiesterase activity. Inhibition was competitive. It was concluded that papaverine relaxed the tone of the smooth muscle through a rise in cellular cyclic 3', 5' AMP.

Because blockade of adrenergic β-receptors strongly reduced the coronarodilator effect of papaverine [1868], the drug has been thought to have a stimulant effect upon the coronary β-receptors which would partially explain the vasodilator action.

Papaverine diminished the extent of the experimental infarct produced in the dog by occlusion of a main coronary artery when it was administered for several weeks after the operation [1310]; it also reduced the mortality occurring within 24 hours [1249].

In rabbits whose left coronary artery was ligated 3 or 4 days previously, papaverine speeded up normalization of the ECG and development of collateral coronary vessels [1295]. In dogs with a gradually occluded anterior descending coronary artery as a result of chronic implantation of an Ameroid ring for 2 months, papaverine (0.5 mg/kg i.v.) increased blood flow (measured by calorimetry) in the infarcted area in 9 out of 12 animals, while irrigation improved, in all cases, in the normal myocardial areas [928]; the rise in the infarcted zone was only half of that in the normal muscle.

The effect of papaverine on the heart includes also depression of intramyocardial conduction and of cardiac irritability, and this increases the refractory period of the cardiac muscle. The drug is therefore indicated in the treatment of auricular and ventricular extrasystoles, particularly when these arrhythmias are secondary to coronary insufficiency or occlusion as it is possible that the resultant coronary vasodilatation assists in the production of a therapeutic effect in these cases [692 p. 252; 485].

In normal man as well as in coronary patients, the coronary flow, which was measured by the BING's technique [165, 339] did not change significantly after the i.v. injection of 32 mg of papaverine completed in one minute [1192].

The beneficial employment of papaverine in the anginal syndrome goes back to PAL [1405] and to MACHT [1202] in the case of the intravenous route and to BOEHM [194] by the oral route. As these early observations involved only a limited number of cases, EVANS and HOYLE [514] attempted an exact evaluation on about a hundred patients, using a critical method of appraisal: administered by mouth in a daily dose of 75 mg, papaverine brought only slight clinical improvement. These unfavourable results were due, according to ELEK and KATZ [485], to the fact that the dosage employed was much too low, as 300—400 mg daily was highly effective in 75% of the latter's cases, which were observed with the same care and assessed by the same standards as those adopted by EVANS and HOYLE. SWANSON [1859] is also enthusiastic in his appraisal. These large doses produced only some somnolence. Accordingly, ELEK and KATZ strongly recommended papaverine in large doses as a prophylactic agent for the anginal syndrome, especially since it increased the "coronary reserve" of the heart by reducing overloading [1669].

On the other hand, certain clinicians have concluded from an investigation which, it is true, concerned only a limited number of patients, that papaverine is incapable of modifying the subjective and objective signs of coronary ischaemia [712, 1755]. RUSSEK and his school [1614, 1616, 1619] have developed a more shaded opinion: whereas the usual therapeutic doses had only a negligible effect, papaverine is capable, in large doses (100 mg intravenously or 200 to 500 mg by mouth), of preventing anginal pain induced in patients with coronary arteriosclerosis by execution of the Master's test and also, in 50—70% of cases, the appearance of the ischaemic electrocardiographic abnormalities caused by this exertion. The minimum active dose by mouth is therefore 200 mg three or four times daily, but this produces undesirable secondary reactions (nausea, headache, anorexia, constipation, possibly slight ebriation) which reduce the therapeutic utility of the drug.

From the standpoint of therapy, papaverine is in fact predominantly of historical interest [120 c].

Because the natural alkaloid is classed as a narcotic and is very expensive, the chemists have tried to produce synthetic analogues of papaverine. One is known under the name of Paveril; it is the Dioxyline phosphate or 6,7-dimethoxy-1-(4'-ethoxy-3'-methoxybenzyl)-3-methyl-iso-quinoline. According to HENDERSON [810], Paveril has an activity in the anaesthetized dog equal to that of papaverine on the coronary flow and on the systemic arterial pressure. LU et al. [1182] consider Paveril to be as active but not for as long as papaverine on the isolated rabbit heart, while it is less active in the dog (isolated heart and heart *in situ*).

Paveril had a favourable effect on the subjective symptoms of angina and on the ischaemic electrocardiographic abnormalities due to exercise [151]; it reduced nitroglycerin requirements and proved effective in some patients in a daily dose of 800 mg by mouth [1710]. RUSSEK [1616, 1619] is of the opinion that Paveril is much less active than papaverine; its effect is of short duration even with massive doses [1620].

Other clinical reports being likewise more or less unfavourable [604, 1293], some additional larger and more completely controlled investigations would have been necessary before the exact usefulness of Paveril, as compared with papaverine, could be defined. But the drug has been definitely discarded.

Among papaverine derivatives, the ethyl analogue (generic name: ethaverine), which has the formula 6,7-diethoxy-1-(3′,4′-diethoxy-benzyl)-isoquinoline and which is known under the trade names of Diquinol or Perparin or Barbonin, is generally credited with a systemic spasmolytic effect two to four times as powerful as that of papaverine; it is not more active at coronary artery level [748, 2018] but its vasodilator effect is more persistent so that its overall effect is superior to that of papaverine [2018].

BERKESY [136] claimed that ethaverine had greater therapeutic effect in angina pectoris than papaverine, but the medication is no longer in use.

GRÜN et al. [748] think that it would be worthwhile to test ethaverine again in clinical trials because, according to the results of their experimental study on guinea pigs, the substance would appear to associate a coronarodilator effect with a certain β-receptor blocking activity, as they found that the effects of injected isoproterenol on heart rate and blood pressure were neutralized by ethaverine. It should, however, be noted that such β-blocking activity required the very large dose of 14 mg/kg, and the antagonism was apparently not competitive. It is thus difficult to accept that ethaverine is effectively endowed with β-blocking properties. It is evident that the investigators base their opinion as to the possible usefulness of ethaverine in angina on the modern conceptions of the treatment of chronic coronary insufficiency, according to which neutralizing the undesirable haemodynamic effects of β-adrenoceptors stimulation could be beneficial.

Xanthines

Three methylxanthines (caffeine or 1-3-7-trimethylxanthine, theobromine or 3-7-dimethylxanthine and theophylline or 1-3-dimethylxanthine) were classical medications in angina pectoris.

As early as 1895 ASKANAZY [58] drew attention to the possibility of using xanthines in the treatment of angina and reported cases of coronary disease treated with theobromine — sodium salicylate (Diuretin).

SAKAI and SANEYOSHI [1628] appear to have been the first to observe that the xanthines increase the coronary blood flow which was collected from the sinus by means of Morawitz' method. BOYER and GREEN [205] have shown that these three substances dilate the coronary vessels by direct action, but that they increase the work of the heart so that, despite the increased coronary flow, there cannot be any increase in the coronary reserve. Theophylline is more active than theobromine and the latter is superior to caffeine [692 p. 340]. Theophylline is insoluble in water; the addition of ethylene diamine renders it soluble and increases its vasodilator activity [881]. This is the reason why theophylline ethylene diamine (aminophylline) has been used more and investigated more than theophylline itself.

1. Aminophylline[1]

The intravenous injection of a mean dose of 10—20 mg/kg increases for a variable time, sometimes exceeding 20 min the coronary blood flow in the un-anaesthetized dog, as measured by means of the thermostromuhr [509]. With the same technique, the rise in blood flow was small and inconstant in anaesthetized and conscious dogs for other pharmacologists [443]. In the chloralosed dog the increase of coronary inflow occurs together with tachycardia and systemic hypotension [468, 717, 1968]. Essentially similar results have been observed on the heart-lung preparation [1844] and in the anaesthetized dog, in which the coronary outflow was measured by Morawitz' method [657, 914, 1390, 1844].

Although unanimous agreement seemed to have been reached on the augmenting effect of aminophylline on the coronary flow, whatever technique was used by experimenters, MAXWELL et al. [1242, 1243] have reported that in healthy unanaesthetized man and in mitral and pulmonary (cor pulmonale) patients this substance, injected intravenously in a dose of 250 mg, reduced the coronary blood flow, a fact which, in the absence of any change in the systemic blood pressure, indicated the presence of an increase of coronary resistance. These observations were even more unexpected in that the cardiac output was also reduced whereas, with the same conditions of dosage and administration, it has been repeatedly described as being increased in man [1840]. The explanation of these curious results may possibly lie in the limitations of the nitrous oxide method employed, in which measurement of the cardiac and coronary outputs required almost 20 min and was only carried out once after the injection.

The mechanisms whereby aminophylline raises the coronary flow are not yet exactly known. As the head of pressure is reduced, the increase in the blood flow arises from reduction of arterial resistance probably due to active vasodilatation [205, 717]. As the stimulation of the myocardium [205, 864] results in elevation of output [1823, 1840] and in the work of the heart [717], the coronary arterial dilatation cannot be attributed with certainty to a direct effect on the vessels as the changes in the cardiac dynamics may cause passive changes in the calibre of the vessels. No more information as to the action mechanisms should be expected from experiments on the isolated heart, all of which report increase of coronary flow, whether the heart be that of the rabbit [793, 1760], the guinea-pig [799] or the resuscitated human heart [1025]. The conditions as arranged in work on the heart of the dog in ventricular fibrillation [957, 1149] as well as on fibrillating isolated rabbit heart [301] allow, however, of the definite conclusion that there is a direct dilator action on the vessel.

On the effect of aminophylline on coronary efficiency, one can accept the conclusion of MELVILLE and LU [1274] that, while increasing coronary flow, the drug also increases the energy requirements of the heart, a fact which explains that the oxygen content of the coronary venous blood is not significantly modified in the dog [1166]; therefore aminophylline is not an entirely satisfactory coronary vasodilator.

In the course of some physiopathological approaches to establish evidence of the efficacy of aminophylline in angina pectoris, FOWLER et al. [574] noted that, in the dog, the substance reduced the zone of myocardial cyanosis produced by experimental occlusion of a coronary artery, an effect which they attributed to action on the collateral circulation. This favourable effect on the extent and

---

1 Several trade names exist for aminophylline: Aminocardol, Androphyllin, Cardophyllin, Carena, Corphyllamin, Diaphyllin, Euphyllin, Inophyline, Tefamin.

colour of the zone of infarction (as well as on the ischaemic electrocardiograms) was a function of the dose administered [1209]; it was unequivocal but of short duration (a few minutes only) with a dose of 50 mg/kg, and it was absent with 25 mg/kg, although this dose was considered active by LAUBRY et al. [1088]. Favourable opinions are also expressed in the works of LE ROY et al. [1105] who found that theophylline (and theobromine) reduced the mortality of dogs with chronic experimental myocardial infarcts produced by ligature of a coronary artery, of BAYLEY et al. [114] in whose hands theophylline abolished the ischaemic electrocardiographic signs produced by surgical occlusion of a main cardiac artery, and of MOKOTOFF and KATZ [1310] who reported reduction in the size of the infarction zone in dogs subjected to the arterial ligation and autopsied after treatment for 8 weeks. These observations could not, however, be confirmed either by WIGGERS and GREEN [1996] or by GOLD, TRAVELL and MODELL [678] in respect of effect on infarct mortality or extent of the ischaemic zone.

Results are likewise discordant in relation to the therapeutic effectiveness of aminophylline in anginal patient. SCHIMERT [1669] described good results which he attributed to coronary vasodilatation and to improved "coronary reserve" resulting from reduction of cardiac overloading. LEVY and his co-workers [1128, 2003] also express a favourable, but more shaded, opinion. After the intravenous injection of 7—8 mg/kg of aminophylline (or of theophylline-sodium acetate) an anoxaemia test 5 min later revealed a 75% prolongation in the inhalation time required for the development of an attack of pain and a reduction of 50% in the extent of the depression of the S-T segment in the electrocardiogram; these facts suggest improvement in the coronary flow. By the oral route, the therapeutic effect of prolonged daily treatment with aminophylline appeared to depend on the size of the dose: while a daily dose of 800 mg increased the delay in the development of the pain induced by the anoxaemia test by 26% and resulted in a reduction of 30% in the average shift of the S-T segment [1128, 1839], a dose of 600 mg had almost the same effect on the electrocardiogram but did not delay development of the anginal attack [2003]. Furthermore, the effect of aminophylline by the oral route is definitely less significant when the patient's clinical state is severe [1128, 2003]. Equally favourable opinions are those of BROWN and RISEMAN [242] and BAKST et al. [75], who report definitely good effects in relation to exercise tolerance, and of LE ROY [1104], for whom aminophylline is effective by mouth in 75% of cases of angina due to coronary arteriosclerosis of luetic origin. On the other hand, at least seven groups of workers are of the opinion that aminophylline, whether by mouth or intravenously, has only a very moderate effect on the frequency and severity of angina attacks [106, 514, 677, 1227, 1232, 1830, 1964], a fact which RUSSEK confirmed by his observations that development of the electrical signs of ischaemia following Master's effort test was unchanged [1616, 1619].

In view of so many diverse opinions with respect to the usefulness of the xanthine bases in the treatment of angina, the Council of Pharmacy and Chemistry (U.S.A.) did not accept the arguments of those who believe them to be effective (see BOYER [204]). Also, quite a number of doctors use them (particularly aminophylline), their attitude being that if they do not do the patients good, they cannot do them any harm. This latter idea calls for correction as the xanthine bases in effective dosage can cause unpleasant reactions, particularly digestive disorders.

According to RUSSEK [1598], who obtained unequivocal objective evidence of the efficacy of aminophylline when administered parenterally, it seems reasonable to assume that the failure with oral therapy may be ascribed to the inadequate blood theophylline levels attained as a consequence of poor absorption from the gastro-intestinal tract. This view promoted the preparation of theophylline in the form of an elixir (hydro-alcoholic solution of theophylline) called Elixophyllin which has been shown to be associated with rapid absorption and attainment of high blood concentrations, mean theophylline blood levels 15 min following oral administration being eight times higher with this preparation than with comparable oral doses of aminophylline [1675]. RUSSEK [1598] found Elixophyllin to be strikingly effective when administered orally to patients with angina pectoris not only in the control of symptoms but in its modifying action on the electrocardiographic response to standard exercise. The effectiveness of this preparation seems to be based not on dosage, since equal amounts of other xanthines have proved of little value, but on the rapid absorption and attainment of high blood levels made possible by the vehicle employed.

2. Choline Theophyllinate

The therapeutic interest of theophylline is marred by the fact that the therapeutic effect is unpredictable because of the uncertainty of intestinal absorption and also by the fact that very large doses must be employed, particularly by the oral route; consequently digestive intolerance is very frequent, while drug tolerance develops rapidly. Although an advance on theophylline by virtue of its solubility, aminophylline is still poorly absorbed by the oral route and is irritant to the gastric mucosa.

Choline theophyllinate or oxtriphylline (Choledyl, Cholegyl) appears not to have these disadvantages. It was synthesized on the hypothesis that a reaction between theophylline and a strong base would yield a more soluble salt, without irritant properties and more readily absorbable by the digestive tract. This salt is stable, much more soluble than aminophylline and considerably less toxic [459]. It has typical but intensified theophyllinic activity — coronary vasodilator, peripheral vasodilator, respiratory stimulant and bronchodilator effects [1654]. Taken by mouth, Choledyl produces a much higher concentration of theophylline in the blood than aminophylline and causes less digestive disturbance [621].

The first clinical trials in the treatment of the anginal syndrome gave excellent results with a dose of 200 mg three or four times daily by mouth, as 72% of the patients were considerably improved, with no signs of digestive disturbances [106, 747]. These favourable observations were confirmed by ARAVANIS and LUISADA [50], who strengthened their results by observation of a parallel series of patients given a placebo and by the employment of electrocardiographic effort tests. The clinical improvement was striking in 50% of cases but it developed only gradually; in a number of patients the electrocardiogram, in which exertion produced deterioration before Choledyl treatment, exhibited no signs of ischaemia when the same exertion followed taking of the drug. On the other hand, however, RUSSEK [1589, 1590] concluded that the drug was ineffective from carefully controlled electrocardiographic effort tests on carefully selected anginal subjects.

3. Various Theophylline Derivatives

Other theophylline derivatives have been synthesized with a view to finding water-soluble substances giving stable and neutral solutions. They include: β-γ-dihydroxypropyl-7-theophylline (by substitution in position 7 of a dihydroxypropyl radicle on the nitrogen of the theophylline), diethylaminoethyl-theophylline (again by substitution in position 7) and the theophylline ethanoate of diethylene-diamine (Etaphylline), prepared by BAISSE [71] by combination of ethano-theophyllinic acid with piperazine. These three substances have been the subject of a comparative study, with aminophylline as reference substance, in respect of their effects on the coronary circulation [914, 1390]. Somewhat unexpectedly, they were, unlike aminophylline, practically inactive. They have not been used in man.

A few other points are worthy of comment.

1. Calcium theophyllinate (Calphyllin) was not considered superior to the placebo as a result of a critical examination of its effectiveness in angina [349].

2. JACOBI et al. [884] considered that the coronary vasodilator activities of hydroxypropyltheophylline, hydroxyethyltheophylline (Cordalin) and dihydroxy-propyltheophylline were in animals respectively three times, three times and six times less than that of theophylline. The increase in coronary blood flow which was brought about by Cordalin in dogs, whether anaesthetized or not, was small [443, 579]; the same kind of effect was reported in the case of dihydroxypropyltheo-phylline [579].

3. Another theophylline salt recommended for treatment of disorders of the arterial circulation in the legs and brain is the 3-(methyloxyethylamine)-2-oxy-propyltheophylline nicotinate, or xanthinol nicotinate (Complamin). Its coronary vasodilator activity on the isolated rabbit heart is very close to that of theophyl-line [85, 301]. There are no indications in the literature of its effects in angina pectoris, although the drug was offered to the physicians some years ago for the treatment of coronary insufficiency, despite its cardiostimulant effects which resulted in man in an increase in cardiac output, stroke volume and heart rate [77a]. It has been confirmed in patients that the intravenous injection of 300 mg of Complamin induces a definite stimulation of heart energetics, as shown by an important increase in cardiac output, stroke volume, heart rate, and velocity of the cardiac contraction [194c]. Following intramuscular injection of the same dose, an initial rise in cardiac output was followed by a slight decrease under the control values [33c].

4. In a cat heart-lung preparation, oxypropyltheobromine, in a dose of 60 mg, antagonized the 30% decrease in coronary blood flow produced by pituitrine; one hour after administration, the level of coronary blood flow was 73% higher than control value [1907]. Taking into account the experimental conditions, this effect can be considered as being due to a decrease in coronary vascular resistance.

5. Two thioxanthines, namely choline-6-thiotheophyllinate and 3-isobutyl-1-methyl-6-thioxanthine cholinate are active at the coronary level [55]: their coronarodilator (dog heart-lung preparation) and peripheral vasodilator (isolated perfused dog hind leg) effects were respectively 2.5 and 15 times more potent than that of choline theophyllinate. They are not specific coronary vasodilators.

6. 1-hexyl-3-7-dimethylxanthine, which is a potent peripheral and cerebral vasodilator, induced an increase in coronary irrigation in isolated rabbit heart at a dose of 0.5 mg; rise in flow was usually preceded by a slight decrease [377].

7. On the isolated rabbit heart, 8-aminotheophylline had a coronarodilator effect equal to that of aminophylline [812].

8. Five alkyl-xanthines, namely, 1-3-dimethyl-8-ethylxanthine, 1-3-diethyl-8-methylxanthine, 1-3-diethylxanthine, 1-3-8-trimethylxanthine and 1-3-8-trie-thylxanthine, which are used in the form of the sodium salts, are less active than aminophylline [1106].

For the present time, the use of xanthines and their several synthetic derivatives for the long-term treatment of angina pectoris is no longer in favour with cardiologists who prefer to rely on recent medications which correspond more closely with present pathogenic conceptions. Reviewing past practices, MODELL states [1307 p. 368] that xanthines provide little for the relief or prevention of an attack of anginal pain and that there is little in their known pharmacological action on which to base such a hope.

Khellin[1]

Khellin or visammin or 2-methyl-5,8-dimethoxyfuranochromone, is one of the biologically active substances which have been isolated from the fruit of Ammi visnaga, a plant which grows in the Mediterranean countries. Its coronary vasodilator activity in the animal and its effectiveness in angina have been the subjects of numerous scientific controversies. We confine ourselves to the most significant papers.

It was SAMAAN [1632] who, in 1932, started the experimental investigations on animals by demonstrating that khellin relaxed all smooth visceral muscles, but ANREP and his group have, since 1945, concerned themselves with the investigation of its effects on the circulatory system, and particularly on the coronary circulation. On the heart-lung preparation of the dog, khellin in a dilution of 10^{-5} increases the coronary outflow three or four times [39]; it is four times more active than aminophylline [37, 38, 45]. ANREP is of the opinion that the coronary vasodilator action of khellin is selective, in that active doses do not modify the systemic arterial pressure in the intact animal.

FELLOWS and KILLAM [534, 983], as well as WEGRIA et al. [1970] have generally confirmed, on the intact anaesthetized dog, the findings of the ANREP school.

Using different techniques for measurement of changes in coronary outflow, JONGEBREUR [908] confirmed the coronary vasodilator activity of khellin in the rat and cat, an effect which was also seen in the guinea-pig [799] and which, in the dog, was about half that of papaverine [1061].

JOURDAN and FAUCON [912, 913] also described the augmentor effect of khellin on the venous outflow from the sinus in the dog, although OLLEON [1390] found its effect as inconstant, varying in intensity and generally transient, in which respects it differs from the action of papaverine which was constant and more powerful. On the other hand, the increase in the coronary outflow was found to be striking and reproducible in the anaesthetized dog by MERCIER and coworkers [1283]. SCHMIDT [1681] suggested that khellin is only active at coronary level because of the solvents employed to dissolve it; the solvent alone (sodium salicylate, for example) was as active as khellin dissolved in this solvent; moreover, a water soluble form of khellin, the sodium salt of khellin-carbonic acid, Khelfren, did not afford experimentally any coronary vasodilator effect. Nevertheless,

---

1 Khellin has been marketed under several trade names: Kellin, Kelamin, Kelicor, Gynokhellan, Kelicorin, Keloid, Norkel, Simeskellina, Vasokellina, Visnagalin, Visnagen, Methafrone, Eskel, Viscardan, Corafurone, Cardio-Khellin, Benecardin, Ammivisnagen, Lynamine, Coronin, Ammicardine, Ammipuran, Ammivin, Visammimix, Rykellin.

careful experimental investigations showed that khellin has a coronary vasodilator activity by itself [1908].

As it increased the coronary flow of the perfused isolated heart without causing
change in the cardiac dynamics, khellin has a direct coronary vasodilator effect
[1112].

BAGOURI [70] found the minimum active khellin concentration to be about
2.10^{-6}, as was also the case in the observations of LU et al. [1182] who assigned it a
coronary vasodilator activity eight times greater than that of aminophylline.

Khellin was much used a number of years ago in the treatment of the anginal
syndrome, particularly after the initial clinical observations of ANREP and his
co-workers, who published reports of beneficial effects in up to 90% of cases [39,
40, 45, 64, 968]. This enthusiastic opinion, which was shared by DEWAR and
GRIMSON [423] and by HEJTMANCIK [803], spurred numerous clinicians to attempt
to define the indications for khellin more exactly, and the conclusions reached,
though always favourable, then limited the effectiveness of the drug to 50—70%
of the cases [54, 150, 353, 1397, 1909]. SCOTT et al. [1708, 1709] found that the
frequency of a beneficial effect from khellin depended on the purity of the form
used; this was also the opinion of NALEFSKI et al. [1339] who employed a khellin
of great purity (Khelloyd) freed from resins, chromones and other impurities, and
obtained good therapeutic effects with small doses (50—100 mg daily).

Although, according to ROSENMAN et al. [1557, 1558], the employment of
khellin would be justified by the fact that it has a very favourable effect on the
ischaemic electrocardiograms that are produced in the anginal subject by Master's
effort test, the cardiological importance of khellin has been considerably reduced,
mainly as a result of the intensive and convincing investigations of GREINER et al.
[738] and HULTGREN et al. [871], who concluded that is was ineffective when care
was taken to check its effect by means of a placebo and the double-blind method.
RUSSEK [1613, 1616, 1619] regarded this drug as devoid of importance for the
patient with angina pectoris. The same opinion was put forward by MODELL in
1966 [1306].

This fall of khellin from favour in the cardiological field may possibly also have
had origin in the digestive side-effects (nausea, vomiting) which supervene
especially after oral administration in close to 60% of cases [353], and may be
dependent on the degree of purity of the form of drug employed [1708, 1709], the
pure form causing much less digestive trouble [1339, 1708] than the impure [1709];
these side-effects could be avoided by use of the intramuscular route [992].

The insolubility of khellin in water has stimulated the synthesis of water-
soluble derivatives. FOURNEAU [573] in 1953 suggested the diethylaminoethoxy-
8-hydroxy-5-methyl-2-furochromone hydrochloride, known commercially under
the name of Nokhel, which he found to have considerable coronary vasodilator
activity on the isolated rabbit heart. BARSOUM and KENAWY [96] found, however,
that it was 10 times inferior to khellin on the heart-lung preparation while JOURDAN
and FAUCON [912, 913], as well as OLLEON [1390], deny all vasodilator activity in
the dog in toto and indeed report a depressor effect on the coronary outflow,
possibly due to a fall in the aortic pressure.

Another hydrosoluble derivative of khellin has been synthesized, 2-methyl-5-
(β-trimethylaminoethoxy-N-theophylline)-8-methoxy-furo-(2',3':6,7)-chromone,
called KCT, which increases the rate of perfusion of the coronary arteries of the
rabbit and which is active against the coronaroconstriction produced by pituitrine
[1794].

Other active principles in addition to khellin extracted from Ammi visnaga
include notably:

1. Visnagin (Visnacorin), or 5-methoxy-2-methylfuranochromone, thus differing from khellin in that it has only one methoxy group instead of two:

2. The glucoside of khellol, khelloside or Khellinin which, although quite without visceral spasmolytic [1633] or coronary vasodilator [45, 70] properties and causing strong stimulation of the myocardium [1634], has been commercialized, mainly as Deltoside, as a coronary vasodilator. Deltoside was abandoned soon after it became available.

3. Visnamine (Provismine, Visnadin, Vibeline, Cardine):

s twice as active as and acts far longer than khellin on the perfused isolated heart of the rabbit or guinea-pig [1631]; it would also appear to be able to increase heart rate and blood pressure considerably. MONIZ DE BETTENCOURT and his co-workers [1314, 1315] considered it to have six times the activity of khellin on the coronary flow of the perfused isolated heart of the cat or rabbit and to produce favourable results in 70% of the anginal patients treated; some interesting therapeutic effects were also reported by MOUQUIN and MACREZ [1325], but its antianginal effectiveness has never been carefully checked.

The drug was abandoned for a few years and then recently reexamined and marketed under the name of Carduben. It has been shown that Carduben increases coronary flow in isolated guinea pig heart [507], being 5—10 times more potent than khellin. Systemic blood pressure was not modified but there was a positive inotropic effect on the heart leading to an increase in cardiac output [507].

A central α-antiadrenergic effect has also been described [755].

Carduben improved a great number of a group of 311 patients presenting degenerative myocarditis [88]. The drug has been reported to be active in angina [982, 1140] regardless of the cause [1057]. According to KRACKE [72a] who reports on 173 coronary patients including 27 cases of post-coronary infarction, 83 of "primary" coronary insufficiency and 63 with "secondary" insufficiency which received Carduben for at least 8 weeks, patients with mild to moderately severe insufficiency were symptom-free after 2—3 weeks, and almost all severe cases showed some degree of relief.

As long as these therapeutic effects are not confirmed by carefully controlled trials, it must be considered that the medication is of only slight interest as an antianginal drug [1792].

As khellin is a furanochromone, a search has been made for the radical to which the coronary vasodilator activity is linked; it would appear that a relaxing effect on the smooth muscle fibre, particularly that of the coronary vessel, is associated with the chromone nucleus. A number of substituted chromones have therefore been synthesized, among them, 3-methylchromone (Diacromone) which would appear to have a coronary vasodilator activity double that of khellin on the isolated rabbit heart [301, 1688].

In the heart in situ in the intact dog, however, the increase in coronary flow is only moderate and is inconstant, although more persistent than in the case of khellin [912, 915, 1390]. Although recommended for the treatment of angina pectoris [1797], 3-methylchromone certainly does not produce any remarkable improvements [324], and its clinical use has been discontinued.

A substance akin to 3-methylchromone, 2-phenylchromone (Cromarile, Chromocor) which JONGEBREUR [908] thinks to have a coronary vasodilator action double that of khellin but which ANREP et al. [41] considered very much inferior, has been used clinically by FERRARI and FINARDI [536], who found it had a beneficial effect in angina pectoris, although the limited number of cases treated does not entitle them to establish its true value. KÖHLER [1011] obtained very good effects in 90% of his patients and HOOGERWERF [858] also expressed himself as satisfied with it.

The drug is no longer in use.

Recordil

$$C_2H_5-OOC-CH_2-O-$$

Recordil, Oxiflavil, or flavone-7-ethyl oxyacetate caused dilatation of the coronary vessels on the beating isolated rabbit heart which could neither be attributed to increase of cardiac metabolism or to changes in cardiac dynamics [1719, 1722].

Of low toxicity and free from any general effects on the cardiovascular system, Recordil has been the subject of clinical trials and it is in consequence of the favourable results published [668, 1819, 1873, 1935] that it has been recommended for the treatment of the anginal syndrome [1221, 1849]. Assessed by the double-blind method, the therapeutic effects afforded by Recordil were however found to be just equal to those of a placebo [424]. RUSSEK's opinion [1594] was also unfavourable because it has no effect on the electrocardiographic signs of ischaemia developing in the subject with angina pectoris after performance of a Master type exercise.

Monoamineoxydase Inhibitors (MAOI)

Iproniazid (Marsilid) was the first MAOI to be used for the treatment of the anginal syndrome as a result of chance clinical observations by CESARMAN [287] who, when administering it to a depressed patient who had also a coronary disease, noted an unexpected favourable effect on the evolution of the angina. CESARMAN then confirmed his initial observation on forty anginal patients [288]. The important clinical contribution of COSSIO [367] upheld this opinion and he suggested that the therapeutic effect was due to a selective analgesic action brought to bear on the muscular pain of ischaemic origin.

The mechanisms which are involved in the antianginal properties of Marsilid have been largely discussed.

It blocks the activity of mono-amine-oxidase [2045, 2046, 2047], the enzyme responsible for degradation of the adrenergic mediators and of serotonin; in consequence, it produces a pronounced and prolonged increase in the levels of catecholamines in the heart muscle [1454, 1457] and in the hypothalamus [1300], an effect which is at the opposite of the result of the therapeutic measures which have been advocated to combat hypersympathicotony.

Iproniazid has a weak effect on coronary haemodynamics: in the rabbit [22, 588] and in the cat [1457] it increases the coronary flow in the perfused isolated heart only for a high concentration, reducing at the same time the amplitude of the cardiac contraction; it is a pituitrine antagonist [588]; on the rabbit heart in situ it reduces, then increases the coronary flow [1457]; injected into the rat in doses of 250—500 mg/kg, it prevents in most instances the development of the electrocardiographic signs of myocardial ischaemia produced by pituitrine [171]; given prior to acute coronary occlusion, iproniazid prevented the onset of the ventricular fibrillation and death that follows acute occlusion of a major coronary artery in the conscious dog [1516]. However, iproniazid did not prevent the S-T segment depression provoked by injection of picrotoxine into the lateral cerebral ventricle in the rabbit [1921]. Since coronary flow increased in the isolated fibrillating rabbit heart, intrinsic coronary vascular resistance was reduced [301]; however the effect was moderate, being only 20 times more potent than that of aminophylline. The weakness of the coronarodilator action of iproniazid has been confirmed by MENDEZ [1279], by PLETSCHER [1456] and by HERMANN and MORNEX [818].

On rabbit heart isolated by the Langendorff method, iproniazid is capable of increasing the resistance to anoxia. This was observed when the drug was perfused at a concentration of 10 mg/litre and also when the animals were given the drug in daily doses of 20 mg/kg for seven days before they were killed for the experiment [1721].

While the mechanism of action of iproniazid appears deceptively to be related to its potency of inhibition of monoamine oxidase, it is difficult to accept that these pharmacological properties can explain the remarkable antianginal effects of the drug. This is particularly true of coronary vasodilator activity which is generally considered to be weak and which can be evidenced in animals only with doses much in excess of the therapeutic dose [1282]. It may be that these various actions are combined [1456], but such considerations are purely speculative. It may be mentioned, in this connection, that HORWITZ et al. [861] reported during such treatment a reduction of the tachycardia and of the rise in blood pressure which appeared in anginous patients during exercise.

The insignificant character of the coronarodilator effect of Marsilid constitutes an indirect argument in favour of the opinion of those clinicians who have suggested a preferential effect of the drug on the mechanism of the anginal pain rather than on its underlying pathophysiological causes. Since antalgic effects have also been reported in some cases of malignant tumours and rhumatoid arthritis, it is likely that Marsilid also acts by blocking the pain pathways in the central nervous system, a suggestion which is rendered all the more acceptable by the fact that the drug has an analgetic effect in animals, which is independent of any accumulation of catecholamines and 5-hydroxytryptamine [491].

The only thing that may be said is that MAO inhibition seems to be the only enzymatic effect which up to now parallels the beneficial action on anginal pain [1455].

On the clinical side, TOWERS and WOOD [1895], after CESARMAN and COSSIO, reported very favourable effects in respect of the frequency and intensity of the anginal pains in forty patients with severe angina due to obliterating coronary arteriosclerosis; for them, iproniazid was much more effective than long-acting nitrites; the electrocardiogram improved in most cases but the observation of patients who retained their electrocardiographic changes of coronary insufficiency (reversible by nitroglycerin) despite considerable clinical benefit led the authors to think that iproniazid acted on the pain and not by improving the myocardial metabolic state. MASTER [1228] and FERRERO [537] expressed the same opinion because the pathological resting and effort electrocardiograms of all the patients who were remarkably improved were unchanged. Nor does RUSSEK observe any improvement in the effort test [1605].

According to other investigators [1, 91, 492, 532], the clinical benefit, which was manifest in almost 70% of the cases treated, was accompanied by a definite improvement of the rest- and effort-electrocardiogram in a proportion of 20—80% according to the study carried out. According to others [1208] the hypoxia and effort tests showed improvement of the ECG in several cases, and occasionally a normalization.

These very favourable subjective results have been checked by a clinical assessment carried out on the double-blind principle [1748].

Although these initial reports claimed a high incidence of improvement and often complete relief of pain, there were however some dissenting voices regarding the efficacy of iproniazid in reducing the frequency and severity of the anginal attacks: the therapeutic effect was doubtful for SCHERBEL [1663] and three carefully controlled trials failed to confirm the good reports as in no trial was the drug more effective than a placebo [424, 546, 1766]. Even in the severer cases, any possible benefit was at best marginal [546]. This drug should always be reserved for very severe and irreducible cases [638, 856, 1170, 1895, 1975]. It is contra-indicated in moderate cases [269] for two reasons: first, the favourable effect on the pain element might lead the improved patient to undertake immoderate exertions capable of precipitating a myocardial infarct, and secondly, undesirable effects are numerous, frequent and unpleasant with effective dosages. Clinicians who have used iproniazid for any purpose are unanimous in drawing attention to these side-effects, which seriously limited its therapeutic value. We refer mainly to headache, constipation, difficult micturition, vertigo, hyperexcitation with insomnia or somnolence, muscular tremors, visual disturbances progressing sometimes to temporary functional blindness [289, 1896] and particularly to three very serious complications: these are sudden acute arterial hypotension, particularly dangerous in the coronary subject in whom it can lead to fatal myocardial infarction [289, 1896]; toxic hepatitis [130, 1462], the number of cases hitherto reported being 230 with 51 deaths, according to a statistical study of July 1959 [907]; and sexual impotence, which develops in a considerable number of cases [289, 1896].

The severity and frequency of these undesirable effects appeared even greater to SCHWEIZER and VON PLANTA [1703, 1705]; of 100 coronary patients in whom the drug proved very effective against the anginal pains in an average dose of 150 mg daily, 89% exhibited undesirable reactions, which necessitated interruption of treatment in 50%; 14% presented grave complications, including four myocardial infarcts (fatal in two cases) and four cases of cardiac decompensation. MASTER [1228], who also reported an impressive percentage of severe undesirable effects, advised that therapeutic trials of iproniazid should only be undertaken in hospitals and under the constant supervision of doctors familiar with the phenomena of intolerance inseparable from the employment of this drug.

One important point which seems to emerge from all the reports is that no therapeutic results are obtained without attendant side-effects. The use of much smaller doses than those usually administered has been said to avoid the development of undesirable reactions, while still giving excellent therapeutic effects [711]. In any case, it is important to bear in mind that even such remarkable symptomatic relief as iproniazid (and other monoamine oxidase inhibitors so far known) may give probably does not affect the underlying coronary arterial disease. Owing to its toxicity the use of Marsilid was discontinued.

Because of the remarkable effects of iproniazid in angina, which for some investigators surpass those of the innumerable drugs which had been recommended before this drug was proposed [544], other mono-amine-oxidase inhibitors, derivatives of iproniazid, have been developed in an attempt to overcome its serious drawbacks. Iproniazid being 1-isonicotinyl-2-isopropyl-hydrazine, the following compounds have been synthesized, experimentally and clinically tested, and consequently advocated for the treatment of angina:

1. 1-benzyl-2-(5-methyl-3-isoxazolylcarbonyl) hydrazine (isocarboxazid, Marplan). Possessing an inhibitor effect on mono-amine-oxidase thirty times greater than that of iproniazid, and preventing partially the cardiac necrosis provoked in the rat by isoprenaline [2043], Marplan was effective in anginous patients [6, 7], producing spectacular improvement in more than 80% of cases [185], although it had no effect on the electrocardiographic signs of cardiac ischaemia [853, 1383]. It has all the undesirable effects of Marsilid [852], possibly in less degree [1330] and its administration should be very strictly supervised.

2. β-phenyl-isopropylhydrazine (generic name: pheniprazine) or JB 516 (Catron, Cavodil). This powerful mono-amine-oxidase inhibitor [859] was very effective in angina [7, 740, 1204] but is apparently as toxic as iproniazid [849, 852] and does not produce any improvement in the electrocardiogram [969]. When therapeutic effectiveness was tested in double-blind, it was only equal to placebo [1638]. This drug has also been withdrawn.

3. Pivaloyl-2-benzyl hydrazine (Tersavid), which was very effective in angina [7, 430, 866] and less toxic than iproniazid according to some authors [6, 430, 911] but equally toxic according to others [852]. The value of Tersavid as an antianginal medication is much lower than that of Marsilid [638]. Tried on a double-blind basis Tersavid did not appear to be valuable [1332, 1439], although the authors of one of these papers had previously reported the results of a non-controlled study ending in favourable therapeutic effects in 70% of the patients [1331].

4. N- [2-(benzylcarbamyl) ethylamino] -isonicotinamide (nialamide, Niamid) increased significantly coronary blood flow in the chloralozed dog for high doses [630]. Side effects in man were negligible and occurred very rarely [741]. Antianginal effects were found to be excellent by some clinicians [1004, 2030] but only equal to placebotherapy by others [21].

5. β-phenylethylhydrazine (phenelzine, Nardil), which is capable of inhibiting monoamine-oxidase for as long as 3 weeks following a single dose [323] and possesses only about one-half the coronary dilator activity of papaverine [129]. Nardil gave relief of pain in almost 80% of the anginous patients treated [556, 842] and clinical evidence seemed sufficient to warrant continued use of the drug in the treatment of such cases particularly when complicated with anxiety and with mental depression.

6. Iproclozide is the isopropylhydrazide of p-chlorophenoxyacetic acid [1135], and is known under the trade name of Sursum. About 60—70% of anginal patients improved by treatment with Sursum [639, 641, 1958]. Orthostatic hypotension frequently occurred [641, 1097, 1958]. As there is as considerable risk of toxic reactions, notably liver damage, the use of Sursum is contra-indicated in patients suffering from hepatic disturbances [639] and also in those having cardiac insufficiency [1097]. The administration of Sursum must be limited to the especially refractory cases and the patients must be carefully and permanently supervised as to their tolerance [1100, 17c]. Treatment should be abandoned if there is no detectable sign of improvement after two weeks [1100]. In a general survey involving 362 angina patients who were treated with iproclozide, BARRILLON et al. [17c] concluded that the medication should be restricted to patients who are unrespon-

sive to conventional therapy and that it is indicated in cases of angina associated with hypertension.

Summarizing the general situation regarding the clinical value of the monoamineoxydase inhibitors for the treatment of angina pectoris, it must unfortunately be concluded that none of the agents introduced to date has been able to match the frequency of symptomatic improvement formerly reported with iproniazid [1599]. Moreover, the clinical data obtained by RUSSEK [1599] indicate that therapeutic effectiveness is roughly proportional to the frequency and severity of untoward reactions.

Certain cardiological centres have remained faithful to their use, subject to the posology being adapted to each case and a close watch being kept on the patient's behaviour in order to take immediate steps in the event of serious adverse reaction [836].

The use of the MAOI's in angina cases cannot be recommended, particularly since it deprives the angina subject of his warning symptom [550], because all that they do is to raise the threshold of wareness of pain and anxiety through an euphoric effect [1307]. Moreover, they potentialise to a dangerous degree too many medications in current use [458]. Their application in angina has been virtually abandoned.

Irrigor

$$\text{phenyl ring}-\underset{\underset{O}{\overset{\|}{N}}}{\overset{\|}{N}}-N-CH_2-CH_2-N(C_2H_5)_2 \quad = NH$$

Basic pharmacological research into Irrigor or LA1211 (generic name: imolamine) has remained elementary. STERNE [1836] has shown that this substance is endowed with properties which are coronarodilator (in the case of an isolated rabbit heart, coronary flow increases threefold at the comparatively high concentration of a 10^{-4}), induces local anaesthesia, is highly analgesic (with half the potency of morphine) and has spasmolytic effects of the papaverine type.

Irrigor counters both the vaso-constrictive effects of pituitrine and barium chloride and the depressive effect on the heart of anoxia. In tests on dogs, it suppresses the electrocardiographic repercussions of ischaemia induced by respiratory anoxia. It produces a slow heart rate and has no effect on blood pressure.

According to DUCHENE-MARULLAZ et al. [456], Irrigor does not alter either coronary venous flow or the oxygen content of the coronary venous blood at doses of 1.25 and 2.5 mg/kg injected intravenously in an anaesthetised dog.

Clinical experiments with Irrigor have been reported by French medical circles [62, 383, 420, 1299, 1835, 1959] who find favourable effects in a variable percentage of cases. The fullest survey is that by KAUFMANN [961] covering 75 patients suffering from angina of coronary aetiology. He is of the opinion that with an average dosage of three 10 mg tablets a day, Irrigor exerts a preventive action in 72% of cases. Since the placebo only achieves improvement in 30% of cases, the author concludes that this medication is in the forefront of preventive treatments for angina pectoris, its side effects being very few and far between and its tolerance excellent.

From the medical viewpoint, and despite these favourable clinical reports, which have not been checked in double-blind, it would appear that, looking back, Irrigor is a relatively ordinary medication and that its use achieves only modest results [329, 1311, 1928]. A similar impression is gained from a very recent clinical report by STROBBIA et al. [304c], who investigated the value of the drug in a group of 31 patients suffering from coronary heart disease and receiving four to six 10 mg tablets a day for a period varying from 10 to 45 days. Taking into account the nature of the clinical criteria which were chosen to assess the therapeutic efficacy of the medication, it can be considered that only half of the patients obtained any benefit.

Very recently, Irrigor has been made available under a new presentation, Irrigor 3, which differs from the initial presentation in that the tablets concentration is 30 mg instead of 10. With this increased dosage, the clinical improvement achieved in angina is said to be excellent but unfortunately it is to be regretted that there are no controlled clinical investigations to substantiate such claims for outstanding antianginal properties.

Segontin

$$CH-CH_2-CH_2-NH-\overset{\overset{\displaystyle CH_3}{|}}{CH}-CH_2-$$

Investigated from the pharmacological angle by LINDNER [1145] in 1960, Segontin or Hostaginan or Corontin (generic name: prenylamine) affects the coronary and peripheral vasomotor functions whilst at the same time developing properties which are sedative for the central nervous system and antagonistic as regards certain functions of the adrenergic system [1146].

Segontin increases coronary flow, but also cardiac output [1145]. In view of the fact that blood pressure drops to a marked extent, it would seem that cardiac work does not increase [according to STAREY (1821) it decreases], since myocardial oxygen consumption does not alter significantly [196] and the oxygen content of the coronary venous blood rises [207]. Nevertheless, Segontin does not appear to act preferentially on the coronary vessels, for blood flow equally increases at the periphery [207].

Fig. 6, arrived at from our observations, shows the extent and temporary character of the increase in coronary arterial flow and of the drop in blood pressure observed at the dose of 5 mg/kg administered intravenously to an anaesthetised dog. Heart rate increases slightly.

However, Segontin makes hardly any difference to coronary flow in a conscious dog when administered orally at the high daily doses of 40—80 mg/kg [887]. According to KUKOVETZ and PÖCH [6e], Segontin, like papaverine, inhibits cyclic-3′,5′ nucleotide phosphodiesterase, this effect resulting in an accumulation of cyclic AMP and being capable of explaining the relaxation of the circular smooth muscle sheath of the coronary arteries.

Segontin has a quinidine-like action since it reduces intracardiac conduction and lessens contraction force whilst at the same time not affecting the adrenergic β-receptors [1661].

The hypotensive effect of Segontin derives from a depression of the vasomotor centre [439] and also from peripheral inhibition of the a-receptors [335]. Segontin lessens the hypertensive effect of adrenaline but not that of noradrenaline [746], contrary to the findings of DONNET et al. [440], this effect being the consequence of the a-lytic activity.

In the case of a normal man, Segontin reduces myocardial oxygen consumption and the noradrenaline content of the plasma when administered for 1 week at a daily dose of 180 mg. By so doing, it reduces the increase in these two parameters induced by nicotine [993].

According to FLECKENSTEIN [562], Segontin inhibits the activity of the cardiac muscle without altering its oxygen consumption. This effect is said to be due to competitive blockade of calcium movements [40a], since the administration of the latter reactivates the use of phosphates by the muscle [561, 563].

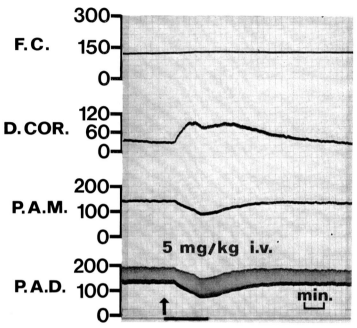

Fig. 6. Effect of prenylamine on heart rate, coronary arterial blood flow, and systemic blood pressure in the anaesthetized dog. From top to bottom: F.C.: Heart rate (beats/min). D.Cor.: Mean blood flow in the left circumflex coronary artery, measured with an electromagnetic probe (ml/min). P.A.M.: Mean blood pressure in the femoral artery (mm Hg). P.A.D.: Phasic blood pressure in the femoral artery (mm Hg). At signal mark: intravenous injection of prenylamine, 5 mg/kg

The incidence of Segontin on the adrenergic nervous system, described in 1960 by LINDNER [1146], was investigated several years later, and the least that can be said is that these investigations are far from having clarified the question. It appears to be established that the drug considerably decreases the noradrenaline content of the peripheral adrenergic tissues [1695, 1696], probably by interfering with the amine storage mechanism in the granules, in a similar manner to reserpine [277]. Although, like reserpine, it causes the liberation of 5-HT from rabbit blood platelets in vitro [98], Segontin does not behave in the same way as reserpine since it does not alter the serotonin content of the brain and merely reduces that of noradrenaline and dopamine, whereas reserpine brings about a very considerable reduction in these three amines [744]. Similarly, as regards the myocardium, high doses of Segontin do not reduce the noradrenaline content by more than 60% [1695]; the amount which remains appears to be localised in the vascular adrenergic nerves and not in the cardiac tissue [1366]. These latter findings suggest to their authors that the antianginal effect of Segontin could be due to a combination of two effects: firstly the preservation of physiological vasodilatation by the coronaries as a result of the releasing of the adrenergic transmitter, and secondly a reduction in cardiac metabolism by "chemical denervation" of the muscle following its partial depletion in catecholamines [1366]. OBIANWU [1382] defends a similar concept when he shows that Segontin abolishes sympathetic transmission by upsetting the mechanism responsible for storing the adrenergic transmitter. However, the same author [1381] describes, alongside the hypotensive and depressive cardiac effect of Segontin, actions on the functions of the adrenergic system which are difficult to reconcile with others. Although he confirms the a-blocking effect, he nevertheless describes a β-blocking effect (opposition to tachycardia, to stimulation of cardiac contraction and to vasodilatation as induced by isoprenaline) which is found particularly *in vitro* but which would seem to be much more modest *in vivo*. According to others, the incidence of Segontin on the sympathetic system is much more complex [745]: it would seem that the drug, along with various antiadrenergic effects which it is difficult to coordinate with each other, possesses adrenergic effects, since amongst other things it behaves like an indirect sympathicomimetic possessing amphetamine-like effects. But LINDNER [1147] denies that Segontin is an indirect sympathicomimetic and a stimulator of the β-receptors because the coronaro-dilator and positive cardiac inotropic effects on an isolated guinea-pig heart are still to be found following reserpine and are not inhibited by a β-blocking agent. It should however be pointed out that according to other authors [746], reserpine cancels out the coronaro-dilator effect of Segontin.

As regards the impact of Segontin on the adrenergic β-system, what OBIANWU describes is the opposite of the phenomena mentioned by SZEKERES et al. [1868]: according to these latter, pharmacological blockade of the β-receptors considerably reduces the increase in coronary flow and accentuates the reduction in myocardial oxygen consumption brought about by Segontin, these facts indicating that the activities of Segontin, according to these authors, take place partly through stimulation of the β-receptors. According to BOISSIER also [198], Segontin has no β-antagonising effect since with dogs it does not alter the tachycardic and hypotensive effects of isoprenaline. From our experiments, we share this view. It does not seem apt to ascribe to a β-antagonist effect the preventive action of Segontin at high doses (250 mg/kg) against extensive disseminated myocardial necrosis which developed in rats following subcutaneous injections of isoprenaline, reported by LEDER et al. [80a]. Calcium antagonism could be involved in the process since calcium ions in excess are known to have a necrosis-promoting or initiating action.

It should also be mentioned that FLATTERY et al. [560], while they confirm that a chronic course of treatment at very high doses causes in rats incomplete depletion of the noradrenaline reserves in the cardiac muscle and the suprarenal, observe that excretion in the urine of adrenaline, noradrenaline and their metabolites is not changed, a fact which suggests that Segontin does not lessen the release of the adrenergic mediators. This observation is supported by the fact that in 6 angina subjects treated for between 3 and 48 months at daily doses ranging from 60—240 mg the same authors find no change in the urine excretion of the catecholamines and their metabolites. This led them to believe that their results do not justify the idea that the antianginal effect mechanism of the drug consists in an inhibition of the sympathetic system. In this connection, they do not agree with the interpretation placed by KUSHKE et al. [1062] on their own results, according to which Segontin increases the urine catecholamine excretion of the angina subject during the first 5 days of treatment. Still dealing with man, SCHMID et al. [1677] find a temporary increase in urine excretion of different acid metabolites, notably 5-hydroxyindolacetic and vanillomandelic acids; this increase occurs during the few hours following a single dose, but disappears in spite of repeated administration. DE SCHAEPDRIJVER et al. [416] hold a more varied opinion, since although they confirm the facts noted by FLATTERY, they point out that his results only partially reflect the liberation of the adrenergic transmitter because he did not quantify the metanephrine and the normetanephrine. Moreover they show that in the case of a healthy man, Segontin lessens the increase in the urine excretion of noradrenaline caused by exercise, and so in their view Segontin does in fact inhibit the adrenergic neurons.

Since Segontin combines with its coronaro-dilator properties sympathicolytic and adrenolytic effects which are found in man [1296], its sponsors felt that it deserved to be applied to the treatment of angina. In fact several clinical reports testify to favourable effects [196, 1089, 1496, 1497, 1627] which are found even under double-blind conditions [1399] and which are accompanied in 40% of cases by significant regression in pathological changes shown on the electrocardiogram [804]. KERTES also describes these favourable effects [971].

According to KRUEGER (1047), the beneficial effect of Segontin on the angina subject increases with the use of high dosages, rising from 64% of cases at a daily dose of 45—90 mg (155 patients) to 72% at a daily dose of 180—360 mg (204 patients); moreover, the combined administration of K-Mg-aspartate enables 82.5% of favourable results to be achieved (102 patients). At the high dose of 270 mg/day for 1 month, Segontin is able to reduce the number of spontaneous attacks and nitroglycerin needs [1795], but this subjective effect could not be objectified by effort tests [112, 1795]. McGREGOR [1251] therefore believes that the drug could act on perception of pain.

Whereas the original pills contained 15 mg of Segontin, their active principle content has been recently increased fourfold and been called Segontin 60 or Synadrin 60. This form has been found active at a daily dose of 180 mg [276, 605, 1843], particularly when it is administered over a period of at least 3 months [649]. The same goes for double-blind experiments [937]. CLOAREC reported on 148 patients who were followed up for five years [2d]. Although no details are given, Segontin 60 at a daily dose ranging from 120 to 180 mg is considered as being one of the most beneficial drugs for the treatment of angina.

After being used by the medical profession for more than a decade, it seems reasonable to admit that the advantages of Segontin are not particularly outstanding. This is the conclusion reached in a clinical investigation carried out under double-blind conditions [885][1].

Amplivix

Answering to the formula:

and dating from 1958, Amplivix (Cardivix, Retrangor, Algocor[2]; generic name: benziodarone) is a coronarodilator substance. From communications which cover research into its pharmacological properties [296, 297, 298, 299, 300, 301, 302, 319], it can be considered as being both of the benign and malignant type, *at least as far as animals are concerned*. In fact it depends on the dose, as will be seen from the experimental data in Table 6 which refer to the changes in coronary arterial flow and myocardial oxygen consumption observed in a chloralosed dog following intravenous administration [303].

---

1 The Russian equivalent of Segontin, known as Diphryl, was used successfully [680].
2 Other synonym: Coronal.

At the dose of 2—3 mg/kg, coronary arterial flow increases, whereas myocardial oxygen consumption is only slightly augmented so that the coronary effect is of the benign type. At higher doses, 5 and 10 mg/kg, the rise in coronary flow is accentuated and is extended, but then myocardial oxygen consumption increases

Table 6

Number of dogs	Dose (mg/kg)	Increase (%) in coronary arterial flow	Increase (%) in myocardial oxygen consumption, after:		
			2 min	10 min	15 min
5	2.5	40	17	8.8	—
6	5	72	45	22	21
4	10	100	61.7	85.2	—

to a marked extent and the oxygen content of the coronary venous blood decreases [303], a fact which has been confirmed by HEISTRACHER et al. [800] and by HIRCHE and SCHOLTHOLT [838], whereas DUCHENE-MARULLAZ [455] finds on the contrary enrichment in oxygen of the coronary venous blood. Under these conditions, the effect is of the malignant type. Two additional proofs are the appearance of an increase in body temperature in dogs [303, 838] and in cats [813], and the fact that, *in vitro*, Amplivix is an uncoupling agent for the oxydative phosphorylations [406, 411].

It must however be emphasised that, whatever the potential drawbacks of Amplivix in the case of animals, at doses of 10 mg/kg and over administered intravenously, the uncoupling phenomena do not occur in man, even under conditions of exceptionally high dosages administered orally or intravenously. For instance, metabolism and body temperature are not altered, even with chronic treatment at comparatively high dosages and following intravenous injection [125]. The reasons for the different behaviour of humans and animals are not known. Furthermore, in spite of the drop in the rate of fixation of I^{131} on the thyroid, which incidentally is reversible after cessation of the treatment, no sign of thyroid dysfunctioning has been observed either in man [126] or in animals [408].

The increase in coronary flow which occurs with Amplivix has been confirmed in dogs [455] and again found in cats [155] and rabbits [1278].

The effect of Amplivix on the coronary vascular bed is fairly preferential, since the dilator action is considerably less or even non-existent in other vascular areas such as those of the skeletal muscle in dogs [208, 296, 301, 1720] and cats [155], and the kidney and brain of cats [155].

Amplivix also makes a favourable change in the symptoms of myocardial ischaemia under various experimental conditions, because:

— It counters the appearance of impairments in the T-wave and the S-T segment of the ECG which reflect the hypoxia due to the coronary spasm occurring after the injection of pituitrine [301];

— In the anaesthetized dog and rat, it causes the electrocardiogram to return to normal when it showed the inversion of the T wave produced by generalized hypoxia due to the inhalation of a low-oxygen atmosphere [319];

— In the heart of the dog, subjected to high ligature of the anterior interventricular coronary artery in the manner described by BECK and LEIGHNINGER [116], Amplivix produces definite improvement in the normal evolution of the ischaemic zone, as it abolishes the electrocardiographic changes that follow this ligation;

— In the dog having an acute experimental infarction produced by ligation of the anterior descending coronary artery, Amplivix increases by 30—50% the blood flow in the infarcted area and in the normal zones as well [1072, 1073];

— Amplivix antagonises the coronary spasm produced in the isolated rabbit heart by two musculotropic coronary vaso-constrictor substances, pituitrine and barium chloride [296].

The aggregate of the pharmacological properties of Amplivix has encouraged various clinicians to undertake investigations on its therapeutic effects in angina pectoris. In 180 patients with anginal syndrome of proved coronary origin, Amplivix when given in an average daily dose of 400—600 mg had a very favourable effect in almost 75% of cases evidenced by spectacular reduction in the frequency of the attacks of pain, with their disappearance in almost 20% of cases [663]. Of these patients 140 had been under observation for at least 2 years before the start of the treatment and had not derived any appreciable benefit from the usual drugs in common use at that time. In 1960, GILLOT [664] had extended his clinical study to 420 cases and reported on beneficial effects which were in accordance with his previous findings.

The effectiveness of Amplivix, its complete harmlessness and absence of undesirable effects led GILLOT to recommend this drug for the preventive treatment of the anginal attacks.

BEKAERT and AUBERT [124] have obtained identical results in 100 patients with angina pectoris, selected on the same aetiological criteria as those selected by GILLOT.

Very good therapeutic results have also been reported by DAILHEU-GEOFFROY and NATAF [382, 384, 385] in about a hundred patients; of these, a large number showed an improvement in electrocardiograph ischaemia patterns.

Another clinical survey is by VASTESAEGER et al. [1929, 1930]: whilst achieving with 120 angina subjects excellent subjective therapeutic results comparable to those of the above authors, these clinicians also provide arguments, based on various cardiovascular examinations, in favour of a specific coronaro-dilator action. They confirm the absence of any undesirable reaction, whether on the digestive system or on various biological constants such as prothrombine levels, cholesterol levels and blood urea.

The efficacy of Amplivix in coronary pain conditions is likewise beyond doubt in the opinion of other clinicians [426, 1292, 1937].

Although its antianginal effect has been denied by certain British authors [425, 1642], especially under double-blind conditions (see later), other clinicians, who investigated Amplivix following publication of the negative results reported by the British authors, claim that this drug is effective as a preventive treatment against anginal attacks [313, 897, 1998], and some consider it as being very effective, by intravenous injection, in the treatment of cardiac pain in particularly painful cases of acute infarction [1260, 1285]. Others again [425], although convinced of its inefficacy when taken orally, even go so far as to consider the intravenous injection of Amplivix as being as effective as taking nitroglycerin or inhaling amyl nitrite, because in 13 out of 18 cases they found that angina attacks in the recumbent position were relieved within 5 min and for an average of 30 min.

As regards the effect of Amplivix on the objective clinical symptoms of effort tests on angina pectoris subjects, one survey shows that it improves the electrocardiograph indications of ischaemia emerging during the monitored hypoxia test [1926].

Other favourable clinical reports are those by MULLER and STRASSBURG [1327] with 80% success in 142 subjects, THIERFELDER [1885] also with 80% success on

70 patients (36% of whom were freed from pain completely), GRUND and WURZ-
BACH [749] with 76% of 103 patients, MARION et al. [1220] who report an interesting functional improvement in two-thirds of cases involving 100 patients,
KLICH [997] with 73% favourable effects with 69 patients, and MALTEZ and
BORGES [1753] in 13 out of 18 cases. On the other hand, JORIS and SCHMETZ [909]
consider that Amplivix is no better than ordinary drugs in use after tests with
58 patients.

Eight clinical tests have been carried out double-blind on Amplivix. Three are
favourable, the other five unfavourable. With 41 patients, HOUTSMULLER [862]
considers that the effect of the drug far exceeds that of the placebo. In the case of
TODESCO and PERMUTTI [1893], Amplivix proved statistically effective in 50
patients, particularly as regards the frequency of angina attacks. The same goes
for JOHNSEN [901] with 21 subjects. On the other hand, five experimenters find
that Amplivix is no better than the placebo: KLOSTER [1001] on seven patients,
BREDMOSE [216] on 14 patients, SANDLER et al. [1642] on 12 angina subjects,
DEWAR and NEWELL [425] on 22 subjects and DAVIES et al. [392] on 36 patients.

Although initial clinical reports [124, 663, 1929] stress the innocuous nature of
Amplivix and above all the rarity of undesirable effects, including dyspeptic
incidence which some authors report as occurring only in 5% of cases [909], and
others 3% [1220], whilst yet others report it as non-existent [997], it is an undoubted fact that with the more widespread use by medical practitioners, the frequency
of digestive disorders (especially diarrhoea) has increased to the extent of representing too high a proportion of cases. More than the features of its therapeutic effect,
the too high frequency of this side effect was the reason for a comparative disaffection of the medical profession to Amplivix. To this must be added the fact that
the antianginal effects cannot be qualified as outstanding, and that many practitioners have given preference over it to other antianginal medications which,
whilst not necessarily being more effective, have the advantage of not causing
digestive upsets.

A further side effect which could possibly be attributed to Amplivix has been
studied by several clinicians. Although the medication can cause a drop in prothrombine rate in certain patients undergoing anticoagulant treatment [124], DAVIES et al.
[392] experienced no difficulty in controlling the dosage of the anticoagulant.
MULLER and STRASSBURG [1327] also report that Amplivix does not modify the effect
of anticoagulants. On the other hand, HOUTSMULLER [862] finds an extension in
the prothrombine time in patients already being treated with anticoagulants, but
adjustment of the anticoagulant doses to a lower level presented no difficulty.
According to PYÖRÄLÄ et al. [1476] who carried out special research into this
question, the anticoagulant effect of certain drugs was not altered by Amplivix,
including that of Dicoumarol and of phenylindanedione, whilst that of other
anticoagulants was considerably potentialised, with particular reference to
warfarin whose posology had to be reduced by 46% to maintain the prothromine
rate. Investigation of the various factors in coagulation showed them that Amplivix causes depression of prothrombine and of factors VII and X.

In view of the fact that because of the presence in its molecule of two iodine
atoms Amplivix considerably decreases thyroid uptake of ^{131}I [126], the possibility
of functional depression of the thyroid has been looked into, but no case of hypothyroid condition has been reported with a specimen group of 180 patients [863]
or another of 100 patients [1220]. In addition, Amplivix is practically entirely
eliminated by the body, and during transit does not give off iodine, or at least not
to such an extent as other iodinated substances [126]. Also, although Amplivix
decreases thyroid uptake of tracer doses of ^{131}I [126], temporary disturbance in

thyroid tests is not accompanied by clinical manifestations of thyroid hypo-
activity, nor by its biological symptoms. Thus it is that neither the basal metabolism nor cholesterolaemia are altered over a series of more than 150 patients,
most of whom had been treated for more than 2 years at an average daily dose of
300 mg [125, 126].

To the picture of side effects must be added others, but their incidence is so
local that they must be taken with some reserves: facial and lower limb oedema in
Japan, and in England a suspected hepatic complication whose clinical symptomatology could not be definitely related to Amplivix, and no case of which has
been reported from Holland [863] or in any other country with a total figure of
over a million patients treated.

Over the past four years, Amplivix has found another clinical application by
reason of the remarkable hypouricaemic properties which it develops in man
[371, 403, 406, 407, 417, 640, 1525].

Isoptin

A german medication, known in Great Britain as Cordilox (generic names:
verapamil, iproveratril), Isoptin, answering to the formula:

$$CH_3O-\begin{array}{c}CH_3O\\\\\end{array}-\overset{\overset{CN}{|}}{\underset{\underset{CH_3\quad CH_3}{\diagdown}}{\overset{|}{\underset{CH}{C}}}}-(CH_2)_3-\overset{}{\underset{\underset{CH_3}{|}}{N}}-CH_2-CH_2-\begin{array}{c}OCH_3\\\\OCH_3\end{array}$$

develops pharmacological effects whose interpretation has given rise to exchanges
in which the various elements put forward and points of view expressed were
thoroughly supported by sound experimental data.

Two basic papers published in 1962 [759, 1672] show that Isoptin increases
coronary flow, stroke volume, cardiac output and heart rate in dogs. Blood
pressure drops to a marked degree. Myocardial oxygen consumption increases less
that myocardial flow, so that there is a rise in the oxygen content of the coronary
venous blood and coronary efficiency is improved. There is no inhibition of myocardial cell respiration [1672]. However, subsequent reports have shown that
Isoptin depresses the myocardium [133, 558] and so brings about a marked drop
in cardiac output [1559, 1892].

Other papers describe the effect of Isoptin on coronary circulation under
various experimental conditions.

For instance, SCHMALL and BETZ [1676] demonstrated the preferential nature
of the dilating effect as regards the myocardial vessels, blood flow scarcely changing at brain level or in the skeletal muscle, liver and kidney. Intracoronary
administration causes, in dogs, a drop in coronary resistance which is accompanied
by a rise in coronary flow during the two phases of cardiac contraction [1560]. It
has been suggested that the coronary dilator effect of Isoptin is due to a muscular
relaxation in consequence of alterations in electrolytic exchanges, notably an
increase in the potassium content of the myocardium [132c].

Fig. 7 provides an example, taken from our personal observations, of the
effect of Isoptin on the coronary circulation of an anaesthetised dog: at the dose
of 0.5 mg/kg administered intravenously, coronary arterial flow shows a marked
increase, return to normal taking place after some 15 min. Systemic blood pressure
drops considerably, and disturbances in heart rhythm, to which we shall be
referring later, occur as soon as the injection is finished.

According to certain authors [628], Isoptin only raises slightly and for a short time the circumflex coronary blood flow in the case of a dog whose anterior descending coronary artery has been occluded. In the case of a conscious dog, daily doses of 40—80 mg/kg administered in food over a period of several weeks have hardly any effect on coronary arterial flow [887].

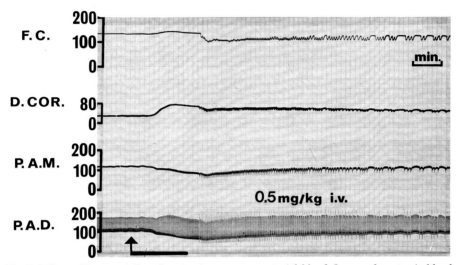

Fig. 7. Effect of iproveratril on heart rate, coronary arterial blood flow, and systemic blood pressure in the anaesthetized dog. From top to bottom: F.C.: Heart rate (beats/min). D.Cor.: Mean blood flow in the left circumflex coronary artery, measured with an electromagnetic probe (ml/min). P.A.M.: Mean blood pressure in the femoral artery (mm Hg). P.A.D.: Phasic blood pressure in the femoral artery (mm Hg). At signal mark: intravenous injection of iproveratril, 0.5 mg/kg

According to HAAS et al. [755, 757], Isoptin possesses inhibitory properties in respect of certain adrenergic β-receptors, notably in the heart: for instance, it counters the positive chronotropic and inotropic effects of adrenaline, and reduces the tachycardia induced by isoprenaline in an anaesthetised animal. According to the same authors, an adrenergic inhibiting effect also occurs with regard to the a-receptors, since there is found a reduction in hypertension due to sympathetic central stimulation obtained in a rat by the administration of physostigmine [757]. It cannot however be accepted that this latter pharmacological agent provides an exact parallel with pure stimulation of the a-adrenergic receptors [67].

This being so, HAAS et al. consider that Isoptin has a blocking action on the adrenergic β-receptors, as for instance with propranolol, although they admit in a subsequent paper [756] that it is not a question of a genuine blocking effect but a partial inhibition of those receptors. Even this latter opinion calls for serious qualification, for if we take account of other pharmacological reports published subsequently it is seen that there is no satisfactory experimental evidence that Isoptin has a β-blocking action on the heart which answers to the generally accepted criteria recently recalled by FITZGERALD [557], viz: (see also p. 205) — a) to develop total and competitive inhibition as regards the positive inotropic and chronotropic cardiac effects of the exogenous catecholamines, of isoprenaline, and of stimulation of the sympathetic cardiac nerves at dosages which do not exert a depressive action on the heart [15, 558, 1892]; and b) to have a high specificity character [502, 1319, 1362].

Incidentally, a thoroughly documented discussion has developed regarding the properties of Isoptin on the adrenergic β-system. It deserves close attention and can be summed up as follows. It is mainly aligned on the findings of MELVILLE's laboratory, i.e. that although Isoptin can in fact, as shown by HAAS [755], reduce the tachycardia induced by isoprenaline in an anaesthetised animal, this inhibitory effect can only be seen at large doses which depress the cardiac muscle [1270, 1277], unlike what occurs in the case of the true β-blocking agents. A comparable reduction in isoprenaline-induced tachycardia can also be observed in the case of procaineamide and pentobarbitone [133], substances which certainly cannot be considered as β-blocking agents. The same objection regarding abnormally high doses can be levelled at HEIM and WALTER [798], who mention an antagonistic action by Isoptin, at a dose of 35 mg/kg, in respect of tachycardia due to the freeing of catecholamines following asphyxia in mice.

We should also point out that, as regards animals, neither SCHMID and HANNA [1678] nor ROSS and JORGENSEN [1559] find any antagonistic effect as regards the tachycardic and hypotensive effects of isoprenaline.

According to GARVEY et al. [628], Isoptin does not affect the increase in the blood flow of the left circumflex coronary artery induced by isoprenaline in a dog whose anterior descending artery has been occluded. Finally, NAYLER et al. [1348] refuse to acknowledge in Isoptin any β-blocking properties because it maintains the tachycardia-inducing effect of isoprenaline in rabbits.

In the case of man, Isoptin is dissociated from the adrenergic β-blocking agents under various experimental conditions: a) No lessening of the tachycardia appearing during exercise or following the administration of isoprenaline has been observed in healthy volunteers after daily oral administration of Isoptin at therapeutic dosage, i.e. three times 80 mg [558, 559], a fact which is in striking contrast to propranolol for instance [710]; b) In the course of a double-blind test, no significant difference was found in heart rate as compared with the placebo [1359], whereas a β-blocking agent always lowers the heart rate; c) The intravenous injection of Isoptin always causes the heart rate of a man to speed up [1298], reported likewise in the case of animals [1672], which does not tie in with the β-blocking agent notion.

Whereas BATEMAN [102] tries to bring arguments to bear in favour of the β-blocking properties of Isoptin, taking as a basis pharmacological research by authors who have used very high dosages, FITZGERALD and BARRETT [559] quite rightly argue against him that certain of the investigations are wide open to criticism as regards the interpretation of the pharmacological facts. SHANKS [1728] for his part refutes BATEMAN's arguments on the basis of carefully documented facts. With GRANT and McDEVITT, SHANKS [710] provides a further demonstration of the difference as regards humans between Isoptin and propranolol in the sense that with healthy volunteers, Isoptin taken orally at therapeutic dosages does not modify the tachycardia which occurs during sustained physical exercise bringing the heart rate up to more than twice its resting value, or during intravenous infusion of isoprenaline, whereas in the same subjects these two forms of tachycardia are suppressed by a therapeutic dose of propranolol. The same inactivity of Isoptin vis-à-vis effort-induced tachycardia has been pointed out in connection with the angina subject by KALTENBACH and ZIMMERMAN [933].

There does not therefore appear to be any doubt regarding the fact that Isoptin is not a β-receptor blocking agent, both in the case of animals and man. The partial inhibition of these receptors noted in animals only occurs at high dosage, and it is the consequence of the highly cardio-depressive effect [558, 1661]. Two recent experimental investigations resulted in similar conclusions. CUNDEY et al. [73 c] showed that in the anaesthetised dog, continuous intravenous infusion of Isoptin increases heart rate, left ventricular work and contractility, and decreases total peripheral resistance and blood pressure. β-blockade did not modify these effects except for an absence of change in myocardial contractility. α-blockade did not prevent the peripheral vascular effects. Predominant effect of Isoptin is thus on smooth muscle, with little effect on adrenergic receptors. FERMOSO et al. [99 c] consider also that the haemodynamic actions of Isoptin are not related to β-adrenergic inhibition.

Incidentally, HAAS has recently admitted that Isoptin differs from the β-blocking agents, because it only antagonises the circulatory disturbances caused by the catecholamines at dosages which themselves bring about depression of the cardiovascular system [16 b][1]. It is this which explains the non-competitive nature of the incidence of Isoptin on the β-receptors [14 a]. The preventive action of Isoptin at high doses (50 mg/kg) against extensive disseminated myocardial necrosis which developed in rats after subcutaneous injections of isoprenaline [80 a] must be ascribed to calcium antagonism rather than to a β-antagonist effect. It has in fact been demonstrated that Isoptin blocks the rise in calcium uptake by the myocardium and the formation of myocardial necrosis induced by high doses of isoproterenol in rats [161 c].

Certain authors take the view that Isoptin is a blocking agent of the adrenergic α-receptors [45 a].

We have personally investigated a few cardiovascular effects of Isoptin.

Selecting in particular the test of tachycardia induced by the intravenous injection of isoprenaline, which by general consensus is still the most selective and most widely used pharmacological criterion for demonstrating blocking properties as regards the adrenergic β-receptors [15, 180, 1120, 1726, 1817], we carried out the following examinations on a dog which was anaesthetised with Nembutal and given atropine: the anti-adrenergic β-effect, the effect on heart rate and on blood pressure, and at the same time checked tolerance to i.v. injection. We give below the essential details of the facts noted.

In the case of a dog (Fig. 8), the intravenous injection of 1 mg/kg of Isoptin causes the heart rate to rise from 165 to 177 beats/min for 2 min. Subsequently, the heart rate returns to its initial level, then drops progressively, readings of 150, 125 and 100 beats/min being noted respectively 10, 90 and 180 min after the injection. The blood pressure, originally 155 mm Hg, is lowered by 55% after 3 min, then slowly rises to an average of 125 mm Hg. A considerable episodic extrasystolic phenomenon is observed. The tachycardia induced by isoprenaline is slightly attenuated at such time as blood pressure remains 30 mm Hg below its original level, i.e. after 10 min (end of the upper curve); but after 3 hours, at a time when blood pressure is back at its control level, the isoprenaline-induced tachycardia is not altered. A second injection of 1 mg/kg of Isoptin 3 hours after the first brings about a considerable drop in blood pressure with severe arrhythmia interspersed with phases of cardiac arrest lasting from 10—15 sec, the animal dying 20 min later.

With a second animal (Fig. 9), the phenomena are comparable. At the dose of 1 mg/kg of Isoptin, the heart rate speeds up at first by 7%, to decrease subsequently by 30% after 20 min (start of the lower trace). Blood pressure drops by over 50% immediately the injection is finished. There then occurs atrio-ventricular

---

1 In a recent paper, HAAS [133 c] further admits that there are important differences between Isoptin and propranolol as regards several modifications of myocardial metabolism which occur in the dog, rat and mouse following experimental cardiac hypoxia due to asphyxia and following administration of dibutyryl-3,5-AMP.

block, interspersed with short phases of cardiac arrest (end of upper trace). The tachycardia induced by isoprenaline is not affected during the 20 and 30 min following the injection (start of lower trace). A subsequent intravenous injection of 1 mg/kg of propranolol intensifies the bradycardia and, unlike what occurs in the case of Isoptin, cancels out the isoprenaline-induced tachycardia within 5 min.

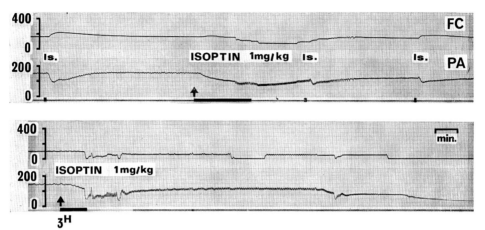

Fig. 8. Effect of iproveratril on heart rate and systemic blood pressure in the anaesthetized dog. F.C.: Heart rate (beats/min). P.A.: Mean blood pressure in the femoral artery (mm Hg). Upper traces: at signal mark, intravenous injection of iproveratril, 1 mg/kg. Lower traces (recorded 3 hours after the first injection): at signal mark, intravenous injection of iproveratril, 1 mg/kg. Is: Intravenous injections of isoprenaline, 0.002 mg/kg

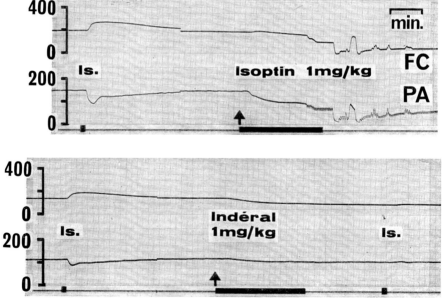

Fig. 9. Effect of iproveratril on heart rate and systemic blood pressure in the anaesthetized dog. F.C.: Heart rate (beats/min). P.A.: Mean blood pressure in the femoral artery (mm Hg). Upper traces: at signal mark, intravenous injection of iproveratril, 1 mg/kg. Lower traces: at signal mark, intravenous injection of propranolol, 1 mg/kg. Is: intravenous injections of isoprenaline, 0.002 mg/kg

The third animal (Fig. 10) is given 0.25 mg/kg of Isoptin: the heart rate shows no marked change, blood pressure drops slightly and the isoprenaline-induced tachycardia is attenuated by some 25% (end of upper trace). There follows a second injection of 0.5 mg/kg: the heart rate drops by 8%, the drop in blood pressure is accentuated, and the attenuation of the isoprenaline-induced tachycardia remains at 25%. Following a final injection of 1 mg/kg (not shown), the heart rate again drops by 10%; blood pressure is almost 50% lower; the isoprenaline-induced tachycardia still remains 25% less; there occurs arrhythmia, less serious than in the case of the first two animals.

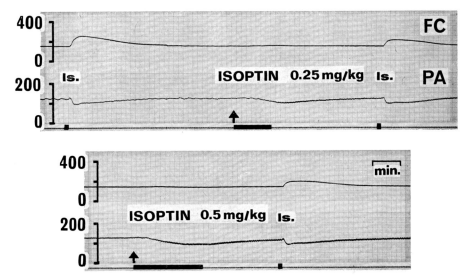

Fig. 10. Effect of iproveratril on heart rate and systemic blood pressure in the anaesthetized dog. F.C.: Heart rate (beats/min). P.A.: Mean blood pressure in the femoral artery (mm Hg). Upper traces: at signal mark, intravenous injection of iproveratril, 0.25 mg/kg. Lower traces (recorded immediately after the end of upper traces): at signal mark, intravenous injection of iproveratril, 0.5 mg/kg. Is: intravenous injections of isoprenaline, 0.002 mg/kg

Our findings agree in several respects with other reports:

1. At average doses, viz. 0.2—0.5 mg/kg, Isoptin does not block tachycardia triggered off by isoprenaline. It depresses it slightly at higher dosages, little more than 3—5 times the proved coronaro-dilator dose. This is in line with the facts described by FITZGERALD and BARRETT [558] who, in the case of a conscious dog, find no change in this tachycardia at doses of from 0.2 to 0.8 mg/kg. The slight β-inhibiting activity of Isoptin in dogs is associated with a considerable depression of the cardiovascular system, a fact which ties in exactly with the ideas put forward by NAYLER et al. [1348] and by SHANKS [1726] who, incidentally, does not find even this slight β-inhibition in the case of cats.

2. Isoptin speeds up and then considerably slows down the heart rate. The tachycardia-inducing effect has been found in conscious dogs at similar doses [558]. The delayed-action bradycardic effect is in line with the findings by SHANKS [1726] who states quite rightly that it is not clear what its mechanism is, since there is no attendant β-blocking effect.

3. The relatively high toxicity of Isoptin in intravenous injection agrees with the facts published by BENFEY [133] who registers the death of the animal at an

12*

intravenous infusion of 4 mg/kg, by FITZGERALD and BARRETT [558] who cause the death of 2 cats out of 3 with an intravenous infusion of 0.1 mg/kg/min, and by DUCHENE-MARULLAZ [456] who reports in all cases involving dogs serious cardiac arrhythmia leading to the death of an animal through heart failure at a dose of 0.25 mg/kg administered intravenously.

There is therefore no experimental evidence in papers by various researchers that Isoptin has a blocking action on the adrenergic β-receptors. On the other hand it is clear that this medication, at doses from three to five times higher than those which are coronaro-dilating, is capable of causing in animals considerable depression of the cardiovascular functions and of upsetting cardiac rhythm by inducing the emergence of polymorphous arrhythmia, found also in cats by FITZGERALD and BARRETT [558] and by BENFEY et al. [133].

A fairly unusual observation is reported by SCHMITT [1684] who shows that Isoptin can protect the myocardium of rabbits in a state of experimental renal hypertension against the muscle damage consequent upon chronic respiratory hypoxia. From the biochemical angle, it should be pointed out that according to FLECKENSTEIN et al. [562] Isoptin exerts a competitive blocking action on calcium movements, since reactivation of the use of phosphate by the cardiac muscle can be obtained by the intravenous injection of excess calcium. This property is held to be the cause of the cardio-depressive action of the drug [561, 563, 40a].

As regards human pharmacology, LUEBS et al. [1192], using an isotopic method, find following the administration of Isoptin an increase in coronary flow in the healthy subject, but not in the patient suffering from coronary heart disease. By means of cineangiography, MIGNAULT [1298] finds no change in coronary flow after intravenous injection of 5 mg of Isoptin either in the healthy subject or in the angina patient. According to BING et al. [2042], Isoptin lowers coronary flow in the atherosclerotic coronary subject.

The effect of Isoptin on the rhythmic nature of the heart contractions calls for a brief survey. It is not clear since, depending on the experimental conditions adopted, this substance appears capable both of disturbing the normal heart rhythm and antagonising existing arrhythmia.

FITZGERALD and BARRETT [558] briefly mention the appearance of cardiac irregularities in a cat which is given an intravenous infusion at a dose of 0.1 mg/kg/min. As far as we are concerned, in the case of the four anaesthetised dogs used, we found at doses from 0.2 — and particularly at 0.5 mg/kg — administered intravenously, disturbances in cardiac rhythm consisting of ventricular extrasystoles followed by atrio-ventricular block leading to bigeminal rhythm, culminating in complete cardiac arrest of an episodic nature lasting for over 15 sec and followed by resumption of contractions, usually with a bigeminal rhythm. DUCHENE-MARULLAZ also emphasises the consistent nature of the arrhythmia in dogs at the doses of 0.25 and 0.5 mg/kg administered intravenously [456].

In the case of humans, such disturbances in rhythm have never been reported with *oral* administration but have occurred following *intravenous* injection of 5 mg in 3 out of 10 angina patients, revealing an arrhythmia of the ventricular type [832].

Despite this potential for exerting a disturbing action on the regularity of cardiac contractions, Isoptin is capable of suppressing existing arrhythmia. For instance, it neutralises the extrasystolic manifestation brought on by adrenaline in the case of a cat given chloroform to inhale, and the arrhythmia occurring in guinea-pigs and rats following the administration of ouabaine and aconitine [758]. In the case of an anaesthetised dog, it eliminates the atrial and ventricular arrhythmia induced experimentally by ouabaine, acetylcholine and aconitine [1549]. It is interesting to find that the authors of these latter observations note, prior to the reversibility, a temporary period of marked impairment of atrio-ventricular conduction, a fact which is in line with that observed on a regular rhythm. They attribute the antiarrhythmic effect to a depression of automatism and of conduction. According to them, Isoptin exerts a quinidine-like effect on the rhythmic character of the cardiac contractions which is reinforced by a remarkable effect on atrioventricular conduction. They attribute the overall antiarrhythmic effect to depressive properties on the cardiac muscle, associated with local anaesthetic properties. The antiarrhythmic activity seems in fact to be due to general depression of myocardial excitability [125a].

NAYLER et al. [1348] show however that Isoptin does not counteract the ventricular extrasystoles and tachycardia induced by electrical stimulation of the stellate ganglion of a rabbit, whereas such arrhythmias are no longer found when the animal is previously treated with true β-blocking agents.

The antiarrhythmic effect of Isoptin also shows up under clinical conditions. BAROUSCH [90] notes that the oral or intravenous administration (5 or 10 mg per day) of Isoptin has a favourable action on various rhythm disturbances such as sinus tachycardia, isolated polymorphous extrasystoles and supraventricular paroxysmal tachycardia, atrial flutter and fibrillation. These findings have been confirmed at doses of 5 and 10 mg administered intravenously in cases of acute arrhythmia with tachycardia [898]. For others [16a], Isoptin (20 mg intravenously) is effective against supraventricular tachycardia and ventricular arrhythmia but has no effect on sinus tachycardia. WOEMEL [40b] considers that, in intravenous administration, Isoptin is quickly effective in various types of arrhythmia with tachycardia. Generally speaking, it merely requires the content of a single ampoule. The injection may be repeated 15 min afterwards. Tolerance is deemed to be excellent. At a dose of 5 or 10 mg intravenously, Isoptin suppressed supraventricular tachycardia in all 60 cases treated [99c]. On the other hand, Isoptin is ineffective, and even counter-indicated, in the case of branch block and atrio-ventricular block where there is feeble heart rate [90]. In the case of humans, Isoptin administered intravenously at the dose of 5—175 mg in 24 hours has no effect on atrial flutter [34a]. It should be mentioned that BAROUSCH finds no sign of arrhythmia in subjects with an even heart rhythm, which confirms the findings of FISCHER [555]. Isoptin was effective in a variety of tachycardias in children [151c].

The opinion of clinicians as regards the antianginal properties of Isoptin is far from unanimous. Several German publications report good effects in angina pectoris [428, 846, 1005, 1173, 1848, 1902]. Two other papers even speak of extraordinary results as regards the frequency of the beneficial effects occurring in almost 95% of cases [555, 847]. BENDA et al. [131] are likewise very satisfied with the use of the drug with 145 angina cases, achieving good and very good results in 72% of the cases. Results are slightly less satisfactory for GUADAGNO et al. [751]. WETTE [1981] for his part reports the disappearance of the electrocardiographic indications of ischaemia in 15 out of 19 patients after a treatment lasting several months. All these surveys were however carried out under uncontrolled conditions.

FISCHER [555] points out the almost immediate disappearance of acute cardiac pain following intravenous injection of Isoptin in the case of all angina subjects where this method of administration was used. HILLS and DOWNES [832] confirm this fact in 8 out of 10 of their patients.

Several double-blind investigations have been reported: NEUMANN and LUISADA [1359] mention a significant reduction in nitroglycerin intake in the case of 30 patients under Isoptin treatment, whilst ATTERHOG and PORJE [60] speak of improvement in the performance of coronary patients placed under treatment with the drug: one patient developed pulmonary oedema after 10 days. Cantor [275] concluded that there was significant improvement in three cases out of eight. According to Phear [1438], on the other hand, the therapeutic effect of Isoptin is no greater than that of the placebo, whilst Sandler [1641 and 279c] finds that at a daily dose of 360 mg there is a significant beneficial effect which can be compared to that provided by 300 mg of Inderal in the same patients.

In the light of all the pharmacological and clinical data at present available, certain British experts [330] consider that it has not been established that Isoptin deserves to be considered as a substitute for the existing β-blocking substances. In their opinion, there remains a doubt as to the efficacy and harmlessness of the medication. Thus they consider at the time (end 1967) that Isoptin cannot be recommended for the angina pectoris subject. Two years later [364] they still hold to their view despite the publication of the favourable clinical report by Sandler [1641] whose conclusions they cannot accept for obvious reasons.

Taluvian, which associates Isoptin with a cardiotonic glucoside, proscillaridine, is stated to give 95% satisfactory results with 105 patients suffering from coronary and cardiac insufficiency [2049]. This very favourable opinion is shared by Eisel and Kaiser [482]. Callsen [271] suggests treating subjects with coronary deficiency by first giving them 120—240 mg of Isoptin per day for from 10 to 14 days, followed by Taluvian at the same dose for 2 weeks.

Side Effects. We have stated earlier that certain clinicians, taking the basic view that Isoptin is a β-blocking agent, advise associating with it cardiotonics in the case of angina subjects displaying latent cardiac insufficiency, since β-blockade can aggravate cardiac deficiency. This opinion appears to be justified by the facts because Hills and Downes [832], using an intravenous injection of 5 mg of Isoptin administered over a period of 5 min to 10 angina patients, report 2 cases of cardiac failure of the congestive type occurring shortly after the injection. They consider that the cardiac risk can be as high as in the case of propranolol. Some clinicians therefore [1892], on observing other similar clinical complications, warn that Isoptin can precipitate or aggravate cardiac insufficiency. Likewise, Singh [114a] considers that Isoptin depresses the myocardium directly, and in this respect the drug appears to be more potent (and dangerous) than β-blocking agents in patients with myocardial disease. Considerable caution is required in the use of Isoptin for patients with cardiac disease, and until the indications for its use are better established it should not be recommended as an agent to be chosen in situations where β-blocking agents are counter-indicated [114a].

A further potential complication consists in cases of arrhythmia, although these have never been reported in humans as a result of oral treatment, but because they have occurred following the intravenous injection of 5 mg in 3 out of 10 patients [832]. This incidence is sufficiently high to urge the authors of these observations to advocate permanent monitoring by E.C.G. in the case of intravenous injection. However, the above-mentioned experts [1892] go even further and recommend that Isoptin should not be administered to human by intravenous injection.

A final important consideration needs mentioning. As pointed out by Wilkinson [2001], the opinion expressed by Bateman that "Isoptin can be administered without danger to patients for whom propranolol might be counter-indicated because of existing cardiac insufficiency" is not backed up by the clinical references which he quotes and which draw attention to the fact that "with patients suffering from circulatory deficiency, Isoptin should be given concurrently with cardiac glucosides since blockade of the β-receptors can aggravate cardiac insufficiency".

The concepts of β-blocking agent and safety as regards the cardiac function are in fact irreconcilable (see p. 43 and 229) and it is essential that those advocating Isoptin decide whether they consider this medication as a β-blocking agent, and accept not only its advantages but also its inevitable drawbacks, or whether it is not a β-antagonist and if so place it in another pharmacological category.

Persantine

Having proved itself to be the most active coronaro-dilator of twelve derivatives of pyrimido (5,4-d) pyrimidine [1281], Persantine (generic name: dipyridamole) or 2,6-bis (diethanolamino)-4,8-dipiperidino-pyrimido(5,4-d) pyrimidine was put onto the pharmaceutical market in 1959.

Persantine increases coronary flow in an anaesthetised dog and its activity is said to be twice that of papaverine and more long lasting, whilst at the same time being three times less potent as regards the peripheral vessels [924]. It slightly increases cardiac output and would not appear to alter myocardial oxygen consumption [924]. Using other methods for measuring coronary flow, GRABNER et al. [703] confirm these observations as to coronaro-dilating activity but note a slight drop in blood pressure and cardiac output, together with a marked reduction in stroke volume because of the tachycardia found. According to later papers [443], the increase in coronary arterial flow caused by Persantine is much greater than that due to papaverine; it is more persistent and more marked in a conscious animal than where there is anaesthesia. Coronary venous flow is considerably increased in dogs [487]. In the case of cats, myocardial flow (measured by calorimetric probe) increases by 118% with a dose of 0.25 mg/kg administered intravenously, at the same time as blood pressure drops moderately [154]. The vasodilator effect is said to be ten times greater as regards the coronaries than for the skeletal muscle vessels [154]. The harmful effect of severe experimental hyoxia on the electrocardiogram of an anaesthetised rat can be reduced or even eliminated by the drug [929].

From these initial pharmacological details, it is difficult to discern the mechanisms responsible for increasing the coronary flow: a direct coronaro-dilator effect appears certain, some modification of the extravascular support is undoubted [632], but it is impossible to say in what way it occurs; an effect on the energy-producing metabolism of the heart is possible [844]. For BRETSCHNEIDER et al. [227], the intervention of the extracoronary factors would appear to be negligible in view of the direct dilating effect.

There is no doubt whatsoever that Persantine is a long-acting coronaro-dilator [227, 924]. It considerably increases the oxygen content of the coronary venous blood [227, 703, 844, 1773, 1977], and has hardly any effect on cardiac output or on the work of the heart [227, 1977]. As for its effect on myocardial oxygen consumption, opinions vary: it appears to be positive for some [1976, 81a], nil for others [924, 1977] and negative for yet other observers.

These pharmacological properties, which achieve a considerable increase in the amount of oxygen supplied to the myocardium [1167], are such that Persantine can be considered as a benign type coronaro-dilator and that its combined qualities should suffice to make it effective for the sufferer from coronary insufficiency.

Since Persantine makes no change in the *collateral* blood flow at the far end from a chronic coronary occlusion in a dog [523], although it considerably increases the *total* coronary flow, FAM and MCGREGOR [522] show that the intravenous injection of a dog with Persantine acts in the opposite way to nitroglycerin, viz. it dilates primarily the small resistance pre-capillary arteries without changing the size of the conductance vessels (this latter fact is in line with the absence of coronary dilatation discernable by X-ray in man and animals, 1093). On the basis of this observation, they suggest that under the conditions of myocardial hypoxia, the ischaemic zone (where there is already maximum physiological dilation of the resistance vessels) is not irrigated any better since the vasodilator effect of Persantine can only be exerted on the resistance vessels of the non-ischaemic zones. Thus only the blood flow of the healthy part of the cardiac muscle would appear to increase, which, in the view of these authors, would explain the absence of antianginal effect in Persantine which they reported in clinical papers [1250. 1360].

The increase in coronary flow due to Persantine occurs in dogs along with a lessening of peripheral resistances, which is a sign of a specific coronaro-dilator action [134]. The fact that pre-treatment with reserpine does not alter the coronaro-dilator effect excludes the possible intervention of an adrenergic mechanism in this effect [1043]. However, phenoxybenzamine blocks the coronaro-dilator effect in the case of an isolated guinea-pig and rat heart [1351].

Persantine increases coronary flow without altering the myocardial oxygen consumption with a dog's heart-lung preparation [1754]. In the case of a conscious dog, it does not change coronary flow at the daily oral dose of 2.5 mg/kg, but considerably increases it at the dose of 40 mg/kg [887]. With a pig treated with 40 mg/kg/day for a week by oral administration, Persantine doubles the coronary flow without changing the nutritional circulation, the increase in blood flow taking place via the non-nutritional vessels [2017].

Following duodenal instillation in anaesthetised dogs at 5—20 mg/kg, Persantine produced a sustained rise in coronary flow and a decrease in arterio-venous oxygen difference [83a].

The effect of Persantine on the coronary irrigation of the animal has further been studied under very diverse special experimental conditions:

a) On dogs with chronic coronary insufficiency due to gradual arterial occlusion by means of a VINEBERG ring applied for a period of two months (66 animals), the intravenous injection of 0.25 mg/kg of Persantine increases coronary flow in every case, both at the infarcted myocardium and in the case of the normal muscle [926, 928], the increase being fifty per cent less in the ischaemic zone than in the normal zone.

b) Persantine increases the blood flow both as regards the acute infarct caused by the ligature of a coronary artery [981] and in the case of a dog suffering from experimental chronic insufficiency [1977]. As regards its effect on the vicarious collateral coronary circulation of a dog suffering from chronic insufficiency, it would appear to be favourable in the eyes of certain authors [1261, 1942] and nil for others [554].

c) In the case of dogs (40 animals) subjected to gradual coronary constriction by means of ameroid rings, one half of them treated with Persantine and the other half with a placebo [1090], complete acute ligature of the left coronary is carried out ten weeks later. The results show that half the animals treated with the placebo survive for over 30 min as compared with 5/7ths of the animals treated with Persantine. Furthermore, the intercoronary collateral coronary circulation is much better in the case of the treated animals than those which were given the placebo.

d) Administered at a daily dose of 150 mg over a period of several weeks, Persantine enables 83% of the 23 animals operated on to survive acute occlusion of the anterior descending coronary artery as against only 9% in the absence of treatment [1680 and 286c]. This would show that Persantine stimulates the formation of intercoronary collaterals to the point where acute occlusion remains without any untoward effect in 83% of cases[1].

e) When given orally for several months, Persantine encourages the development of intercoronary and intracoronary collateral circulation in pigs [766].

f) Oral administration of Persantine causes the dog to develop coronary collaterals whose extent depends primarily on the dosage, being optimum at the dose of 2—3 mg/kg three times a day [1262].

g) With a dog suffering from experimental infarction, Persantine injected intravenously at the dose of 0.5 mg/kg increases the anastomotic coronary flow with effect from 24 hours following the infarct, but in most cases after 48 hours [1506].

h) With a dog subjected to temporary occlusion of the largest collateral of the anterior coronary artery, Persantine injected intra-arterially or intravenously causes, and this despite a marked drop in blood pressure, almost maximum coronary dilatation whilst at the same time increasing the collateral flow [1143]; this latter phenomenon, according to the authors, reflects a genuine dilatation of the collateral vessels surrounding the ischaemic area.

i) In intramuscular injection at the daily dose of 4 mg/kg over a period of 4 months, Persantine increases collateral coronary circulation in rabbits [34b].

Amongst the most interesting studies as to the effect of Persantine on collateral coronary circulation, mention must be made of that by REES and REDDING [1509] who used a group of 10 dogs — 5 of them for control purposes and the other 5 being given 4 mg/kg of Persantine orally three times a day for 3 months. Following this treatment, the animals were anaesthetised and the measurement of coronary flow and oxygen content of the coronary venous blood indicates that these two parameters do not differ from one group to the other. But if acute ligature of the anterior coronary artery is applied, it is found that the collateral coronary blood flow in the treated group is 30% greater than that of the untreated group, and also that X-rays reveal the presence of a denser collateral network.

Investigations have been carried out into the mechanisms of the coronaro-dilator action of Persantine. BRETSCHNEIDER [222, 227] has demonstrated a specific pharmacological fact, namely that Persantine potentialises to a tremendous extent the coronaro-dilator effect of adenosine. The facts shown in Figs. 11 and 12 of our own documentation confirm BRETSCHNEIDER's findings. Figure 11 shows the coronaro-dilator effect of Persantine on two dogs, the upper part at a dose of 0.5 mg/kg and the lower 0.75 mg/kg. The increase in coronary flow is considerable and long-lasting, especially at the higher dose. Blood pressure is fairly markedly reduced, but this hypotension obviously has no harmful effect on coronary irrigation. Figure 12 gives an example of the potentialising of the coronaro-dilator effect of adenosine by Persantine. On the first graph there is shown the increase in coronary flow brought about by the intravenous injection of 0.6 mg/kg of adeno-

---

1 In rats, pretreatment with Persantine does not protect against ventricular fibrillation, size of the ischaemic area and mortality following experimental coronary occlusion [189c].

sine. A dose of 1 mg/kg of Persantine is then administered intravenously. The second graph shows the increase in coronary flow following a dose of adenosine which is ten times smaller than the previous dose, and this increase is very much

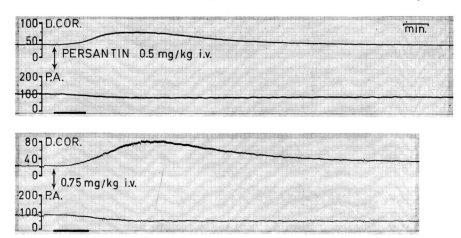

Fig. 11. Effect of dipyridamole on coronary arterial blood flow and systemic blood pressure in the anaesthetized dog. From top to bottom: D.Cor.: Mean blood flow in the left circumflex coronary artery, measured with an electromagnetic probe (ml/min). P.A.: Mean blood pressure in the femoral artery (mm Hg). Upper traces: at signal mark, intravenous injection of dipyridamole, 0.5 mg/kg in one dog. Lower traces: at signal mark, intravenous injection of dipyridamole, 0.75 mg/kg in another dog

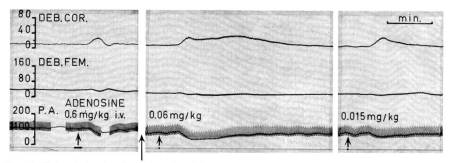

Fig. 12. Potentiation by dipyridamole of the action of adenosine on coronary blood flow in the anaesthetized dog. From top to bottom: D.Cor.: Mean blood flow in the left circumflex coronary artery, measured with an electromagnetic probe (ml/min). D.Fem.: Mean blood flow in the right femoral artery, measured with an electromagnetic probe (ml/min). P.A.: Phasic (and sometimes mean) blood pressure in the left femoral artery (mm Hg). Left tracing: intravenous injection of adenosine, 0.6 mg/kg. Between left and middle tracings: intravenous injection of dipyridamole, 1 mg/kg. Middle tracing: intravenous injection of adenosine, 0.06 mg/kg. Right tracing: intravenous injection of adenosine, 0.015 mg/kg

more marked. This potentialisation can be worked out, since we find in the third graph the increase in coronary flow caused by a dose of 0.015 mg/kg of adenosine; it is largely identical to that which occurs, before the administration of Persantine, at the dose of 0.6 mg/kg. Potentialisation is therefore equivalent to forty times, which is in line with the figures suggested by BRETSCHNEIDER[2].

---

2 There are animal species differences as regards the potentialisation of adenosine by Persantine (and also hexobendine) since the phenomenon was present in guinea-pigs but not in rats [185c].

In connection with the observations by BRETSCHNEIDER, AFONSO and O'BRIEN [12] show with an anaesthetised dog: a) that the combined intravenous infusion of doses of ATP and Persantine, which on their own do not change the coronary venous flow, increases this flow fivefold; b) that the dose of 0.5 mg/kg of Persantine administered intravenously increases the coronaro-dilator effect of ATP by from five to a hundred times depending on the cases; c) that the same dose of Persantine does not alter the coronaro-dilator effect of nitroglycerin, bradykinine and acetylcholine. Phenomenon b) is the result of a saving of adenosine in the blood and cells consequent upon a reduction by Persantine in the membrane permeability of the erythrocytes to adenosine [256, 1021, 1050, 188 c], which slows down the normal process of its destruction by intracellular deaminase [358]. Potentialisation vis-à-vis the coronaro-dilator effect of adenosine (and of ATP) is also found on the isolated heart of a cat [1813].

A further proof that Persantine acts on the metabolism of the nucleotides is provided by the fact that it considerably extends the duration of cardiac block induced by adenosine in a guinea-pig [1814] as also by adenylic acid and by ADP and ATP [1813]. An additional proof lies in the fact that it increases the adenosine and ATP content of the cardiac muscle, especially under the conditions of hypoxia [643, 844, 1751]. Persantine inhibits by 80% the degradation of adenosine nucleotides to inosine in the ischaemic myocardium of the dog by hindering the penetration of adenosine through intracellular membranes prior to its enzymatic deamination [190 c].

It has also been shown that Persantine inhibits the breakdown of adenosine in the blood [256, 1050] and in the cardiac muscle [643], and also that it exerts *in vitro* a competitive inhibitory action on the deaminase of adenosine [422], a fact which, in the view of the authors of these observations, supports the concept that the coronaro-dilator effect of the drug arises from the action of the endogenous adenosine accumulated in the myocardium. In this connection, we should point out that according to MIURA et al. [1302], the intracoronary injection of Persantine potentialises both the coronaro-dilator effect of adenosine (but not that of bradykinine and acetylcholine) and the level of reactive hyperaemia consequent on arterial occlusion.

It has also been shown that the potentialisation of the coronary dilating effect of adenosine by Persantine is attenuated or abolished by aminophylline in dose-dependent fashion [119 a]. In the same context, it must be pointed out that, when infused locally into the anterior descending coronary artery, Persantine considerably potentialised myocardial reactive hyperaemia induced by temporary occlusions. Increases were due to lengthening of hyperaemia duration while peak flow rates remained unchanged [12 a].

It may well be, therefore, that all the pharmacological effects of Persantine, and particularly its action on coronary circulation, arise from its capacity to allow the accumulation of adenosine or adenine nucleotides in the tissues or cells. For a series of pyrimidopyrimidine derivatives, including Persantine, there is a reasonable correlation between the rank orders of potency in potentiating heart block produced by adenosine in the guinea-pig and in eliciting coronary vasodilatation. Such facts are compatible with the concept that Persantine owe its coronary dilator activity to potentiation of endogenous adenosine [237 c].

At the moment, the opinion prevails that the inhibition of adenosine uptake is likely to be the most important pharmacological effect of Persantine [96 a]. Since Persantine reduces the uptake and inactivation of adenosine by the lung [1437], its potentialising effect could arise from a considerable accumulation of adenosine in the arterial blood. Persantine prevented the uptake of adenosine by the heart, lungs and the whole body, an effect which is thought to be more important than the adenosine-saving effect in the blood [2a]. PFLEGER et al. [21b, 30b] reported that when ^{14}C-labelled adenosine was added to the perfusion fluid of isolated guinea-pig hearts, there was a specific uptake by the heart cells which was powerfully inhibited by Persantine.

Experiments were performed to determine whether intravenously administered aminophylline inhibits the coronary vasodilating effects of intravenous or intracoronary administration of Persantine or adenosine and whether aminophylline locally administered in the coronary artery inhibits the vasodilating action of adenosine given intravenously or injected into the coronary artery [5c]. Intravenous aminophylline was found to inhibit coronary vasodilatation induced by intravenous or intracoronary Persantine or adenosine. Aminophylline injected locally into the coronary artery was also effective in inhibiting coronary vasodilatation induced by intravenous and intracoronary adenosine. The mechanism of this inhibitory phenomenon has not been elucidated. It was also found that aminophylline does not influence coronary vasodilatation induced by nitroglycerin and acetylcholine and thus it seems that the interaction between aminophylline and adenosine or Persantine is a selective one. On the basis of this observation, a likely suggestion is that aminophylline acts on the smooth muscle of the coronary vascular bed to antagonize the action of adenosine at this site.

On in vitro preparations of cat papillary and left atrial muscles, Persantine had no effect on the oxygen consumption of resting muscles, but increased both the contractility and the oxygen consumption of electrically stimulated muscle, the increase in contractility occurring before oxygen consumption changed. Persantine did not alter the tissue content of either glycogen or energy-rich phosphate compounds [139a]. From these data, it was concluded that the increase in oxygen consumption following Persantine is a consequence of the increased contractility, and furthermore that the drug increases contractility through an adrenergic mechanism, since β-adrenergic blocking drug and reserpine pretreatment were found to block the inotropic effect of Persantine.

The pharmacological effects of Persantine have also been examined in humans. In the case of the subject free from cardiovascular disease, it is generally accepted that Persantine raises the coronary flow [436, 1976]. As regards its effect on myocardial oxygen consumption, this would appear more debatable, being positive according to some [1976, 81a] and zero to others [436, 1582].

When injected intravenously at the high dosage of 150 mg, Persantine increases coronary flow and the oxygen content of the coronary venous blood in the normal subject and in the angina patient. The same dose administered orally provides identical results, but these are less consistent and less pronounced [436]. This oxygen-enriching of the coronary venous blood also occurs at the dose of 20 mg administered intravenously [436, 1693], whereas it is markedly less or imperceptible at 10 mg [827], which leads the authors to recommend, in the case of i.v. administration, a higher dose than that which is normally used. This is also the view of KUBLER et al. [1051] who, after making comparative studies both with dogs and humans as to the distribution of Persantine between the plasma and the myocardial cell, consider that the normal dose should be trebled for intravenous administration in order to ensure in human subjects a coronary-dilating effect comparable to that found with dogs. In point of fact, extremely high dosages of Persantine (2 mg/kg/hour as an intravenous infusion) resulted, in the case of normal subjects, in an average maximal increase of 340% in coronary blood flow and 250% in patients with coronary sclerosis [35a].

A double-blind investigation carried out on a group of old people treated for more than three years has made it possible, by examining post-mortem coronaro-angiograms to detect a highly significant difference as regards the development of collateral intercoronary circulation and as regards mortality as a result of acute coronary occlusion [1542]. Following 6 months continuous treatment by oral administration, coronarography shows the increase in collateral circulation[464].

In 6 healthy subjects and 10 with heart disease, an intravenous infusion of 150 mg of Persantine for one hour decreases the part played by lactate in the oxydative metabolism of the heart, but increases that of the free fatty acids [974], without any disturbance of cardiac metabolism [975], which confirms similar findings at lower dosages [1582].

From the therapeutic angle, the first publications relative to the antianginal effect of Persantine were, as is usual, extremely favourable [283, 374, 335, 554, 773, 774, 776, 921, 1358, 1807, 2025]. Then several subsequent investigations cast doubts on this beneficial effect, whether on the frequency of angina attacks, on tolerance to exercise, or on electrocardiographic tests [401, 986, 1250, 1428, 1773, 2051].

Various clinicians concluded that Persantine was ineffective when tested under double-blind conditions [401, 572]. In 1964, the American Council on Drugs stated that additional clinical investigations were needed to determine whether or not Persantine is effective for sufferers from angina pectoris [891]. But later research did not clarify the problem. Indeed, an investigation carried out on patients treated for more than a year led its authors to consider the antianginal effect of Persantine as being very relative [1360]. FISCH [551] places its activity on a level with that of the placebo. SBAR and SCHLANT [1647], using the high daily dose of 150 mg divided into six separate intakes over a period of 6 months with 23 patients, and comparing results with those obtained with the placebo on 24 patients, consider that there is no statistical difference between the effects of the two treatments. BECKER [118] and others [653, 1731, 1971] consider, however, that the results by SBAR cannot be qualified as negative, but rather as being an inadequate investigation for the objective aimed at, and that it does not lend itself to a statistical conclusion. According to FRIEDEMANN [600] who uses the very high dosage of 300 mg in three separate doses, Persantine provides in 30 angina patients favourable results which differ statistically from those obtained with the placebo. They could be subsequently maintained at a reduced posology. IGLOE [18b] also stresses the need for a high dosage and an adequate length of treatment. Thus the average administration for 20 weeks of a daily dose of 200 mg enables him to conclude in favour of Persantine following a double-blind investigation carried out on 48 patients: marked clinical improvement is reflected in a considerable reduction in the number of angina attacks and nitroglycerin requirements and in a significant increase in tolerance to effort.

In spite of this diversity of opinions, there is still no doubt that Persantine is often used by the practitioner for the prophylactic treatment of angina attacks.

Posology has recently been increased by the appearance of a "strong" form, the tablets containing 75 mg of active substance instead of 25 mg, but it seems that the frequency and severity of the side effects have greatly increased [1018, 1289].

In acute myocardial infarct, Persantine administered from the day of admission to hospital and for a period of four weeks, at the daily dosage of 400 mg, has no beneficial effect and does not alter normal mortality rates, according to a double-blind check made on 120 patients [636].

Persantine has been associated, at the rate of 25 mg per pill, with 20 mg of Adumbran (tranquilliser) to produce Persumbran. This has formed the subject of several particularly eulogistic clinical reports. ALGAN and KIELE [20] report over 90% favourable cases with 227 patients suffering from coronary insufficiency treated with 2—3 pills a day. HIRSCH and WOSCHEE [840] obtain 81% positive results with 169 angina subjects treated with 2—6 pills a day. The same dosage achieves 79% favourable results for KANDZIORA [934] and KLEVER [996], and 75% for DORNAUS [442]. HEHENKAMP [142c] obtained also satisfactory results in a group of 96 patients with clinical signs of coronary failure who were treated over a period of 18 months. With the exception of two patients who complained of giddiness necessitating drug withdrawal after a fortnight of treatment, the medication was on the whole well tolerated.

Intensaine

$$C_2H_5-COO-CH_2-O \underset{\text{with } CH_3, CH_2-CH_2-N(C_2H_5)_2}{}$$

Intensaine (generic names: carbochromene, chromonar) has a coronary-dilating effect on dogs with doses of from 1 mg/kg administered intravenously [1369]. This activity is considerable and of particularly long duration [531, 1369, 1577]. Intensity and duration of rise in coronary flow increases with the doses up to a certain limit, after which a drop in blood pressure is liable to limit to some extent myocardial hyperirrigation.

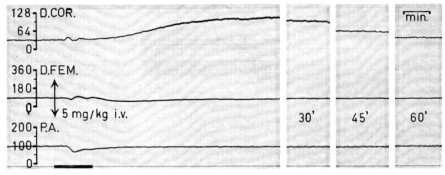

Fig. 13. Effect of carbochromen on coronary arterial blood flow, femoral arterial blood flow and systemic blood pressure in the anaesthetized dog. From top to bottom: D. Cor.: Mean blood flow in the left circumflex coronary artery, measured with an electromagnetic probe (ml/min). D.Fem.: Mean blood flow in the right femoral artery, measured with an electromagnetic probe (ml/min). P.A.: Mean blood pressure in the left femoral artery (mm Hg). At signal mark: intravenous injection of carbochromen, 5 mg/kg. Parts of tracings recorded successively 30—45 and 60 min after injection

Figure 13 shows that at the dose of 5 mg/kg i.v., coronary flow quadruples after 5 min, to drop back very slowly to its initial level which it does not reach even after an hour. At this time, blood pressure remains 20% lower. It is also seen that there is hardly any effect on peripheral circulation, which confirms reports by NITZ [1369]. LOCHNER and HIRCHE [1164] round off the spectrum of the haemodynamic effects by showing that neither the heart rate, nor cardiac output nor the work of the heart are altered and that the oxygen content of the coronary venous blood increases. Oxygen enrichment of the coronary venous blood has also been reported by other authors [531, 1370, 1577, 1691]. Since in the course of experiments by LOCHNER the coronary arterio-venous oxygen difference decreases as myocardial flow increases, it can be deduced that oxygen consumption by the cardiac muscle, although it was not measured, does not change to any significant degree under the effect of Intensaine [226, 1164], a fact which has indeed been subsequently proved [530, 531, 1577].

FAUCON et al. [529] report that a slow and continuous intravenous infusion of Intensaine in a dog results in a considerable and lasting increase in coronary irrigation but at the cost of sub-toxic effects which, after a dose of 30 mg/kg administered in 3 hours, are reflected in tachycardia, hypotension and marked depression of the cardiac function [530].

According to GRAYSON et al. [714], Intensaine is capable of raising the blood flow in the ventricular apex previously rendered ischaemic by acute ligature of the anterior interventricular coronary artery of an anaesthetised dog.

In the case of conscious dogs, the oral administration of daily doses of Intensaine has no effect on coronary flow at doses less than 40—80 mg/kg; it is only at this considerable dosage that flow increases, but to minor extents [887]. These findings may be grouped with the observations of LORENZ et al. [83a] showing that after duodenal instillation in anaesthetised dogs at 5—20 mg/kg, Intensaine did not modify coronary flow or arterio-venous oxygen difference. Intensaine appears to be rapidly hydrolysed in the liver, and the acid being tested in dogs had no coronary action. The therapeutic effect found in the drug must therefore depend on other mechanisms.

The possibility of an effect of the oxidative phosphorylations-uncoupling type or that of cellular respiratory inhibition at the myocardium has been excluded [226, 1164]. It should also be pointed out that Intensaine increases tolerance to anoxia in a rat's heart-lung preparation [1056], and that when administered chronically, it induces the development of a collateral coronary circulation which is sufficiently effective to alleviate the consequence of acute coronary constriction [1370, 1371].

Speaking fundamentally, it is especially interesting to analyse other reports tackling the investigation into the action mechanisms of Intensaine. An initial concept is that it does not potentialise the coronary-dilating effect of adenosine [226, 1694]. Furthermore, its coronary-dilating effect is not changed either by reserpine [1043] or by blockade of the adrenergic β-receptors [267].

BRETSCHNEIDER and colleagues [226] believe that the effect of Intensaine calls for the intervention of a "sympathine" specific to the coronaries, whose metabolic degradation could be slowed up or fixation on the receptors prolonged. This "sympathine" could be isopropylnoradrenaline and might be released physiologically by the adenosine leaving the myocardial cells.

This hypothesis appears acceptable at first sight, since isopropylnoradrenaline, a stimulant of the adrenergic β-receptors, is a direct-acting coronary-dilating substance, because the increase in blood flow which it brings about is not due to additional myocardial oxygen demands [837, 1087]. However, HIRCHE [837] throws some doubt on the hypothesis of any intervention by the β-adrenergic system in the metabolic regulation of the coronary circulation, since the placing of these receptors out of action by a β-antagonist agent does away with the coronary-dilating effect of isopropylnoradrenaline but does not alter that of adenosine. Moreover, Intensaine probably does not act through this mechanism because its coronary effect is not modified by blockade of the β-receptors [267].

A further effect, examined *in vitro*, consists in a reduction in the break-down of the 3′, 5′-adenosine monophosphate [1697] by competitive inhibition of phospho-diesterase similar to that caused by theophylline [1372].

Intensaine thus attacks the adenylcyclase system: it does not affect the synthesis of 3′, 5′ AMP but it does affect its degradation, which is slowed up by inhibition of phosphodiesterase. This latter effect naturally entails the enriching of the tissues in 3′, 5′ AMP, which according to the authors [1697] would provide a biochemical explanation of the sensitisation which Intensaine brings to bear on the coronary-dilating effect of isoprenaline observed in various investigations [226, 1369].

In the case of man, Intensaine has been the subject of haemodynamic research on healthy patients and on patients suffering from coronary heart disease [1446]: when injected intravenously, it does not modify blood pressure nor affect the heart rate; cardiac output increases to a moderate extent. Oxygen consumption by the cardiac muscle does not vary, and there is no sign of any effect of the type which causes hypoxia or uncouples the oxidative phosphorylations [1583].

Intensaine increases coronary flow in the normal man but not in the patient suffering from coronary atherosclerosis [1192]. BING et al. [2042] show by an accurate method of measuring coronary flow that this is reduced in the coronary patient when Intensaine is administered.

In the case of an angina subject treated orally for 6 months, the coronarography showed an increase in collateral circulation [464].

From the clinical viewpoint, reports are in favour of there being a satisfactory antianginal effect. This is the opinion of MAASSEN [1200] in a limited survey, of KLIGGE [998] over a larger number of cases, and of ASCHENBECK [57] and FRIESE [603].

Two investigations by FIEGEL et al. [543, 544] carried out on over 500 coronary subjects enabled them to set the optimal dose at 3 times 2×75 mg tablets a day. According to GILLE and RAUSCH also [661], posology should be high and treatment prolonged, failing which there is inadequate therapeutic effect. No major side-effect has been reported [1920] except by BELL et al. [127] who speak of the appearance of arthralgia which can sometimes compel the patient to discontinue the treatment.

In a double-blind investigation, BELL et al. [127] consider that Intensaine is useful in angina pectoris since, as compared with the placebo, it significantly lessens the severity of attacks and increases *subjective* tolerance to exercise. They admit however that this is only a question of improvement in subjective para-meters, and that neither the number of attacks nor the number of times nitro-glycerin was taken were affected by the medication.

In another double-blind experiment, STORCK [1845] demonstrates that the effect of Intensaine considerably exceeds that of the placebo. He also reports the disappearance of the electrocardiographic indications of ischaemia during the Master test, this in 68% of cases after intravenous injection and in 80% of cases given prolonged oral treatment.

It would therefore seem that the efficacy of Intensaine as an antianginal medication is a genuine fact, although it does not appear to have any special advantage over the drugs in current use. This indeed is the impression gathered from several French clinical papers published altogether in a special issue of "Semaine des Hopitaux": in oral administration, favourable results range from 75% [325, 821] and 60% [252, 1157, 1442] without it being possible to exclude the part played by resting in bed [1157]; when administered intravenously, the immediate effect on the heart pain (infarct or angina pectoris) can be complete and final in 60% of cases [1407], in 44% [1205] or in 1 case in 10 only [1157]. Developments in the electrocardiogram would seem to be favourable in the majority of cases [1477]. The patient suffering from acute coronary insufficiency is stated to be dependent on the medication [294].

CONWAY et al. [360] were unable however to objectify the subjective beneficial effect of Intensaine on the angina subject: in a double-blind test, they show that intravenous injection of the dose of 40 mg which is subjectively effective in the case of other authors does not improve tolerance to exercise in any of the 14 patients treated. Along the same lines, HUNSCHA et al. [872] find no beneficial effect from an intravenous injection of 40 mg on the electrocardiograph indications of effort-induced cardiac ischaemia.

Quite recently, a special section of Arzneimittel Forschung (1970, 20, 3a, p. 421—470) was devoted entirely to reports on a symposium held in Moscow in November 1968 and whose subject was the application of Intensaine to the treatment of coronary diseases.

Most of the 19 papers presented concern clinical investigations of a therapeutic character carried out in the U.S.S.R. Since these investigations were made on different types of coronary subjects, with varied methods of administration and dosages, and widely differing durations of treatment, a systematic analysis of each paper would not seem to be indicated. We have felt it preferable to draw from them a few general ideas.

From the haemodynamic angle, HILGER et al. (p. 441)[1] show that in the case of heart patients who are not necessarily suffering from angina the intravenous injection of 80 mg Intensaine does not alter coronary flow. On the other hand, the intravenous injection of 200 mg over a period of 15 min doubles this flow. Neither heart rate nor blood pressure are altered. However, according to SAVENKOV et al. (p. 461), the low dose of 40 mg i. v. doubles coronary flow in a group of 43 angina patients.

From the therapeutic viewpoint proper, the combined ten papers presented covered about a thousand patients [we are not including the 500 patients of HAIAT (p. 465) since this is a question of clarification of investigations carried out in France which have been dealt with earlier]. The essential facts which emerge from these clinical reports are as follows:

1. All the authors consider that the effect of Intensaine on angina attacks is satisfactory and that this medication has a place as a long-term treatment for angina pectoris.

2. In severe cases of angina, it would seem that the most advantageous application of Intensaine consists in starting off with intravenous administration of 40 mg once or twice a day for 3—4 weeks, and then changing over to oral administration (FRIESE, p. 451).

3. In the acute phase of myocardial infarction, the intravenous injection of Intensaine at a dosage of 80—120 mg twice a day for the first ten days is very effective as regards cardiac pain and seems to improve the electrocardiograph signs (KIPSIDZE et al., p. 456). There is no drop in blood pressure providing the injection is made slowly.

4. When administered orally as a chronic treatment, Intensaine does not modify cardiac output in angina subjects (SAVENKOV et al., p. 461).

5. Stress is laid by several authors, notably RAJEVSKAJA and ERSOVA (p. 464), on the fact that the posology should be high and adapted to each case. The therapeutic effects achieved by oral administration are better at a high dosage, i.e.

---

1 The page numbers refer to the section of Arzneimittel Forschung in question.

450 mg per day. SAVENKOV et al. (p. 461) also show that the increase in coronary flow is considerably higher following a 3-week course of treatment at a daily dose of 450 mg than following a course of the same length at 225 mg.

It is probably in the light of these facts, and also with a view to reducing the number of doses taken by the patient, that the content of the tablets has recently been doubled, thus bringing it to 150 mg; this is the Intensaine 150 presentation.

There is a sedative form, Sedo-Intensaine (Intensaine in association with phenobarbitone), which does not achieve better clinical results than those of the non-sedative form [637].

A cardiotonic form, Intensaine-Lanicor (an association of Intensaine and digitoxine) has been investigated with 22 angina patients and 88 patients suffering both from coronary and cardiac insufficiency: the efficacy of this preparation was demonstrated in 86% of the cases [1822]. HOHENSTEIN [848] with 50 cases, and LORDICK [1177] with 197 patients arrive at an identical conclusion.

Recently, Intensaine has been associated with INPEA, a β-blocking drug (see p. 248), under the name of Beta-Intensaine 150, which contains 150 mg Intensaine, 100 mg INPEA and 10 mg hydroxyzine per capsule. Some theoretical considerations concerning this association can be found in a paper by DREBINGER [84c].

Ustimon

$$CH_3O-\underset{\underset{CH_3O}{|}}{\overset{\overset{CH_3O}{|}}{\bigcirc}}-\overset{O}{\overset{\|}{C}}-O-(CH_2)_3-\overset{CH_3}{\overset{|}{N}}-(CH_2)_2-\overset{CH_3}{\overset{|}{N}}-(CH_2)_3-O-\overset{O}{\overset{\|}{C}}-\underset{\underset{OCH_3}{}}{\overset{\overset{OCH_3}{}}{\bigcirc}}-OCH_3$$

A drug for treating angina, perfected in Austria, Ustimon or Reoxyl (generic name: hexobendine, hexabendin) increases the coronary blood flow in dogs whilst at the same time raising the oxygen content of the coronary venous blood and reducing correspondingly the coronary arterio-venous oxygen difference [802]. It increases the heart rate, raises cardiac output, and considerably increases the work done by the heart [1037, 1042]. Blood pressure is lowered. Since the increase in coronary blood flow is proportionally much greater than the increase in oxygen consumption, cardiac efficiency would appear to be increased [1042].

Despite the statement by the authors of these observations as to a specific action on the coronary vessels, the increase in heart work is certainly responsible in part for the myocardial hyperirrigation. In the case of rats [282], the drop in blood pressure is accompanied by a slowing up of the heart rate.

Our own experience (Fig. 14) would indicate that at the dose of 0.5 mg/kg administered intravenously, Ustimon increases considerably, and for over an hour, the coronary arterial flow of anaesthetised dogs, without any marked change taking place in blood pressure. The considerable and prolonged increase in the myocardial blood flow also occurs in cats with an intravenous dose of 0.25 mg/kg, which reduces at the same time the production of cardiac metabolic heat without affecting either blood pressure or cardiac contractility [1256]. At higher dosages, the drug lessens myocardial contractility, an effect which would appear to be the cause of the sustained hypotension observed [1256].

According to McINNES and PARRATT [1256], Ustimon does not however increase blood flow in the myocardial ischaemic zone experimentally induced in dogs. Since the oxygen content of the coronary venous blood simultaneously increases to a considerable extent, these authors consider that the blood flow is only increased in those zones of the myocardium not affected by the artificially induced ischaemia.

Following duodenal instillation in anaesthetised dogs at 5—20 mg/kg, Ustimon caused a sustained rise in coronary flow and a decrease in coronary arterio-venous oxygen difference [83a].

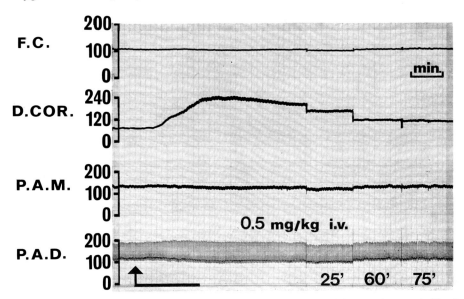

Fig. 14. Effect of hexobendine on heart rate, coronary arterial blood flow, and systemic blood pressure in the anaesthetized dog. From top to bottom: F.C.: Heart rate (beats/min). D.Cor.: Mean blood flow in the left circumflex coronary artery, measured with an electromagnetic probe (ml/min). P.A.M.: Mean blood pressure in the femoral artery (mm Hg). P.A.D.: Phasic blood pressure in the femoral artery (mm Hg). At signal mark: intravenous injection of hexobendine, 0.5 mg/kg. Parts of tracings recorded successively 25—60 and 75 min after injection

A fairly unexpected fact was the observance of an inversion of the arterio-venous difference in lactates in the coronary circulation, which would allow of the assumption that the limit had been reached of an effect of the cell respiration inhibiting type. In support of this idea there is also the fact that myocardial oxygen consumption drops considerably [1041] whereas a rise would be expected since the work of the heart increases.

Antifibrillatory properties have also been described [801] and antagonism with regard to the indications of hypoxia appearing on the electrocardiogram following the administration of vasopressine [247]; there has also been mentioned a dilating effect on the cerebral vessels, which would seem to be of secondary importance [801]. According to SCHMITT et al. [1685], Ustimon causes the development of collateral coronary circulation in rabbits provided it is administered for 8 weeks at a daily dose of 20 mg, a shorter treatment or one with a lower dosage having no effect. Using their observations as a basis, these authors recommend a considerable increase in the posology generally recommended for humans so as to ensure the setting up in the angina patient of a collateral circulation which, as shown by GIESE and MULLER-MOHNSSEN [656], enables the myocardium to remain functional where there is coronary stenosis and arterial obstruction.

From the biochemical angle, Ustimon retards the metabolic degradation of adenosine [1846], an effect which could explain the potentialisation of the coronary-dilating effect of adenosine reported by SPIECKERMANN et al. [119a]. Introduced

13*

by intraduodenal route in the anaesthetised dog, Ustimon enhances the coronary dilator action of adenosine administered by intravenous or intracoronary injection [262c].

According to PFLEGER et al. [30b], Ustimon strongly inhibits the specific uptake of adenosine by heart cells when ^{14}C-labelled adenosine was added to the perfusion fluid of isolated guinea-pig hearts. Furthermore, Ustimon causes a significant increase in ATP in the myocardium without changing the glycogen, lactate or pyruvate content, facts which are the opposite of those found where there is anoxia [1039]. These findings, according to the authors, would argue in favour of the intervention of an increase in ATP content in the coronary-dilating effect of the drug [1040]. According to KUKOVETZ et al. [73a], Ustimon owes its coronary-dilating effect to an intracellular accumulation of cyclic AMP, because it competitively inhibits the activity of phosphodiesterase of isolated coronary vessels in the same way as does papaverine (see p. 150).

The possibility of a dilating effect via the adrenergic system is excluded because the reduction in coronary arterio-venous oxygen difference caused by Ustimon is identical in a reserpine-treated dog and in a dog which has not been previously treated with reserpine [1043]. In the opinion of KRAUPP et al. [1036 and 261c] one of the factors in the reduction in coronary arterial resistance is primary metabolic acidosis which causes a change in the intracellular pH and tension of the CO_2. Similarly, the increase in coronary blood flow in man may be a consequence of metabolic acidosis [276c]. It has also been reported that Ustimon considerably reduces in animals the marked rise in plasmatic free fatty acids caused by the intravenous infusion of noradrenaline [1368].

In the case of humans free from coronary disease, HILGER et al. [826] consider, on the basis of observations made on 10 patients given an intravenous injection of 10 mg of Ustimon, that this drug ensures a marked but short-lived increase in coronary circulation, because they find a considerable but only temporary (15 min) rise in the oxygen content of the coronary venous blood, a fact which goes hand in hand with considerable, but also fleeting, increase in blood flow. They also find a speeding up of the heart rate by 13.5%. Rather high doses are necessary to attain an optimum increase in coronary blood flow in man [148c].

Still with normal men, Ustimon causes a rise in cardiac output and rate, and a reduction in peripheral vascular resistance [1194].

RUDOLPH and his colleagues published three interesting reports on the actions of Ustimon in man. The effects of the drug on coronary blood flow and oxygen uptake of the heart were studied with various modes of application and different dosages in a total of 54 patients with congenital and acquired heart disease [276c].

Following intravenous infusion of 10 and 15 μg/kg/min, the myocardial blood flow measured by means of the ^{133}Xe method showed a marked rise in all patients, the maximum recorded being 123%. Concomitantly, the myocardial oxygen consumption exhibited only minor alterations and the arterial oxygen content remained nearly constant, thus allowing also the assessment of the elevation in coronary blood flow from the coronary arterio-venous oxygen differences. The elevation of the coronary blood flow computed from changes in these differences rarely reached values beyond 100% when doses of 8 μg/kg/min were applied, but with higher doses of 10—15 and 19 μg/kg/min respectively, these values were regularly exceeded. This increase persisted throughout the entire period of infusion.

After single i.v. injections of Ustimon a mean rise in coronary blood flow of 37%, 110% and 128% was respectively observed for the doses of 0.085—0.15 and 0.2 mg/kg. This increase occurred within 3 min of the beginning of the injection and had almost completely ceased after 5 min.

Measurable rises in coronary blood flow were regularly accompanied by a decrease in the general vascular resistance which may lead to a fall in arterial blood pressure but was mostly compensated by an increase in heart rate. On the contrary, oral administration of Ustimon had no influence on the coronary arterio-venous oxygen differences, and thus had no effect on the coronary blood flow in spite of high doses and extensive premedication with the drug. Similar results were recorded either after application of the drug with stomach-resistant coating, or by duodenal or gastric tube instillation of the pure substance in solution. Following parenteral application of the drug many patients reported side effects, such as headache, dizziness, sensations of warmth and nausea. No physical discomfort was experienced after oral administration.

Comparison with experimental findings in animals showed good correlation with regard to the extent of the coronary-dilatory action of Ustimon following parenteral administration. However, the duration of action after injection of the drug was considerably shorter in man than in animal studies. This finding is probably attributable to different experimental conditions and to the differences in strength and rapidity of the plasma-protein bound of the drug in man and animal. In contrast to findings in animals, Ustimon given by oral route fails to influence the coronary and systemic circulations in human subjects, which may also be due to the inactivating mechanism mentioned.

In the second paper, the carbon dioxide content of the arterial and coronary venous blood, and the behaviour of the respiratory quotient were studied in the same patients following application of Ustimon in varied doses by infusion, intravenous injections, oral route and by gastric and duodenal instillation [274c]. The carbon dioxide concentrations in the arterial blood fell markedly within the first 5 min after injection and during the entire 1 h infusion. This finding is interpreted as an increased carbon dioxide expiratory elimination due to the formation of H^+ ions and CO_2 in the organism. The coronary venous blood also showed a decrease in carbon dioxide concentration. Therefore, a decrease in the coronary venous-arterial CO_2 differences was observed, which did not reach the values expected from the elevation of the coronary blood flow. This results in a distinct increase of the respiratory quotient during the first few minutes after the beginning of the injection, and pronounced deviations with a transitory tendency to rise during infusion. These findings may be attributed to enhanced myocardial CO_2 liberation under the influence of Ustimon supposedly originating from an increased intracellular acidity. After oral administration of the drug, the alterations of the respiratory quotient are within the usual ranges of variation.

In the third report, the metabolism of the human heart was studied in 11 patients following intravenous infusion of Ustimon in doses of 8—10 and 15 $\mu g/kg/$ min [275c]. A rise of myocardial glucose extraction occurs at the 30th min after the beginning of the infusion, particularly with higher doses. This leads to a considerable elevation of the oxygen extraction ratio and utilisation of glucose. In spite of a slightly raised glucose level in the arterial blood, there was also a rise of the percentual extraction. The degradation of glucose is presumably induced by an enhanced glycolysis probably due to activation of phosphofructokinase. Further anaerobic degradation appears to take place through reductive pyruvate carboxylation.

The myocardial lactate and pyruvate extraction and the oxygen extraction ratio are initially decreased, and this was ascribed to an enhanced glycolysis in the heart muscle with temporarily increased lactate formation. Later on, a rise of these values and of the lactate utilisation above control levels is observed, which can be explained essentially by an elevation of the arterial lactate concentration.

The myocardial extraction of the nonesterified fatty acids is relatively higher. The myocardial uptake of the ketone bodies β-hydroxybutyrate and acetoacetate as well as the arterial concentration of these substrates were not directly influenced. The oxygen extraction ratio of all the myocardial substrates rose above 100% during the administration of Ustimon. As the substrates taken up by the heart cannot be all oxydatively utilised, an anaerobic degradation offers a logical explanation for these biochemical findings.

In the case of men with symptoms of coronary disease, a 2-week course of treatment at a daily dose of 180 mg improves the hypoxia tests by an increase in myocardial blood supply [987].

Various unchecked experiments [1003, 1071, 1094, 1700, 1702, 1866, 2034] with Ustimon have concluded that there are favourable effects on the anginal subject. This opinion however calls for the test of time and confirmation of its accuracy by experiments of the double-blind type.

Ustimon has brought marked improvement to 80% of the 230 patients treated by three authors [120, 506, 2050] and 61% of the cases treated by another [811]. The antianginal effect appears to be very rapid [506, 2050]. The pathological E.C.G. is reported to be improved in 51% of the cases treated [811], and in 65% of cases according to others [506].

Ustimon is stated to increase significantly the favourable results provided by kinesitherapy for angina subjects [448]. It is also an excellent adjuvant to cardiotonic therapy by shortening the duration of insufficiency and allowing the dose of cardiotonics to be reduced.

Ustimon has satisfactory tolerance [448]. No allergic reaction has been found [120]. No side effects have been found on the haemogram and on the renal functions [120]. No potentialising of anti-coagulants has been reported [506].

Certain clinicians consider that Ustimon can also be very useful for treating cerebral circulation disorders [1440], as suggested by the speeding up of the blood flow observed in animals by KRAUPP et al. [1038], and which is said to be due to metabolic acidosis whose result is to lessen cerebral vascular resistance [102a].

Ildamen

Considered from the angle of its pharmacological effects, Ildamen is a hydroxyphenylisopropylamino-propiophenone whose suggested use in the treatment of angina pectoris might give rise to some astonishment. With a structure of the phenyl-ethylamine type, fairly closely resembling ephedrin (generic name: oxyfedrin), Ildamen in fact has the essential property of stimulating the β-adrenergic receptors, which should lead to an increase in myocardial oxygen needs, i.e. effects which are the very opposite of those looked for in the light of our existing pathophysiological concepts of coronary angina.

There is no doubt that Ildamen, which has a low toxicity level [760], does increase coronary flow in an isolated heart and in a dog in toto [1882]. This effect is shown on Fig. 15 drawn from our personal observations: coronary arterial flow increases appreciably for a relatively short time, whilst at the same time blood pressure shows a marked drop. But this increase in coronary flow is the direct consequence of the stimulating effects which Ildamen exerts on the heart and which are reflected in tachycardia (seen on the Fig.), a marked increase in cardiac output, increased heart work, and in consequence a rise in myocardial oxygen consumption. In other words, it is the increase in the heart's oxygen requirements which induces the myocardial hyper-irrigation. The evidence that it

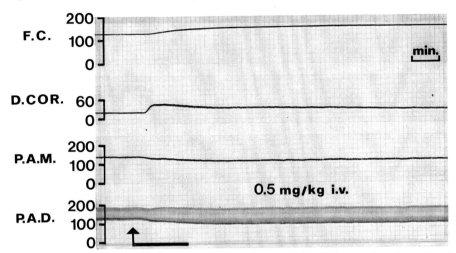

Fig. 15. Effect of oxyfedrin on heart rate, coronary arterial blood flow, and systemic blood pressure in the anaesthetized dog. From top to bottom: F.C.: Heart rate (beats/min). D.Cor.: Mean blood flow in the left circumflex coronary artery, measured with an electromagnetic probe (ml/min.). P.A.M.: Mean blood pressure in the femoral artery (mm Hg). P.A.D.: Phasic blood pressure in the femoral artery (mm Hg). At signal mark: intravenous injection of oxyfedrin, 0.5 mg/kg

is this mechanism which is involved, and also that the coronary blood flow does not entirely adapt itself to the extra work of the heart, lies in the fact that Ildamen lowers the oxygen content of the coronary venous blood [303]. This clearly shows that the limit of a hypoxia-inducing effect has been reached, the increase in myocardial oxygen needs exceeding the additional oxygen supplied to it by the arterial blood. It follows that, unlike the view taken by STERNITZKE [1837], the coronary reserve does not increase but in fact diminishes.

The coronary-dilating effect of Ildamen would appear to affect both the extramural vessels and the capillary vessels [762]. KUKOVETZ considers that this effect is papaverine-like because there is an inhibition of the activity of phosphodiesterase [191c]. Ildamen caused a 75% restitution of blood flow in the region of an experimental infarction resulting from ligation of a branch of the left coronary artery in dogs [135c].

STERNITZKE [299c] expresses the opinion that Ildamen is a β-stimulating agent because the increase in cardiac output and stroke volume which occurs after the administration of the drug does not appear when the animals are pretreated with propranolol. But Ildamen has no effect on the α-receptors and thus does not belong to the group of typical sympathicomimetics [300c]. It should also be noted that the inhibition of the effects of Ildamen provoked by β-blocking agents is not competitive [134c] whereas it is competitive in the case of isoprenaline.

From the biochemical viewpoint, Ildamen does not interfere with monoamine oxydase nor does it change the catecholamine content of the heart and the surrenal [1883]. The positive inotropic effect of Ildamen, which is related neither to that of the cardiotonic glucosides nor of the endogenous sympathicomimetic amines [1880, 74a], should be compared, according to KUKOVETZ [1054], to that of isoprenaline and results from direct stimulation of the cardiac β-receptors and not from a discharge of noradrenaline. This β-stimulating effect has been found by others [14a] and would appear to be at the root of the calorigenic effect of Ildamen on rats, whose general oxygen consumption increases according to the dose administered [70a]. The heart-stimulating action of the drug is accompanied by an increase in the ATP and creatine phosphate supply to the myocardium [1884], a fact which the authors consider to be favourable since it is necessary for a physiological increase in cardiac performance. The effect of Ildamen has been studied on different enzymes forming part of the aerobic and anaerobic glycogenolysis cycles in the isolated heart of a guinea-pig in whom a state of anoxia has been induced [1324]: amongst other things, it has no effect on the degradation of the energy-rich phosphates arising from this ischaemia. Using dogs, the infusion of Ildamen at the rate of 0.02 mg/kg/min for 30 min increased the free fatty acids and ketone bodies concentration in the arterial blood whilst increasing their extraction by the myocardium. Simultaneously, there was a drop in arterial level and myocardial uptake of lactate and pyruvate [92a].

Although what was possibly a metabolite was prepared and endowed with coronary-dilating activity [1881], it is not known whether it was in fact the active metabolite.

In the case of a healthy man, Ildamen causes no change in urinary excretion of the metabolites of the catecholamines [1045] or any increase in free fatty acids and glucose in the serum, so that the existence of sympathicomimetic properties could be brought into question according to the authors of these observations [569]. The heart stimulating effect is reflected in man by and increase in systolic and cardiac outputs [1010].

Ildamen is a comparatively recent antianginal medication. Despite its special pharmacological properties, which in the light of our present concepts do not conform to its application in the treatment of angina, Ildamen is said to be particularly effective if we look at clinical reports now available [839, 865, 737]. According to this latter report [737], 80% of the 156 patients treated responded favourably or excellently, being reflected in the disappearance of or reduction in pain attacks and by a considerable reduction in the number of doses of nitroglycerin taken. Since by the end of the treatment renal excretion of adrenaline, noradrenaline and vanillino-mandelic acid had dropped by 45, 19 and 35% respectively, the authors conclude that the beneficial effect of the drug is not due to the release of catecholamines. They also report 5 cases which, out of 7 patients tested, saw the disappearance, after double-blind treatment, of the electrocardiographic indications of myocardial ischaemia consequent on exertion on the upright bicycle. Checked throughout the treatment, the hepatic and renal functions were not impaired. According to the documents emanating directly from the pharmaceutical firm, Ildamen has proved effective in 84% of a total of 7000 patients split up between 700 doctors.

MOLL and PETZEL [1312] investigated the effects of an intravenous injection of Ildamen on the changes in certain cardiovascular parameters resulting from ergometric bicycle exertion by 30 patients suffering from angina pectoris or from myocardial infarction. At the dose of 2 mg administered to 15 patients, the severity and earliness of the anginal pain, and the extent of the electrocardiographic indications of cardiac ischaemia were reduced in half the cases; the proportion was $^2/_3$ rd at the dose of 4 mg administered to the other 15 patients. No effect was observed on the level of blood pressure nor on the heart rate.

A double-blind clinical investigation was carried out on 59 angina cases [737]: at the dosage of 3×2 tablets per day, the favourable effect of Ildamen on attacks and the taking of nitroglycerin proved much better than that of the placebo. The authors of these investigations consider that it is basically more logical to stimulate the β-receptors than to block them, because this latter approach can only aggravate coronary insufficiency if account is taken of the fact that it is accompanied by a considerable reduction in the noradrenaline and adrenaline content of the myocardium [326]. Another double-blind test on 76 patients ended up with 80% very favourable results [1815].

In a very recent report [2e], CARLIER states that he has obtained a favourable therapeutic effect in 70% of 34 angina patients who were treated for at least three months at a daily dose of six 8 mg tablets of Ildamen. However, according to HAKKINEN et al. [5e], the beneficial effect of Ildamen on the clinical symptoms of angina is not striking because in a double-blind study involving 43 patients who were treated at a daily dose of 48 mg in two 3-week courses, they recorded an average reduction in the number of anginal attacks of only 28% and only a slight decrease in the consumption of nitroglycerin tablets. Moreover, the patients' subjective evaluation of the intensity and duration of painful attacks as well as their total impression was not favourable.

CARLIER further reports that he had the opportunity of testing the effect of a special form of the product which is not available on the market [2e]. In this instance, the form used was that of pearl-like coated tablets to be crushed between the teeth, each tablet containing 16 mg of active substance and to be taken by the patient when the angina attack occurs. According to this author, the effectiveness of this particular form is equal to or even superior to that of nitroglycerin.

There is a sedative form, known as Ildamen-S, which associates Ildamen with an original substance of the phenothiazine type, which has sedative and tranquillising effects.

Ildamen is too recent a medication to be able to judge of its actual advantages in the hands of the medical practitioner. It is to be hoped that it will in fact render great service, since despite its individual action mode which entails cardiac stimulation, it could take a useful place amongst the usual antianginal drugs whose pharmacological properties conform to the orthodox nature of our existing concepts.

Clinium

Offered to the medical profession in 1969, Clinium (generic name: lidoflazine) is a coronary-dilating agent which is characterised by its exceptional long-lasting action, at least at the highest doses of 5 mg/kg. At this dosage, coronary flow increases by 4 or 5 times in the case of anaesthetised dogs, i.e. to exactly the same extent as that found where there is respiratory anoxia [1660]. TAKENAKA and TACHIKAWA [39b] have also shown that, with dogs, the i.v. administration of Clinium at doses of 0.5—1 and 2 mg/kg causes a marked rise in the coronary flow of the venous sinus whilst at the same time considerably reducing the coronary arterio-venous oxygen difference.

From our personal observations with anaesthetised dogs, Clinium increases coronary arterial flow in a marked and lasting manner: Fig. 16 shows that the dose of 2 mg/kg in intravenous administration almost trebles the blood flow, which has not returned to its original level more than 40 min after the injection. It is also seen that the heart rate is reduced for a short time (it returned to its original level after 15 min) and that blood pressure drops sharply for a long period. These effects on pressure and rate have also been reported by DUCHENE-MARULLAZ [456]. It should be pointed out that since Clinium is not soluble in water, it had to be used

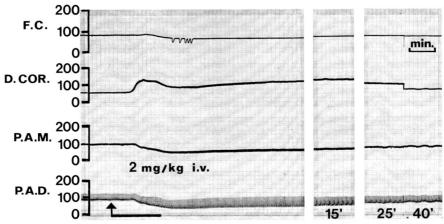

Fig. 16. Effect of lidoflazine on heart rate, coronary arterial blood flow, and systemic blood pressure in the anaesthetized dog. From top to bottom: F.C.: Heart rate (beats/min). D.Cor.: Mean blood flow in the left circumflex coronary artery, measured with an electromagnetic probe (ml/min). P.A.M.: Mean blood pressure in the femoral artery (mm Hg). P.A.D.: Phasic blood pressure in the femoral artery (mm Hg). At signal mark: intravenous injection of lidoflazine, 2 mg/kg. Parts of tracings recorded successively 15—25 and 40 min after injection

in accordance with the instructions supplied by the makers, i.e. in the form of an acid solution with a pH of 3.2, and that under these conditions, this solution without any Clinium has haemodynamic effects which are identical and very comparable in intensity. This fact has, incidentally, just been confirmed by TAKENAKA and TACHIKAWA [39b] who have shown that in the case of dogs the acetic acid solution recommended for dissolving Clinium causes a considerable increase in coronary venous flow and reduces by two-thirds the coronary arterio-venous oxygen difference.

A further fact which also emerged from our tests is the severe myocardial depression caused by the intravenous injection of Clinium in anaesthetised dogs. Figure 17 clearly shows that at the dosages of 2 and 4 mg/kg, Clinium causes a profound drop in the systolic ventricular pressure and in the dp/dt, for which the acidity of the aqueous solution is largely responsible.

Clinium is active when administered orally to non-anaesthetised dogs, coronary flow increasing by from 2 to 6 times after a few hours [887]. It was, however, inactive in the unanaesthetised mini-pig with chronically implanted electro-magnetic flowmeters when given oral doses of 2—40 mg/kg onwards. The drug caused coronary dilatation only at 80 mg/kg, and the degree of dilation was only very mild [111a].

SCHAPER [1660] has also demonstrated the oxygen enrichment of the coronary venous blood with Clinium, a phenomenon which has been confirmed by DUCHENE-MARULLAZ [456], together with the absence of any change in arterio-venous lactate difference in the myocardium. Although SCHAPER interprets the coronary effect as a selective activity, it should be mentioned that the peripheral vessels also dilate [1888] as do the cerebral vessels likewise [1660], although in the latter case at higher doses than the coronary-active doses. Blood pressure drops because of peripheral vaso-dilatation associated with depression of the myocardium (confirmed on Fig. 17).

Although it has not been measured with any precision, myocardial oxygen consumption does not appear to change to any marked extent [1660].

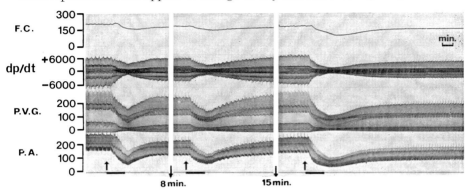

Fig. 17. Effect of lidoflazine on heart rate, rate of rise in left ventricular pressure, left ventricular pressure and systemic blood pressure in the anaesthetized dog. From top to bottom: F.C.: Heart rate (beats/min). dp/dt: Rate of rise in left ventricular pressure (mm Hg/sec). P.V.G.: Left ventricular pressure (mm Hg). P.A.: Phasic blood pressure in the femoral artery (mm Hg). Left tracing: at signal mark, intravenous injection of lidoflazine, 2 mg/kg. Middle tracing: at signal mark, intravenous injection of a volume of solvent corresponding to a dose of 4 mg/kg of lidoflazine. Right tracing: at signal mark, intravenous injection of lidoflazine, 4 mg/kg

According to THOMSEN et al. [1888], Clinium is a substance of the benign type, in the sense given to it by GREGG and SABISTON [732], because while it increases coronary flow it would not appear to change the myocardial oxygen requirements, although the rate, output and work of the heart rise by 33, 55 and 41% respectively. The rise in heart rate (16%) and in cardiac output (31%) has also been reported by AFONSO et al. [13]. Also SONNTAG has pointed out that the effect of lidoflazine in increasing cardiac output and work, as shown by THOMSEN and by AFONSO, is a pharmacological phenomenon which is at variance with the changes brought about by clinically acceptable antianginal substances [1792]. However, according to TAKENAKA and TACHIKAWA [39b], Clinium does not alter myocardial oxygen consumption when administered to dogs intravenously at doses of 0.5—1 and 2 mg/kg. Nevertheless, it must be pointed out that the myocardial oxygen consumption was calculated by multiplying the coronary arterio-venous oxygen difference by the coronary *venous* flow, whereas it is currently accepted that, at the risk of grave sources of error, the venous flow cannot be used instead of the arterial flow in arriving at this consumption.

Clinium is said to speed up in dogs the formation of the collateral circulation which appears in the normal way with dogs suffering from chronic coronary insufficiency as a result of fitting an Ameroid type constrictor ring [1659]. A sustained rise in coronary flow, together with a decrease in coronary arterio-venous oxygen difference has been reported in anaesthetised dogs after the duodenal instillation of Clinium at 5—20 mg/kg [83a].

At the dose of 5 mg/kg injected intravenously, Clinium antagonises the coronary spasm produced by pitressin in rats and lowers the heart rate; it produces an atrio-ventricular block at higher dose [291c].

From the biochemical angle, Clinium, which *in vitro* is an antagonist of angiotensine [674], serotonine [1904], histamine and prostaglandin [1905], powerfully potentiates the effect of adenosine and ATP on the coronaries [13]: the vaso-dilator effect of these two substances is increased by from 20 to 150 times. This potentialisation phenomenon is greater and longer lasting than is the case with Persantine [13]. It occurs in the conscious dog at low oral doses which are inactive in themselves as regards coronary circulation [888]. It would seem to be due either to interference with the uptake of adenosine by the red corpuscles, or to direct inhibition of adenosine deaminase [13]. Lidoflazine prevented the uptake of adenosine by the heart, lungs and entire body [2a], an effect which is thought to be more important than the adenosine sparing effect in blood. Mention must be made of the fact that Clinium provided marked inhibition of the specific uptake by heart cells of adenosine when ^{14}C-labelled adenosine was added to the perfusion fluid of isolated guinea-pig hearts [30b].

Given orally to dogs at doses as low as 0.31 mg/kg, Clinium significantly de-creased the rate of disappearance of adenosine in blood [318c]. Thus, low oral doses result in blood levels sufficiently high to inhibit the uptake and thus the degradation within the blood corpuscles of adenosine. There is a striking parallelism between these results and the potentiation of the effect of exogenous adenosine by low oral doses of Clinium [888][1].

The increase in coronary flow caused by artificial tachycardia and by hypoxia is not affected by Clinium [11]. On the other hand, the reactive hyperaemia induced by temporary occlusion of the anterior descending branch of the left coronary artery in an unanaesthetised mini-pig is intensified and prolonged during the 24 hours following the oral administration of a single dose of Clinium [889, 111a]; this effect should be related to the potentialisation of the coronary-dilating effect of adenosine. Yet it would appear [248] that Clinium does not alter the coronary flow in the pig since the heart of this animal is adenosine-free.

According to WINBURY et al. [2013], Clinium — unlike the nitro derivatives which cause prolonged vasodilatation of the *large* coronary arteries — would appear mainly to dilate the *arterioles*. In their opinion, the fact of greatly incre-asing myocardial irrigation would seem to prove that Clinium (like all the non-nitro coronary dilating agents) interferes with coronary auto-regulation. Its exclusive effect on the small arteries could lead to malajusted distribution of the myocardial blood flow, marked by an excess in those areas where it is undesirable at the expense of ischaemic areas.

From the therapeutic viewpoint, DZIUBA [466] in an open investigation achieves 72% of good and excellent results out of a total of 261 angina subjects with a daily dose ranging from 3×10 to 3×30 mg.

BATLOUNI et al. [103] studied the effect of Clinium at a daily dose of 180 mg under double-blind and cross-permutation conditions, drug and placebo being administered to 40 patients over a period of 45 days. In 25 cases, the effect of Clinium proved superior to that of the placebo. The authors consider that there is significantly greater improvement with Clinium than with the placebo. Their judgment is open to criticism, since the figure of 25 patients improved out of 40 is not significant if these results are processed statistically by the sign test.

The effect of Clinium has been double-blind investigated in five centres applying a new procedure which was referred to on p. 114. Ignoring such objections as may be directed at this type of procedure (see p. 115), these clinical investiga-tions taken as a whole [400, 412, 1670, 1925, 1938] provide an impressive percen-tage of cases which benefitted from the medication from the subjective point of view. Account must be taken, however, of the comments made on p. 115 in order

---

1 The effect of Clinium on the rate of disappearance of adenosine in blood is species dependent [319c].

to reduce to their proper value results which might have been involuntarily influenced by the type of method adopted[2].

In three of these investigations, it is shown that the work capacity tested by ergometric-bicycle loading tests was markedly increased when under Clinium treatment. As usually, the electrocardiographic patterns show a decrease in the ischaemic configuration, but this was neither so regular nor so marked as the clinical improvement [400, 1670].

Finally, the tolerance of *healthy* subjects to work is reported to be increased by taking Clinium [886]. Safety of chronic treatment has been outlined [39c].

The action mechanisms suggested by Clinium for its favourable effects on the development of collateral coronary circulation in animals and in humans are worthy of special discussion because of the possibility of new vistas which they open up in the treatment of angina pectoris. Clinium speeds up transformation of the practically non-functional interarterial anastomoses into functional collateral arterioles because, when administered orally at the rate of 20 mg/kg per day to a conscious dog suffering for the past 8 weeks from chronic coronary insufficiency induced by the fitting of an Ameroid constrictor ring, it increases to a significant degree the coronary quotient (retrograde coronary pressure divided by aortic pressure) as compared to untreated animals [1659]. The reason for this effect lies in the coronary-dilating action of long duration which the treatment reveals in the dog [1659]. The development of collateral circulation would seem to result from a speeding up of the histological growth process, transforming the arteriolar anastomoses into collateral arteries [1657] along the lines of a mechanism outlined on p. 46 et seq. An analysis of the results reported in dogs [1659] shows that these conclusions must be accepted with caution in view of the difficulties which arise in the comparison between treated animals and untreated controls (see also p. 46). True, the coronary quotient is significantly higher in the treated batch than in the control batch, but account must be taken of two variables which could have played an unforeseeable part, namely: a) since Clinium speeds up a process of arteriolar neoformation which is normally set in action by the myocardial hypoxia resulting from gradual occlusion of the circumflex coronary artery, it is vital that the extent and speed of development of this hypoxia should be the same in both the control batch and the treated batch. These factors were not checked, nor can they be (see also p. 46). b) The animals were allowed to take of their own accord a certain amount of daily physical exercise which was not measured and which in fact differed from one animal to another [1659] since it was not prescribed nor was it set at a given level (e.g. using an endless belt). This involves a second variable, therefore, which is even more likely to falsify the results in that, as the author himself shows [1659], physical exercise encourages the development of collateral circulation under his experimental conditions.

As regards the fundamental concept of the action mechanism advanced for the effect of Clinium on the development of the collaterals, it must also be stressed that, in view of the physical mechanisms called upon for the neoformation of functional arterioles by myocardial hypoxia (see p. 46), it must be agreed that any speeding up of this normal process by Clinium should provide a very finely adjusted

---

2 In a recent double-blind study on 12 patients [39c] the improvement achieved in the open phase was maintained or increased in 9 patients who were consequently kept for 6 months in the double-blind study. There was a relapse in the clinical condition in 3 patients. It was predicted, before breaking the code, that the patients who had deteriorated had been receiving placebo, while those who had completed the study successfully were on lidoflazine therapy. In fact, 7 of them did receive lidoflazine whereas 5 were under placebo. Hence treatment prediction was correct in ten instances.

regulation of the degree of hypoxia induced by coronary occlusion. Indeed, should this speeding up process bring the harmful state of hypoxia to a benign level, not only does the physiological stimulus to neoformation of collateral arterioles advanced by SCHAPER [1657] disappear, but also the physiological adjustment dilation of vessels still capable of dilation is enough to ensure satisfactory conditions of myocardial oxygenation. On the other hand, should this speeding up fail to correct severe hypoxia to a sufficient extent, such hypoxia entails irreversible myocardial lesions. As long as definite proofs are not provided, it is difficult to accept that such a finely adjusted regulator mechanism, capable of keeping myocardial hypoxia within such strict limits, can be the work of a medication, whatever that medication may be.

If we take a look at what is said to occur in the angina subject, where the therapeutic benefit is likewise ascribed to the speeding up of normal development, by hypoxia, of coronary collaterals, it should be emphasised at the outset that such a fact has not been demonstrated up to now. For the time being, the explanation put forward is therefore only an assumption justified by the extrapolation to the angina subject of the observations made in animals. Here again this opinion must be taken with caution, because the mechanism invoked in the animal to explain the speed-up in development of the collaterals, namely prolonged coronary vaso-dilatation [1659], cannot apply to humans since, as far as we are informed [248, 282 c], Clinium does not alter the coronary flow in man. Must it therefore be accepted that Clinium is able, by reason of its chemical structure, to set up localised tissue neoformation on the vascular walls of the anastomoses leading to the production of elastic and muscular tissue which, from the histological viewpoint, is arterial tissue ? There lies the question.

A final comment is called for. In the case of the anginal subject who has benefitted from the administration of the drug, the suspension of the treatment or its replacement by a placebo means the relapse of the patient [39 c]. This being so, it must be taken that the newly-formed arterioles degenerate and so deprive the patient of the benefits of the collateral circulation which has developed. Although this degeneration is possible in dogs, it still has not been demonstrated in man (see p. 47).

Clinium is also reported as having interesting properties for the treatment of certain conditions of arrhythmia. This is especially the case for chronic atrial fibrillation. Thus MIYAHARA et al. [26 b] were able to restore the normal sinusal rhythm in 7 out of 12 cases. PIESSENS et al. [31 b] confirmed this anti-arrhythmic effect in the case of chronic atrial fibrillation over a larger number of patients. Treating 26 cases at a daily dosage of 240 mg, split up into 4 separate doses, they observe a return to the sinusal rhythm in 11 cases, and they emphasise the fact that this therapeutic effect is often experienced at an early stage, since normal rhythm was restored in 7 cases within 36 hours. They do however point out the appearance of various rhythm disturbances in most of the unsuccessfully treated subjects, namely ventricular extrasystoles, bouts of ventricular tachycardia, and even ventricular fibrillation in one instance. Experimental details at present available provide no explanation for the appearance of these forms of arrhythmia which, in the view of the authors, deserve more thorough investigation. VAN CAUWENBERGE [9e (bis)] also reports the frequency of these rhythm disorders wich can occur in the form of sudden attacks of ventricular tachycardia or even of ventricular fibrillation. Since such disorders are observed more particularly amongst patients presenting extrasystoles, VAN CAUWENBERGE considers that myocardial infarction constitutes a contraindication to the use of lidoflazine of wich the exact role in the treatment of angina still remains to be defined.

β-Adrenergic Blocking Drugs[1]

A new and original pharmacological concept, applied in particular to the treatment of angina pectoris, has dominated the past decade: that of the blockade of the adrenergic *β*-receptors.

Since the papers by AHLQUIST [14], the category of adrenergic *β*-receptors has included in particular those through whose medium the adrenergic-induced stimulation of the cardiac muscle takes place. From the haemodynamic angle, stimulation of the cardiac *β*-receptors is marked by a speeding up of the heart rate and an increase in the energetics of cardiac contraction, both as regards its force and its velocity. It results *in fine* in a considerable increase in the oxygen requirements of the cardiac muscle.

In view of the fact that the clinical picture of the anginal syndrome is dominated by hypersympathicotony (see p. 35), it seemed logical to expect a beneficial effect from medications likely to antagonise this exaggeration of adrenergic tonicity. It was this idea which gave rise to the *β*-receptor antagonising drugs. Synthesis tended towards substances whose chemical structure is very close to that of the specific *β*-agonist, isoprenaline (isoproterenol). First came dichloroisoproterenol [1464] which was not used clinically because it is not a pure blocking agent but also possesses sympathicomimetic properties [447, 1320]. Then followed pronethalol [180] which was abandoned as being cancer-forming [1404], quickly succeeded by propranolol [178] whose *β*-antagonising effect is ten times greater than that of pronethalol and which does not produce *β*-stimulating effects [179]. The therapeutic success of propranolol encouraged the production of other medications whose chemical structure is more or less similar and which all include the same radical which is responsible for the *β*-antagonising biological activity, namely the sequence OCH_2—CHOH—CH_2—NHCH $(CH_3)_2$ [2] grafted onto a benzene ring.

A *β*-blocking agent is one which develops a competitive, selective and reversible antagonism vis-à-vis the *β*-adrenergic receptors [557].

The general haemodynamic consequences of specific blockade of the adrenergic *β*-receptors are easy to forecast if we refer to the basic notions of physiology which govern the role of these receptors as regards the cardiovascular system.

Stimulation of the *β*-receptors, *as regards the heart*, produces two basic types of effect: a positive chronotropic effect and a positive inotropic effect. The former is seen in the speeding up of the heart rate, the latter being reflected in an increase in the velocity of cardiac contraction and a rise in tension in the ventricular wall. *As regards the arterial vascular wall*, it is known that the *β*-receptors only play a secondary role since their activity is normally masked by the potency of the *α*-receptors. The permanent sympathetic tonus ensures that these haemodynamic parameters maintain a certain level.

The suppression of this tonus by pharmacological blockade will quite obviously entail a decrease in the heart rate[3], and a reduction in the cardiac contraction

---

1 Since, in the short period of time since they were introduced into clinical practice, almost 1000 scientific papers have been written on the subject of *β*-receptor blocking agents, it is strongly recommended to read the recent review by DOLLERY et al. [36a] which, while not covering the whole of this literature, does deal particularly with the effects of *β*-blocking drugs in man.

2 This sequence is symbolised by the letter R in the structure formulae which follow.

3 Part of the bradycardic effect of propranolol arises from the central nervous system [197c]: direct application of the drug in powdered form into different structures of central nervous system (especially the anterior hypothalamus and reticular formation) is followed by a decrease in heart rate.

velocity and in the tension in the ventricular wall. From the vascular angle, the freeing of the a-tonus causes vasoconstriction and thus brings about an increase in overall vascular resistance, which is due to the suppression of a tonic vasodilator activity mediated by the β-receptors [123 c]. The haemodynamic consequences of β-blockade will therefore be:

a) a decrease in cardiac output by the reduction of heart rate and stroke volume, this latter arising from a drop in contraction velocity and in ventricle wall tension;

b) a decrease in heart work basically due to the reduction in cardiac output;

c) a reduction in myocardial oxygen consumption (it will be seen that this is at the cost of increased oxygen extraction, see p. 209 and 210), in which several factors play a part:

— a reduction in the external work of the left ventricle
— a reduction in contraction velocity
— a reduction in ventricular wall tension;

d) a drop in systemic blood pressure, despite an increase in overall vascular resistance, mainly due it would seem to cardiac depression[4];

e) some coronary vasoconstriction because the β-receptors have a dilating action on the myocardial vessels [999, 1280] (see p. 63), and their blockade frees the vasoconstrictor a-tonus;

f) broncho-constriction for the same reasons as in the case of the coronary vascular system.

We shall be examining in turn the main substances which are antagonistic to the adrenergic β-receptors, starting with propranolol which is at the head of the list and which is always taken as the reference substance in the very great majority of experimental and clinical investigations into other β-blocking agents.

1. Inderal (Dociton, Avlocardyl)

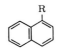

Propranolol

The disclosure of the blocking properties of Inderal in respect of the adrenergic β-receptors was the work of the Imperial Chemical Industries pharmacologists [178, 1724, 1725, 1726]. These researchers provide experimental evidence of the neutralising of the cardiac stimulating effects of the catecholamines and of the peripheral vasodilator effect of isoprenaline [1727]. The position is one of *competitive*, and therefore pharmacologically reversible, blockade [183, 502]. They also demonstrated with anaesthetised cats and dogs that Inderal reduces heart rate, cardiac contraction force and blood pressure; these phenomena are due, at least in part, to the suppression of the sympathetic β-tonus during resting, since they do not appear following pre-treatment with syrosingopine.

Inderal also possesses local anaesthetic properties which are double those of procaine [1318], i.e. five times those of cocaine [1783, 1954], and which are independent of the β-blocking effect [1123].

The β-antagonist effect of Inderal has also been demonstrated in man. When administered intravenously or orally, it reduces *effort tachycardia* in a normal man

---

4 There is a central component in the hypotensive effect of propranolol which is independent of the β-blocking properties [173 c].

[291, 785, 1545]. Since this type of tachycardia is primarily due to increased sympathetic activity [293, 1545], the antagonist effect of Inderal can be attributed to its β-blocking effect. In the case of a normal man, the oral administration of 20 mg Inderal considerably reduces [4] and of 40 mg abolishes [710] *tachycardia resulting from isoprenaline*. Since the effective dose in angina often far exceeds the β-blocking dose, it must be admitted that the antianginal effect of Inderal is also due to other actions [1892], one of these being a cardio-depressive effect (see p. 215).

The application of Inderal to the treatment of angina pectoris seems logical if the opinion of RAAB [1481, 1489, 1490] is accepted; he attributes an important role to the catecholamines in the origin of the anginal phenomena, through the medium of an excessive increase in myocardial oxygen consumption (see p. 36). Most of these cardiac effects of the catecholamines are due to a stimulation of the β-receptors, and so it was reasonable to believe that the fact of blocking these effects provided a new method of approach to the treatment of angina [2007]. Since Inderal abolished the cardio-stimulating effects of the catecholamines, it could be assumed that there would be an antianginal effect in the case of human treatment.

Various British clinicians did in fact start reporting favourable effects [659, 769, 966]. Then, as the application of Inderal spread, definite limits were recommended for its use in angina following cases of outright heart failure or aggravation of latent hyposystolic conditions [1467, 1764, 1841]. Reports of cases of cardiac dysfunction also prompted pharmacologists to look more closely into the effects of Inderal on the coronary vasomotor function and on haemodynamics. As a result, PARRATT and GRAYSON [1424] reported a considerable reduction in coronary flow in animals due to a sharp increase in coronary vascular resistance which was immediately confirmed by MCKENNA et al. [1258]. It was also shown that the contractile force of the myocardium is reduced [1333], as also is aortic flow [1724], cardiac output [622, 1258, 1336, 1800, 1982], the work of the heart [1258, 1800] and its oxygen consumption [1258]. Another major effect is the increase in peripheral arterial resistance [1258, 1336, 1982].

The reduction in myocardial irrigation, the lowering of cardiac performance and the marked increase in total arterial resistance are the three factors which explain cardiac decompensation in clinical observations. For these three effects of Inderal are also found in man. For instance, GEBHARDT and his co-workers [633] showed that a dose of 60 mg of Inderal administered orally for three days is enough to reduce cardiac output in the healthy subject by 25% and to cause a considerable increase in arterial resistance. They consider that these effects are capable of rapidly causing cardiac insufficiency in a balanced heart case. This drop in cardiac output has been confirmed in man on several occasions [378, 505, 785]. It also occurs during exercise, when it is put down to the combined effect of a sharp drop in the heart rate and inhibition by β-blockade of the increased cardiac contraction force which normally occurs during exertion [505].

Such in brief are the basic details of experimental and clinical pharmacology which were originally published on Inderal. Later on, this medication was the subject of a considerable amount of research which, for clarity of information, we have grouped under various headings.

Primary Cardiac Effect

The *primary* cardiac effect of Inderal consists in a reduction in the velocity of cardiac contraction [768, 1406, 227c], the decrease in myocardial contractility being independent of any fall in heart rate [136c]. When administered during exercise to a healthy man, Inderal blocks the reduction in ventricular volume at the end-systole and end-diastole point and also the increase in myocardial contractility [1406, 1789]. When injected intravenously into a healthy man [503, 505], Inderal reduces by 40% the effort capacity for violent exercise and reduces by 22, 15, 34 and 21% respectively the increases in cardiac output, blood pressure, ventricular work and heart rate caused by exercise. All these haemodynamic changes have been confirmed by other authors [379]. Similarly, the drop in cardiac output and heart rate has been found in the subject with coronary insufficiency when exercising [770].

According to the authors of these observations [503, 505], such cardiovascular disturbances reflect a weakening of the cardiac function and indicate that Inderal has the potential for precipitating cardiac decompensation in patients who depend to a critical extent on their sympathetic system for keeping cardiac compensation within limits[1].

According to others [1543], when intravenously injected at the dose of 5 mg in the case of the subject with or without coronary heart disease, Inderal reduces the velocity of cardiac contraction, pulse rate and heart work.

In the case of the coronary subject, left ventricular end-diastolic pressure rises, which in fact indicates that the β-system is supporting the cardiac function of the coronary subject. These haemodynamic effects of Inderal lead to impairment of myocardial cell oxydation, as shown by the drop in myocardial oxydo-reduction potential [1543], which testifies to a reduction in myocardial oxygenation. This effect of Inderal on the angina subject, which is the opposite of what occurs in the case of nitroglycerin, is not found in the healthy subject. However, according to LEWIS and BRINKE [1132], Inderal sets up favourable changes in the intermediate metabolism, notably a decrease in the costly process of oxidative catabolism in favour of preferential use of glucose, which entails a reduction in cell hypoxia and a corresponding increase in aerobiosis. It would seem that this observation can be compared to the fact that, with dogs, the intravenous administration of 1 mg/kg decreases by almost 50% the amount of free fatty acids taken up by the myocardium, whilst consumption of glucose, lactate and pyruvate remains unchanged [88a].

Effect on Coronary Flow

Under various experimental conditions, Inderal lowers coronary blood flow to considerable extents. This fact has been demonstrated on an isolated rabbit heart [1223, 1224] and on an anaesthetised dog [1347, 1349]. In the latter case, coronary flow is reduced by 32% at the (blocking) dose of 0.1 mg/kg administered intravenously [292], by 22% and 37% respectively at intravenous doses of 0.05 and

---

1 This should be compared with observations made on an unanaesthetised dog whose ventricular beating rate is speeded up: comparison of the changes in coronary flow, cardiac output and blood pressure caused by this artificially induced tachycardia before and after the administration of Inderal indicates that β-blockade seriously endangers the physiological haemodynamic adjustments [336, 24a], because it counters the maintenance of aortic flow and reverses the normal coronary dilatation reaction [337]. Highly indicative also is a study by KEROES et al. [69a], ventricular function curves of cardiac output and stroke volume versus left ventricular end-diastolic pressure having been obtained during rapid infusion of Tyrode's solution in dogs standing at rest and during near-maximal exercise both before and after administration of propranolol. Propranolol negated the increase in contractility associated with exercise (which reflected the heightened sympathetic activity) and the plateaus of ventricular function curves were then not significantly different from those obtained at rest, while these plateaus were significantly higher during exercise than at rest prior to the administration of propranolol.

1.25 mg/kg, with corresponding rises in coronary resistance [763], and by 24%
(with a 26% increase in coronary resistance) after an intravenous dose of 0.3—0.6
mg/kg [1828, 1829]. In these experiments, the reduction in coronary flow is not
accompanied by any change in myocardial oxygen consumption. The cardiac
muscle must therefore meet its needs by raising its oxygen extraction coefficient,
which is revealed by a drop in the oxygen content of the coronary venous blood
[1258]. Figure 18 gives two examples, taken from our own publications, of the
effect of Inderal on coronary arterial flow in an anaesthetised dog: the reduction
is noticeable at the intravenous dose of 1 mg/kg; it is considerable (over 50%) and
permanent at the dose of 2 mg/kg (upper graph). At the same time, blood pressure
drops sharply, also in a permanent manner.

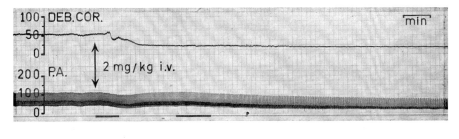

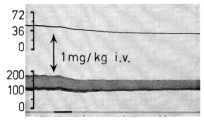

Fig. 18. Effect of propranolol on coronary arterial blood flow and systemic blood pressure in
the anaesthetized dog. From top to bottom: D.Cor.: Mean blood flow in the left circumflex
coronary artery, measured with an electromagnetic probe (ml/min). P.A.: Phasic blood
pressure in the femoral artery (mm Hg). Upper traces: at signal mark, intravenous injection of
propranolol, 2 mg/kg in one dog. Lower traces: at signal mark, intravenous injection of
propranolol, 1 mg/kg in another dog

The drop in coronary flow caused by Inderal has its origin therefore in an
increase in coronary vascular resistance, a phenomenon which has again been
described by other authors [1989] and which is observed both in dogs and monkeys
[1422]. The mechanism of this effect is still disputed. Whilst certain authors [1424]
are of the opinion that the β-blocking effect frees the a-receptors, thus bringing
about an increase in vascular resistance, the coronary effect is largely due, according to others, to the slowing up of the heart rate, because pre-treatment with
reserpine, which eliminates the role of the a- and β-receptors, does not prevent
constriction [1989]. Others again [394], who compare the changes in a series of
cardiovascular parameters recorded simultaneously, consider that the reduction
in coronary flow is not conditioned by a drop in perfusion pressure or in heart rate,
nor by the rise in ventricular volume or systole duration. In their opinion, it is the
consequence of the lessening of cardiac work. Moreover, the fact that, after
administration of propranolol, sympathetic stimulation does not bring about any
reduction in coronary flow, and that the administration of phentolamine does not

cause any increase in flow, excludes in their opinion the suggestion put forward by PARRATT and GRAYSON [1424] that the reducing effect of propranolol on coronary flow is a result of a liberation of active vasoconstriction of the adrenergic a-type. It is interesting to note that Inderal at an intravenous dose of 1 mg/kg failed to alter significantly coronary or systemic haemodynamics in the unanaesthetised dog [97a, 32b], a result which suggests that in the supine unanaesthetised animal at rest, β-adrenergic receptor activity is minimal in the coronary arteries.

It must be pointed out that although *total* coronary flow is reduced following the administration of Inderal, blood flow does not appear to alter in those myocardial zones which are made experimentally ischaemic by partial coronary occlusion [375], but blood flow to non-ischaemic areas is selectively decreased in the same experimental conditions [252c]. These authors therefore believe that selective flow maintenance, associated with the reduction in cardiac oxygen requirements, would explain the beneficial clinical effect. Inderal significantly increases myocardial oxygen tension at a time when there is no change in coronary venous oxygen content. Inderal thus appears to augment myocardial oxygen availability by decreasing the oxygen requirements of the heart [228c]. It should also be mentioned that following the administration of Inderal, adrenaline and noradrenaline cause coronary vasoconstriction in the animal instead of vasodilatation [616].

The reduction in coronary flow which occurs in animals following the administration of Inderal is also found in man. In the case of the angina subject, for instance, Inderal brings about a 25% reduction in coronary flow and in myocardial oxygen consumption [2033]. A particularly interesting paper on this subject by WOLFSON et al. [2032] reports both the haemodynamic changes induced by Inderal in normal and anginal subjects, and suggests the possible mechanisms governing its therapeutic effects. From the haemodynamic viewpoint, these authors show that an intravenous dose of 5 mg induces, after 20 min, in 13 patients (4 normal and 9 with obstructive coronary disease) a marked slowing up of the heart rate, a drop in cardiac output, a 25% reduction in myocardial oxygen consumption and a decrease in coronary flow. This latter indicates the existence of vasoconstriction, because it goes hand in hand with an increase in arterial oxygen extraction and is greater than the reduction in myocardial oxygen consumption. As for the therapeutic effects which, at the oral dose of 160—280 mg per day on 37 patients, result in significant improvement in 30 cases, or 81%, these could be explained, on the basis of haemodynamic observations, by three possible mechanisms: very probably a decrease in cardiac metabolic requirements, perhaps interference with the awareness of pain, and exceptionally in certain patients possible blockade of the adrenergic coronary constriction. In a subsequent paper, the same authors confirm that, at an intravenous dose of 5 mg with 27 subjects, 18 with coronary atherosclerosis and 9 without, Inderal lowers coronary flow at rest and during exercise, whilst at the same time reducing the oxygen needs of the heart. The antianginal activity is due to the second effect [138a].

Effect on Cardiac Output

Just as it reduces coronary flow, Inderal considerably lowers cardiac output under various conditions. Firstly with the anaesthetised dog after an intravenous dose of 0.2 mg/kg [1738] and in the case of the *conscious* dog following the intravenous administration of 0.3 mg/kg [1763], both at rest and during exercise. Figure 19 shows the observations we made on four anaesthetised dogs: at the intravenous dose of 1 mg/kg, the drop in cardiac output is 30% half an hour after the injection.

In the case of the *healthy* subject, cardiac output drops by 20% following an intravenous injection of 5 mg [1493] and 10 mg [1911], the cardiac index dropping sharply after 5 mg i.v. [379]. In other studies, cardiac index decreases by 31% following an intravenous injection of 5 mg [335c], and cardiac output diminishes by 23% following an intravenous injection of 10 mg [308c].

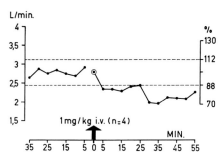

Fig. 19. Effect of propranolol, 1 mg/kg i.v., on cardiac output in the anaesthetized dog (mean values for 4 animals)

With the *anginal* subject, cardiac output and work decrease after an intravenous dose of 0.1 mg/kg [1743]. The dose of 10 mg administered intravenously causes [59, 465]: a) at rest, a 22% drop in cardiac output, a 25% drop in the dp/dt, a 25% drop in heart work; b) during exercise, a 13% reduction in the increase of cardiac output, a 25% reduction in the speeding up of the dp/dt, and a 10% drop in the increase in heart work and 7% of tachycardia. According to these authors [465], the subjective improvement brought about by Inderal in the anginal patient is due to the drop in oxygen consumption, which has its main roots in the partial inhibition of increase in dp/dt and tachycardia.

In the case of man, atropine reduces inhibition of the cardiac response to exercise resulting from Inderal [379].

It is especially interesting to note that cardiac output is also reduced in patients with a fixed heart rate (complete A-V block and implanted pacemaker), which proves that the cardio-depressive effect is independent of the heart-slowing effect [186, 441].

We shall be considering later the probable mechanisms behind the cardio-depressive effect (see heading "Effect on the cardiac function").

Antianginal Effect[2]

From the therapeutic viewpoint, it is accepted that Inderal increases the anginal subject's tolerance to exercise [170, 771] and that it has genuine anti-anginal properties [660, 1492, 1547, 2032], although the favourable effect noted in a double-blind test [666] was at first disputed [1812].

Inderal is undoubtedly beneficial for the angina pectoris subject. According to certain authors, it proved effective, with groups of 30—50 patients, in almost 90% of cases [1031, 1079], whilst others speak of 80% even at the comparatively low daily dose of 80—120 mg [1063].

This clinical effect has been confirmed in various reports on double-blind tests. Whilst certain authors [783, 1303, 1356] simply state that their investigation

2 A review dealing with the clinical use of propranolol in angina pectoris has recently been published by ELLIOTT and STONE [37a].

achieved very favourable results, others mention that clinical improvement is accompanied by a reduction in myocardial oxygen consumption, calculated by the Robinson heart rate x blood pressure index [354].

In another investigation [651], 15 out of 19 patients showed improvement: lessening or disappearance of cardiac pains, reduction in nitroglycerin intake, and increased tolerance to exercise, without however any prolongation of the time after which the ischaemic S-T appears; the heart rate and Robinson index drop sharply, which would suggest a reduction in myocardial oxygen consumption. For certain authors, the treadmill exercise capacity is not significantly improved despite decrease in incidence of attacks of angina and in number of nitroglycerin tablets consumed [115c].

In another, equally favourable, test [794], effectiveness appeared to depend on the dosage, 40 mg being without effect, 80 mg being significantly active and 160 mg being active to a very significant degree. Finally, other authors [1323] state that with a daily dose of 160 mg the favourable effect is achieved in 53% of cases. Checked double-blind, Inderal increases by 70% the tolerance to exercise of an anginal subject, and reduces the maximal depression of the S-T segment of the ECG appearing during effort [48a].

The quality of the antianginal effect of Inderal does appear to be in direct relation to the dose used, for PRICHARD [1466] achieves maximum benefit with a daily dose of 400 mg, the therapeutic effect lessening linearly with the reduction in dosage (200 — 100 — 50 mg per day) to become insignificant at the dose of 50 mg. In the same way, ZSOTER and BEANLANDS [141a] report that in a double-blind trial, a low dosage of propranolol (80 mg/day) failed to reduce the frequency of anginal attacks, whilst 160 mg/day decreased the number of pain episodes and the amount of nitroglycerin consumed with the same patients.

According to MIZGALA et al. [89a and 90a], who were concerned with 15 patients suffering from acute coronary insufficiency without evidence of acute myocardial infarction, Inderal at a daily dose of 160—400 mg given during 32—120 weeks effectively reduced intractable anginal symptoms and stabilised the course of the disease in 13 patients. It appeared to reduce also the high incidence of acute myocardial infarction associated with this syndrome.

The most obvious objective effect of Inderal on the anginal subject is the reduction in effort tachycardia [444], which would perhaps explain why, according to some authors [615], the medication develops its maximal activity in the case of the anginal subject with a high heart rate.

Inderal is reported to improve the short-term prognosis of the anginal subject assessed 18 months after the start of applying a continuous course of treatment [28, 2031]. This very prolonged type of treatment at a daily dose ranging from 80 to 480 mg achieves a considerable therapeutic effect (reduction by a half in attacks and nitroglycerin intake, going hand in hand with a persistent symptomatic improvement) in 87% of cases, over half of them suffering from side effects, mainly gastro-intestinal upsets, which can be remedied by reducing the dosage [29]. Cardiac decompensation appeared in 7% of the cases treated.

The same authors state in a subsequent paper [27] that the effectiveness was maintained throughout 29 months of continuous treatment, but stress the fact that provided there are no side effects the daily dose should be increased in stages in order to achieve the optimum effect. Thus over two-thirds of their patients were given from 160 to 240 mg per day.

After two years treatment at the daily dose of 100—160 mg, KARGES [940] achieved with 58 anginal subjects similar therapeutic results to those just described.

A similar clinical benefit following two years treatment, and a like incidence of cardiac decompensation have been reported by ZEFT et al. [2044] who feel that the medication is incapable of changing the natural course of severe coronary heart diseases since 12.3% of the patients treated died either from infarction or sudden collapse.

A study has been made of the clinical effect of an association of Inderal with nitro-derivatives in the hope of improving the therapeutic effects by thus combining different pharmacological effects, with the idea of neutralising the coronary and peripheral vasoconstrictive properties of Inderal by the reverse activity of the nitro-derivatives, and at the same time associating two types of drugs which, although pharmacologically dissimilar, both lead to a reduction in heart work by different mechanisms. Thus, according to RUSSEK [1607, 1609, 1610, 1611], the simultaneous use of Isordil and Inderal achieves a remarkable degree of synergy which enables an impressive antianginal effect to be obtained in 90% of severe cases of angina pectoris. The doses are 40 mg Inderal 4 times a day *before* meals and 5 mg Isordil taken sublingually 4 times a day *after* meals. RUSSEK confirmed his findings in a double-blind test [1618] on 115 patients who were comparatively recalcitrant to the two medications when they were administered separately. BATTOCK et al. [109] state that, as compared with each of these two drugs, this medicinal association increases clinical effectiveness but does not improve performance with effort. But ARONOW and KAPLAN [56] do not share the enthusiastic opinion of RUSSEK because 44% of their patients had less attacks with the placebo than during the administration of the active drugs, and also because they find no significant difference in tolerance to exercise in 50% of their patients, 40% of them on the contrary showing a deterioration in their capacity for effort. ARONOW and KAPLAN therefore consider that this medicinal combination can be as harmful as beneficial to the anginal subject. According to HARRISON [786], this lack of harmony between the results of two similar investigations carried out under double-blind conditions could be explained primarily by the fact that the severity of the angina is certainly not comparable from one test to the other, that the activity criteria chosen are not strictly the same, and also by the impossibility of checking the interplay of certain psychic factors in the effect of the treatment. GOLDBARG et al. [52a] express yet a different opinion following an investigation covering 14 anginal patients treated double-blind and with cross permutation with the two drugs separately or in association, at the daily dose of 4×10 mg of Isordil and 4×40 mg of propranolol. They note a significant reduction in the frequency of anginal attacks with propranolol alone and in association, but Isordil on its own is no more active than the placebo. Furthermore, there is no significant difference between the effect of propranolol alone and that of the association. The beneficial action of propranolol is in relation to a significant lowering of the heart rate at rest and during effort. However, the symptomatic effect is not accompanied by an improvement in the effort capacity of the patients. These authors therefore draw the conclusion that Isordil on its own brings no improvement, and that association with propranolol does not increase the latter's beneficial effect. The same conclusions were reached by the authors in question in a subsequent paper [53a] dealing with 21 patients, each patient receiving placebo, Isordil, propranolol, and the combination of the two drugs for one month each in a random sequence over a period of 4 months. These findings were confirmed by DAVIES et al. [31a] in a double-blind trial carried out on 23 patients: beneficial effects from combined treatment appeared to be due to propranolol, response to Isordil and placebo being similar.

Despite these discordant views, RUSSEK maintains his judgment according to a very recent study he made in 115 patients with severe angina pectoris relatively resistant to propranolol or nitrate therapy when administered alone. He found [277 c] that the average maximum S-T segment depression following exercise was 3.2 mm with placebo, 1.9 mm with Isordil, 1.6 mm with propranolol and 0.4 mm with propranolol and Isordil combined (p < .001). The average increase in exercise tolerance with propranolol or Isordil alone was approximately 24%, whereas the increment with combined therapy was more than three times this value, averaging more than 83%. In 106 of the 115 patients, striking clinical improvement was recorded on combined therapy. Success in treatment was however dependent upon the administration of a sufficient dose of propranolol to produce a relative resting bradycardia of 55—60 beats per min. The daily dosage varied from 20 mg to 520 mg. Propranolol was administered before meals and Isordil after meals because of differences in time of onset of action. On long-term propranolol-Isordil therapy, disability, recurrent infarction and mortality during a three year follow-up period have been found to be significantly lower than in a comparable series subjected to myocardial revascularization procedures and followed for a similar period of time (p < .001).

The adjunction of nitroglycerin to Inderal is said to increase considerably its beneficial effect on tolerance to effort in the anginal subject [25]. The major advantages of this association are due to the fact that the increases in cardiac index, rate and work, and in dp/dt brought about in man by nitroglycerin are antagonised by Inderal [1993] so that, by associating these two medications, heart rate, tension-time index and dp/dt are reduced at the same time as the ventricular function improves as a result of nitroglycerin. LICHTLEN et al. found that in patients with severe coronary insufficiency, nitroglycerin, 0.8 mg sublingually, partially restored to control values the left ventricular function curve which was strongly depressed by Inderal, 5 mg intravenously, during exertion [206 c].

Mechanisms of the Antianginal Effect

The mechanisms governing the antianginal effect of Inderal have given rise to various views which are not always reconcilable. According to EPSTEIN and BRAUNWALD [504], the improvement of the angina condition is due to a reduction in the oxygen requirements of the heart, which in turn is due to the lowering of various haemodynamic parameters: heart rate, general blood pressure, myocardial contractility, stroke velocity and the degree of shortening of the cardiac muscular fibres. Inderal also reduces the increase in the heart's oxygen needs in the case of the anginal subject given exercise to do [108]. PARRATT [1420] suggests that Inderal could, because of its local anaesthetic properties [1318, 1727], exert this effect on the coronary and cardiac receptors involved in pain, thus acting on the perception of pain and not on the metabolism and dynamics of the myocardium. In his view, this concept could also explain why the coronary-dilating effect of anoxia is reduced by Inderal [568], since it could involve the anaesthetising of the myocardial chemo-receptors whose stimulation causes a reflex coronary dilatation [1006] which is, for example, inhibited by the anaesthetising action of procaine on these receptors [1686]. This is not the view taken by SHANKS [1728] who is of the opinion that the antianginal effect of Inderal is the consequence of the haemodynamic modifications brought about by the blocking of the β-receptors. This is also the opinion of clinicians who feel that the therapeutic benefits are due to the suppression of untoward cardiac hyperactivity resulting from the sympathetic excitation (to which the ischaemic myocardium is particularly susceptible) occasioned by emotion and by effort [1492, 9 b]. There also militates in favour of the role of the β-blockade and against that of local anaesthetic properties the fact that the two isomers, racemic and dextrogyre, although being equally active as local anaesthetics [435] are clearly dissociated from the β-blocking effect angle, the dextrogyre isomer being without effect on the β-receptors in animals at doses 16 times higher than those which are active in the case of the racemic form [92]. In PARRATT's opinion [1422], it could well be that the part played by the anti-adrenergic effect in the antianginal activity consists in an antagonism which Inderal exerts as regards the increase in production of metabolic heat due to the catecholamines, an effect which he observed in dogs [1424] and monkeys [1422].

As we have earlier stated (p. 210 et seq.), the general view which prevails is that of a reduction in myocardial oxygen requirements. We will not labour the point further.

Effect on the Cardiac Function

It has been stated earlier that the haemodynamic disturbances caused by Inderal in man reflect a weakening of the cardiac function and have an unfavourable effect potential which can manifest itself in the appearance or precipitation of cardiac insufficiency [503, 505]. A certain number of cases have in fact been reported [28, 361, 1195, 2044] and as long ago as 1966, STEPHEN [1832] records 13 cases out of 5000 subjects treated where Inderal is clearly responsible for the cardiac decompensation which occurred. Its appearance cannot be foreseen, primarily because it is not linked to the dosage since it could occur after 4—5 days of administration of doses as low as 20 mg per day [1652]. The potential cardiac risk is therefore a real one. It provides justification for the drug being contra-indicated where there is cardiac insufficiency [564] and for the recommendation that digitalis should be administered simultaneously to prevent the cardio-depressive effect [1537] and strictly enforced in the case of patients having to be treated with Inderal who have or have had overt cardiac insufficiency [1304,1652]. In these cases the initial doses of Inderal must be very low. Even so, the combined administration of digitalis does not always prevent insufficiency, and the present consensus of opinion is that existing cardiac insufficiency should be considered as a definite contra-indication for the use of Inderal.

In the view of certain authors [1738], Inderal is contra-indicated where there is merely an enlarged heart, even in the absence of indications of congestive failure. They support their opinion by the fact that they find in mice the emergence of myolytic lesions of the myocardium [1856] whose origin they cannot at present trace: it could either be the consequence of a reduction in coronary flow or a direct cardio-toxic effect.

The origin of the cardio-depressive effect of Inderal has given rise to extensive research work. It appears in closed-chest dogs [646]. It is a *direct* effect, independent of β-blockade [1123, 1125, 1255, 1318] and of the noradrenaline content in the myocardium, for pre-treatment of the animal with reserpine or guanethidine does not prevent it [1124]. According to certain authors [1255], the cardiac depression only occurs at a much higher dosage than the β-blocking dose, but in our view this opinion calls for correction. For proof of this we only need the experimental facts illustrated in Fig. 20 gathered from experimentation with an anaesthetised dog. The intravenous dose of 0.5 mg/kg of Inderal is necessary to block the β-receptors completely, as is shown by the persistance of a very weak accelerating effect on heart rate by the injection of isoprenaline 5 min later (1st graph). Now this dose is sufficient to produce a sharp reduction by almost 50% in velocity of cardiac contration (2nd graph). At the same time, left ventricular systolic pressure drops to a marked extent (3rd graph) and ventricular end-diastolic pressure rises gradually, this weakening of the power of the heart contraction being sufficient to bring about a slight drop in blood pressure (4th graph). By following the phenomena over a period of time, it is seen that cardiac depression is progressively accentuated. It is spontaneously irreversible. It increases still further with the subsequent i. v. injection of doses of 1 and 2 mg/kg.

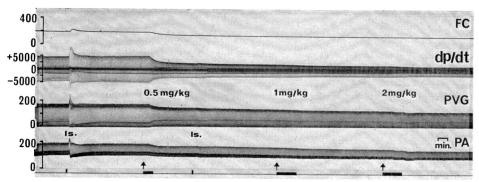

Fig. 20. Effect of propranolol on heart rate, rate of rise in left ventricular pressure, left ventricular pressure and systemic blood pressure in the anaesthetized dog. From top to bottom: F.C.: Heart rate (beats/min). dp/dt: Rate of rise in left ventricular pressure (mm Hg/sec). P.V.G.: Left ventricular pressure (mm Hg). P.A.: Phasic blood pressure in the femoral artery (mm Hg). At first signal mark: intravenous injection of propranolol, 0.5 mg/kg. At second signal mark: intravenous injection of propranolol, 1 mg/kg. At third signal mark: intravenous injection of propranolol, 2 mg/kg. Is: intravenous injections of isoprenaline, 0.002 mg/kg

The actual mechanism of the direct cardio-depressive action of Inderal is not known. It is not due to the activation of the cholinergic receptors. It also appears that it cannot be related to the local anaesthetic effect, because other β-blocking agents such as MJ 1999 [1159] and INPEA [1783] are cardiodepressors [3, 1255] whilst at the same time having no local anaesthetic effect. The fact that Inderal exerts a quinidine-like depressive action on the maximal velocity of depolarisation of the cardiac cell membrane [1318] could signify, according to certain authors [1125], that this effect causes depression of the contractility by interfering with the excitation-contraction coupling mechanism. It is known that the link between membrane depolarisation and contraction, viz. the excitation-contraction coupling, calls for the presence of ionised calcium [1342]. The level of cardiac contraction is proportional to the influx of the calcium ions from the extra-cellular phase to the myocardial cell [1364, 2019]. This translocation of calcium takes place by passage through the hydro- and liposoluble layer of the cell membrane. Now Inderal depresses the rate at which the myocardium accumulates calcium ions [1342]. Since its negative inotropic effect is in parallel with the inhibiting effect which it exerts on the lipidic transport of the calcium ions, and since the activity of ATP-ase of the myofibrillae is not modified at the same moment [1352], it has been suggested that the cardio-depressive effect depends primarily on the obstruction of the lipidic transport [1352], this inhibition being reflected in the fact that uptake of the calcium by the cardiac sarcoplasmic reticulum is sharply depressed [824, 1649, 1988]. ENTMAN et al. [38a] have also demonstrated that Inderal abolished both the activation of adenylcyclase and the increase in microsomal calcium accumulation produced by epinephrine in a microsomal fraction of canine myocardium thought to represent sarcoplasmic reticulum. FLECKENSTEIN [561] expresses a similar view, since he found that Inderal inhibits the Ca-dependent myofibrillary ATP-ase, and the activity of the enzyme could be re-established by administering calcium.

Recommendations for the Treatment of Angina Pectoris

In view of the side effects of Inderal, the current attitude of clinicians is to use it *only advisedly and prudently* for treating angina, and at all events to avoid it with subjects with suspected latent cardiac insufficiency and even more so those suffering from incipient or overt cardiac insufficiency, for whom it is strictly contra-indicated [659, 1068, 1467, 1683, 1841] because, in a review covering 5000 cases treated in 1966, STEPHEN [1832] reports some twenty cases of cardiac decompensation occurring mainly in major heart disease cases and leading to death in eleven cases. Some clinicians recommand to associate digitalics to Inderal in order to avoid the cardiac risk [287 c].

It seems that the therapeutic efficacy of Inderal in angina depends strictly on the posology [453, 709, 1466] and that to achieve a favourable effect it requires a relatively high daily dose (400 mg) which is often the maximum dose tolerated [502, 660, 1466]. This being so, the clinician has to use a daily dose which is often in the region of that at which cardiac side effects occur [1492], so that its use must be subject to special precautions and it is recommended that the posology should be constantly adjusted so as not to exceed the minimal dose at which an anti-anginal effect is obtained [709]. The handling of Inderal is therefore particularly delicate, especially for the general practitioner, the more so since it is recommended to keep the patient under close medical surveillance as a matter of general practice [453]. The greatest caution is required as regards the patient suffering at the same time from bronchial asthma [502], which is explained by the fact that Inderal sharply increases resistance in the respiratory tract in the case of the asthmatic [156], and causes bronchial constriction in normal people [195 c] and also in asthmatics [146 c, 195 c, 219 c].

Ineffectiveness of Inderal in Acute Myocardial Infarction

From the experimental viewpoint, immediate mortality following acute ligature of the circumflex coronary artery of an anaesthetised dog is significantly reduced by Inderal administered intravenously at the dose of 0.08 mg/kg during the 3 min preceding the ligature [1429]. As compared with the untreated group, heart rate, cardiac output and work, and the tension-time index are lowered. The favourable effect observed is attributed to the lessening of myocardial oxygen consumption (which minimises the hypoxia-inducing effect of the ligature) and also perhaps to the anti-arrhythmic effect.

SNOW [1765] has noted that the administration of 20 mg of Inderal every 8 hours to 52 patients suffering from acute infarction reduces mortality to 13% whereas it was 29% in the case of 55 untreated patients. It would however seem that this is an exceptional finding since it has been invalidated on several occasions. For instance, according to BALCON et al. in a double-blind experiment [79], when administered daily at a dose of 80 mg for 28 days to 114 patients, Inderal does not alter mortality from acute infarction. The same opinion is expressed by CLAUSEN et al. [333] in respect of a group of 110 cases treated with 40 mg. This ineffectiveness is largely confirmed by DOTREMONT and DE GEEST [445] with some sixty cases, and especially by NORRIS et al. [1377] who, in the course of a double-blind test on 536 cases treated for 3 weeks at the daily dose of 80 mg, find no difference in the mortality rate between the treated group and the control group. This investigation justifies the conclusion of a multicentre investigation [1069] that the use of Inderal is not indicated in the normal treatment of myocardial infarct, an opinion shared by others [877]. In addition, NORRIS found no favourable effect on the incidence of post-infarct cardiac pain, confirming in this the findings of

BALCON [79] and of CLAUSEN [333]. The use of Inderal in this indication should
be accompanied by the greatest possible precautions since it brings about a drop
in cardiac output under these conditions [113]. Its intravenous use in acute
infarct must be rejected because of the risks of a fatal outcome [1762].

Inderal has other clinical applications than for angina pectoris. It is indicated
in the treatment of sub-aortic hypertrophic idiopathic stenosis, especially with
angina complications, because it considerably increases tolerance to exercise on an
endless belt [214, 342] and improves the permanent clinical condition of the
patient [322, 1554, 1555], probably by reducing the extent of the functional
obstruction of ventricular ejection (an obstruction which is accentuated by effort)
and of the oxygen needs of the heart, by lowering the heart rate and reducing both
ventricular parietal tension and cardiac contraction velocity [343]. Long-term
oral Inderal therapy is considered the treatment of choice for patients with latent
or labile outflow obstruction due to muscular sub-aortic stenosis because it has
been of significant symptomatic benefit in all the patients treated [11b]. Inderal
would merit being applied in such cases before considering any surgical operation
[343].

Inderal is also active in the hyperkinetic heart syndrome [199, 647, 1197], and
in the circulatory disturbances arising from hypersympathicotony [405, 607],
exerting a regulatory effect by reducing pulse rate [46a]. ROSENBLUM and DEL-
MAN [108a] believe that Inderal may be effective in the control of hyperdynamic
β-adrenergic states, but its administration calls for a careful appraisal of possible
side effects.

The Use of Inderal in Cardiac Arrhythmia

Besides angina pectoris, Inderal has a major therapeutic indication: that of
arrhythmia.

As is usual, this indication is based on pharmacological observations on animals.

The fact of having available a drug possessing specific β-blocking properties
logically had to lead to investigations as to an anti-arrhythmic effect on animals,
and this for two reasons: firstly the existence of a slowing-up effect on the heart
rate, and secondly the fact that hyperactivity of the adrenergic β-receptors
appears to be the cause of certain upsets in cardiac rhythm, although it is rather
felt now that cardiac arrhythmia originates more from the activity of certain
specific intracardiac receptors, different from the β-receptors (see p. 220). Whatever
may be the pathogeny, still imperfectly understood, of rhythm disorders, physiologists have reported in animals various properties possessed by Inderal as regards
the intrinsic conduction system of the heart. It lowers the frequency of the automatic activity of the sinusal node [599]. It also acts on the atrio-ventricular node
[923, 1990], for it reduces its automatism, prolongs the refractory period of A-V
transmission (even in the case of an animal with a denervated heart, 1955) and
increases A-V conduction time, all effects which are almost entirely due to β-
blockade. As regards the A-V node, Inderal competitively blocks the positive
chronotropic effect of the catecholamines and counters their shortening effect on
the refractory period [923]. In the anaesthetised dog, Inderal blocks the atrio-ventricular junctional tachycardia produced by direct perfusion of the septal artery
or the atrio-ventricular node artery with noradrenaline or isoproterenol [160c].

Obviously all these effects cause a slowing up of the rhythm which was foreseeable since the heart beat rate is, amongst other things, subject to the tonic activity
of the β-receptors, not only as regards the sinusal node but also the atrio-ventricular node, as demonstrated by LINHART et al. [1151] using an original technique

enabling the refractory period of the atrio-ventricular conduction system to be measured in man. They found that isoprenaline shortens this refractory period, a fact which they interpret as an activation of the adrenergic β-receptors located in the atrio-ventricular conduction system. Furthermore, they find that the effects of any stimulus on the rhythmic nature of the sinusal node are exerted in the same direction as regards the atrio-ventricular system, and that in many cases the relative effect on this latter is greater than at the sinusal node. It follows that cardiac acceleration due to sympathetic stimulation is due to the combined effect of an acceleration of the rhythmicity of the sinusal node and a shortening of the refractory period of the atrio-ventricular conduction system.

Inderal also has a quinidine-like effect [599, 1317], that is to say, like quinidine, it exerts a negative dromotropic effect (lessening of the velocity of conduction) and reduces the excitability of the cardiac muscle, thereby extending its refractory period. These properties would seem to be independent of the local anaesthetic activity of the drug [1932]. Indeed, there is no correlation between the relative potency of the local anaesthetic effect and of the extending effect on the refractory period [1495]. The cardiac actions are due to membrane stabilising properties, because certain analogues of propranolol, which have no β-antagonising effect, are anti-arrhythmic probably as a result of a membrane stabilising effect which, according to certain authors, is in relation to the local anaesthetic effect [1188].

VAUGHAN-WILLIAMS [1931] has pointed out that, like quinidine, Inderal does not change the resting potential nor does it extend the myocardial cell repolarisation period, but does considerably decrease the height and speed of the rise in intracellular action potentials, and prolongs the refractory period[3]. These effects, which are also found at the ventricle [7b], have therefore been called quinidine-like. But since, unlike Inderal, sympathetic stimulation increases the action potential height and the speed at which it rises [1931], it does not seem necessary to KERNOHAN [970] to speak of the "quinidine-like" effects of Inderal (an expression similarly rejected by other authors [125a]), and it seems logical to him to consider them as manifestations of the β-blocking effect which form the basis of the anti-arrhythmic properties. Conversely, PITT and COX [1451] think of a direct effect, independent of the anti-β properties, on the cells of the auricle, because they display a quinidine-like effect on the transmembrane action potential consisting in a significant slowing down of depolarisation speed and an extension of the refractory period. Finally, according to LUCCHESI [1186], the situation is more complicated. He showed that the dose of Inderal necessary for suppressing arrhythmia induced by ouabaine in the isolated rabbit heart is much higher than the β-blocking dose. Similarly [1190], he noted in the case of an anaesthetised dog that the anti-arrhythmic activity is independent of the isomeric form, whereas Inderal (which is the racemic form of propranolol) is 50 times more active as a β-blocking agent than is the dextrogyre form. There come within the same context the findings of THOMPSON and LETLEY [1887] who examined the quinidine-like activity of Inderal from the angle of two criteria: a) the extension, quinidine-like, of the P-R interval of a rat's ECG, which calls for high dosages of Inderal; b) the reversibility to the sinusal rhythm of ventricular tachycardia brought on by barium chloride. By comparing the active doses over the two anti-arrhythmic

---

3 It has been confirmed that Inderal significantly decreases the rate of rise of the action potential in human ventricular tissue with no significant effect on other electrophysiological events [66c]. There is a similar effect on dog ventricle [66c], in agreement with the work of DAVIS and TEMPTE [7b]. There was no increase in rate of rise at low concentrations in either species, contrary to the observations of SHEVDE and SPILKER [13d] who found an increase in the rate of rise in a similar preparation but only at low concentrations.

activity tests and the β-blocking doses, these authors find that the blocking dose is not anti-arrhythmic and that it must be increased tenfold to achieve a significant anti-arrhythmic effect. They thus confirm the dissociation between the two doses as shown by LUCCHESI, and they infer from this that there are in the heart two types of receptors which can be influenced by Inderal, the β-receptors which can be blocked with low doses, and some receptors of a different kind which can be affected by substances whose structure is much less specific as regards the anti-β effect, but only at a high concentration. According to LUCCHESI et al. [1190], the anti-arrhythmic effect of Inderal therefore arises both from a specific anti-β effect (it is this which intervenes in the case of the adrenergic type arrhythmia conditions) and a non-specific action of the quinidine type (which comes into play in the case of digitalis-induced arrhythmia).

A more complex view is taken by SHINEBOURNE et al. [1745]. They compare four anti-arrhythmic substances as regards some of their activities (Table 7).

Table 7

Substance	Cardio-depressive effect	β-blocking effect	Antagonising effect as regards Ca ions	Local anaesthetic effect
Lidocaine	0	0	0	+
Tetracaine	0	0	0	+
Quinidine	+	+	+	+
Propranolol	+	+	+	+

In the light of this information, they believe that the anti-arrhythmic activity of propranolol (and of quinidine) can be independent of β-blockade because lidocaine and tetracaine, which are anti-arrhythmic, are not β-blocking agents and therefore do not oppose the uptake of Ca ions by the cardiac sarcoplasmic reticulum. VAUGHAN-WILLIAMS however [1933] advances very pertinent arguments in favour of the role played by the anti-β effect, for, taking as a basis the comparative effects of the levogyre and dextrogyre derivatives of propranolol, he points out that these two isomers have a local anaesthetic effect and an effect on the action potential depolarisation phase which are quantitatively identical. Yet the dextrogyre derivative is 100 times less active on the β-receptors and also much less active as regards cardiac arrhythmia.

When administered to patients in clinically effective doses (0.1 mg/kg i.v.), propranolol prolongs atrio-ventricular conduction and has no effect on intra-ventricular conduction [11a].

As far as experimental arrhythmia in animals is concerned, Inderal neutralises the adrenergic-type ventricular extrasystoles [1189, 57a] and those caused by barium chloride [1198, 1411]. It also counters the disturbing effect of adrenaline on a dog whose anterior coronary artery has been ligatured [1729]. As regards ouabaine-induced arrhythmia, certain authors consider it to be inactive [1189] while others believe it to be active [1009]. The apparent lack of harmony between these latter results could be explained in the light of the data published by RAPER and WALE [1495]: they show that Inderal (as also Trasicor and Sotalol) is active against adrenaline-type and digitalis arrhythmia, but they do emphasise that the ouabaine-countering effect calls for doses 20—50 times higher than in the case of adrenaline. The explanation they give is that the anti-arrhythmic effect as regards adrenaline is ascribable to a specific β-antagonising effect and only calls for low doses, whereas the anti-arrhythmic properties vis-à-vis ouabaine can be ascribed to a quinidine-like cardio-depressive effect, and for this reason call for very much stronger doses. Their interpretation thus lines up with that of LUCCHESI.

In the case of cats, a blocking dose of Inderal reduces the frequency of the ectopic rhythms which appear following vagal stimulation [104a].

All these experimental findings justify the clinical research undertaken with Inderal into cardiac rhythm disorders. They have made it possible to specify the therapeutic indications in this sphere. Inderal is effective in cases of sinusal tachycardia, whatever the reason for it [1652], and in all instances of rapid ventricular rhythm [599, 1032]. Active for supraventricular tachycardia [1903], it provides a means for controlling the rapid ventricular rhythm of atrial fibrillation which is recalcitrant to digitalis [153, 361, 1193, 1579, 1758, 1867] and of atrial flutter [502, 1193, 1758, 1962]. Inderal is the drug of choice for the treatment of recurrent supraventricular tachycardias which satisfy the criteria for reciprocating tachycardia, because it prevented tachycardia in five patients out of seven and slowed it in one [112c]. Certain authors believe, however, that it is risky to use Inderal where there is cardiac decompensation, even when combined with a suitable digitalis treatment [361], the risk being particularly grave where there is valvular heart disease. It should not be used in latent or overt heart failure [113c]. Its intravenous administration as a very slow injection at the maximum dose of 0.1 mg/kg is recommended, because of its almost immediate favourable effect, for ventricular tachycardia of atrial origin, whether fibrillation or flutter [1130], and for digitalis-induced arrhythmia [1130], but caution must be taken in the case of patients with low cardiac output.

Inderal is also effective against ventricular arrhythmia of a digitalis nature where it is held to be the best treatment to select [652, 878], but it is not very active as regards non-digitalis ventricular arrhythmia [213, 503]. It is also useful in paroxystic atrial tachycardia [652, 878] and is said to be effective in cases of paroxystic tachycardia with a history of over two years [650].

Inderal is effective in cases of arrhythmia occurring during the halothane anaesthesia preparatory to cardiovascular surgery [876, 893, 1247], and also those which appear during and after open heart operations [1239, 1246]. When combined with quinidine, it can ensure the reconversion of chronic atrial fibrillation to the sinusal rhythm [1834], normally recalcitrant to any type of therapy, but this favourable result has not been confirmed by others [831] who draw attention to the many side effects of this medicinal association. A combination of Inderal and Digoxin is capable of restoring sinusal rhythm in atrial flutter [337c].

Inderal is, however, inactive as regards the very frequent arrhythmia conditions which occur in the course of myocardial infarction [79, 333, 445, 1091]. Despite unanimity on this point, LEMBERG et al. [1099] claim the opposite, because they were able to reestablish the sinusal rhythm by slow intravenous injection of Inderal in the course of 16 incidents of arrhythmia occurring in 12 patients who, during the first five days of acute infarction, suffered either from atrial fibrillation or flutter or from atrial or nodal tachycardia. That these authors should have succeeded in every case to reestablish the sinusal rhythm in these types of arrhythmia is astonishing enough, but what is even more so is the fact that, unlike all their predecessors, they found that the moderate or severe cardiac decompensation from which all the patients suffered, was improved. Prudence is therefore advisable before falling in with their conclusion that Inderal can be used without risk in cases of tachyarrhythmia occurring during acute infarct and without taking into account the possible presence of overt heart failure.

Inderal is counter-indicated in cases of complete A-V block and of idio-ventricular rhythm [502][4].

Since 1970, and more especially as a result of the clinical investigations performed by PRICHARD [257c, 258c] and by ZACHARIAS [344c], Inderal has been advocated for the control of hypertension. As the recommended dosage regimen, beginning with 20 mg four times daily, can attain in most patients a daily maintenance dose of 240—320 mg by the 5th week of treatment in order to control the diastolic pressure and keep it below 100 mm Hg, a special presentation, Inderal-80, has been made available.

2. Trasicor

Synthesised by WILHELM et al. [1999], Trasicor (generic name: oxprenolol) or Ciba 39089-Ba is a medication recommended in two major clinical indications: angina pectoris and disturbances in cardiac rhythm. Basically it is a β-blocking agent whose structure is very similar to that of propranolol:

$$R \qquad\qquad R$$
$$\qquad\qquad -OCH_2-CH=CH_2$$

Propranolol   Oxprenolol

Such an analogy explains why most of the investigations carried out into it are mainly of a comparative character with propranolol, with the object of bringing out any advantages it might offer as compared with the latter substance.

BRUNNER et al. [249] show that the β-blocking properties of Trasicor in the case of animals are equivalent to those of propranolol in the conventional tests, and that it has no anti-adrenergic α-properties. Trasicor has the pharmacological side effects inherent in the β-antagonists since it reduces coronary flow, lessens cardiac contraction force and increases the oxygen extraction coefficient of the myocardium, with as a consequence an increase in coronary arterio-venous oxygen difference. As regards cardiac output, this would not appear to be reduced.

A comment is called for in this connection: the authors provide no detailed figures for their experiments. This fact is the more regrettable in that the purpose of their paper was also to show that the cardio-depressive properties of Trasicor are less accentuated than those of propranolol, the negative inotropic cardiac effect of this latter being, as we know, its main side effect. The authors therefore bring no definite arguments forward to support their conclusion that the non-specific side effects, peculiar to all β-blocking agents, are less pronounced in the case of Trasicor.

FERUGLIO et al. [542] publish a purely haemodynamic paper covering dogs, in which they conclude that Trasicor increases coronary arterial resistance by 22%, reduces coronary flow by 22%, lowers myocardial oxygen consumption by 11%, slows down cardiac contraction velocity by 40%, and differs from propranolol in the fact that it does not reduce cardiac output.

The decrease in coronary flow has been confirmed in dogs [1346], although in the same animal species, a dose of 0.07 mg/kg of Trasicor administered by intravenous route did not alter coronary blood flow whereas 0.25 mg/kg of propranolol reduced it [85c].

According to MAXWELL [1241] also, Trasicor sharply reduces coronary flow in dogs, a phenomenon which he ascribes to the reduction in coronary perfusion

---

4 GIBSON and SOWTON recently summarized up the available facts concerning the clinica use of propranolol and other β-blockers in arrhythmias [49a].

pressure because it runs parallel to a drop in systemic blood pressure. The reduction in blood flow must however be contributed to by an increase in coronary arterial resistance, a fact which has been demonstrated in dogs [1350]. Handled by us also, Trasicor considerably reduces coronary flow: Figure 21 relates to an anaesthetised dog, where the intravenous administration of a dose of 0.5 mg/kg of Trasicor reduces by almost 50% the coronary arterial flow. The development of this effect, and of the drop in heart rate and blood pressure, are strikingly reminiscent of what is observed in the case of Inderal (see Fig. 18).

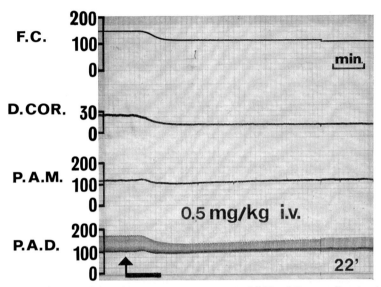

Fig. 21. Effect of oxprenolol on heart rate, coronary arterial blood flow, and systemic blood pressure in the anaesthetized dog. From top to bottom: F.C.: Heart rate (beats/min). D.Cor.: Mean blood flow in the left circumflex coronary artery, measured with an electromagnetic probe (ml/min). P.A.M.: Mean blood pressure in the femoral artery (mm Hg). P.A.D.: Phasic blood pressure in the femoral artery (mm Hg). At signal mark: intravenous injection of oxprenolol, 0.5 mg/kg. Part of tracings recorded 22 min after injection

According to NAYLER [1343], Trasicor reduces the work of the left ventricle of a dog to a lesser extent than does propranolol, but in a subsequent paper [1346] this difference between the cardio-depressive effect of the two medications does not emerge clearly. The negative inotropic effect of Trasicor is reported to be considerably lower than that of propranolol on human and dog heart atrial and papillary muscle specimens [1345] and on an isolated heart [1225].

Finally, KOROXENIDIS et al. [1019] report, following intravenous injection of Trasicor in an anaesthetised dog, a moderate slowing up of heart rate, a slight drop in cardiac output and in contraction velocity, and a marked reduction in cardiac work.

This diversity of opinions regarding the cardio-depressive effect of Trasicor prompted us to carry out some experiments on anaesthetised dogs. Figure 22 shows that an intravenous dose of 0.25 mg/kg of Trasicor, insufficient in the case of this animal to block the cardiac stimulating effect of isoprenaline administered 5 min later (start of graph C), is already cardio-depressive since cardiac contraction velocity is reduced by 20% (compare graph B with the start of graph C). An additional dose of 0.5 mg/kg of Trasicor, which blocks the heart-stimulating effect of isoprenaline (end of graph C), accentuates the decrease in cardiac contraction velocity, this now being only 68% of its control value, and reduces the left ventricular systolic pressure sufficiently to cause the general blood pressure to drop.

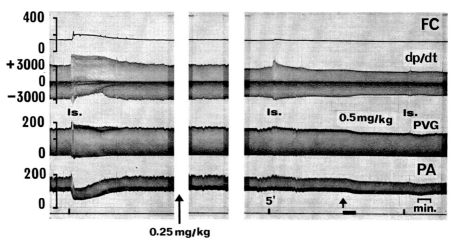

Fig. 22. Effect of oxprenolol on heart rate, rate of rise in left ventricular pressure, left ventricular pressure and systemic blood pressure in the anaesthetized dog. From top to bottom: F.C.: Heart rate (beats/min). dp/dt: Rate of rise in left ventricular pressure (mm Hg/sec). P.V.G.: Left ventricular pressure (mm Hg). P.A.: Phasic blood pressure in the femoral artery (mm Hg). Left tracing: intravenous injection of isoprenaline, 0.001 mg/kg. Between left and middle tracings: intravenous injection of oxprenolol, 0.25 mg/kg. Right tracing: at signal mark, intravenous injection of oxprenolol, 0.5 mg/kg. Iso: intravenous injections of isoprenaline, 0.001 mg/kg

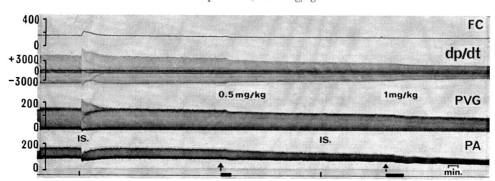

Fig. 23. Effect of oxprenolol on heart rate, rate of rise in left ventricular pressure, left ventricular pressure and systemic blood pressure in the anaesthetized dog. From top to bottom: F.C.: Heart rate (beats/min). dp/dt: Rate of rise in left ventricular pressure (mm Hg/sec). P.V.G.: Left ventricular pressure (mm Hg). P.A.: Phasic blood pressure in the femoral artery (mm Hg). At first signal mark: intravenous injection of oxprenolol, 0.5 mg/kg. At second signal mark: intravenous injection of oxprenolol, 1 mg/kg. Is: intravenous injections of isoprenaline, 0.002 mg/kg

With another animal (Fig. 23), the intravenous dose of 0.5 mg/kg of Trasicor, which ensures complete blockade of the β-receptors (as witness the inactivity of isoprenaline injected 10 min later), straight away brings about a marked and progressive drop in cardiac contraction velocity, left ventricular systolic pressure and blood pressure, these three parameters being reduced by 29, 23 and 21%

respectively within 15 min following the injection. A subsequent intravenous injection of 1 mg/kg of Trasicor considerably accentuates at this point the depression of the three haemodynamic parameters. In the case of a third animal (Fig. 24), the cardio-depressive effect of Trasicor at the intravenous dose of 0.5 mg/kg establishes itself more slowly than in the previous animal, but it is no less marked after 30—45 min when the β-receptors are progressively freed, as witness the slight cardiac stimulation which reappears with the injection of isoprenaline. Two subsequent intravenous injections of 1 and 2 mg/kg of Trasicor accentuate the depression of the myocardial functions.

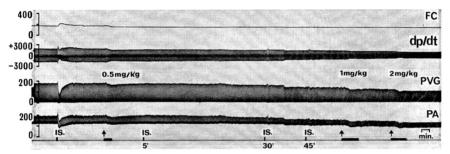

Fig. 24. Effect of oxprenolol on heart rate, rate of rise in left ventricular pressure, left ventricular pressure and systemic blood pressure in the anaesthetized dog. From top to bottom: F.C.: Heart rate (beats/min). dp/dt: Rate of rise in left ventricular pressure (mm Hg/sec). P.V.G.: Left ventricular pressure (mm Hg). P.A.: Phasic blood pressure in the femoral artery (mm Hg). At first signal mark: intravenous injection of oxprenolol, 0.5 mg/kg. At second signal mark: intravenous injection of oxprenolol, 1 mg/kg. At third signal mark: intravenous injection of oxprenolol, 2 mg/kg. Iso: intravenous injections of isoprenaline, 0.002 mg/kg

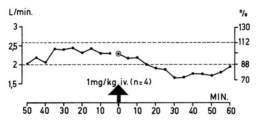

Fig. 25. Effect of oxprenolol, 1 mg/kg i.v., on cardiac output in the anaesthetized dog (mean values for 4 animals)

These experiments demonstrate the cardio-depressive effect of Trasicor, whose intensity appears to us to be difficult to distinguish from that of Inderal. This action by Trasicor can also be demonstrated by measuring cardiac output. Figure 25 illustrates four experiments which we carried out on anaesthetised dogs: with an intravenous dose of 1 mg/kg, cardiac output is reduced by almost 30% within the following half hour. If we compare this figure with Fig. 19, which relates to the behaviour of cardiac output measured by the same technique following the intravenous injection of 1 mg/kg of Inderal, we see the striking similarity between the two graphs.

Trasicor has anti-arrhythmic properties as regards animals. This is particularly so as regards conditions of arrhythmia induced by adrenaline, where its action is equal to that of propranolol [1495], and in the case of digitalis-arrhythmia which calls for considerable dosages for the reasons given earlier (see p. 220). It increases the refractory period of an isolated auricle to the same extent as does propranolol

15*

[1495], and it has local anaesthetic properties five times lower than those of propranolol [1495]. As is the case with this latter drug, there is no correlation between the cardiac effect and the local anaesthetic effect [1495]. Trasicor counters the fibrillating effect of fatal doses of ouabaine in the case of guinea-pigs, this property being perhaps attributable in part to the β-blocking action. There is also a quinidine-like effect on the action potential of the cardiac cell, which can be qualitatively superimposed on that of propranolol [1412].

The results of several investigations into human pharmacology have been published. BENDER and SCHMIDT [132] observe that in a man at rest and with sinusal rhythm, the reduction in heart rate achieved by Trasicor is less marked (at an identical dose) than is the case with propranolol, a fact which has been confirmed by BENDER et al. [10a]. On the other hand, a given increase in heart rate resulting from the intravenous injection of isoprenaline is countered by a lower dose of Trasicor than of propranolol.

REALE et al. [1502] show that at the intravenous dose of 5 mg, Trasicor reduces coronary flow by 30%. In another test with 41 patients subjected to cardiac catheterisation for diagnosis purposes, REALE et al. [1503] confirm the reduction in myocardial irrigation. They also observe a drop in cardiac output and in cardiac contractility [1500], the latter giving rise to an increase in end-diastolic ventricular pressure; aortic pressure rises, as also does peripheral arterial resistance.

According to VORIDIS et al. [1950], Trasicor does not appear to have an inhibiting action on the cardiac function under basal conditions; but where there is cardiac overloading (injection of macromolecular dextran), the adaptation response of the heart appears to be inadequate following administration of Trasicor.

In a haemodynamic survey carried out on 34 patients suffering from left cardiopathy, GRANDJEAN and RIVIER [708] compared the haemodynamic effects of Trasicor and propranolol administered intravenously at the dose of 5 mg. In their view, the two drugs are equi-active as regards the degree of slowing up of the heart rate. They are unlike, however, in the following respects:

1. pulmonary blood pressure does not change with Trasicor whereas it rises sharply with propranolol; 2. whilst they both reduce the resting cardiac output, a rise in the stroke volume offsets the slowing down of rhythm in the case of Trasicor, whereas this compensation is not found with propranolol.

It should however be pointed out that the compensating increase in stroke volume which appears under resting conditions in the case of Trasicor is much lower during exercise, which would explain why the drop in cardiac output caused by Trasicor is greater during exercise than in the resting state. GRANDJEAN and RIVIER, whose clear intention it was to assess the risks of precipitating cardiac insufficiency by using Trasicor and propranolol, conclude that the negative inotropic cardiac effect of Trasicor is less marked than that of propranolol.

This conclusion does not agree with those of BURGIN [260] nor of LEKOS et al. [1098]. BURGIN carried out a comparative haemodynamic survey on Trasicor, propranolol and a placebo with 8 healthy volunteers and 6 coronary subjects who were given orally the two active drugs at the same dosage. He finds in the case of Trasicor a drop in cardiac output which is roughly the same as that found with propranolol. According to him, there is no significant difference between the haemodynamic effects of the two medications. In his view, Trasicor offers no advantage over propranolol, and "in the long run, it is the cost which will determine the choice as between these two drugs". LEKOS, for his part, reports a marked drop in cardiac output and myocardial contraction velocity in the case of a man receiving an intravenous injection of 5 mg of Trasicor, these two phenomena being especially marked during physical effort. In his view, these haemodynamic changes can be superimposed on those brought about by propranolol. For GER-HARD et al. also [642], Trasicor injected in a normal man at the dose of 10 mg i.v. reduces cardiac output in the same way as does propranolol. Regarding the effect of Trasicor on cardiac output, BENSAID et al. make a distinction between subjects with absolutely normal cardiac functioning and patients suffering from cardiopathy. Following an intravenous injection of 0.1 or 0.2 mg/kg, the cardiac index is not significantly altered in the healthy subject, which means that there is no cardiodepressant effect under these conditions [25c]. On the other hand, the cardiac index falls by 20% in cardiac patients presenting a certain degree of insufficiency, and the myocardial depressant effect of Trasicor appears to be similar to that of propranolol [24c].

By measuring the heart rate of ski jumpers by telemetry, and carrying out the double-blind and cross-permutation test, it has been shown [64a] that when administered orally at the dose of 40 mg prior to the test, Trasicor reduces to a greater extent the emotional tachycardia (prior to descent) than the effort tachycardia (during the jump).

Clinical Application

In a preliminary survey, RIVIER [1537] mentions the favourable results which he obtained over a limited number of angina pectoris patients. BIANCHI [158] reports the results of a multi-centre investigation carried out double-blind with 62 patients. Each patient was treated for two weeks with Trasicor at a daily dose of 120 mg (3 × 40 mg) and for two further weeks with the placebo. The criteria for the effect on the anginal syndrome are conventional: number and gravity of the anginal attacks, number of doses of nitroglycerin taken, and physical potential of the patient. A statistical analysis of the results shows that Trasicor proved more active than the placebo for these three criteria.

A second survey by the same authors, spread over several months of treatment, confirm these results, whilst at the same time demonstrating that in certain cases the daily dose of 60 mg is sufficient to achieve a good therapeutic effect [159].

When administered at the dose of 60 mg intravenously to the angina subject, Trasicor significantly extends the duration of an exercise on the ergometric bicycle [10]. For his part, ROOKMAKER [1551, 1552] points out that in the case of 15 patients suffering from angina pectoris, the Master type effort test is considerably improved by Trasicor in 11 cases insofar that the drop in the level of the S-T segment of the electrocardiogram is considerably less where there is chronic treatment than prior to treatment. According to the author, the activity of propranolol (5 cases improved out of 15) is much less marked. WILSON and TURNER [2005] publish four observations of anginal patients who found the number of their attacks considerably reduced under treatment with Trasicor. In a later paper [2006], they report their opinion of a double-blind test, unfortunately limited to only 12 patients: Trasicor proved to be active. In their view, treatment should never be suddenly interrupted once the therapeutic effect is obtained, but the dosage should be gradually reduced because half the patients suffered a serious return of their symptoms when put on the placebo, a phenomenon which they attribute to an extended rebound of sympathetic hypertonicity of a β-character. In a double-blind study, Trasicor at the oral dose of 40 mg tds reduced the incidence of anginal attacks and the number of nitroglycerin tablets consumed [250c]. Forty five angina patients who were followed up over two years received a starting daily dose of 40 to 60 mg, the dosage being gradually increased until a clinical response or a maximal amount of 240 mg daily was reached. 34 patients showed

definite clinical improvement sustained over two years, 14 of them becoming
symptom-free. Cardiac failure occurred in two cases [19 c].

Various clinical publications dealing with Trasicor speak of its effect in cardiac
rhythm disorders.

GRANDJEAN [707] reports that in sinusal tachycardia during rest, an oral dose
of 40 mg returns the heart rate to its normal value, and that sinusal tachycardia
due to muscular exercise is considerably reduced following the injection of 5 mg
into the vein. In the case of atrial fibrillation, the intravenous injection of 5 mg of
Trasicor sharply slows down the rate of ventricular rhythm, both at rest and under
effort. Finally, in the case of atrial flutter, Trasicor is inactive, as is usual with the
β-blocking agents, but can in certain cases slow down the rate of the ventricular
rhythm. With RIVIER et al. [1538], he confirms the essentials of these observations
with 112 patients with whom he had only 14 failures.

FUCCELLA and IMHOF [612] publish the results of a combined investigation by
28 Swiss doctors on about a hundred walking patients suffering from disorders of
cardiac rhythm. The course of treatment lasted for three weeks at an oral dose of
an average of 60 mg. Trasicor proved very effective in cases of sinusal tachycardia
and the rapid ventricular rhythms of atrial fibrillation. Furthermore, it either
eliminated altogether or sharply decreased the frequency of ventricular and supraventricular paroxystic tachycardia attacks.

A further investigation carried out by PINTO [1445] with a hundred or so
patients suffering from the most varied forms of cardiac arrhythmia led to results
which are largely in line with those of the above-mentioned authors.

VETTORI et al. [1940], reporting a survey made on 30 patients suffering from
chronic atrial flutter or fibrillation, find a return to the sinusal rhythm obtained in
4 cases by the use of Trasicor. In 16 other cases, sinusal rhythm was only re-
established by the addition of quinidine.

Finally, CORCONDILAS et al. [362] treated an unspecified number of patients
suffering from cardiac arrhythmia which was recalcitrant to the usual treatments.
These cases consisted of isolated ventricular extrasystoles or various types of
supraventricular tachycardia. Sinusal rhythm was re-established by Trasicor in
all cases after an average of 12 days, the dose required being 90 mg per day on
average. Similar good results were recorded in 39 patients suffering from several
types of cardiac arrhythmia [19 c].

According to ROJAS [1550], the anti-arrhythmic effect of Trasicor is exerted
rather on the ventricular stage than on the atrial stage.

Fundamentally, it seems to be generally accepted that, at equal dosage, the
negative chronotropic effect of Trasicor is superimposable on that of propranolol.
In other words, at a given dosage, the slowing down of heart rate caused by the
two drugs is roughly the same, both in animals and humans. Similarly, the doses
necessary for blocking the tachycardia induced by isoprenaline in animals are very
similar for both substances. Looked at from this angle, it can therefore be considered that the blocking properties of Trasicor and propranolol vis-à-vis the
adrenergic β-receptors are comparable in intensity.

If we try to compare the two drugs from the point of view of their *negative
inotropic* effect on cardiac dynamics, there is profound disagreement between
authors. It does however seem that the majority of them consider that the cardiac
depression induced by Trasicor can be likened to that produced by propranolol.
Our tests lead us to a similar conclusion.

For the reasons expounded on p. 43, the potential cardiac risk presented by
Trasicor seems to be superimposable on that of propranolol. In point of fact, it is
not so much the direct cardio-depressive effect of the β-blocking agents which

entails cardiac risk, but above all *the fact that the adrenergic β-receptors are neutralised by these drugs*, because this blockade deprives the subject with cardiac insufficiency of the compensating adrenergic mechanism which he normally brings into play to combat his circulatory deficiency [620]. Incidentally, RIVIER et al. [1538] reported two cases of acute cardiac insufficiency following intravenous injection of Trasicor. They consider that this possible risk should be taken into account, which leads them to associate digitalis in all cases where the possibility of myocardial impairment is suspected. This attitude lines up with what ROJAS [1550] has shown and according to whom the cardiac output in man decreases with a daily dose of 240 mg, higher doses being capable of setting up cardiac insufficiency. JUCHEMS and WERTZ also observed a significant fall in cardiac index and heart rate, associated with a rise in peripheral resistance, after an intravenous injection of 5 mg of Trasicor in normal individuals. The stroke volume was slightly decreased [65a]. A reduction of 27% in cardiac output has also been reported in the subject with high blood pressure following the intravenous injection of 0.2 mg/kg of Trasicor over a period of 6 min [36b].

All the known β-blocking agents entail the risk of causing heart failure in patients suffering from left ventricular heart disease [451]. As mentioned by FITZGERALD [557], every β-blocking substance can cause cardiac decompensation with sufficient dosage and also in situations where the tonus of the sympathetic system should be maintained because of the role which it plays in the homeostasis of the cardiac function. Now it is just this sympathetic tonus which is the limiting physiological factor in heart failure in the cardiac insufficiency subject. The fact of suppressing this tonus upsets the homeostatic response and precipitates the insufficiency. In terms of heart safety, there is as yet no convincing evidence that the β-blocking agents at present available are any different from each other. Additional clinical research is required before being able to claim the superiority of one over the other. There can however be degrees of risk, depending amongst other things on the active dosage used with man. This has been very well put by WOLLHEIM [2035] in the case of propranolol: moderate doses entail no cardiac risk but are inactive as regards angina pectoris, whereas high dosages which are active in the anginal patient involve decompensation incidents.

According to WAAL [1951], Trasicor has the advantage over propranolol of being somewhat of a central stimulating agent, whereas propranolol often causes depression. In the opinion of BEUMER [156], Trasicor only slightly raises the resistance of the respiratory tract in the asthmatic, whilst Inderal considerably increases it.

Like propranolol, the use of Trasicor has been advocated for the treatment of the hyperkinetic heart syndrome, characterised in the majority of patients by a resting tachycardia and an excessive increase in heart rate in response to exercise [84a].

3. Aptin

Synthesised by BRANDSTROM et al. [210], Aptin, Gubernal or H 56/28 (generic name: alprenolol) has a structure formula extremely close to that of the foregoing compound, Trasicor, differing only from it by the absence of the oxygen in position 2:

So it is not at all surprising that it is also an antagonist of the β-receptors. According to its originators, Aptin is dissociated from the other β-blocking substances, however, including Inderal and Trasicor: it is said to be a unique β-antagonising agent in the sense that it *also has an intrinsic stimulating effect on these receptors*. We shall be seeing later what to think of this curious association of inhibiting and stimulating effects.

Cardiovascular investigations carried out on animals indicate that the β-blocking properties of Aptin are equivalent to those of propranolol: in particular, it antagonises the positive inotropic and chronotropic effects of isoprenaline in *vivo* [3] and *in vitro* [128], and those of electrical stimulation of the sympathetic system [3]. In anaesthetised cats, Aptin (1 mg/kg intravenous) markedly reduced the increasing effect of adrenaline, noradrenaline and isoprenaline on myocardial blood flow and myocardial heat production [95a].

ABLAD et al. consider that Aptin also has a slight stimulating effect on the β-receptors [3] because it brings about a moderate degree of stimulation of the heart rate and myocardial contraction force in a reserpine-treated cat, these stimulating effects being eliminated by prior treatment with propranolol.

A further argument in favour of a slight β-stimulating effect is said to be the fact that, in men, the intra-arterial injection of Aptin does not reduce blood flow in the forearm [904] and that the intravenous injection of a blocking dose does not cause any drop in cardiac output, which would seem to reflect the existence of a slight cardiac stimulating effect [571].

According to PARRATT, it is only very occasionally that there occurs in the anaesthetised cat a very fleeting increase in the dp/dt (the actual existence of the phenomenon is, incidentally, debatable on the basis of the illustration which he gives, because of its insignificant nature), which could suggest, in his view, the existence of an initial β-stimulating effect of a slight and highly transitory character [1425]. In the same context, the findings by PROCTOR et al. [100a] do not line up with those of ABLAD [3]: using a reserpine-treated and open chest anaesthetised dog with doses of 0.1 — 0.3 — 0.6 — 1.2 and 2.4 mg/kg intravenously injected at successive intervals of 10 min, they note a slight speed-up in the heart rate, but the dp/dt is not stimulated and cardiac output is reduced. These results would therefore appear to limit the sympathicomimetic effect of the low dosages of Aptin to cardiac rate, since the inotropism is not increased. PROCTOR et al. quite rightly point out that this dissociation cannot be explained, since according to BLINKS [13a] the adrenergic β-receptors which operate as intermediaries for the two cardiac effects appear to be pharmacologically identical, a fact which has been confirmed later by BRISTOW and GREEN [47c]. Again, such β-agonist activity could not be consistently demonstrated by WASSERMAN et al. in reserpined dogs nor in humans since cardiac index fell by 26% [130a]. The question may reasonably be asked therefore whether this effect actually does exist.

In order to have a personal opinion based on experimental facts, we studied the effects of Aptin, in four anaesthetised and atropinised dogs, on several cardiovascular parameters. Heart rate, phasic left ventricular pressure, left ventricular dp/dt and phasic systemic blood pressure were measured in two dogs, while heart rate, blood flow in the circumflex coronary artery, and mean and phasic systemic blood pressure were recorded in the other two animals. In the four experiments, there was no initial acceleration in heart rate following Aptin at the dose of 0.5 or 1 mg/kg in intravenous administration, the heart rate decreasing as soon as the injection started, as shown in Figs. 26 and 27. Figure 26 also demonstrates that there was no increase in dp/dt since velocity in ventricular contraction decreased sharply during the injection, this effect being strikingly comparable with what was seen in the case of propranolol and oxprenolol in the same experimental conditions. We were thus unable to detect any sign of a stimulating effect on the cardiac β-adreno-ceptors in the case of Aptin.

According to ABLAD et al. [3], Aptin, unlike propranolol, does not reduce either the resting heart rate or the myocardial contraction force in animals except at very high dosages or in the case of animals with very considerable sympathetic tonicity.

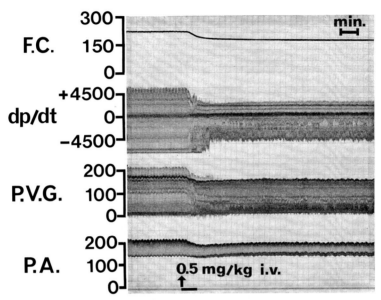

Fig. 26. Effect of alprenolol on heart rate, rate of rise in left ventricular pressure, left ventri-cular pressure and systemic blood pressure in the anaesthetised dog. From top to bottom: F.C.: Heart rate (beats/min). dp/dt: Rate of rise in left ventricular pressure (mm Hg/sec). P.V.G.: Left ventricular pressure (mm Hg). P.A.: Phasic blood pressure in the femoral artery (mm Hg). At signal mark: intravenous injection of alprenolol, 0.5 mg/kg

It seems that it is only at a high dose, far exceeding the blocking doses, that Aptin directly depresses the cardiac function, this effect being much more short-lived than the inhibition of the β-receptors. The mechanism of the cardio-depressive action is not yet known, but it could be related to the local anaesthetic properties of the substance [3]. Again these facts are not confirmed by PROCTOR et al. [100a] who regularly find a reduction in heart rate and output and in the dp/dt at the very low dose of 0.1 mg/kg administered to a chloralosed dog. Similarly, according to PARRATT and WADSWORTH [1425], the cardio-depressive effect occurs at the β-blocking doses, for in the case of anaesthetised cats, Aptin (0.5 and 1 mg/kg administered intravenously) reduces the systemic blood pressure, heart rate, ventricular systolic pressure and dp/dt, the latter effect reflecting myocardial depression. Coronary flow (measured by thermo-couple) drops by 17% and the production of metabolic heat remains unchanged. In PARRATT's view, such haemodynamic effects would seem to justify the application of the drug in the treatment of angina pectoris. In confirmation of PARRATT's findings, our experi-mental studies on anaesthetised and atropinised dogs show that there is a reduc-tion in coronary blood flow (Fig. 27) following an intravenous injection of Aptin, at the dose of 0.5 mg/kg. It seems however that the diminution in myocardial irrigation is smaller than in the case of propranolol and oxprenolol (compare with Fig. 21) under the same experimental conditions.

By studying the action of Aptin on cardiac intracellular potentials, Singh and Vaughan-Williams [35b] demonstrated that the most striking effect of the drug was to reduce the rate of rise in the action potential, the duration of the action potential not being extended and resting potentials remaining the same. Aptin

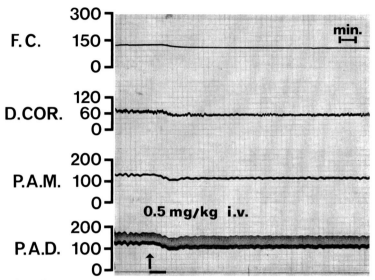

Fig. 27. Effect of alprenolol on heart rate, coronary arterial blood flow, and systemic blood pressure in the anaesthetised dog. From top to bottom: F.C.: Heart rate (beats/min). D.Cor.: Mean blood flow in the left circumflex coronary artery, measured with an electromagnetic probe (ml/min). P.A.M.: Mean blood pressure in the femoral artery (mm Hg). P.A.D.: Phasic blood pressure in the femoral artery (mm Hg). At signal mark: intravenous injection of alprenolol, 0.5 mg/kg

was also shown to be a powerful local anaesthetic, four times more potent than procaine, and thus marginally more active than propranolol. Surface anaesthesia properties (rabbit cornea) of Aptin are four times more potent than those of propranolol [18c].

Like the other β-blocking agents, Aptin antagonises the lipolytic effect of the catecholamines in animals [177]. It also eliminates the ventricular tachycardia caused in dogs by ouabaine [454], and its anti-arrhythmic effect is thought to be due to blockade of the β-receptors [1155, 1176]. At doses of 0.125 mg/kg and above in intravenous administration, Aptin protected anaesthetised guinea-pigs against ouabaine-induced ventricular fibrillation [35b]. In the unanaesthetized dog, ventricular arrhythmias produced by ligation of the anterior descending branch of the left coronary artery were also abolished by an intravenous injection of 3.5 mg/kg of Aptin [86c]. Myocardial depressant properties rather than antagonism of sympathetic influences are thought to account for this antiarrhythmic activity. Both dextro and laevo isomers of Aptin are effective against ventricular arrhythmias produced by coronary artery ligation or by Strophantine [210c]. Since the dextro isomer has only 1/100th the β-adrenoceptor blocking activity of the laevo isomer, the antiarrhythmic action appears therefore to be independent of β-receptor antagonism [210c].

Human pharmacology studies indicate that the β-blocking properties of Aptin are equivalent to those of propranolol in intravenous injection [571, 905] but 50% less with oral administration [4]. Furthermore, at an identical dosage (10 mg i.v.),

Aptin makes practically no change in heart rate and output, whereas propranolol reduces them by 15 and 22% respectively in the same subjects [571]. However, BENDER et al. [10a] found with 88 healthy subjects that at a 5 mg dose intravenously injected, Aptin was almost as active as propranolol in reducing heart rate.

In a very recent study made on nine patients with normal heart function, Aptin was found to decrease cardiac index in all subjects ten minutes after the infusion at a dose of 10 mg [130a]. The average drop was 26%. These haemodynamic findings are consistent with the data previously obtained with dogs by the same investigators [99a] and provide evidence of a cardio-depressive action by Aptin which does not appear to differ from the effect of propranolol. Similarly, stroke index decreased in eight of the nine patients. The effect of Aptin on haemodynamics was studied in 14 patients with various types of acquired heart disease following the intravenous injection of 0.2 mg/kg: the drug had a significant negative inotropic action and a consequent deleterious effect on cardiac performance [176c].

From the clinical angle, BJORNTORP [175] treated 13 anginal subjects under double-blind conditions at the high doses of 400 mg per day. He reports significant favourable results, and mentions the absence of indications of cardiac decompensation, although two of the patients were decompensated subjects stabilised by means of digitalis. A certain inclination to fatigue was observed. It is the levogyre derivative which is active in angina, for in a double-blind survey the dextrogyre derivative proved inactive, unlike the racemic form [176]. Elaborating upon his preliminary observations, BJORNTORP showed that frequency of attacks and nitroglycerin consumption decreased significantly within 1—3 weeks in about $^2/_3$ of the patients and these effects were well sustained after 1—3 years. There was only a small increase in maximal physical capacity [32c].

In another clinical trial [8a], 21 angina patients took part in a double-blind cross-over comparison between Aptin (100 mg four times daily), Peritrate (30 mg four times daily) and placebo. Two-thirds of the patients were clinically improved on Aptin, which was found to be significantly better than Peritrate and placebo. There was also an indication of reduced severity of anginal attacks. No serious complications or side effects occurred during treatment. However, in a double-blind cross-over test on nine angina patients, WASSERMAN et al. [130a] were unable to demonstrate any beneficial effect with 160—400 mg daily doses of Aptin over a 3—4 week period. Reporting the results of a double-blind multicentre trial of Aptin involving 50 angina patients, who received a daily dose of 200—400 mg of Aptin during 10 weeks, HICKIE [147c] showed that there was a significant difference between the drug and the placebo, Aptin producing a 69% reduction in attacks and a 60% reduction in nitroglycerin consumption, compared with reductions of 40% and 29% respectively in the case of placebo.

The effect of Aptin on the exercise performance in angina patients has been examined in two clinical trials. Following an intravenous injection of 0.1 mg/kg or an oral administration of 50—200 mg before bicycle exercise tests, total work and time until onset of angina pain were increased, and the time for ischaemic ECG changes to normalise was shortened [290c]. In the second investigation, Aptin prolonged significantly the ergometer exercise duration by 40% but did not augment the 80 % increase brought about by erythrityl tetranitrate [74c].

Just as was done with Inderal, the effect of an association of Aptin and Isordil was tested on patients suffering from coronary insufficiency. Taking as a criterion the amount of work possible with standard exercise, it is seen that at the dose of 100 mg Aptin is more active than Isordil at a dose of 5 mg, and also that the combination of the two medications results in a synergy [4a].

Aptin is also effective for certain cardiac functional disorders of a sympathico-tonic origin [1048, 1375], reducing tachycardia and effort hypertension [1375]. Aptin was administered by intravenous route in doses of 0.125—0.3 mg/kg in patients with atrial arrhythmias. It appears to be an effective and relatively safe agent for the treatment and prevention of such rhythm disorders because ventricular rate was reduced and reversion to sinus rhythm was obtained in several cases of paroxysmal atrial tachycardia [175c]. By intravenous injection, Aptin (5 and 10 mg) reduced heart rate in patients with hyperthyroidism, but was less effective than propranolol for the same doses [317c].

Fundamentally, it is difficult to grasp what advantage there might be in the very slight stimulating effect of Aptin on the adrenergic β-receptors demonstrated under very specific conditions, i.e. following pre-treatment of animals with reserpine. The authors of these observations [3] see a possible advantage from the clinical angle in that this stimulating property could counter the cardio-depressive effect inherent in the β-blocking agents, which, as we know, is their main side effect. It goes without saying that the β-stimulating effect can no longer take effect on blocked receptors. Its existence can therefore only be imagined under two conditions, either following complete depletion of the catecholamines by reserpine, a situation which is never experienced under clinical conditions in the treatment of angina, or at low dosages which are not sufficient to block the receptors (yet the authors report no β-stimulating effect at these doses with animals), and consequently the patient is no longer able to benefit, as regards his anginal conditions, from the haemodynamic effects resulting from the blockade of his β-receptors.

Furthermore, Aptin reduces the cardiac contraction force (and heart rate) as does propranolol in animals with high sympathetic tonus [3], which provides a clear indication that the β-stimulating effect of the drug does not play any role in these cases; this, incidentally, is in line with the cardio-depressive effect observed at high dosages, which the authors consider as "the third fundamental action of the drug" [3]. Knowing that the angina pectoris subject is in fact distinguished by an excessive sympathetic tonus, it could be expected, as the authors point out, that under such circumstances the blocking effect should be predominant, with the consequent risks of cardiac depression. It is also significant to note that the originators of Aptin [49] consider cardiac insufficiency as a formal contra-indication to its use because symptoms of aggravation of decompensation have appeared. It is obvious that in these cases the insignificant β-stimulating effect could not occur where there was β-blockade as a result of the large doses used.

In the same context must be placed the possible unfavourable effect of Aptin on the subject suffering from obstructive bronchopneumopathy because of the possible appearance of a bronchospasm, although, according to BEUMER [156], the drug only moderately increases the resistance of the respiratory tract in the asthmatic subject. However, Aptin reduces vital capacity by 10.5—18% and forced expiratory volume/sec by 10.2—24.4% in patients with obstructive pulmonary disease, whereas it has no effect in healthy subjects [15d]. Since broncho-spasm appeared occasionally in asthmatic patients, Aptin is considered to be contra-indicated in obstructive pulmonary disease.

It is difficult to see, therefore, under what clinical conditions could occur the slight β-stimulating effect of Aptin, which is essentially a β-blocking agent. Such clinical benefit as Aptin might provide for the patient suffering from angina pectoris calls for inhibition of his sympathetic β-system; this being so, the drug obviously cannot exert its stimulating action on the same system. Although, pharmacologically speaking, the β-stimulating effect which Aptin exerts on a reserpined animal marks it as differing from propranolol (which does not have this effect), scepticism can be expressed as to the advantages which this action is likely to offer from the clinical angle. In this connection, we can refer back at this point to the considerations propounded as regards Trasicor (see p. 229) on the question of cardiac safety: as things stand at present, there is no convincing clinical evidence of the fact that Aptin presents no heart risk. Furthermore, LARSEN and SIVERTSSEN [85a] recently stressed the danger of Aptin in patients in whom cardiac contractility may be adversely affected. It is worthy of note that there was some intrinsic sympathetic stimulation, but this was not considered as being sufficient to overcome the β-adrenergic blocking effects which resulted in a fall in cardiac index. We can therefore only be entirely of the opinion of GAULT [629] who recommends caution in the use of this medication.

Aptin is effective in humans in certain types of cardiac arrhythmia [1156], notably ventricular extrasystoles [46], and in paroxystic sinusal tachycardia [1048, 1656]. It is unable to maintain in sinusal rhythm those patients whose arrhythmia has first been eliminated by electroconversion [830]. Aptin was found to be effective in intravenous administration (12—20 mg) with patients with various types of supraventricular and ventricular tachyarrhythmia: there was a slowing down of ventricular rate and conversion to normal sinus rhythm in several cases [130a]. The cardio-depressive effects may however limit the usefulness of the drug as an anti-arrhythmic [130a].

Aptin may be useful in the hyperkinetic heart syndrome [84a].

Unlike the levogyre derivative, the dextrogyre derivative whose β-blocking activity is forty times less has only a minor and short-lived anti-arrhythmic effect [1176].

4. Eraldin

Taking propranolol as a basis, the ICI research workers synthesized ICI 50.172[1] or Eraldin (generic name: practolol) which has the following structure:

This modification in the chemical structure of propranolol essentially resulted in limiting the β-blocking properties to the heart; therefore, practolol may be considered as being a *selective cardiac β-blocking drug*. Endowed in the anaesthetized animal with a β-blocking activity which is roughly 40% that of propranolol [93], practolol effectively antagonizes the chronotropic and inotropic positive cardiac effects of isoprenaline, without modifying neither its hypotensive action [93, 266, 1121], or its coronarodilator properties [93]. When perfused in dogs at a constant rate into the left coronary artery at doses of 0.1 up to 5 mg/min, which are devoid of any significant effect on cardiac contractile force and coronary vascular resistance, practolol blocked the increase in cardiac force due to intracoronary injections of adrenaline, noradrenaline and isoprenaline [23a]. The adrenergic coronary vasodilation was reversed in the case of noradrenaline, and unaffected or only slightly lowered in the case of adrenaline and isoprenaline.

In the unanaesthetized dog, the i.v. injection of practolol reduces by 50% the tachycardia due to physical exercise and also, but to a lesser extent, the isoprena-

---

1 Also coded as AY 21011 in U.S.A.

line-tachycardia [93]. For a given dose, the β-antagonism is weaker in the conscious dog than in the anaesthetized dog [463].

WALE et al. [128a] confirmed the cardiac selectivity of the blocking effect in the cat since the dose which abolished the isoprenaline-tachycardia did not modify the hypotensive effect. In this animal species, the β-blocking activity of practolol was seven times weaker than that of propranolol.

In a dose which had little effect on blood pressure, heart rate, myocardial blood flow or myocardial vascular resistance (see p. 237), practolol markedly reduced the positive effects of isoprenaline infusions on heart rate, aortic dp/dt, myocardial blood flow and cardiac effort index in the anaesthetised cat [246c], the isoprenaline-induced vasodepression being unaffected. LUCCHESI and HODGEMAN also showed that practolol blocks myocardial and coronary vascular β-receptor responses but not the β-receptor-induced dilatation in the peripheral vascular bed in the anaesthetised dog [208c]. LUCCHESI and HODGEMAN [7e] further demonstrated that practolol significantly reduced the positive inotropic and chronotropic responses to left stellate ganglion stimulation in the anaesthetised dog, and changed the coronary vascular response to stellate ganglion stimulation and to the intracoronary injection of catecholamines from a vasodilatation to one of vasoconstriction.

In the isolated supported heart preparation of the dog, SOMANI et al. [9e] showed that an intracoronary infusion of isoprenaline produced, along with the usual cardiac stimulant effects, a decrease in the extraction of Rb^{86} by the heart, in the calculated values for Rb^{86} clearance and in the capillary transport coefficient. These effects are considered as indicative of a decrease in nutritional circulation, e.g. effective capillary flow. SOMANI et al. consider that such a decrease in nutritional blood flow may be an important factor in aggravating the ratio of oxygen demand to oxygen supply when the total coronary blood flow is fixed, and therefore may also be involved in the mechanism of precipitation of angina in patients with arteriosclerotic coronary artery lesions. Since they show that pretreatment with 0.25 mg/kg of practolol (and also with 0.2 mg/kg of dl-propranolol but not with 2 mg/kg of d-propranolol) significantly reduced these effects of isoprenaline, SOMANI et al. suggest that the clinical effectiveness of β-blocking agents in the treatment of angina may be due not only to blockade of the cardiac stimulant effects of catecholamines but also to an antagonism of the reduction in nutritional myocardial circulation due to catecholamines.

The β-antagonism induced by practolol seems to be competitive. In effect, in healthy subjects who were given intravenously progressively increasing doses of practolol, 5—20—80 and 160 mg, there was gradual reduction in the tachycardia induced by isoprenaline and by endogenously induced sympathetic activity (VALSALVA manoeuvre or physical exercise) and log/dose response curves suggest competitive inhibition by practolol both in response to challenge by isoprenaline and endogenously liberated catecholamines [4c]. On rabbit isolated atria, practolol produced a parallel shift in the log dose-response curve of isoprenaline, without a decrease in the maximal response, suggesting that the β-antagonism was competitive [332c].

It has been demonstrated by DUNLOP and SHANKS [463], who incidentally confirmed the observations of BARRETT [93], that practolol has also some intrinsic sympathomimetic properties since heart rate was increased in the cat which had been pretreated by syrosingopine. Because of its intrinsic sympathomimetic activity and its myocardial selectivity, practolol might conceivably, in the opinion of Ross [272c], prove a more suitable drug than propranolol when cardiac β-adrenergic blockade is considered desirable in patients with angina.

Practolol is devoid of the local anaesthetic and quinidine-like properties of propranolol [463] (an opinion that is not shared by others, see p. 242), while decreasing, as propranolol, the rate of rise of the action potential of the cardiac cell [435]. Practolol is not a direct cardiac depressant [463] in the cat, and a dose which effectively blocked the β-receptors did not depress the myocardium in the blood-perfused isolated supported dog heart preparation [116a], a fact which SOMANI and LADDU consider as bearing a possible advantage for clinical application with regard to propranolol. In another paper by the same investigators [117a], it has been reported that in the same heart preparation, pretreatment with 0.25 mg/kg of practolol effectively blocked the myocardial effects of isoprenaline in a competitive manner (increase in heart rate, left ventricular contractile force, left ventricular systolic pressure and myocardial oxygen consumption, and decrease in coronary artery perfusion pressure). Practolol reduced the myocardial oxygen consumption of the same preparation, with little or no effect on myocardial contractility or heart rate, suggesting an improved myocardial efficiency.

The possibility for a β-blocking drug to affect selectively the cardiac β-receptors without influencing the vascular β-receptors is not unexpected when some physiological aspects of the adrenergic system, which have been recently reported by LANDS et al. [76a], are taken into account. They demonstrated that the β-receptors have not the same receptivity through the whole organism, and that some of them likely correspond to different "biochemical structures". LANDS showed that there are at least two distinct β-adrenergic receptor types, on one side those which are concerned with cardiac stimulation and lipolysis (β_1-receptors) and on the other side those by which bronchodilation and vasodepression are subserved (β_2-receptors). This concept of dual β-receptor has recently received additional evidence by COLLIER and DORNHORST [26a], and by KOFI EKUE et al. [184c]. The possibility of fundamental differences between cardiac and vascular β-adrenoceptors is also well supported by studies which describe the ability of butoxamine to block selectively vascular but not cardiac β-adrenoceptors [1121]. Therefore, the concept that β-adrenoceptors can be divided into β_1- and β_2-receptors is gaining wider acceptance.

According to BUSSMANN et al. [266], practolol diminished cardiac output and dp/dt in the anaesthetized dog, but increased coronary blood flow and content of oxygen in the coronary venous blood [5b], a finding which, in their opinion, could represent an advantage with respect to propranolol for the treatment of angina. PARRATT [1426] however did not oberve in the anaesthetized cat any increase in coronary blood flow, which he considered to remain unchanged. In a subsequent paper [246c], PARRATT confirmed that practolol has no effect on myocardial blood flow or myocardial vascular resistance in the anaesthetised cat. He also showed that practolol produced slight but not significant reductions in aortic dp/dt, cardiac output and in the calculated cardiac effort index. CLARK et al. also found that right coronary blood flow remained unchanged in anaesthetised dogs following intravenous administration of practolol [61c].

Having obtained some ampoules of practolol[2], we examined the effect of this substance upon several cardiovascular parameters in the anaesthetised dog by measuring heart rate, systemic blood pressure, phasic left ventricular pressure, rate of rise in left ventricular pressure (dp/dt), mean blood flow in the left circumflex coronary artery, tension-time index and cardiac output. In order to be able to compare the results obtained in the case of practolol with those afforded by propranolol in other experiments, equiactive β-blocking doses were chosen. This

---

2 For which we express our thanks to Drs Fitzgerald and Malcolm.

means that doses of 1 and 2 mg/kg by intravenous administration were used. The results were as follows:

— There was a regular reduction in the coronary blood flow following the dose of 1 mg/kg in three experiments. An example is illustrated in Fig. 28.

— Left ventricular dp/dt significantly decreased in four other experiments, two of which are illustrated by Fig. 29.

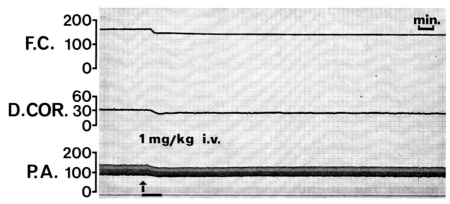

Fig. 28. Effect of practolol on heart rate, coronary arterial blood flow, and systemic blood pressure in the anaesthetised dog. From top to bottom: F.C.: Heart rate (beats/min). D.Cor.: Mean blood flow in the left circumflex coronary artery, measured with an electromagnetic probe (ml/min). P.A.: Phasic blood pressure in the femoral artery (mm Hg). At signal mark: intravenous injection of practolol, 1 mg/kg. There is a slowing in heart rate and a moderate decrease in coronary flow

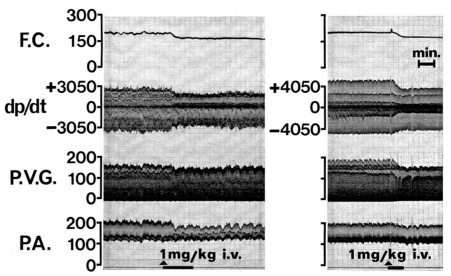

Fig. 29. Effect of practolol on heart rate, rate of rise in left ventricular pressure, left ventricular pressure, and systemic blood pressure in the anaesthetised dog. From top to bottom: F.C.: Heart rate (beats/min). dp/dt: Rate of rise in left ventricular pressure (mm Hg/sec). P.V.G.: Left ventricular pressure (mm Hg). P.A.: Phasic blood pressure in the femoral artery (mm Hg). At signal mark: intravenous injection of practolol, 1 mg/kg, in two dogs. The fall in heart rate is accompanied by a distinct decrease in the systolic ventricular pressure and in the rate of rise in pressure

— Following both doses of 1 and 2 mg/kg, practolol markedly lowered the tension-time index (Fig. 30).

— As far as cardiac output is concerned, the intravenous injection of 1 or 2 mg/kg of practolol resulted in a progressive, conspicuous and longlasting reduction (Fig. 31).

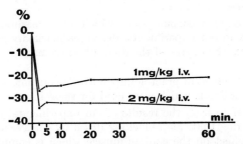

Fig. 30. Effect of practolol on the tension-time index in the anaesthetised dog. The changes in tension-time index are expressed in % of control values. Intravenous injection of practolol, 1 mg/kg in one dog, and 2 mg/kg in another dog. There is a conspicuous and long lasting reduction of tension-time index

These overall effects call for the following remarks:

a) The regular reduction in myocardial irrigation which was observed following the administration of practolol does not line up with the findings of PARRATT [246c] who reported that there was no alteration in the myocardial blood flow (measured by calorimetry) in the anaesthetised cat following intravenous injection of practolol at doses up to 10 mg/kg, nor with the observations of BUSSMANN [266] who found an augmentation in venous coronary flow in the anaesthetised dog. However, ADAM et al. [1e] have found a similar fall in blood flow in the left coronary artery measured by the same technique as in our own trials. It appears however that the decrease in coronary blood flow observed in all our experiments is less marked than that obtained with propranolol in equiactive β-blocking doses.

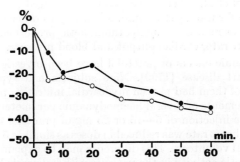

Fig. 31. Effect of practolol on the cardiac output in the anaesthetised dog. The changes in cardiac output are expressed in % of control values. Intravenous injection of practolol, 1 mg/kg in three dogs, and 2 mg/kg in three other dogs. There is a marked and long lasting reduction of cardiac output

b) In all our trials, heart rate was steadily reduced (see Figs. 28 and 29) but we have confirmed PARRATT's findings [246c] that for equivalent β-blocking doses, the fall in heart rate is considerably less than in the case of propranolol.

c) In the same way as propranolol, practolol reduces dp/dt, which indicates a diminution in cardiac contractility. We therefore confirm BUSSMANN's [266] and

ADAM's [1e] observations but our results are not consonant with PARRATT's findings [246c] who did not observe any significant modification of the aortic dp/dt in the anaesthetised cat even with high doses. However, as in the case of the bradycardic effect, we consider that the reduction in velocity of the cardiac contraction induced by practolol is less pronounced than in the case of propranolol for equiactive β-blocking doses.

d) Myocardial oxygen consumption, which was measured by means of the tension-time index in our experiments, decreases markedly and remains reduced for at least 2 hours. The degree of the diminution seems to be related to the dose (see Fig. 30).

e) As regards the effect of practolol upon cardiac output, there was a considerable fall in the six animals which were used for these investigations.

It follows therefore from the results of our experimental trials carried out in the anaesthetised dog that, at β-blocking doses by intravenous route, practolol has a depressant effect on the cardiac muscle which is comparable with that of propranolol. Myocardial irrigation is reduced as in the case of propranolol, although it could be that the restricting effect of practolol on coronary blood flow is less marked than that of propranolol for equiactive β-blocking doses.

In healthy volunteers, practolol seems to be four times less effective as a β-blocker than propranolol when given by i.v. route [52]. Doses ranging from 5 to 20 mg i.v. produced little change in pulse rate or blood pressure, but reduced by about 50% the isoprenaline-tachycardia without altering vasodepression [229]. Thus, the selectivity of the antagonistic properties against cardiac β-receptors appear also in man, this activity remaining however partial since isoprenaline-tachycardia could never be reduced by more than 50% for larger doses [229].

Another proof of the cardiac selectivity of the β-blocking effect of practolol is given in the paper by HARRISON and TURNER [787], who showed that in normal man 200 mg of practolol by oral administration significantly reduced the tachycardia but not the increase in skin temperature produced by isoprenaline inhalation, while a dose of 80 mg of propranolol abolished both responses in the same subjects. THOMPSON et al. [311c] have also demonstrated that the β-blockade by practolol is specific for the heart in man. According to other investigators [1744], practolol develops in man some sympathomimetic properties, while reducing in the same time heart rate, cardiac output and blood pressure.

The haemodynamic effects of practolol have been investigated in 14 patients with coronary heart disease [1799]. Nine subjects had typical severe angina pectoris while five of them had proved myocardial infarction from one to six days previously. Measurements of several haemodynamic parameters were taken before and 5 min after the injection of 5—15 or 25 mg of practolol into the pulmonary artery. The resting heart rate was reduced in doses as small as 5 mg, an effect which is not seen in normal volunteers. This difference may be explained by a higher level of resting sympathetic activity in the patients with ischaemic heart disease, which is antagonized by a β-adrenergic blocking effect of the drug. Cardiac output did not change, except for the dose of 25 mg which induced a significant reduction. Thus, there was in the 5 mg group of patients an increase in stroke volume without any increase in systolic ejection time. These findings suggest that, in the 5 mg dose, practolol had a positive inotropic effect on the heart, perhaps due to an intrinsic sympathomimetic action. This effect was not seen with a higher dosage; in fact with 25 mg there seemed to be a negative inotropic effect in that the left ventricular end-diastolic pressure was raised and the cardiac output reduced. Although these facts could indicate a therapeutic advantage with respect to propranolol, the authors think that, as with propranolol, caution should be used when giving equivalent doses to patients with evidence of myocardial dysfunction.

In other clinical observations which have been made on 8 patients with good cardiac function, practolol was given i.v. at a dose of 5 mg during exercise on a bicycle ergometer [655]: there was a fall in heart rate of 16%, but stroke volume increased so that cardiac output remained constant. Furthermore, no significant changes were found in left ventricular work, aortic pressure, pulmonary artery pressure and pulmonary capillary wedge pressure. All these effects differ from those of propranolol at the same dose which produces a drop in pulse rate, in cardiac output and in blood pressure; in addition there is an increase in the pulmonary arterial pressure [1800]. It was therefore concluded that practolol may have therapeutic value from an ability to antagonize the tachycardia produced by catecholamines without seriously impairing left ventricular function.

The circulatory effects of practolol have been studied in 15 patients during the acute phase of myocardial infarction [162c]. A negative chronotropic effect followed doses of 5 and 25 mg given intravenously. In five patients who received the 5 mg dose, the fall in heart rate was not associated with any significant change in cardiovascular function (cardiac output, stroke volume) and only a modest negative inotropic effect (significant fall in cardiac output and prolongation of the systolic ejection time) was observed in the 10 patients who were given 25 mg. Comparison with the known effects of propranolol suggests that practolol possesses an important advantage when used as an antiarrhythmic agent for treatment of arrhythmia complications in patients with myocardial infarction.

In anginous patients, the prolongation of a cycloergometric exercise is particularly evident after an i.v. injection of 160 mg of practolol over a period of 5 min [10]. Again in anginous patients, practolol increased the tolerance for an exercise test for a single i.v. injection of 20 mg and also after a fortnight oral treatment at the daily dose of 200 mg [52]. This favourable objective effect has been confirmed by other investigators [135a] who furthermore reported that, in the same patients, a comparable benefit was achieved by propranolol, whereas dexpropranolol (the dextro-derivative of propranolol) was inactive. Taking these clinical observations into account, and considering also the fact that propranolol and dexpropranolol both have the same local anaesthetic properties, an effect which is not shared by practolol, these investigators concluded that the antianginal effect of propranolol must be ascribed to its β-blocking and not to its local anaesthetic properties.

Six patients with long-standing angina pectoris were exercised on a treadmill to assess the effect of intravenous administration of practolol (0.3 mg/kg), propranolol (0.15 mg/kg) or a placebo on their exercise tolerance [65c]. The same procedure was repeated after oral administration of practolol (100 mg three times a day), propranolol (50 mg three times a day) or a placebo. There was a significant increase in exercise tolerance in the oral and intravenous study with both propranolol and practolol. No distinction could be made on the basis of exercise tolerance between either the drugs or their mode of administration. Thus a beneficial effect on exercise tolerance is observed in angina pectoris from β-adrenoceptor blockade by practolol.

The therapeutic effect of the oral administration of practolol in angina is to be assigned to a reduction in cardiac work which is due to a decrease in the velocity of heart contraction and to a fall in mean systemic blood pressure [52].

As far as the controlled clinical evaluation of practolol in angina pectoris is concerned, the drug was given at doses ranging from 200 to 600 mg b.d. to 15 patients in a double-blind study, and compared with propranolol 80 mg q.d.s. [280c].

Though practolol did not significantly affect the subjective criteria, including the number of attacks recorded by the patient or the nitroglycerin intake, it did significantly improve the more objective indices of myocardial ischaemia such as the amount of exercise possible in exercise tests[3] and the degree of ischaemic S-T depression in the radiocardiogram during exercise. In this respect, practolol was superior to propranolol which did not significantly alter the amount of S-T depression induced by exercise. Unlike propranolol, practolol did not produce any adverse effects on bronchial smooth muscle. Hence, it was concluded that practolol is an effective drug in treating angina, and in the dosage used is of potential value in patients with asthmatic bronchitis and angina. It should however be used cautiously in anginal patients when myocardial dysfunction is present since there is as yet no convincing evidence that it can be given with impunity to patients with cardiac failure. In another double-blind trial [110 c], 24 patients were treated by a daily dose ranging from 400 to 1200 mg: 17 patients experienced less angina and consumed fewer nitroglycerin tablets. It was considered that the existence of well-controlled cardiac failure is not necessarily a contraindication to practolol.

Like propranolol, practolol is endowed with antiarrhythmic properties. For example, it suppressed in the dog the ectopic ventricular rhythms which occur after the acute ligation of a large coronary artery [286] and those which appeared after an i.v. injection of adrenaline [93], as in the particular case of general anaesthesia by halothane [1735]. Practolol prevented also ventricular fibrillation due to i.v. injection of ouabain in the guinea-pig, but the active dose was three times larger than in the case of propranolol [1412]. Practolol has the same quinidine-like effect as propranolol on the action potential of the cardiac cell [1412]. Since its local anaesthetic effect was found to be only hundred times weaker than that of propranolol, PAPP and VAUGHAN WILLIAMS [1412] express the opinion that the anti-arrhythmic action of practolol against ouabain is partly dependent on the specific β-blocking activity of the drug. WALE et al. [128 a] confirmed the existence of anti-arrhythmic properties in the cat against dysrhythmias provoked by adrenaline.

LADDU and SOMANI [75 a] specified that in the dog heart-lung preparation, practolol prevented the ventricular fibrillation resulting from a combination of halothane and adrenaline for a dose of 0.5 mg, but a total dose of 2 mg was needed to antagonize the multifocal ventricular tachycardia produced by a combination of halothane, adrenaline and mechanical elevation of the aortic pressure. Since pretreatment with 25 mg of practolol did not modify the dose of ouabain necessary to induce multifocal ventricular tachycardia and the drug was also ineffective in doses up to 50 mg against ouabain-induced ventricular tachycardia, it was concluded that practolol can selectively antagonize adrenergically induced cardiac arrhythmias in the heart-lung preparation.

However, NAYLER et al. [1344] reported that arrhythmias induced in the rabbit by a combination of Strophantine and adrenaline were not suppressed by the drug. According to BOISSIER et al. [37 c], practolol slows down the dromotropic function in the dog by suppressing the β-sympathetic drive and also by a direct depressive action.

With 19 patients suffering from impaired cardiac function, not responding to other anti-arrhythmic substances and for whom propranolol was contra-indicated because of the heart condition, an intravenous injection of 5—25 mg of practolol allowed ventricular rhythm to be controlled in most of the cases (atrial fibrillation

---

3 Exercise-tolerance test applied by SANDLER was a modification of the two-step technique he used previously for the clinical evaluation of pheniprazine [1638].

or supraventricular tachycardia), without side effect on blood pressure or on the clinical symptoms of cardiac insufficiency [654]. The authors consider this drug as better for this type of patient than propranolol. They point out that, basically speaking, it is interesting to find an anti-arrhythmic effect under clinical conditions in the case of a β-antagonising substance with no local anaesthetic properties. This fact would therefore also suggest that in the case of Inderal these properties are only called upon to play a minor part in its anti-arrhythmic effect, and this latter is primarily due to the β-blocking properties.

Because it does not bring about any drop in cardiac output in the patient suffering from acute myocardial infarction [899], unlike what occurs in the case of Inderal [1832], and also because it would be an advantage to have available an anti-arrhythmic medication of the β-blocking type which presented no hasard for the failing heart [284], practolol could be used to replace Inderal in the treatment of angina, but above all for treating ventricular and supraventricular arrhythmia occurring during the critical period of acute infarct. This fact emerges from the report by JEWITT et al. [899] who find with 47 patients suffering either from ventricular tachycardia or ventricular extrasystoles that the slow intravenous injection of 5—25 mg results in the rapid return to the sinus rhythm in the majority of cases. The effect is much more prolonged than that of lignocaine. The authors attribute the anti-arrhythmic effect to the β-blockade, since acute myocardial infarct is accompanied by sympathetic hyperactivity [1915]. They consider that practolol has major advantages over Inderal because of the absence of cardiodepressive effect [899] and peripheral vascular effects [228]. Later on, JEWITT and his colleagues [163 c] reported their results obtained on a group of 75 cases of acute myocardial infarction presenting different types of cardiac arrhythmia. They confirmed that at doses of 5 to 25 mg by intravenous injection, practolol is a valuable drug in the management of supraventricular tachycardia and ventricular extrasystoles. Practolol has advantages over alprenolol (10 mg) since it causes less cardiovascular depression.

A like anti-arrhythmic effect has been reported in the case of the supraventricular tachycardia which occurs during the post-operative period after fitting intracardiac valves [654]. Practolol was used to treat supraventricular dysrhythmias (atrial fibrillation, atrial flutter and supraventricular tachycardia) in 32 patients with a rapid ventricular rate and with heart disease of varied aetiology. Heart failure was present in 22 patients. Practotol was injected intravenously at a dose of 2 mg/min until a therapeutic effect was noted or a total dose of 20 mg had been administered. In 26 patients, the average reduction in ventricular rate was 75 per min, while immediate reversion to sinus rhythm occurred in 3 patients. The slowing effect was mainly due to a direct action on the atrio-ventricular node. No serious adverse clinical effects were noted, and the risks of haemodynamic deterioration are probably less than with propranolol [47 a].

Similar antiarrhythmic effects have been reported by two other teams. VOHRA et al. [329 c] treated 26 episodes of various cardiac arrhythmias occurring in 20 patients. At a dose of 4 to 40 mg in intravenous injection, reversion to sinus rhythm was observed in 40% of cases of supraventricular arrhythmias and atrial tachyarrhythmias. Practolol was less effective in ventricular tachycardia. BRAY et al. [45 c] treated arrhythmias which were present in 60 patients suffering from heart failure and serious bronchospasm. Intravenous injections or oral route were used. There was a reduction in frequency of ventricular ectopic beats. Practolol slowed heart rate in supraventricular tachycardia and frequently reverted cardiac rhythm to normal, and also reduced ventricular rate in atrial fibrillation. Practolol was often active when other conventional drugs had failed or were contraindicated.

They pointed out that practolol did not produce any deterioration in cardiac dysfunction and induced some increase in bronchospasm only in a small proportion of cases.

The specific character of the β-blockade as regards the heart is reflected in the benign nature of respiratory impact since, unlike Inderal, practolol administered intravenously at treble dosage to an asthmatic subject only slightly increases the resistance of the respiratory tract without involving any clinical manifestation [1201]. This advantage of practolol over propranolol has been confirmed by BEUMER [156] who only finds a slight increase in the respiratory resistance of asthmatics given aerosols of the drug to inhale, and by PALMER et al. [93a] who report that at the intravenous dose of 20 mg practolol does not significantly reduce the broncho-dilating effect of isoprenaline on asthmatics.

BERNECKER and ROETSCHER [28c] have investigated the effect of practolol on bronchial function in 22 asthmatic patients, who were accustomed to inhaling isoprenaline, but had not used it for several hours before investigation. The peak expiratory flow and the non-forced vital capacity were used as measures of lung function during the introduction of a practolol aerosol added to the inspired air. In 18 patients, there were no signs of bronchial obstruction and no dyspnoea, but there was a marked fall in both respiratory criteria in four subjects, thus demonstrating a bronchospastic effect. This suggests the need for caution in the use of practolol in patients with asthma or chronic bronchitis. Commenting the report by BERNECKER and ROETSCHER that practolol, when given by inhalation, causes a fall in vital capacity and peak expiratory flow in some asthmatic subjects, KERR and PATEL [177c] stress that the rapid reversal of the fall in ventilation by isoprenaline contrasts with the observations reported by McNEILL [219c] that the fall in ventilation produced by intravenous propranolol in similar subjects was not reversible with isoprenaline. Taken together, these observations suggest that either practolol is not affecting the β-receptor sites on bronchial smooth muscle and its effect on ventilation is nonspecific, or the β-receptor blockade produced by practolol on bronchial smooth muscle is "surmountable" and the receptor site is still capable of being stimulated by isoprenaline. Although KERR and PATEL agree that caution is required in the use of practolol in patients with obstructive airways disease, it would appear to be a safer preparation to use than propranolol in view of the rapid reversal of its effect by isoprenaline.

Confirming the prospects which could be deduced from the advantages which it presented over Inderal, practolol has in fact been offered in mid-1970 to the medical profession for the treatment of angina pectoris and of cardiac arrhythmia.

Probably of importance from the clinical viewpoint is the discovery of such a β-adrenergic blocking drug that blocks cardiac stimulation by isoprenaline without affecting bronchodilatation. This finding may lead eventually to the availability of a β-adrenergic blocking agent that does not carry the risk of precipitating asthmatic attacks in susceptible individuals.

Although it has not yet been demonstrated in multicentre controlled clinical trials that practolol does reduce both the frequency of anginal attacks and the consumption of nitroglycerin tablets, and does increase in chronic oral administration the tolerance to effort, it can be held as capable to help in angina pectoris [30c], although some patients may require high doses, more than 2 g daily, to produce symptomatic improvement in angina. As practolol has potentially serious side-effects, it should be used with great caution [30c]. According to a recommendation to practitioners issued in 1971 [8e], practolol should be used cautiously where cardiac function is impaired and it is better to use practolol where propranolol is likely to precipitate heart failure or bronchospasm.

5. ICI 45763 or Kö 592

Another specific antagonist of the adrenergic β-receptors was synthesised by two different laboratories under the names of ICI 45763 [1730] and Kö 592 (generic name: doberol). It answers to the formula:

When examined under the ICI 45763 form, this substance can be considered as equi-active to propranolol when administered intravenously to man and animals [1726], but it is three times less active in oral administration. In the case of an anaesthetised cat, it does not alter the heart rate at the intravenous doses which induce bradycardia in the case of propranolol [1726]. It has an intrinsic sympathicomimetic activity because it increases the heart rate of a cat treated with syrosingopine [1730).

ICI 45763 is effective in animals for rhythm disturbances caused by adrenaline and ouabaine [1777, 1778], but ineffective against arrhythmias occurring as a result of ligaturing the coronary artery [1778].

Tested in the form of Kö 592, this substance is an antagonist of the β-receptors [494], has an equal activity to propranolol according to certain authors [1123] but less according to others [133, 1622]. It has local anaesthetic properties [1123] which are better than those of cocaine, but three times less than those of propranolol [1954]. Its cardio-depressive effect is said to be relatively low [1123], less than that of propranolol but greater than that of Trasicor on human and canine heart fragments [1345]. As in the case of propranolol, this effect is probably due to the competitive antagonism which Kö 592 exerts on the calcium ions [561, 1352].

Kö 592 reduces coronary flow in the isolated rabbit heart [1223] by increasing coronary resistance [1350].

In the case of man, it slows down the heart rate and reduces cardiac output at the intravenous dose of 5 mg, at the same time blocking isoprenaline-induced tachycardia [1493]. It is almost as active as propranolol in reducing heart rate in healthy subjects [10a]. Another clinical investigation carried out with 15 patients suffering from congenital or acquired heart disease, but without an anginal condition, shows that intravenous injection of 5 or 15 mg of Kö 592 brings about a 13% reduction in heart rate and lowers cardiac output by 10% [1825].

We do not know of any clinical research concerning antianginal properties carried out with this β-antagonist, but it has been shown that a daily dose of 100 mg brings about the appearance in a healthy subject during physical exercise of the premonitory signs of slight cardiac insufficiency, which disappear after stopping the intake of the drug [44a]. They occur however later than is the case with propranolol administered at the same posology.

HAMM et al. [137c] studied the effect of Kö 592 on respiration. 39 subjects including 8 healthy subjects, 12 patients with bronchial asthma and 19 patients with chronic bronchitis and emphysema received 5 to 10 mg of Kö 592 by intravenous injection. Vital capacity, expiratory secondary capacity and compliance were only slightly reduced in the healthy subjects but there was a marked reduction of these functional pulmonary tests in the patients suffering from respiratory diseases. Furthermore 7 of the 12 asthmatic patients suffered asthmatic attacks. Therefore, the authors recommend caution in treating patients with asthma or ventilatory obstructions.

6. Visken (LB 46)

LB 46 (generic name: pindolol) is another β-blocking substance whose chemical structure is closely related to that of propranolol:

The potency of its β-antagonising effect is 5 times greater than that of propranolol [1185, 1622], whereas its negative inotropic cardiac activity is 15 times less [1622]. Like propranolol, it has quinidine-like properties but to a lesser extent [1185, 1623]. LB46 competitively blocks the positive inotropic effect of isoprenaline in the isolated supported dog heart preparation [9d]. It has minimal overt myocardial depressant effect since, although producing a significant decrease in myocardial oxygen consumption at the dose of 0.25 mg/kg by intravenous route, it does not depress left ventricular peak systolic pressure [9d].

According to NAYLER [1343], LB 46 at the blocking doses has no cardio-depressive effect on a whole dog nor on human papillary and atrial muscle fragments. This has been confirmed on an anaesthetised dog [195]. At a higher dose there appears cardiac depression which, as in the case of propranolol, is probably due to inhibition of the passage of calcium ions through the myofibril membrane [1352].

LB 46 counters adrenergic arrhythmia conditions [195]. In the case of digitalis-induced arrhythmia, it is only antagonistic at a dose 60 times greater than that which brings about β-blockade [195]. BOISSIER et al. have shown that LB46 depresses the dromotropic function in the anaesthetised dog by suppressing β-sympathetic drive [37c].

In humans, LB 46 exerts its antagonistic properties vis-à-vis effort-induced tachycardia and the tachycardia brought on by isoprenaline at an oral dose forty times lower than propranolol [829] without basic heart rate being changed. This absence of reduction in pulse could be due to the presence of an intrinsic sympathicomimetic activity [829, 1622].

By intravenous injection in healthy subjects, the β-blocking effect of LB46 against the tachycardia induced by intravenous infusion of isoprenaline is significantly higher than with propranolol, alprenolol and oxprenolol [20c].

The effect of LB46 on cardiac output in man has been studied in different conditions. Whereas KOEHLER reported a decrease in cardiac output together with a slight reduction in stroke volume and an increase in peripheral resistance in healthy subjects [183c], WIRZ et al. have shown that in patients with various cardiopathies but without heart failure, LB46 administered intravenously at the dose of 0.01 mg/kg did not alter cardiac index or maximal dp/dt, whereas there was a marked decrease in both parameters in the case of propranolol at the dose of 0.1 mg/kg [340c]. McCREDIE [218c] reported that, in normal subjects, an intravenous injection of 0.02 mg/kg of LB46 decreases cardiac output by 18%, with no change in stroke volume owing to the fact that heart rate is reduced. The systemic vascular resistance rises by 17% and left ventricular work falls by 16%. GURTNER et al. [131c] also found a reduction in cardiac index and a significant decrease in dp/dt in thirty subjects following intravenous injection of doses ranging from 0.005 to 0.4 mg/kg; they concluded that LB46 has a negative inotropic effect. Finally, RIVIER et al. [269c] showed that an intravenous injection of 1 mg of LB46 reduced cardiac output by 12% in cardiac patients, an effect which was smaller than in the case of 5 mg of propranolol. There was no significant modification of the pulmonary arterial resistance.

The behaviour of coronary blood flow following the administration of LB46 has also been investigated. A decrease has been reported by GURTNER et al. [131 c] in a group of thirty subjects after the intravenous injection of doses ranging from 0.005 to 0.4 mg/kg. Similarly, LICHTLEN et al. [204 c] demonstrated that 30 min after an intravenous injection of 0.01 and 0.02 mg/kg in atherosclerotic coronary patients, coronary blood flow had decreased by 28% and coronary resistance increased by 34%. They consider that there was no difference as compared with propranolol.

With his colleagues [203 c and 205 c], LICHTLEN made an important clinical investigation into the haemodynamic changes which occur in eight normal subjects and in 17 patients with coronary insufficiency following an intravenous injection of 0.01 or 0.015 mg/kg of LB46. The phenomena were similar in both groups of patients. Left coronary blood flow was reduced and coronary resistance increased. Myocardial oxygen consumption decreased, as well as cardiac index as a consequence of a negative inotropic effect. There was a rise in peripheral resistance. As in the same time dp/dt, left ventricular stroke work and heart rate were only slightly reduced, LICHTLEN et al. consider that this suggests an additional mild β-stimulating activity preventing an excessive reduction in myocardial contractility.

A study has been carried out on the antianginal effect of LB 46 given orally at the dose of 5 mg three times daily to 14 patients [110a]. Results were assessed on the basis of the subjective data supplied by the patients regarding their consumption of nitroglycerin and tolerance to exercise, and also on the basis of serial ECG examinations at rest involving 5 patients with abnormal resting graphs, and following exercise in the case of 9 patients with abnormal Master test. Consumption of nitroglycerin was lowered with 10 patients, and tolerance to exercise was improved subjectively in all patients. This improvement could be verified by the Master test in 8 cases, and resting ECGs were improved in 4 cases. Slight and transitory gastro-intestinal irritation occurred in half of the cases. There was no accentuation of cardiac failure.

In 28 patients treated with 5 to 15 mg daily for 6 weeks [343 c], there was a marked reduction in the number of anginal attacks and in consumption of nitroglycerin. The electrocardiogram was normalized in some cases. In 11 out of 14 cases, the clinical benefit afforded by LB46 was superior to that obtained with nitrate, verapamil and dipyridamole. In 48 angina patients, LB46 administered at a daily dose of 7.5 to 15 mg for 4 to 40 weeks induced a significant improvement in all but 7 patients. There was a case with pulmonary oedema [9 c]. In a double blind study, LB46 was effective against angina when given during 15 days in a non-specified number of patients [77 c].

In 20 patients with confirmed longstanding angina, an oral dose of 2 mg of LB46 improved the ischaemic response to effort as demonstrated by a definite reversal of the S—T segment depression [169 c]. In 11 patients with angina, LB46 significantly delayed the appearance time of S—T changes in the exercise-ECG compared to placebo, prolonged total work time and reduced the magnitude of S—T depression. ECG returned to normal more quickly [301 c]. There was no synergetic effect between LB46 and isosorbide dinitrate on these parameters [301 c]. In angina patients and coronary atherosclerotic cases, LB46 at the daily dose of 15 mg reduced the S—T segment depression due to exercise [281 c].

As in the case of other β-blocking agents, LB46 was found to be effective against cardiac arrhythmia. This has been demonstrated in two trials. In a group of a hundred patients with various types of arrhythmias, MICHEL [221 c] used an oral daily dose of 15 to 50 mg. He showed that LB46 is effective in supraventricular extrasystoles and in 50% of cases of supraventricular paroxysmal tachycardia; in atrial fibrillation, ventricular rate was slowed. In a double blind investigation, KEULEN found that when administered for 25 days at a daily dose of 14 mg, LB46 had the same antiarrhythmic effectiveness as propranolol at a daily dose of 90 mg; the tolerance of LB46 was considered to be better because there was no occurrence of cardiac insufficiency [178 c].

In patients with obstructive pulmonary disease LB46 reduces vital capacity by 10.5—18% and forced expiratory volume/sec by 10.2—24.4%, whereas it has no effect in healthy subjects [15d]. Since bronchospasm appeared occasionally in asthmatic patients, LB46 is considered to by contraindicated in obstructive pulmonary disease.

7. Ro 3-3528

Another antagonist of the adrenergic β-receptors [761], whose activity is roughly the same as that of propranolol and is accompanied by local anaesthetic and anti-arrhythmic properties [761], Ro 3-3528 does not slow down the heart rate in a conscious animal at an oral dose of 3 mg/kg [761].

In the case of a healthy man, the ingestion of the drug causes a slowing down in heart rate which is not proportional to the dose [828] and an intravenous infusion at the rate of 0.02 mg/kg/min for 30 minutes decreases heart rate, stroke volume, heart work and cardiac efficiency [233 c].

Ro 3-3528 must be administered at a dose 10 times higher than that of propranolol to inhibit the tachycardia induced by isoprenaline [828], but at a dose only $2^1/_2$ times higher to inhibit exercise-induced tachycardia.

8. INPEA

Answering to the chemical structure [1877]:

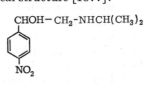

INPEA is a β-antagonising substance [736, 1263, 1783] which is said to have an unusual specific action since it has no local anaesthetic [1123, 1329] and quinidine-like [763] properties.

In the case of animals, INPEA antagonises the positive inotropic [1263, 1783] and chronotropic [1783] cardiac effects of adrenaline. It has a negative inotropic effect [86, 1783] and potentialises the hypertensive effect of adrenaline [1783]. Intravenous injection of 5 mg/kg of INPEA lowers coronary flow by 19% by increasing coronary resistance, causes no change in heart rate, or cardiac work, or cardiac output or blood pressure, and reduces by 12% myocardial oxygen consumption [541]. At doses ranging from 2.5 to 12.5 mg/kg administered intravenously to an anaesthetised dog, coronary flow is reduced, but unlike what occurs in the case of Inderal, a drop is noted in global vascular resistance [763].

The β-blocking effect of INPEA when administered orally to a conscious dog is 20 times less than that of propranolol [763] and 40 times less when given intravenously to an anaesthetised dog [763]. It is not cardiodepressive as regards an anaesthetised dog [763].

INPEA counters adrenergic arrhythmia [1783, 1784]; as regards the rhythm disturbances caused by the digitalics, they are not eliminated by the action of

INPEA [1783, 1784] but could be prevented by pre-treatment in the case of cats [1119]. It prevents the ventricular fibrillation produced in cats in a state of profound hypothermia [1365], a condition in which the adrenergic mechanisms play a major role in the development of this cardiac arrhythmia.

In the case of normal man, the intravenous administration of 2 mg/kg of INPEA changes neither heart rate nor blood pressure [1452]; it blocks the tachycardia resulting from the intravenous infusion of adrenaline, but sharply increases its hypertensive effect [1452]; it considerably inhibits the tachycardia-inducing and hypotensive effects of isoprenaline [1452]. According to other authors, the intravenous injection of 50—75 mg of INPEA, whilst reducing the tachycardia-inducing effect of isoprenaline, lowers the basic heart rate and output [1493].

In the case of the coronary subject at rest, the dose of 2 mg/kg of INPEA changes neither the heart rate nor blood pressure, but it does neutralise the tachycardia resulting from the intravenous infusion of adrenaline [1452]. In the case of the coronary subject given the Master test, INPEA reduces exercise-induced tachycardia and hypertension, attenuates the electrocardiographic indications of myocardial ischaemia, and counters the appearance of angina pain in patients where it occurred during the test carried out prior to treatment [1452]. It improves tolerance to effort in the anginal subject [86] and the symptomatic results in angina pectoris would appear to be encouraging [1291, 1750]. According to DOTTI et al. [446], this drug, active in the case of the anginal subject, it the β-blocking medication to choose since it causes neither slowing down in rhythm, nor has it a cardio-depressive effect. They admit however that their clinical experimentation must be extended in order to provide a better assessment of the therapeutic benefit and possible limitations of the medication.

Like the other β-blocking agents, INPEA slows down the heart rate in cases of sinus tachycardia [1291]. By intravenous administration, INPEA reduces sinus rate in man, decreases ventricular rate in atrial flutter and fibrillation, is only slightly active in atrial tachycardia and ineffective against ventricular extrasystoles and tachycardia [54c].

9. Sotalol (M.J. 1999)

With the structure formula:

$$CHOH-CH_2-NHCH(CH_3)_2$$

$$NH-SO_2-CH_3$$

M.J. 1999 has β-antagonising properties [1159] which are selective because they are not accompanied by any β-stimulating effect and activity as regards the a-receptors [462, 25a]. It is 10—20 times less active than Inderal against isoprenaline-induced tachycardia [1726], only 2—4 times less potent according to other authors [2, 525, 526]. With dogs, it counters the cardiac stimulation resulting from the injection of isoprenaline and the stimulation of sympathetic trunks. With a perfused isolated dog heart, it competitively blocks tachycardia, increase in ventricular contractile force and in myocardial oxygen consumption, and also the drop in coronary perfusion pressure brought about by isoprenaline [1779]. It also lowers the tachycardia and the speed-up in dp/dt caused by hyperthermia in the case of a conscious dog [1914]. According to BROOKS et al. [17a], who report a bradycardia-inducing and cardio-depressive effect at the dose of 1—6 mg/kg in an anaesthetised dog, Sotalol at a low dose (1 mg/kg) exerts a selective blocking action vis-à-vis the chronotropic effect of isoprenaline, since the positive inotropic effect of this latter is not changed whereas the two effects of the β-stimulant are blocked by larger doses.

M.J. 1999 depresses cardiac contraction force and reduces heart rate, but it does not alter coronary vascular resistance in dogs [1817]. However, other authors find that it increases coronary resistance in the whole dog [1350] and reduces coronary flow in an isolated rabbit heart [1223]. It lowers the heart rate of an anaesthetised cat [1726] but at a much larger dose than is the case with Inderal.

On isolated rat- and guinea pig hearts perfused with the Langendorff technique, M. J. 1999 did not decrease left ventricular pressure or maximum dp/dt, in contrast to propranolol. The vascular coronary resistance was increased [315c]. Equiactive β-blocking doses of M.J. 1999 and propranolol were given to anaesthetised dogs by intravenous injection. M. J. 1999 caused a lesser reduction in dp/dt and a lesser increase in left ventricular end-diastolic pressure than did propranolol. Comparison of responses between normal and reserpinised animals suggested that M. J. 1999 possesses less non specific depressant action on the myocardial contractility than propranolol [119c].

LEVY demonstrated that Sotalol at an intravenous dose of 5 mg/kg produced a significant decrease in myocardial oxygen consumption in anaesthetised open chest dogs [23b]. Compared to the action of 1 mg/kg of propranolol, the effect was greater in magnitude and persisted longer. The lowering of myocardial oxygen consumption can be attributed largely to the negative chronotropic effect. Coronary sinus blood flow was also decreased, Sotalol having a greater effect than 1 mg/kg of propranolol.

M.J. 1999 counters adrenergic arrhythmia [1784]. As regards digitalic arrhythmia, it is inactive according to certain authors [1782, 1784] and active according to others [1495]. It protects guinea-pigs against ouabain-induced ventricular fibrillation [293c].

As in the case of Inderal, this variance in opinion only seems to emerge for the same reasons as those outlined earlier (see p. 220), although the potency of the anti-arrhythmic activity of M. J. 1999 is less than that of Inderal [1495]. According to SOMANI and WATSON [1785], the anti-arrhythmic effect of M. J. 1999 is the consequence of its specific anti-β activity, and this substance does not have the non-specific anti-arrhythmic effects of propranolol because it is inactive against digitalis-induced arrhythmia, a fact which has been confirmed [2, 33b]. In the case of cats, a blocking dose of Sotalol lowers the frequency of the ectopic rhythms caused by electrical vagal stimulation [104a].

M.J. 1999 has no adrenergic stimulating properties [1818]. According to certain authors, there are no local anaesthetic properties [525, 1123, 1159], whilst others consider it to be active, but 50 times less so than propranolol [1495]. It increases the refractory period of the isolated auricle [1495], the extent of this activity only being one tenth of that of propranolol [1495]. This quinidine-like property, which some say does not exist [2, 504, 525], explains why M.J. 1999 has a potential cardio-depressive effect [1818], although certain authors find no decrease in cardiac output in cats at a dose which in the case of Inderal does reduce it [2]. According to SINGH and V. WILLIAMS [293c], M. J. 1999 reduces the rate of rise of intracellular action potentials of isolated rabbit atria and greatly prolongs the duration of the action potential of atrial and ventricular muscle, an effect which would contribute to antiarrhythmic activity. M. J. 1999 has been shown to have little effect on resting potential on dog and rabbit cardiac tissue [303c]. As membrane responsiveness is a principal determinant of cardiac conduction at lower transmembrane voltages, the drug should not depress cardiac conduction, even when transmembrane voltage has been decreased by myocardial damage. In the light of the fact that M. J. 1999 has been shown to have less cardiac depressant effect than propranolol [2, 260 c], STRAUSS et al. [303 c] suggest that an agent like M. J. 1999, having less negative inotropic effects and less depressive effects on cardiac conduction would have fewer detrimental effects to the patient with myocardial infarction, and that M. J. 1999 might be preferred to propranolol in the treatment of patients with angina pectoris in whom the risk of myocardial infarction while on therapy is great.

Like all the β-blocking agents, M.J. 1999 counters hyperglycaemia and the increase in plasmatic free fatty acids caused by the catecholamines [1066]. With rats it accentuates insulin hypoglycaemia without being itself hypoglycaemia-producing [798].

It is the levogyre derivative which is active — the dextrogyre is not so [1779, 1780].

In the case of a healthy man, an intravenous dose of 0.06—0.08 mg/kg is needed to counter the tachycardia induced by isoprenaline [581], but this dose only reduces, without cancelling out, the stimulating effect on cardiac output and work. The dose which blocks the stimulating effects of isoprenaline causing no drop in cardiac output, these authors consider that M.J. 1999 presents no heart risk. According to FITZGERALD [557], this opinion is misleading, because the dose of M.J. 1999 used in this survey depended on the dose of isoprenaline chosen, so that if this latter had been higher it would have necessitated, for its effects to be countered, a larger dosage of M.J. 1999 which might well have been cardio-depressive.

With the healthy subject, Sotalol at the oral dose of 40 mg reduces the stimulating effects of isoprenaline on the heart rate and on the general oxygen consumption. The level of this activity is the same as for propranolol at an identical dosage, but the duration of the inhibiting effect is far longer in the case of Sotalol [122 a]. On the other hand, a different ratio has been found by RICE et al. [106 a] in normal men who were given both drugs in a cross-over pattern, the dose being doubled each day from 5 to 1280 mg by mouth. Antagonism of heart rate increase and blockade of the fall in diastolic blood pressure induced by isoprenaline infused daily were used to measure β-blockade. The propranolol/Sotalol potency ratio was found to be 2:1 for heart rate and 1:3 for blood pressure.

In another study carried out on healthy volunteers [71 a], Sotalol was found, in i.v. administration, to be three times less active than propranolol in reducing by 50% the tachycardia induced by the intravenous infusion of isoprenaline. Sotalol reduced resting heart rate in the standing position and exercise-induced tachycardia, being equal in potency to propranolol. In oral administration, Sotalol decreased resting heart rate and exercise-induced tachycardia, being slightly less active than propranolol.

In healthy subjects, Sotalol does not alter cardiac output following an intravenous dose of 40 mg [308 c]. Doses of 10 and 40 mg by the same route do not decrease cardiac output whereas an injection of 10 mg of propranolol caused a marked reduction in the same subjects [309 c]. There was, in consequence, a significant difference in the haemodynamic effects of propranolol and Sotalol at doses exerting a similar β-blocking action.

Haemodynamic effects of Sotalol were investigated in cardiac patients by BROOKS et al. [18 a]. Sotalol was injected intravenously at a dose of 0.2—0.6 mg/kg to ten heart disease cases, four of whom had chronic heart failure as indicated by elevated left ventricular end-diastolic pressure and low cardiac index, stroke index and dp/dt. It was concluded that Sotalol has no adverse haemodynamic effects in man even in the presence of heart failure, because there were no significant changes in stroke index, mean blood pressure or left ventricular end-diastolic pressure, although cardiac index and dp/dt were decreased in the same time as heart rate dropped significantly. To demonstrate that changes in cardiac index and dp/dt were primarily rate-dependent and could not be ascribed to myocardial depression, further studies were performed in which heart rate was held constant by atrial pacing in normal and catecholamine-depleted dogs. Sotalol, at the dose of 1 mg/kg i.v., which is much higher than the minimal β-blocking dose, did not change stroke index, blood pressure, left ventricular end-diastolic pressure, or estimated maximal velocity of isotonic shortening, confirming that myocardial contractility was unaffected. As the same clinical results were further obtained in ten other patients with heart disease, four of whom had clinical and haemodynamic evidence of chronic heart failure [49c], BROOKS et al. concluded that Sotalol-induced β-blockade had no observable myocardial depressant action in dogs or adverse haemodynamic effects in cardiac patients, even when advanced chronic heart failure was present. From these studies with Sotalol, it appears evident for them that acute β-blockade, in the absence of associated nonspecific myocardial depression, does not sufficiently impair cardiac function to produce observable deleterious changes in the resting haemodynamics of patients with advanced chronic heart failure.

In the case of the anginal patient, the intravenous injection of 60 mg of M.J. 1999 significantly increases the duration of an exercise on the ergometric bicycle [10].

In a cross-over single-blind investigation on 6 patients with angina and documented coronary artery disease, Sotalol was compared with propranolol. Patients received increasing doses of Sotalol and propranolol until they had maximal objective exercise improvement, which was not reached until daily doses of 480 mg of Sotalol or 160 mg of propranolol. Both drugs increased exercise tolerance to pain and onset of S—T segment depression in some patients but considerably higher doses of Sotalol were necessary to obtain the beneficial effect [13c]. In a double blind cross-over trial on 9 patients, there was a marked reduction in frequency of angina attacks which was not significantly different from that obtained with placebo, but pain was less severe under Sotalol than under placebo. Patients took fewer nitroglycerin tablets when treated with Sotalol [314c].

10. Recetan

$$\text{CHOH}-\text{CH}_2-\text{NHCH}\overset{\displaystyle CH_3}{\underset{\displaystyle CH_2-CH_3}{}}$$

An antagonist of the β-receptors, considerably less potent than propranolol [1218], and possessing no sympathicomimetic properties [1218], Recetan (generic name: butidrine) has greater local anaesthetic effects than lidocaine [540], and prevents the ventricular fibrillation caused in a rat by $CaCl_2$ administered intravenously [540]. It neutralises the arrhythmia induced by ouabaine [1945] and by aconitine [1944] in rabbits; it prevents in the case of this animal the ectopic ventricular rhythms appearing after adrenaline [1944].

Butidrine causes bradycardia and is cardio-depressive in animals [148]. It reduces coronary blood flow in the anaesthesised dog [212c].

In the case of normal man, the intravenous injection of 150 mg of butidrine reduces heart rate, raises diastolic blood pressure and slightly lowers cardiac output [201]; the tachycardia induced by intravenous infusion of adrenaline is neutralised [201].

This medication had a favourable antianginal effect on 46 patients [87]. It is also effective in certain cardiac rhythm disorders, particularly those resulting from digitalis intoxication [201].

Associated with Peritrate, under the name Butidrate (50 mg of butidrine and 20 mg of Peritrate), it is said to provide better therapeutic results than those achieved by the separate use of either of these two medications [1498]. BORRONI reported that the administration of one tablet of Butidrate three times daily for 15 days improved 80% of the 31 angina patients treated [38c]. The same dosage for the same length of time produced very good results in 30 patients [60c]: the anginal attacks disappeared in 22 patients and were greatly reduced in the other 8 cases; nitroglycerin was no longer needed in 23 patients. Heart rate was reduced in half of cases but atrial fibrillation was not affected.

11. PhQA 33

HERMANSEN has shown [819] that PhQA 33

is a *non-selective* β-antagonist because, although it blocks the β-receptors at a high dosage (its activity being roughly that of propranolol), it has a very slight β-stimulating effect at a weak dose.

Using the SEKIYA and WILLIAMS technique [1714], he also shows [820] that PhQA 33 increases the guinea-pig's tolerance to the fibrillating toxic dose of ouabaine, its activity being 50% less than that of propranolol but three times that of INPEA. According to HERMANSEN, this anti-arrhythmic effect is in correlation with the local anaesthetic effect of the substance, whose surface and conduction anaesthetic properties are respectively equal to and three times less than those of propranolol.

12. AH 3474

One of the most recent of the β-antagonists, AH 3474 has a structure which differs widely from the foregoing substances:

It is between 2 and 4 times less potent than propranolol in parenteral administration, but almost equivalent when taken orally by dogs [182]. It has no β-stimulating effect, nor has it any quinidine-like properties. However, SINGH and V. WILLIAMS reported that AH 3474 reduces the rate of rise of intracellular action potentials of isolated rabbit atria without altering the duration of the potential [293c]. It protects guinea-pigs against ouabain-induced ventricular fibrillation [293c].

13. D 477 A

D477A, which is a phenylbutylamine derivative

$$COO-\underset{\underset{NH_2}{|}}{\overset{\overset{OH}{|}}{C}}-CH_2-CH_2-\underset{NH_2}{\overset{}{CH}}-CH_2-CH_2-\text{(phenyl)}$$

(with phenyl rings bearing NH_2 and OH substituents)

produced at low dosages β-adrenergic blocking effects which were proved by the antagonism against the stimulating properties of isoprenaline on isolated guinea-pig atrium preparations [56a]. Larger doses, however, brought about a positive inotropic and chronotropic effect which was dose-dependent and about a thousand times less marked than the effect of isoprenaline.

14. USVC 6524

This agent differs structurally from propranolol in that it possesses an indane rather than a naphthyl group:

(indane structure with substituent R)

According to the experimental study by LEVY and WASSERMAN [202c], USVC 6524 inhibits the positive inotropic, positive chronotropic and vasodilator responses to isoprenaline in the dog in a dose of 0.01 mg/kg injected intravenously. USVC 6524 is approximately 10 times more potent as a β-adrenoceptor antagonist than propranolol.

Cardiac depressant effects produced by USVC 6524 are relatively mild and occurred only after the onset of a strong β-adrenoceptor blockade, since there was no significant negative inotropic effect until after 1 mg/kg of USVC 6524, which is a dose 30—100 times its β-adrenoceptor blocking dose. Results obtained in this study thus show this compound to be a β-adrenoceptor antagonist of considerable potency with relatively weak cardiac depressant properties.

15. S-D/1601

FERRINI et al. compared S—D/1601

(OCH_3-substituted ring with substituent R)

to propranolol with a view to evaluating β-blocking action and some other pharmacological properties [100c]. The results show that S—D/1601 is endowed with a slightly greater β-blocking activity than propranolol. Endoduodenal absorption also seems more favourable with S—D/1601 than with propranolol. However, the two drugs proved to have some interesting differences in their general pharmacological properties. In fact, S—D/1601 possesses a lesser degree of myocardial depressant action than propranolol. It also seems to be endowed with a more limited anaesthetic and antiarrhythmic action. Moreover neurodepressant effects are much less evident with S—D/1601 than with propranolol. In conclusion, S—D/1601 is slightly more active on the whole than propranolol in terms of β-blocking action, while at the same time non-specific side effects, such as myocardial and neurodepressant actions, are much less evident than in the case of propranolol.

16. Bunolol

Answering to the formula:

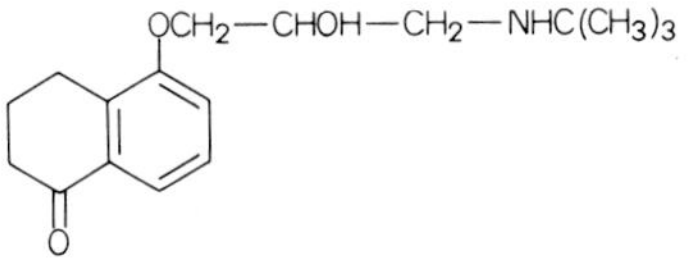

OCH$_2$—CHOH—CH$_2$—NHC(CH$_3$)$_3$

bunolol is a new β-adrenergic blocking agent, selected from a series of substances as the compound most warranting detailed pharmacologic studies from the viewpoints of good oral efficacy and separation between β-receptor antagonist and direct myocardial depressant properties in dogs [8d, 11d]. Bunolol is approximately three times as potent as propranolol by intravenous administration in suppressing the positive chronotropic action of isoprenaline, but is estimated to be approximately twenty times as potent as propranolol when both agents are compared by oral administration in dogs.

Bunolol is devoid of β-sympathomimetic activity. The β-adrenoceptor blockade by bunolol appears to be competitive in nature, is highly specific and has a persistent action. There appears to be a uniform susceptibility to blockade of β-receptors at different sites since bunolol is equally effective at β-receptors of the myocardium and the smooth muscle of the coronary arteries and femoral vasculature. At doses much higher than those producing β-adrenergic blockade, bunolol causes direct myocardial depression. When evaluated in dogs for activity against the arrhythmias induced by adrenaline, ouabain and coronary artery ligation, bunolol prevented adrenaline-induced ventricular tachycardias in both normal anaesthetised and adrenaline-sensitive, coronary ligated, unanaesthetised dogs. Bunolol is considerably less effective than propranolol against ouabain-induced ventricular tachycardia in anaesthetised and conscious dogs and is ineffective against the ventricular arrhythmias in dogs 24 hours after coronary ligation.

Cordarone

Cordarone[1] (generic name: amiodarone) or 2-butyl-3-(3,5-diiodo-4-β-diethylaminoethoxybenzoyl)-benzofuran, L. 3428:

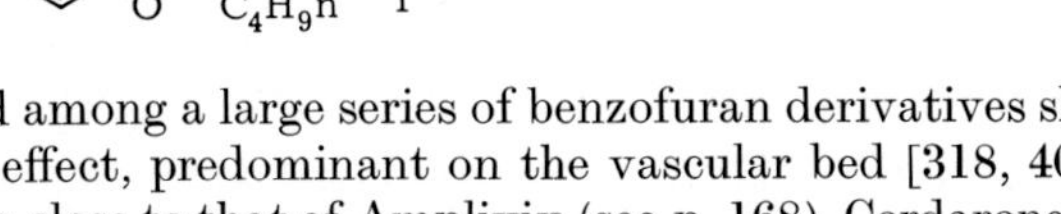

I

—CO—⟨ ⟩—O—CH$_2$-CH$_2$-N⟨C_2H_5 / C_2H_5⟩   · HCl

C$_4$H$_9$n   I

has been selected among a large series of benzofuran derivatives showing a smooth muscle relaxing effect, predominant on the vascular bed [318, 409]. Although its structure is quite close to that of Amplivix (see p. 168), Cordarone displays haemodynamic and metabolic properties which differ radically from those of Amplivix. This arises from the facts that Cordarone reduces the normal oxygen requirements

---

1 Synonyms: Trangorex, Angoron.

of the heart by alleviating its work and furthermore protects the myocardium against the excessive metabolic demands induced by stimulation of the sympathetic drive.

1. Pharmacological Properties

Most of the haemodynamic effects of Cordarone have been evidenced in the anaesthetized dog with an electromagnetic bloodflowmeter [728, 977, 979, 1014, 1016]. Mean blood flow has been measured in several vessels: aorta and left (or left circumflex) coronary, femoral, renal, hepatic, splenic and superior mesenteric arteries. Some other haemodynamic parameters have been calculated from the simultaneously measured parameters: cardiac output by additioning aortic flow and coronary flow[2], left ventricular work by multiplying cardiac output by mean systemic blood pressure[3]. Coronary vascular resistance was computed as the mean systemic blood pressure divided by coronary flow, whereas overall vascular resistance was calculated by dividing the mean systemic blood pressure by cardiac output.

For some biological reasons which will appear clearly later on (see p. 266), the various haemodynamic effects of Cordarone can be grouped into two series. The first one includes the "intrinsic" properties i.e. those pharmacologic effects in which the adrenergic system is not involved. The second comprises the antiadrenergic effects.

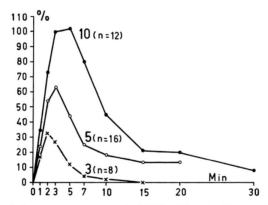

Fig. 32. Effect of amiodarone on coronary arterial blood flow in 19 anaesthetized dogs. Blood flow has been measured in the left (or left circumflex) coronary artery with an electromagnetic probe. 3: intravenous injection of amiodarone, 3 mg/kg. 5: intravenous injection of amiodarone 5 mg/kg. 10: intravenous injection of amiodarone, 10 mg/kg. n: number of injections. The average increases are in % of control-values

1.1. Intrinsic Effects

Cordarone increases coronary arterial blood flow [310][4]. Intensity and duration of the effect are dose dependent. The maximal rise in coronary flow is by 44—89 and 134% respectively with doses of 3—5 and 10 mg/kg. The duration of the augmentation of blood flow is not exceptionally long since blood flow returns to initial values within 30 min with the largest dose (Fig. 32). Coronary vascular

---

2 See p. 92.
3 See p. 92.
4 A similar increase in coronary blood flow has been reported in the anaesthetised cat by HENSEL who measured myocardial blood flow by calorimetry [244c]. All the intrinsic effects of Cordarone have been recently confirmed by PETTA and ZACCHEO [8e bis].

resistance falls by respectively 39—51 and 64% for the doses of 3—5 and 10 mg/kg. Aortic flow and cardiac output are not significantly modified, a fact which has been confirmed by MORET with the same procedure [1322].

On the other hand, the work of the left ventricle is diminished by 12% with 3 mg/kg, 23% with 5 mg/kg and 25% with 10 mg/kg, whereas total vascular resistance is reduced respectively by 10.5—15 and 20%, systemic blood pressure being lowered in the same order of magnitude.

It has been confirmed by the thermodilution method (see p. 91) that cardiac output does not change significantly after injection of Cordarone (Fig. 33). Heart

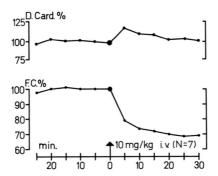

Fig. 33. Effect of amiodarone, 10 mg/kg i.v., on cardiac output (upper trace) and heart rate (lower trace) in the anaesthetized dog. Data are average values of 7 experiments, and changes are expressed in % of control values

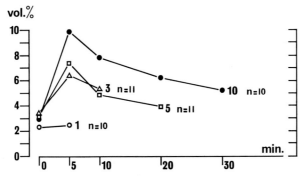

Fig. 34. Effect of amiodarone on oxygen content of coronary venous blood (expressed in vol. %) in 15 anaesthetized dogs. 1: intravenous injection of amiodarone, 1 mg/kg. 3: intravenous injection of amiodarone, 3 mg/kg. 5: intravenous injection of amiodarone, 5 mg/kg. 10: intravenous injection of amiodarone, 10 mg/kg. Data are average values for n injections

rate is reduced by Cordarone, by 10—19 and 30% with 3—5 and 10 mg/kg respectively (Fig. 33). This bradycardia is not antagonized by atropine. The morphology of the ECG is not changed by Cordarone, the P-R interval not being modified even at doses which induce bradycardia, but the electric systole is lengthened when bradycardia is present [110].

Myocardial oxygen consumption is reduced by Cordarone. The results obtained by the FICK method at doses of 3—5 and 10 mg/kg on 15 dogs show that oxygen consumption by the myocardium diminishes proportionally to the dose level. The same graduation is observed for the oxygen content of coronary venous blood which increases by 87—133 and 220% with 3—5 and 10 mg/kg Cordarone respectively (Fig. 34). Since arterial oxygen content does not change, oxygen coronary arterio-venous difference is lowered, proportionally to the dose and to the increase in coronary blood flow (Fig. 35). All the haemodynamic changes which have been observed for an i.v. injection of 10 mg/kg of Cordarone have been summarized in Fig. 36 [317].

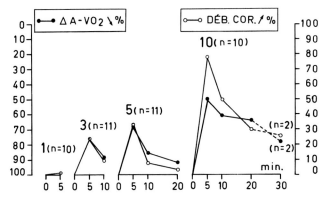

Fig. 35. Effect of amiodarone on oxygen coronary arterio-venous difference and arterial coronary blood flow in 15 anaesthetized dogs. $\triangle$A-VO$_2$: oxygen coronary arterio-venous difference (decrease in % of control values). DEB. COR.: arterial coronary blood flow (increase in % of control values). 1: intravenous injection of amiodarone, 1 mg/kg. 3: intravenuos injection of amiodarone, 3 mg/kg. 5: intravenous injection of amiodarone, 5 mg/kg. 10: intravenous injection of amiodarone, 10 mg/kg. Data are average values for n injections

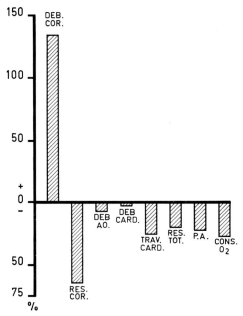

Fig. 36. Haemodynamic effects of amiodarone, 10 mg/kg i.v., in the anaesthetized dog. DEB. COR.: Arterial coronary blood flow. RES. COR.: Coronary vascular resistance. DEB. AO.: Aortic blood flow. DEB. CARD.: Cardiac output. TRAV. CARD.: Work of the left ventricle. RES. TOT.: Total vascular resistance. P.A.: Systemic blood pressure. CONS. O$_2$: Myocardial oxygen consumption. Data are average values of 20 experiments. Changes are expressed in % of control values

Calculation of myocardial oxygen consumption by the Tension-Time Index method (see p. 93) gives the same results as there is a reduction of 25% with 10 mg/kg i.v. (mean decrease for 15 experiments).

The decrease in myocardial oxygen needs has been evidenced also on unanaesthetized dogs receiving Cordarone daily by oral route during several weeks. Ten dogs have been trained to remain still on an operation table for periods allowing measurements. Three of them were not given any Cordarone and were used as controls. The remaining seven dogs received 10 (two dogs), 15 (three dogs) and 20 (2 dogs) mg/kg Cordarone twice a day for seven weeks in succession. Determinations of the tension-time index were made on each animal once a week for fourteen weeks i.e. twice before the beginning of the administration, seven times during, and five times after interruption of Cordarone. Figure 37 shows that during the seven weeks treatment, tension-time index, heart rate and blood pressure were

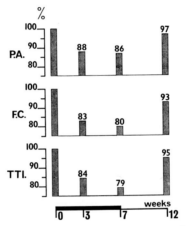

Fig. 37. Effects of amiodarone on blood pressure, heart rate and Tension-Time Index in the conscious dog. Amiodarone has been given by oral route every day during 7 weeks at a daily dose of 20 mg/kg in two experiments, of 30 mg/kg in three experiments and of 40 mg/kg in two experiments. P.A.: Systemic blood pressure. F.C.: Heart rate. T.T.I.: Tension-Time Index. Although the three haemodynamic parameters have been measured every week, values are only given, in this schematic drawing, after 3 and 7 weeks of treatment, and also after amiodarone has been discontinued for 5 weeks. Data are average values of 7 experiments. Changes are expressed in % of control values

significantly smaller (P < 0.01, t test) than in control animals during the same period [309]. When the treatment was discontinued, the three parameters slowly returned towards their control levels. These experiments also indicate that the reduction in heart rate and, to a lesser extent, the decrease in blood pressure play a part in the reduction in myocardial oxygen consumption (see Fig. 37).

Left intraventricular pressure is not modified when 3 or 5 mg/kg of Cordarone are injected intravenously to dogs; with 10 mg/kg, a slight negative inotropic effect can be seen (Fig. 38), which does not last over 5 min, whereas an i.v. injection of 1 mg/kg propranolol induces an important and progressive fall in left intraventricular pressure together with a lasting drop in systemic blood pressure. In the case of Cordarone, the maximal decrease in left ventricular systolic pressure is by 10%, which is attained 1 min after the end of the injection. Systemic systolic and diastolic blood pressures being respectively lowered by 6.5 and 21% at the same moment (see Fig. 38), this suggests that the negative inotropic effect accoutns for the diminution in systolic pressure while the larger reduction in diastolic pressure is chiefly due to the decrease in total vascular resistance, which was calculated in other experiments as amounting to 20% of control values (see p. 257).

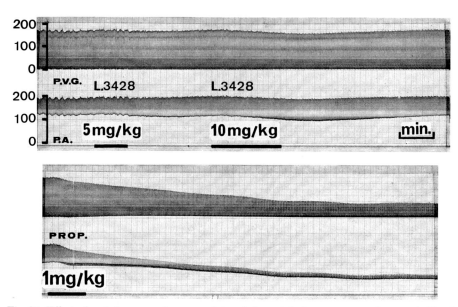

Fig. 38. Effect of amiodarone and propranolol on left ventricular pressure and systemic blood pressure in the anaesthetized dog. P.V.G.: Phasic left ventricular pressure (mm Hg). P.A.: Phasic femoral blood pressure (mm Hg). The lower tracing is the immediate continuation of the top tracing. At signal marks: successive intravenous injections of amiodarone (L. 3428), 5 mg/kg and 10 mg/kg, and of propranolol, 1 mg/kg

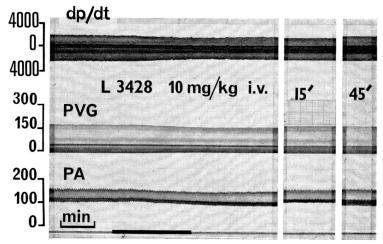

Fig. 39. Effect of amiodarone on rate of rise of left ventricular pressure, left ventricular pressure and systemic blood pressure in the anaesthetized dog. From top to bottom: dp/dt: rate of rise of left ventricular pressure (mm Hg/sec). P.V.G.: Phasic left ventricular pressure (mm Hg). P.A.: Phasic femoral blood pressure (mm Hg). Left tracing, at signal mark: intravenous injection of amiodarone (L. 3428), 10 mg/kg. Middle and right tracings: respectively 15 and 45 min after injection

Cordarone induces a moderate diminution in left ventricular dp/dt which disappears after fifteen minutes (Fig. 39), whereas 0.5 mg/kg of propranolol i.v. irreversibly reduces dp/dt to 50% of its initial value (see p. 215 and Fig. 20).

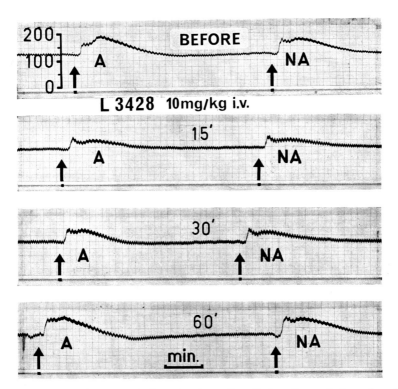

Fig. 40. Effect of amiodarone on the hypertensive action of adrenaline and of noradrenaline in the anaesthetized and vagotomized dog. Recording of mean blood pressure in the femoral artery (mm Hg). A: intravenous injection of adrenaline, 0.002 mg/kg. NA: intravenous injection of noradrenaline, 0.002 mg/kg. From top to bottom: First trace: before intravenous injection of amiodarone, 10 mg/kg. Second trace: 15 min after injection of amiodarone. Third trace: 30 min after injection of amiodarone. Fourth trace: 60 min after injection of amiodarone

LOCHNER [1163] confirmed that dp/dt and left ventricular systolic pressure are diminished in dogs after the i.v. administration of Cordarone, but he showed that this effect cannot be considered as reflecting a cardiodepressant action similar to the negative inotropic effect of β-blocking agents. In his opinion, the slight reduction in cardiac dynamics due to Cordarone is secondary to the fall in systemic blood pressure since it does not appear in animals in which there is exceptionally no decrease in blood pressure after the i.v. injection of the drug. Furthermore, such diminution in ventricular performance does not occur when systemic blood pressure is artificially maintained at a constant level after the i.v. injection of Cordarone or when the drug is injected into a coronary artery, a mode of administration which does not lead to any fall in blood pressure.

Variations of blood flow in various territories have been checked after the i.v. injection of Cordarone: data obtained for spleen, liver, kidney, intestine and hind leg in dogs show that blood flow is only slightly affected in any of these territories [110], in striking contrast with the myocardium where the increase is considerable.

1.2. Antiadrenergic Effects

Cordarone exhibits inhibiting properties against several adrenergic phenomena of the a- as well as of the β-type.

1.2.1. a-antiadrenergic Effects

The a-antiadrenergic effects of Cordarone were evidenced by studying the vasoconstriction induced by adrenaline and noradrenaline in several experimental conditions.

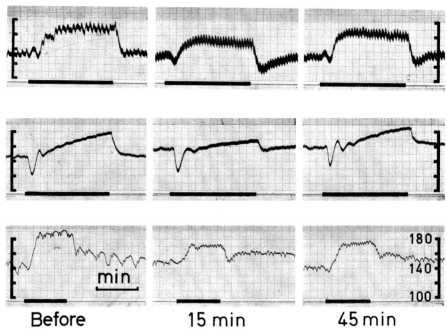

Before   15 min   45 min

Fig. 41. Effect of amiodarone on the hypertensive effect of electric stimulation of the splanchnic nerve (freq: 5 s/sec; duration: 6 msec; tension: 5 mV) during two min in 3 anaesthetized and vagotomized dogs. Recording of mean blood pressure in the femoral artery (mm Hg). Left traces: control splanchnic hypertension in the 3 dogs. Between left and middle traces: intravenous injection of amiodarone, 10 mg/kg. Middle traces: splanchnic hypertension 15 min after injection of amiodarone. Right traces: splanchnic hypertension 45 min after injection of amiodarone

Cordarone reduces the hypertensive effect of these catecholamines injectde i.v. to chloralosed vagotomized dogs. This effect is moderate with 3 and 5 mg/kg but conspicuous with 10 mg/kg (Fig. 40). The phenomenon wears off within 1 h. This antiadrenergic effect has also been observed in the anaesthetized cat.

Cordarone reduces the rise in blood pressure induced by splanchnic electric stimulation [316]: in each of the four dogs used the increase in blood pressure was reduced by 50% within 15 min. Splanchnic hypertension returned to its initial levels one hour later (Fig. 41). Similar results have been obtained in the cat.

Cordarone reduces the vasoconstrictor effects of adrenaline and noradrenaline injected intra-arterially via a polyethylene catheter inserted into a collateral branch of the femoral artery and through the main trunk of the vessel in such a way that the tip was proximal to the flow transducer. After an i.v. injection of

10 mg/kg of Cordarone, the drastic decrease in blood flow due to both catecholamines was appreciably reduced; the phenomenon reached its peak within the first 5 min following injection, and then gradually disappeared so that 30 min after administration of Cordarone the reduction in blood flow was almost identical with that occurring during control-reaction [309].

In the spinal cat, the increase in blood pressure due to an i.v. injection of adrenaline was reduced by two-thirds within 3 or 4 min following a 10 mg/kg i.v. dose of Cordarone [309], and adrenaline-hypertension reverted to nearly normal level only within 30 min. In the pithed rat, Cordarone reduced by 60% the rise in blood pressure due to an i.v. injection of noradrenaline made five minutes thereafter [309]. This inhibition progressively regressed later on and completely disappeared after 30 min.

1.2.2. β-antiadrenergic Effects

Three haemodynamic phenomena relevant of the stimulation of β-adrenoceptors have been studied.

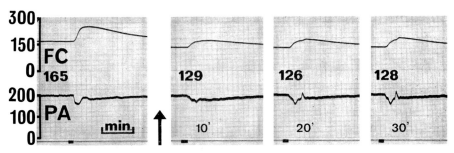

Fig. 42. Effect of amidarone on the tachycardia and hypotension induced by isoprenaline in the anaesthetized and atropinized dog. F.C.: Heart rate (beats/min). P.A.: Mean femoral blood pressure (mm Hg). At signal marks: four intravenous injections of isoprenaline, 0.002 mg/kg, made respectively (from left to right) before, and 10—20 and 30 min after an intravenous injection of amiodarone, 10 mg/kg (at arrow)

a) Tachycardia induced by isoprenaline in the dog is reduced by Cordarone (Fig. 42): 10—15 min after a dose of 10 mg/kg i.v. of Cordarone has been injected, isoprenaline increased the heart rate by only 50% compared with control tachycardia. This effect disappeared slowly thereafter.

b) Hypotension induced by isoprenaline is also reduced by Cordarone in the chloralosed dog. The drop in systemic blood pressure provoked by isoprenaline was reduced by two thirds within the 5 min following an i.v. injection of 10 mg/kg of Cordarone [309]. This inhibition vanished with time and completely disappeared within 60 min.

c) Cordarone reduces the maximal acceleration of the rise of left intraventricular pressure (dp/dt) brought about by adrenaline in the anaesthetized dog [309]. The damping of the maximal acceleration was by 50% after the injection of Cordarone (Fig. 43); control acceleration was again attained within 45 min after Cordarone. On the other hand, the i.v. injection of 0.5 mg/kg propranolol blocked the acceleration in dp/dt induced by adrenaline in the same animals, a result which is consonant with the observations of BENFEY et al. [133].

From the previous results, it appears that Cordarone reduces, but does not block, several haemodynamic effects of catecholamines, whether of the α-type (increase in blood pressure) or of the β-type (tachycardia and stimulation in heart energetics). Catecholamines are known to increase myocardial oxygen consump-

tion [478, 685, 739, 960] probably through their three aforementioned haemodynamic effects [645, 1000, 1034]. As these phenomena, when considered separately,
are largely reduced by Cordarone, it could be expected that augmentation in oxygen needs of the myocardium induced by catecholamines be also partially inhibited
by Cordarone. Such an effect has been evidenced. Myocardial oxygen consumption
has been measured by the FICK procedure in ten experiments on six atropinized
dogs at the peak of the increase in blood pressure induced by i.v. injection of adrenaline. Twenty minutes after the i.v. injection of 10 mg/kg of Cordarone, adrenaline
was injected again at the same dose as that for control injection, and myocardial
oxygen consumption measured again. The results are summarized in Fig. 44: in

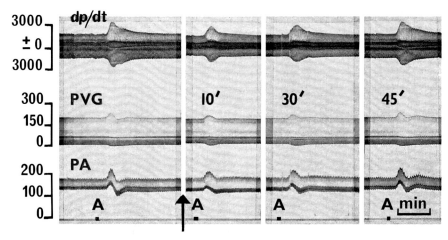

Fig. 43. Effect of amiodarone on the actions of adrenaline on rate of rise in ventricular pressure
and left ventricular pressure in the anaesthetized and atropinized dog. From top to bottom:
dp/dt: Rate of rise of left ventricular pressure (mm Hg/sec). P.V.G.: Left ventricular pressure
(mm Hg). P.A.: Phasic femoral blood pressure (mm Hg). At signal marks: four intravenous
injections of adrenaline (A), 0.002 mg/kg, made respectively (from left to right) before, and
10—30 and 45 min after an intravenous injection of amiodarone, 10 mg/kg (at arrow)

every instance, Cordarone either strongly diminished or inverted the effect of
adrenaline on myocardial oxygen consumption. The arithmetic mean of the data
indicates that oxygen consumption increased by 48% by adrenaline before Cordarone, whereas it decreased by 9% after a previous administration of Cordarone.

Similar findings were obtained when myocardial oxygen consumption was
measured by the tension-time index method. Figure 45 shows the partial inhibiting effect of Cordarone in 15 anaesthetized atropinized dogs towards the increase
in tension-time index induced by adrenaline and noradrenaline. Recorded heart
rates and blood pressures during these experiments indicate that tachycardia as
well as arterial hypertension were both reduced to the same extent.

It seems even more relevant to mention that chronic assays in which Cordarone
has been given per os daily for seven weeks to 7 unanaesthetized atropinized dogs
provided the same results. The protocol of the experiment was close to the assay
previously described (see p. 259) except that after each control of the basal tension-
time index, the animals received an i.v. injection of adrenaline, the dose of which
was chosen so that their normal blood pressure would increase by more than 75%.
Tension-time index was measured at the time when the increase in blood pressure
was maximal. The values of tension-time index under adrenaline were measured

each week and expressed in % of the mean of the two control values. The same procedure was adopted for the expression of the rises in heart rate and in blood pressure. The results (Fig. 46) show that during the seven week period of treatment with Cordarone, the increase in the three measured cardiovascular parameters induced by adrenaline is significantly smaller than in control animals during the same period (P < 0,01, test t). These parameters revert slowly to their initial

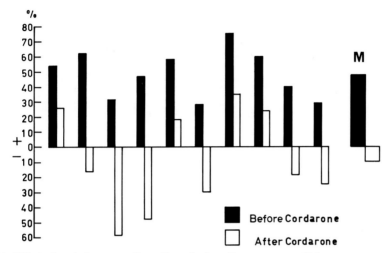

Fig. 44. Effect of amiodarone on the action of adrenaline on myocardial oxygen consumption in the anaesthetized and atropinized dog. Changes induced by adrenaline (intravenous injection of 0.003—0.008 mg/kg according to the experiment) in ten experiments, before (black columns) and 15 min after (open columns) an intravenous injection of amiodarone, 10 mg/kg. Changes are expressed in % of control values. M: arithmetic average data of the 10 experiments

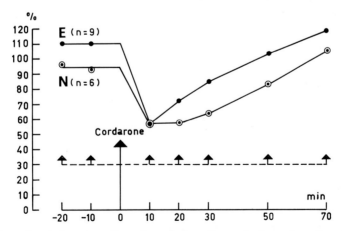

Fig. 45. Effect of amiodarone on the action of adrenaline and of noradrenaline on Tension-Time Index in the anaesthetized and atropinized dog. Changes induced by adrenaline (intravenous injection of 0.003—0.01 mg/kg according to the experiment) in 9 experiments, and by noradrenaline (intravenous injection of 0.003—0.01 mg/kg according to the experiment) in 6 experiments, two times before an intravenous injection of amiodarone, 10 mg/kg (at long arrow) and 10 — 20 — 30 — 50 and 70 min after amiodarone. Increases in Tension-Time Index are expressed in % of control basal values measured before the injection of catecholamines. ●——● E: Adrenaline. ⊙——⊙ N: Noradrenaline

values when Cordarone is discontinued. Hypertension and tachycardia induced by adrenaline are reduced by Cordarone to the same extent (see Fig. 46).

In other experiments, it has been demonstrated that Cordarone does not modify the coronarodilator effect of adenosine but the action of bradykinine on the coronary circulation is enhanced [310]. Cordarone does not depress vasomotor center and has no effect on coagulation process. The fonctions of the kidneys and of the central nervous system are not altered. There is no incidence upon the thermoregulation center, even for high doses.

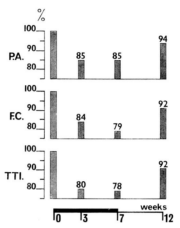

Fig. 46. Effect of amiodarone on the actions of adrenaline on blood pressure, heart rate, and Tension-Time Index in the conscious dog. Amiodarone has been given by oral route every day during 7 weeks at a daily dose of 20 mg/kg in two experiments, of 30 mg/kg in three experiments, and of 40 mg/kg in two experiments. An intravenous injection of adrenaline, 0.003—0.01 mg/kg, according to the animal, has been made every week. P.A.: Systemic blood pressure. F.C.: Heart rate. T.T.I.: Tension-Time Index. Although the three haemodynamic parameters have been measured every week, values are only given, in this schematic drawing, after 3 and 7 weeks of treatment, and also after amiodarone had been discontinued for 5 weeks. Data are average values of 7 experiments. Changes are expressed in % of values measured before each injection of adrenaline

1.3. Action Mechanisms and Therapeutic Deductions

At this stage of our investigations the intrinsic effects and the antiadrenergic effects of Cordarone cannot be attributed to a common mechanism. In effect, Cordarone still caused bradycardia and a fall of total vascular resistance in a dog pretreated with reserpine intraperitoneally. The heart rate decreased by 25% in these conditions (Fig. 47), a finding which demonstrate that the main intrinsic effects of Cordarone are independent of the endogenous adrenergic mediators [307, 314][5]. The two kinds of effects will thus be discussed separately.

1.3.1. Intrinsic Effects

Intrinsic effects of Cordarone comprise essentially reduction of cardiac work with reduction of myocardial oxygen consumption, slowing in heart rate and relaxing effect on vascular smooth muscle. This last phenomenon is particularly marked

---

5 It is noteworthy that chronic deprivation of the thyroid gland does not affect the pharmacological properties of Cordarone since decrease in heart rate and in blood pressure occur also in animals which were deprived of their thyroid gland by surgical procedure or by administration of labelled sodium iodide [78 c].

as regards coronary circulation, resulting in a fall in coronary resistance and therefore in an increase in myocardial irrigation. Decrease in vascular resistance occurs also, but to a minor extent, in the general circulation, where the diminution of total vascular resistance is mainly responsible for the slight and transient reduction in systemic blood pressure.

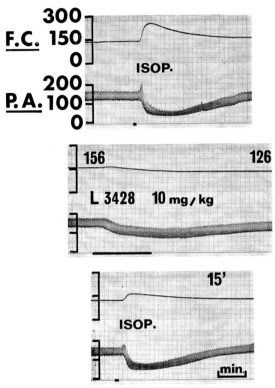

Fig. 47. Effect of amiodarone on heart rate and systemic blood pressure in an anaesthetized and atropinized dog, pretreated with reserpine (0.5 mg/kg intraperitoneally 48 and 24[H] before the experiment). F.C.: Heart rate (beats/min). P.A.: Phasic femoral blood pressure (mm Hg). Upper tracings: at signal mark, intravenous injection of isoprenaline, 0.0005 mg/kg. Middle tracings: at signal mark, intravenous injection of amiodarone, 10 mg/kg. Lower tracings: at signal mark, intravenous injection of isoprenaline, 0.0005 mg/kg, made 15 min after amiodarone

The reduction in the work of the left ventricle provoked by Cordarone may be attributed to the fall in total vascular resistance and to the slowing in heart rate. This diminution of cardiac load is in harmony with the view of ROWE [1571] who considers that this kind of biological effect should be beneficial in angina pectoris, provided that cardiac output is either maintained or only slightly reduced (Cordarone does not depress cardiac function), a strong reduction in cardiac output leading, among other phenomena, to a reduction in coronary irrigation [144].

The reduction in myocardial oxygen consumption provoked by Cordarone is due to four factors: slowing in heart rate, decrease in blood pressure (both parameters have been shown repeatedly to be of importance in governing the oxygen consumption of the heart [644, 1316, 1355, 1644]), slight reduction in left intraventricular systolic pressure and decrease in ventricular dp/dt, both these parameters having been shown to be important determinants of myocardial oxygen consumption [1791], as the first one expresses the tension developed by cardiac contraction and the second one the velocity of that contraction [1511, 1585]. It is relevant to recall that the reduction in myocardial oxygen requirements and in heart rate have also been evidenced in conscious dogs receiving Cordarone by oral route in chronic administration at daily doses which are only twice the dosage recommended in patients.

Biochemical investigations have shown that Cordarone increases the lactate/pyruvate ratio in the coronary venous blood in dogs [234] and in myocardial tissue in rats [235]. This effect cannot be ascribed to a relative hypoxia since, would it be the case, there should be a definite production of lactate by the myocardium; lactate production has never been found after administration of Cordarone. Lactate/pyruvate ratio increases by diminution of pyruvate content, indicating a decrease of oxydation rate but not in oxydising possibilities: the myocardium behaves as if less oxygen was needed [233, 410]. A respiratory impairment can thus be excluded [233]. There is no uncoupling effect on oxydative phosphorylations [1297].

Cordarone increases coronary arterial blood flow without augmenting myocardial oxygen consumption. This coronarodilating effect, which is dose related, is due to a direct reduction of coronary wall resistance. The decrease in coronary resistance is probably mainly due to a direct myolytic action, but a reduction of the extravascular component of the resistance may come into play as an additional factor, since reduction in myocardial contractility, in rate of development of isometric tension and in systolic ejection (these effects have been evidenced in the case of Cordarone) may permit an increase in coronary flow during systole [1393]. The vasodilating effect of Cordarone bears predominantly on the myocardial vessels, since there are only minor variations in blood flow in various other territories (see p. 261) and since total vascular resistance is proportionally strongly less diminished than coronary resistance.

However, Cordarone is not the most active or long-acting coronary vasodilator, but since coronary flow rises without any increase in myocardial oxygen consumption, Cordarone can be considered as a primary dilating agent. Consequently, Cordarone increases coronary efficiency (,,Güte der Koronargefässdurchblutung", 686), which expresses the relation existing between coronary arterial blood flow and myocardial oxygen consumption. This effect may be of interest to compensate cardiac hypoxia due to pathological reductions in coronary flow, and to widen the margin of autoregulation of coronary flow, which is still present during myocardial ischaemia but to a much smaller degree than in the normal heart [217]. The pharmacological features of Cordarone suggest also that coronary reserve, as described by RUSHMER [1584], is improved. As the oxygen content of arterial blood does not change while the coronary arterio-venous oxygen difference decreases, myocardial oxygen utilization coefficient is also reduced.

Cordarone thus differs completely from uncoupling agents of the dinitrophenol type, the "malignant" coronary dilating effect of which is well documented [222, 223, 1168].

The rise in coronary flow concomitant with the absence of increase in myocardial oxygen consumption provides an enrichment in the venous coronary oxygen concentration, a fact which has been repeatedly confirmed [456, 1163, 1322]. This correlation between hyperoxygenation and hyperirrigation is such that the increase in oxygen level is proportional to the augmentation in blood flow. These characteristics seem to fit in with the type of drug which has been described as "benign" coronarodilator [732, 2007]. Although the coronary dilating effect of Cordarone can certainly not explain by itself the pharmacological and/or therapeutic effects of the drug, it must not be neglected. In fact it has been stressed that, in many pathological situations, the normal regulating mechanisms of coronary flow are not always able to adapt myocardial irrigation to the demands of the myocardium, within the limits of the anatomical and physical possibilities [217, 225, 226]. Nevertheless, some clinical and anatomo-pathological observations suggest that a sclerosed coronary artery can still — at least partially — retain some functional possibilities. Atheromatous coronary degenerescence bears predominantly on the larger coronary vessels, the resistance of which is considered as insignificant for the variations of vasomotricity [488], whereas the smaller intramyocardial vessels, where essential resistance changes take place [488], are not invaded by this process, leaving some coronary "reserve" [656, 1690]. In the central zone of an anoxaemic region, local regulation provokes a vasodilation which is probably of maximum intensity, whereas in the peripheral area there still exist unemployed coronary "reserves". It seems therefore possible that pharmacological agents, capable of reducing coronary bed resistance, as in the case of Cordarone, could ameliorate the irrigation of the heart in the peripheral zone of previously stenosed regions [218]. Such an event takes place effectively in both healthy man and anginous patient, a decrease in coronary vascular resistance having been evidenced [1322]; but the share of this mechanism in the therapeutic effect of Cordarone in angina is still open to question.

In order to determine the mechanisms involved in the main intrinsic haemodynamic effects of Cordarone — slowing in heart rate, moderate diminution in systemic blood pressure, reduction in oxygen needs of the myocardium —, and also to investigate the biological findings capable of showing that Cordarone does not act as a β-blocking agent, any possible interference with these three phenomena by certain pharmacological agents acting at various levels of the adrenergic system (hexamethonium, guanethidine, propranolol and phentolamine) was examined by measuring the three parameters with the Tension-Time Index technique: none of these substances modified the main effects of Cordarone. Furthermore, when both a- and β-receptors were blocked at the same time by phentolamine and propranolol in the anaesthetized atropinized dog, the subsequent i.v. injection of Cordarone still diminished the three parameters studied as in an untreated animal [309]. It is also unlikely that the bradycardia induced by Cordarone involved any effect on the β-adrenoceptors. Indeed, as shown in Fig. 48, propranolol was given i.v. to an anaesthetized atropinized dog and reduced heart rate from 204 to 156 beats/min. A second and third injection of 0.5 mg/kg of propranolol again slightly decreased heart rate, but a fourth dose had no additional effect. Cordarone 10 mg/kg i.v. however, given at this point, reduced the heart rate by a further 23% [307, 314].

The intrinsic pharmacological effects of Cordarone are thus not mediated through the adrenergic and parasympathetic systems, but are dependent on a direct action on vascular and cardiac cells. In view of this fact, slowing in heart rate induced by Cordarone in the intact animal could be due partially to inhibition of the β-adrenoceptors controlling the impulses of the sinusal and the atrio-ventricular nodes, thereby reducing the basal β-sympathetic drive, and mainly to an effect on more peripheral structures belonging to the cardiac excitation-conduction system and on the cardiac muscle itself. Direct action upon the cardiac muscular cell has, in fact, been demonstrated by VAUGHAN-WILLIAMS [1934]. He showed that, although having no effect on the *resting* potential of isolated rabbit atrial or ventricular muscle fibers, Cordarone caused a considerable prolongation of the *action* potential in both tissues, without any significant change in the height and in the rate of rise of the action potential.

Although Cordarone did not depress thyroid function, it has effects on cardiac potentials which are similar to those which, according to FREEDBERG et al. [101c], occur after thyroidectomy. VAUGHAN-WILLIAMS states that Cordarone has an

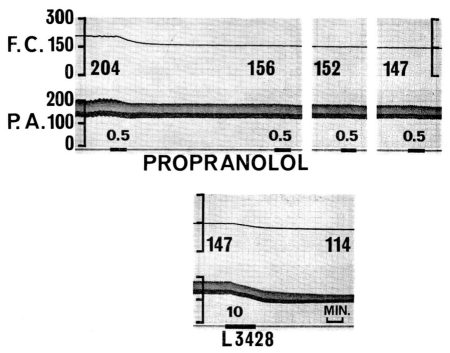

Fig. 48. Effect of amiodarone on heart rate and systemic blood pressure in an anaesthetized and atropinized dog, pretreated with propranolol. F.C.: Heart rate (beats/min). P.A.: Phasic femoral blood pressure (mm Hg). Upper tracings: at the four signal marks, intravenous injections of propranolol, 0.5 mg/kg. Lower tracings: at signal mark, intravenous injection of amiodarone (L. 3428), 10 mg/kg

unusual action on cardiac intracellular potentials in that it interferes with repolarising currents to a much greater extent than it affects depolarisation, whereas quinidine and propranolol, for instance, do the reverse. Tentatively, VAUGHAN-WILLIAMS concluded that Cordarone exerts a depressant effect on metabolic turnover which has some cardiac specificity. It may be added that, according to VAUGHAN-WILLIAMS [1934], Cordarone does not modify significantly the conduction velocity and electrical threshold, and has no local anaesthetic action.

Very recent advances in experimental studies of the mechanisms involved in the cardiac effects of Cordarone [48c] show that there is an inhibiting effect on the calcium ions pump of the sarcoplasmic reticulum. According to the hypothesis arising from such an experimental finding, administration of calcium ions should antagonise the reducing effect of Cordarone upon the velocity of ventricular contraction but not the slowing down effect on heart rate. As shown in Fig. 49, this is what has been found in the dog. Cordarone was injected into the vein at a depressive dose of 20 mg/kg on ventricular dynamics, as witnesses the reduction in dp/dt. CaCl$_2$ was subsequently administered at a dose of 10 mg/kg i.v.: diminution in dp/dt was immediately antagonised whereas bradycardia was not affected.

1.3.2. Antiadrenergic Effects

Although Cordarone antagonizes conspicuously several cardiovascular reactions brought about by pharmacologic stimulation of a-adrenoceptors (hypertension) and of β-adrenoceptors (tachycardia and increase in heart energetics), these

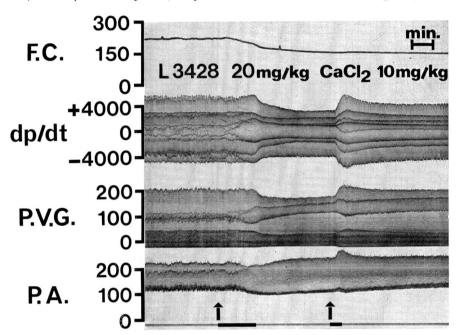

Fig. 49. Effect of high doses of amiodarone on heart rate, rate of rise in left ventricular pressure, left ventricular pressure and systemic blood pressure in the anaesthetised dog. Antagonistic effect of calcium ions. From top to bottom: F.C.: Heart rate (beats/min). dp/dt: Rate of rise in left ventricular pressure (mm Hg/sec). P.V.G.: Left ventricular pressure (mm Hg). P.A.: Phasic blood pressure in the femoral artery (mm Hg). At first signal mark: intravenous injection of amiodarone, 20 mg/kg. At second signal mark: intravenous injection of CaCl$_2$, 10 mg/kg

reactions are never blocked even at extremely high doses. For instance, tachycardia induced by isoprenaline and hypertension due to epinephrine are only partially inhibited in anaesthetized dogs receiving up to 70 mg/kg Cordarone i.v. at a rate of 10 mg/kg every 15 min. In this context, the inhibition of isoprenaline-tachycardia induced by a first i.v. injection of 10 mg/kg of Cordarone was not more pronounced after a second injection of the same dose had been given, whereas a further injection of 1 mg/kg of propranolol abolished the tachycardia (Fig. 50).

It is advisable to point out that Cordarone cannot be regarded as an a-blocking drug or more especially as a β-blocking agent. Experimental evidences are the following:

a) Repeated i.v. doses of 10 mg/kg of Cordarone up to a total of 70—80 mg/kg, interspersed with challenges by isoprenaline and adrenaline, never abolish the adrenergic reactions, the responses to both catecholamines after the last dose of Cordarone being no smaller than after the first [309].

b) When heart rate has been reduced by successive i.v. injections of propranolol to a point where a further dose has no additional slowing effect, Cordarone injected subsequently diminishes the heart rate by a further 23% [314].

c) After isoprenaline-tachycardia and maximal acceleration of velocity of cardiac contraction induced by adrenaline have been reduced by 50% by a dose of 10 mg/kg i.v. of Cordarone, both phenomena are blocked after a subsequent administration of propranolol [309].

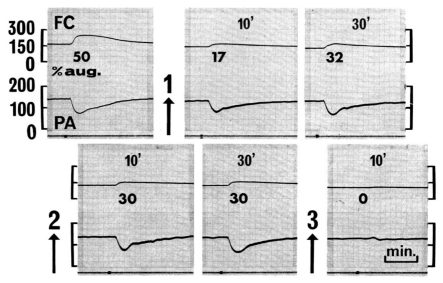

Fig. 50. Effect of amiodarone and of propranolol on tachycardia and hypotension induced by isoprenaline in the anaesthetized and atropinized dog. F.C.: Heart rate (beats/min). P.A.: Mean femoral blood pressure (mm Hg). At signal marks for the six tracings, intravenous injections of isoprenaline, 0.002 mg/kg, made at times (minutes) indicated on the traces. At arrow n° 1: intravenous injection of amiodarone, 10 mg/kg. At arrow n° 2: intravenous injection of amiodarone, 10 mg/kg. At arrow n° 3: intravenous injection of propranolol, 1 mg/kg

d) Peripheral vascular resistance is reduced by Cordarone [317] but is increased by the β-blocking agents [1258, 1336, 1982].

e) Cordarone does not depress cardiac dynamics [317] whereas propranolol reduces cardiac output [308] (see also p. 210).

f) Coronary blood flow is enhanced by Cordarone [317] but is reduced by propranolol [304].

g) Cordarone reduces the hypertensive response to adrenaline, whereas propranolol increases the pressor effect of adrenaline [1725].

h) The effect of Cordarone upon the cardiac intracellular action potential differs radically from the effect of propranolol (see p. 269).

i) Cordarone has no local anaesthetic effect [1934], contrary to propranolol.

On the biochemical plane also, certain properties of Cordarone differ from those of β-blocking agents [233]. Sharp rise in blood lactate and lactate/pyruvate ratio induced by adrenaline is not modified by Cordarone but is completely inhibited by propranolol. Increase in basal metabolic rate provoked by theophylline is not influenced by Cordarone whereas propranolol abolishes it. Propranolol blocks adrenaline-induced lipolysis in vivo (serum free fatty acids) and in vitro (fat pad test) but Cordarone does not affect these adrenergic phenomena.

From all the above evidence, it may be concluded that Cordarone does not act by competitive β-receptor blockade. Thus, Cordarone can be considered as a new pharmacological type of adrenergic antagonist which does not produce any competitive blockade. It is proposed to term it an *adrenomoderator* agent [306].

Another experimental finding is worth reporting as it demonstrates also that it cannot be assigned to a competitive blockade of the β-adrenergic receptors.

It is known that glucagon increases heart rate, systolic left ventricular pressure and its rate of increase (dp/dt) in perfused isolated rat hearts [196c] and when given intravenously to anaesthetized animals [673, 1187]. These cardiac stimulant effects are due to an activation of adenylcyclase [1114]. Since this type of activation has been assimilated to the stimulation of adenylcyclase by catecholamines [1187], it was interesting to test the incidence of Cordarone upon the cardio-stimulating properties of glucagon [308]. Glucagon, 4—5 and 25 μg/kg i.v. respectively, was injected into anaesthetised dogs in three experiments, after records had been taken of heart rate and femoral blood pressure, and, in the third experiment, of the rate of change of left ventricular pressure also. The results are presented in Table 8, and it is evident that Cordarone reduced both the size and the duration of chronotropic responses to glucagon, as well as the positive effect of glucagon on left ventricular pressure and its first derivative (Fig. 51). Propranolol 1 mg/kg i.v., on the other hand, did not modify the tachycardia induced by glucagon (Fig. 52), in confirmation of the findings of other investigators [1187, 1831].

Table 8. *Effect of Cordarone, 10 mg/kg intravenously, on the chronotropic responses to intravenous glucagon in anaesthetized dogs*

Expt. No.	Dose of glucagon (μg/kg)	Maximum heart rate in response to glucagon		Time taken for 50% of effect to wear of (min)	
		Control	After Cordarone	Control	After Cordarone
1	4	+ 25%	+ 13%	25	15
2	5	+ 14%	+ 6%	20	12
3	25	+ 33%	+ 18%	38	20

These findings suggest that the mode of action of Cordarone on the adenylcyclase system must be different from that of propranolol. It is now recognized that the stimulating effects of glucagon on the heart are independent of the β-adrenoceptors [1187]. Since propranolol blocks the cardiac effects of isoprenaline and noradrenaline, without modifying those of glucagon, existence has been proposed of two different types of receptors in the adenylcyclase system, one which is activated by catecholamines, the other being stimulated by glucagon [673]. A similar opinion is held by LEVEY and EPSTEIN [1114] who consider that there are at least two sites of receptors in the myocardium which are responsible for the activation of adenylcyclase, one which is sensitive to glucagon and the other to noradrenaline. These facts suggest that glucagon might act beyond the site of the adrenergic β-receptors [1831], but such a suggestion still remains hypothetical.

Since Cordarone strongly reduces the cardiac actions of glucagon, it is clear that its action must bear upon other structures than propranolol. This also suggests that the depression of the cardiostimulant consequences of stimulation of the β-receptors provoked by Cordarone could be due not to a direct interference with these receptors but to a reduction in the production of $3'$—$5'$ cyclic AMP. Some preliminary biochemical observations have shown that 0.1 mM Cordarone inhibits the activation of adenylcyclase by adrenaline in rat heart homogenates, whereas 0.01 mM propranolol abolishes the activation [232]. Further studies are in progress in order to obtain more precise informations.

18*

Since it increases coronary flow and does not modify cardiac output significantly, Cordarone is devoid of the two main possible sources of pharmacological
side-effects induced by β-blocking agents i.e. reduction in heart muscle irrigation
[1258, 1424, 2033] and decrease in cardiac output [1258, 1336, 1800, 1982].

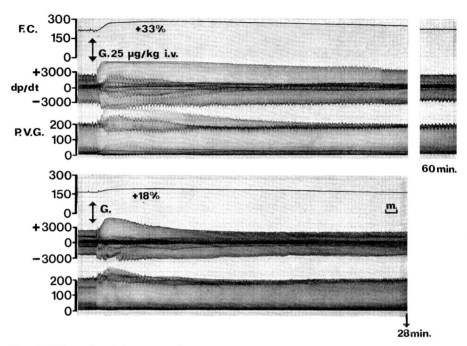

Fig. 51. Effect of amiodarone on the actions of glucagon on heart rate, rate of rise in left
ventricular pressure and left ventricular pressure in the anaesthetized and atropinized dog.
F.C.: Heart rate (beats/min). dp/dt: Rate of rise of left ventricular pressure (mm Hg/sec).
P.V.G.: Left ventricular pressure (mm Hg). Upper tracings: at arrow, intravenous injection
of glucagon (G), 0.025 mg/kg. Between upper and lower tracings: intravenous injection of
amiodarone, 10 mg/kg. Lower tracings: at arrow, intravenous injection of glucagon (G),
0.025 mg/kg, made 15 min after amiodarone

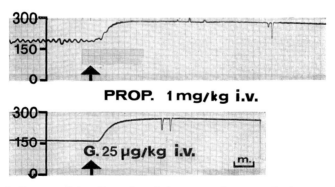

Fig. 52. Effect of propranolol on the action of glucagon on heart rate in the anaesthetized and
atropinized dog. Heart rate in beats/min. Upper tracing: at arrow, intravenous injection of
glucagon, 0.025 mg/kg. Between upper and lower tracing: intravenous injection of propranolol,
1 mg/kg. Lower tracing: at arrow, intravenous injection of glucagon, 0.025 mg/kg

The increase in myocardial oxygen consumption induced by adrenaline and noradrenaline was strongly diminished by Cordarone when given as a single i.v. injection into anaesthetized dogs or by oral chronic administration in conscious dogs. This finding (and especially the fact that Cordarone has been found to have an effect on endogenous catecholamines as well as exogenous) may be of clinical interest in view of the alleged role of the adrenergic system in the increase in myocardial oxygen needs due to several stress situations leading to acute angina pectoris (see p. 36).

The importance of adrenergic hyperactivity in angina led some authors [48, 1483, 1485, 1523] to assume that therapeutic means which are apt to reduce hypersympathicotonic states could be beneficial to anginal patient, as a consequence of reduction in the oxygen wasting increase in contractility produced by excessive sympathetic stimulation.

Table 9. *Angina pectoris*

Pathogenesis	Pathophysiology	Effects of Cordarone
Predisposing cause		
Coronary atherosclerosis	Permanent latent myocardial ischaemia	— Decrease in myocardial oxygen requirements due to reduction of cardiac work (slowing in heart rate and fall in overall vascular resistance). — Increase in oxygen supply by improvement in myocardial irrigation.
Releasing causes		
(Effort, emotion, cold, digestion, decubitus, spontaneous, nocturnal)	Sympathetic stimulation → excessive increase in myocardial oxygen needs (and occasionally coronary vasoconstriction) due to: — hypertension (generalized vasoconstriction) — tachycardia — increase in heart contraction velocity — increase in ventricular wall tension, resulting in acute myocardial ischaemia.	Inhibition of all adrenergic haemodynamic perturbations, including the excessive increase in oxygen myocardial consumption.

The presumed interest of the pharmacological properties of Cordarone for the long term treatment of the clinical manifestations of coronary insufficiency appears clearly when these biological effects are correlated with the present pathogenic conceptions of angina, which were recently summed up by CONDORELLI [352]. In short, two types of causes for the anginal syndrome are now recognized:

— a predisposing cause represented by permanent latent myocardial ischaemia, as a consequence of the obstructive and/or stenosing atherosclerotic alterations of the coronary arteries, and resulting in myocardial chronic hypoxia [345, 1288, 1842, 1953];

— a releasing cause of angina attacks (whatever their origin: effort, emotion, cold, digestion, decubitus) which consists of a sympathetic stimulation (see p. 35) finding clinical expression in elevation of blood pressure and of heart rate, preceding the cardiac pain. Hypertension and tachycardia increase in excess the oxygen needs of the ischaemic cardiac muscle, so that chronic ischaemia turns into acute ischaemia, productive of angina attack.

The overall pharmacological properties of Cordarone meet to this multicausal pathogenesis of angina pectoris (see Table 9), and suggest that coronary insufficiency syndromes may benefit to a considerable degree from the drug through several haemodynamic factors, which are the following. First, Cordarone may correct the pathophysiological functional consequence of the predisposing cause of angina, i.e. myocardial hypoxia, by reducing ventricle's work and thus lowering the oxygen requirements of the heart, and by increasing coronary blood flow which augments the supply of oxygen to the heart. Furthermore, the antiadrenergic properties of Cordarone fit in well with modern pathogenic concept of angina pectoris, as the haemodynamic manifestations of sympathetic overstimulation, i.e. tachycardia, hypertension and increase in myocardial oxygen demands, are largely antagonized.

It may also be anticipated that coronary vasoconstriction occurring during some anginal attacks could be counteracted by the relaxing effect of Cordarone on myocardial vessels.

1.4. Anti-Arrhythmic Properties

Cordarone is also endowed with anti-arrhythmic properties in animals. In the dose of 10 mg/kg i.v., it suppresses almost immediately various experimental cardiac arrhythmias: 1. spontaneous ventricular extrasystoles and ventricular extrasystoles induced by i.v. injection of adrenaline in the anaesthetized dog [315], multifocal ventricular ectopic beats induced by i.v. administration of barium chloride in the anaesthetized dog and rabbit, and ventricular extrasystoles occurring after acute occlusion of the anterior descending coronary artery in the anaesthetized dog [311, 312]; 2. atrial fibrillation induced in the anaesthetized dog by application of a solution of acetylcholine on the anterior wall of the right atrium [311, 312]; 3. ventricular tachycardia induced by placing a crystal of aconitine nitrate on the anterior wall of the right ventricle in the anaesthetized dog or by i.v. injection of a large dose of Strophantine in the morphinized dog [311, 312]. In the guinea pig, a larger dose of i.v. ouabain was needed to kill the animals from ventricular fibrillation when they were pretreated with Cordarone [1934]. According to VAUGHAN-WILLIAMS [1933], these properties of Cordarone exactly come up to the criteria of action he expects with regard to the effect on the cardiac action potentials in the case of a reliable anti-arrhythmic drug. In his opinion, the unusual effect of Cordarone on the cardiac action potentials (see p. 269) would lead to a reduced probability of cardiac arrhythmias.

2. Therapeutic Properties

Details of clinical surveys carried out with Cordarone can be grouped under six headings: 1. therapeutic effects in open tests; 2. therapeutic effects under double-blind conditions; 3. effects on the symptomatology of cardiac overload tests; 4. effects on the pathological electrocardiogram of coronary angina; 5. effects in cases of rhythm disturbances; 6. clinical tolerance and side effects.

2.1. Antianginal Effects in Open Tests

Some thirty clinical studies were aimed at defining the therapeutic activity of Cordarone in open administration.

The group covered by VASTESAEGER, GILLOT and RASSON [665 and 1927], the largest of the groups, involves 1014 angina pectoris cases, 980 of whom could be kept under regular observation. This survey is spread over more than seven years. It includes patients suffering from true angina, effort-induced or spontaneous, with characteristic localisation and irradiation of pain, which is relieved by nitroglycerin, and found in the pure state, i.e. with no digestive or vertebral complications. Split up according to electrocardiographic criteria, the patients are grouped as shown in Table 10.

Table 10

	Failure	Moderate improvement	Very great improvement	Excellent result
Subjects with normal ECG	60	31	71	38
(200 cases)	(30)	(15.5)	(35.5)	(19)
Subjects with ischaemia- and ischaemia-lesion-ECG	54	60	182	302
(598 cases)	(9)	(10)	(30.5)	(50.5)
Subjects with symptoms of left ventricular strain (57 cases) . .	14	6	26	11
	(28)	(10.5)	(45.6)	(15.9)
Subjects with myocardial infarction ECG (97 cases)	15	43	21	18
	(15.3)	(44.4)	(21.6)	(18.7)
Left branch block (14 cases) . . .	4	5	4	1
	(28.6)	(35.7)	(28.6)	(7.1)
Right branch block (14 cases) . .	0	0	6	8
			(42.9)	(57.1)

N. B. The figures in brackets show the percentages in each group.

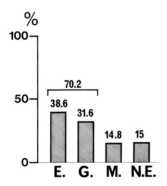

Fig. 53. Therapeutic results obtained, in 980 anginous patients, following administration of amiodarone. Results are expressed in % of cases. E.: Excellent result. G.: Good result. M.: Moderate result. N. E.: No effect

Cordarone was administered orally at a daily dose of 600 to 300 mg over a period of from 6 months to several years depending on the subjects[6].

The results achieved are given in Fig. 53.

Table 10 shows the response of the patients in the light of the ECG criteria[7].

6 Intravenous injection was used very exceptionally and only in the case of 10 patients suffering from particularly severe angina of an evolutive character with attacks occurring frequently when resting. One or two 150 mg ampoules were used every day or every two days for two consecutive weeks.

7 Of the 10 coronary subjects in the evolutive phase treated by intravenous injections of 150 mg, 5 were very rapidly improved subjectively and their evolutive stage ended in less than a week.

The action of Cordarone often declared itself after the first 72 hours of administration. The persistence of the favourable effect following cessation of treatment is felt on an average for 3 weeks.

The dosage of 600 mg per day was the one most commonly active, *at least as regards the initial treatment*. However, during evolutive bouts of angina pectoris, the dose of 900 and even 1200 mg was prescribed exceptionally for several weeks without any ill effects. Once initial improvement is obtained and stabilised, a maintenance treatment of 200 to 400 mg per day was usually very satisfactory. VASTESAEGER et al. conclude in favour of the considerable antianginal activity of Cordarone, its ease of handling for therapeutic purposes and the rarity of minor side effects which make it a particularly useful and effective medication.

BARZIN and FRESON [100] carried out a survey covering 109 anginal patients of whom 44 were pure coronary cases, 39 suffering from sequelae of infarction, 22 left or right ventricular hypertrophy subjects with or without overload complications, 3 recent evolutive cases of infarct and 1 calcified pericarditis case. Cordarone was administered at the rate of 600 mg per day, split up into three doses of 200 mg, for a period of 20 days.

86% of the patients treated found a considerable attenuation of their pain syndrome; attacks became more rare and sometimes disappeared altogether during the course of treatment. In the case of 55 patients who were in the habit of taking 3—10 capsules a day of nitroglycerin, 40 were able to do without it after a few days treatment, i.e. immediately on attenuation or the disappearance of the anginal syndrome. The remaining 15 considerably reduced the number of nitroglycerin doses.

SOLVAY and VAN SCHEPDAEL [1776] treated 65 proved cases of coronary disease suffering from regular anginal attacks; the presence of coronary insufficiency was confirmed in 57 of them by characteristic ECG changes showing up as a result of effort.

Cordarone was administered at the attacking dose of 400—600 mg per day, subsequently reduced to a holding dose of 300—500 mg depending on the results achieved. Eight patients did not carry on with the treatment for a sufficient length of time to allow for a valid assessment of the drug's activity, although their anginal attacks were almost completely eliminated. Six of them ended the treatment prematurely because of side effects, and two others died as a result of infarction during the early weeks of treatment. Of the remaining 57 cases, the authors report the complete elimination of angina attacks in 41 patients, and a considerable improvement with a marked reduction in the frequency and intensity of attacks in the other 16.

The therapeutic effect often appears from the third or fourth day, and always in under a week. The initial improvement can progressively increase to reach its full effect several months after starting treatment, when the patient has been able little by little to resume regular physical activity.

HUEBER and KOTZAUREK [868] report on 100 patients treated at the daily dosage of 600 mg. They obtain a very satisfactory result in 75% of the cases which is reflected from the third or fourth day in a marked reduction in, or the disappearance of, the anginal attacks, a very significant reduction in the nitroglycerin doses taken, and a sharp increase in walking distance possible, which can be increased 100 times for certain patients.

In order to avoid irksome repetition, we have summarised in Table 11 the essential details relating to 30 further clinical studies.

The combined clinical surveys covering some 2500 cases would indicate that the percentage of good and excellent results amounts to over 80%. These cardiologists are unanimous in acknowledging in Cordarone a remarkable antianginal effect, even where there are involved patients with a severe angina condition recalcitrant to the usual treatments. They consider that the therapeutic results achieved with Cordarone are vastly superior to those obtained with the other existing antianginal medications.

Table 11

Authors	Country	Number of cases	% of favour- able results	References
DELEIXHE and DELREE	Belgium	80	77	404
BERNAL and ABITEBOUL	France	160	$\pm$80	138
FACQUET and NIVET	France	$\pm$100	$\pm$70	516
FAIVRE et al.	France	40	75	519
TATIBOUET	France	25	80	1874
WAREMBOURG and JAILLARD . .	France	100	80	129a and 1960
BROUSTET and LAPORTE . . .	France	44	70	238 and 239
JOUVE et al.	France	32	80	920
VON PLANTA	Switzerland	15	73	1949
PESCADOR	Spain	15	90	1434
BALAGUER	Spain	46	70	76
BERTEAU	France	30	80	149
GOMEZ	Mexico	10	70	687
DETRY et al.	France	38	74	421
ARMAND et al.	France	38	76	53
AUDIER	France	27	80	61
KAPPERT	Switzerland	36	64	938
REYMOND	Switzerland	40	80	1520
JURY	France	50	80	66a
ISHINOSE	Japan	30	85	880
FOUCAULT and OLIVIER	France	63	73	41a
TEODORINI and SERBAN	Rumania	17	87	123a
DENIS et al.	France	33	84	32a
HARDEL et al.	France	30	66	58a
AMEUR et al.	France	48	67	3a
PERROT et al.	France	100	85	29b
LESBRE et al.	France	30	77	200c
IZBICKI	Switzerland	20*	95	157c
ALIX et al.	France	125	80	6c
GAZAIX and ALZEARI	France	51	82	108c

* All very old patients

2.2. Antianginal Effects in Double-Blind Tests

Eight clinical investigations have been carried out under double-blind conditions, involving a total of 252 patients.

VASTESAEGER et al. [1927] made an investigation of this type on 60 anginal subjects. Three had to quit the therapeutic test because of digestive intolerance. Of the 57 subjects showing good tolerance to the drug, 41 (or 71.9% of the patients on whom the test was satisfactorily completed) obtained a favourable result with Cordarone at the dose of 600 mg/day for one month, but 13 of them (22.8%) also had a favourable effect from the placebo. The remaining 16 (28.1%) showed no improvement either with the active product or the placebo. In other words, 49.1% of the coronary patients were therefore helped exclusively by Cordarone and were able to distinguish it from the placebo.

Seven other double-blind experiments all returned significant results. We will restrict ourselves to listing them in Table 12.

Table 12

Authors	Number of cases	References
BERNAL and ABITEBOUL	42	138
DELEIXHE and DELREE	10	404
FACQUET et al.	30	516, 518, 1373
LEUTENEGGER and LÜTHY	34	1113
SCEBAT and MAURICE	35	1653
BALAGUER	15	76
ZELVELDER	26	2048

2.3. Effects on the Symptomatology of the Cardiac Overload Tests

Several clinicians have attempted to assess the therapeutic effects of Cordarone by applying tests which impose an overload on the anginal patient's cardiovascular system. These experiments can be split up into two categories: those which use the respiratory hypoxia test, and those which use physical effort either by means of the ergometric bicycle or by applying the Master technique, whether in its original or in a modified form.

2.3.1. Hypoxia Test

VASTESAEGER et al. [1927] used a hypoxia test on anginal subjects whose ECG was normal at the outset and for whom the test proved positive during the check-test.

The electrocardiographic criteria governing the positive nature of the test were as follows: a) the total of S-T downward shifts at leads I, II, III and V_4 exceeds 3 mm; b) the negativing of T at lead V_4; c) the marked flattening out of T at lead I or V_4 with at least 1 mm drop in level of S-T in at least one of these leads. The appearance of a single one of these three types of deterioration constituted in itself a criterion of the positive character of the test.

The controlled hypoxia tests before and after Cordarone administration were carried out under strictly superposable conditions.

Of the 21 patients with a positive check-test result, 8 were arbitrarily selected and given a further hypoxia test after 2—4 weeks treatment at the daily dose of 600 mg. The selection of these 8 subjects was purely a matter of willingness on the part of those agreeing to undergo this test, no other selection method being adopted.

The 8 individuals subjected to this test all showed improved tolerance to this experience following treatment in that deteriorations in the electrocardiogram were less marked or occurred later and the 5 subjects suffering from anginal pain prior to the treatment no longer did so during the second test.

2.3.2. Ergometric Bicycle Test

VASTESAEGER et al. [1927] got together a group of 19 patients suffering from undoubted effort-induced angina. They carried out a fundamental test as to the maximum effort capacity of the patient by working out exactly in kilogramme-metres or metabolic units the amount of physical effort required, and reproducing on the ergometric bicycle efforts whose intensity is in line with those of daily life: walking, washing and dressing, driving a car, taking part in sporting activity, etc. The cyclo-ergometer test provides a guide-line as to the acceptable effort capacity of each coronary subject.

The 19 patients were given the test prior to administering Cordarone, then after one month's treatment at 600 mg/day. Of these 19 subjects, 14 considerably improved their performance, i.e. their cardiac effort capacity, since the electrocardiograph deteriorations[8] only appeared at a loading far higher than that which they had previously endured. Compared with the initial test, the improvement varied, depending on the cases, from 6 to 96.7%. The average improvement over the 14 cases was 26.8%. The remaining 5 cases merely repeated the cyclo-ergometric test which they had managed prior to treatment. After treatment, none of these patients produced a test result inferior to that achieved during the check-test. For the 19 cases examined, the overall average improvement was 19.7%.

BARZIN and FRESON [100] subjected to a similar test 7 patients treated for a month with Cordarone at a daily dosage of 600 mg. From the electrocardiographic criteria adopted, 5 patients showed an improvement in their response after treatment as compared with the check-test.

Analysing the readings for heart rate and blood pressure before and at the end of the effort, both prior to and after treatment, the authors find that the rises in blood pressure during effort cannot be considered as differing from one test to another. It is quite a different matter as regards heart rate. In point of fact: 1. over the 7 patients as a whole, the average increase in heart rate due to effort during the two tests is less after treatment than before treatment, 25.9% as against 31.6%; 2. effort-induced tachycardia is sharply reduced by the end of the treatment, since the absolute values for heart rate under effort conditions are 97 and 82 beats/minute respectively before and after treatment, i.e. a decrease of 15.5%.

Despite the small number of subjects taking part in this experiment, the authors conclude from their observations that Cordarone enables the angina patient, with improvement from the subjective angle, to react to effort with a lesser degree of tachycardia than prior to treatment. These beliefs will be enlarged upon later in the light of the following investigation.

The third clinical investigation, likewise applying the cyclo-ergometric test [1776] assumes particular importance, not so much so in that it involves a larger number of cases (65 patients), but because by adopting the combined and simultaneous measurement of heart rate and the drop in level of the *dynamic* (i.e. during the effort) ischaemic S-T segment, these authors were able to assess the changes brought about by Cordarone in the patient's coronary reserve and in the call made on that reserve during a standard effort (see p. 99). The heart rate and blood pressure levels reached at the moment the effort is halted are carefully recorded in 19 cases. Cordarone was administered at the attacking dose of 400—600 mg per day, then reduced to a maintenance dose of 300—500 mg. Over the 65 coronary subjects treated, these results are as follows:

a) of the first 41 cases where, in answer to questions, the disappearance of any angina pain was noted, there is seen:

— in 12 cases, the disappearance of the dynamic anomaly arising from the effort test when under treatment. Here the reduction in heart rate is 30 beats on average;

---

8 The criteria chosen by these authors are the same as those which they adopted for the hypoxia test (see p. 280).

— in 13 cases, regression of the dynamic anomaly with an average reduction in effort-induced heart rate by some 20 beats;

— the absence of any valid conclusions in 16 cases where comparative efforts could not be carried out after treatment (7 cases) or before treatment (3 cases) or again before and after treatment (6 cases).

b) of the 16 cases where the anginal condition improves without disappearing, there is seen in 12 cases a regression in the dynamic anomaly, going hand in hand with a slight reduction in the rise in heart rate (about 10 beats). In 2 cases the dynamic anomaly and heart rate resulting from effort show little change from one test to the other. In the remaining 2 cases, the effort-induced heart rate is reduced, but there is no change in the dynamic anomaly.

c) in 8 cases suffering from a long-standing infarct without angina pectoris, who have no dynamic anomaly during the effort tests, the exercise-induced tachycardia is considerably less high.

SOLVAY and VAN SCHEPDAEL conclude from their investigation that, under the effect of Cordarone, speeding up of effort-induced heart rate is less marked in spite of identical muscular loading. This reduction in effort-induced tachycardia varies with the individual, but may be estimated as an average of 30 beats when the anginal attacks and the dynamic anomaly disappear, 20 beats when the anginal condition disappears despite the persistence of a lesser degree of dynamic anomaly, and finally 10 beats where the effort-induced angina and the dynamic anomaly persist.

In their opinion, the prime therapeutic effect of Cordarone is to reduce this effort-induced tachycardia and consequently to enable the anginal subject to call on his coronary reserve to a lesser extent, so that the degree to which the coronary subject uses his individual coronary reserve during effort is less marked.

Individual reasons can be advanced when we analyse the report by SOLVAY [1776] and that of BARZIN [100] who also found with 7 patients given the cyclo-ergometric test a marked reduction in effort-induced tachycardia as compared with that which occurs during the same test applied before starting the Cordarone treatment.

These two authors in fact measured not only the rises in heart rate during effort, but also those in systolic blood pressure. The multiplication of these two parameters gives ROBINSON's index (see p. 29). This author has demonstrated [1544] that an improvement, for whatever reason, in the clinical condition of the angina pectoris subject means that the patient can effect, *without experiencing any pain*, the standardized physical effort which triggered off the painful attack when the effort in question was accomplished before clinical improvement. The reason for this is that, as a consequence of his improved clinical condition, the patient does not reach the index which had been obtained by multiplying the two parameters found at the moment he experienced pain during the same effort exerted previously when his clinical condition was less satisfactory (see also p. 30). It follows that the improved subject is able to exceed the limits of the usual angina-producing effort, and also that it is only at a considerably greater effort that he will get his heart pain, the heart rate x blood pressure index being at that moment identical to that which is found during the lesser angina-producing effort exerted during the clinical phase preceding the improvement (see p. 30).

If we compare these heart rate and blood pressure factors in the 26 angina subjects examined by BARZIN and SOLVAY, we get the individual figures appearing in Table 13.

Calculated mean values of heart rate and of Robinson index for the 26 patients and their variations, expressed in %, are given in Table 14.

Table 13. *Effort test with bicycle ergometer. Effect of Cordarone (600 mg daily for 1 month)*

No of cases	Before Cordarone				After Cordarone			
	Rest Heart rate	Rest Robinson index	Effort Heart rate	Effort Robinson index	Rest Heart rate	Rest Robinson index	Effort Heart rate	Effort Robinson index
1	80	1280	120	2160	37	666	45	810
2	95	1615	120	2160	97	1358	115	1725
3	58	1102	140	3080	57	1083	111	1998
4	71	923	135	1755	75	788	115	1265
5	77	1386	130	2600	62	992	109	2180
6	75	900	130	2080	65	845	122	1830
7	72	756	130	1690	64	928	100	1600
8	72	1080	145	2900	60	900	105	2310
9	90	1800	140	2800	70	1050	113	1808
10	57	884	130	2145	53	689	110	1760
11	66	726	140	1820	59	678	100	1400
12	60	750	120	1440	53	689	81	1053
13	67	938	85	1275	65	975	97	1552
14	65	1105	110	1980	65	975	110	1980
15	85	1360	130	2730	69	1173	120	1800
16	65	748	130	1820	75	788	130	1365
17	95	1235	100	1300	80	1040	100	1300
18	75	1425	120	2640	63	1008	100	1650
19	80	1200	140	2520	57	912	120	1920
20	63	819	76	1216	72	864	78	1092
21	84	1428	94	1833	70	1260	80	1520
22	84	1386	120	2520	69	1173	102	2040
23	67	905	96	1728	65	910	90	1710
24	77	1617	108	2592	63	1260	73	1825
25	63	1197	77	1694	50	850	65	1430
26	78	1053	108	1944	67	1005	88	1496
	73,9	1139	118,2	2093	64,7	956	99,2	1631

Table 14

Haemodynamic parameters	Before Cordarone		After Cordarone	
	Rest	Effort	Rest	Effort
Heart rate	73,9	118,2	64,7	99,2
Robinson index	1139	2093	956	1631
	←———————————— 88			
Heart rate (%)	←——————— 160			
		←——————— 153		
		←————————— 84		
	←———————————— 84			
Robinson index (%)	←——————— 184			
		←——————— 170		
		←————————— 78		

The following conclusions can be drawn from this Table:

a) the Robinson index during the effort test following treatment is 22% less than what it is prior to treatment;

b) as compared with the resting conditions, the index rises as a result of effort to a lesser extent after treatment than before, viz. by 70% instead of 84%;

c) during the resting period preceding the effort test, this index after treatment only reaches 84% of its pre-treatment value;

d) heart rate, under resting conditions, is 12% less after treatment than what it was prior to treatment. During the effort exerted, it speeds up less after treatment than before, the increase only reaching 84% of the basic increase.

Since ROBINSON places the heart rate x blood pressure index on the same footing as a given level of myocardial oxygen consumption, an analysis of the variations found in these 26 patients would indicate that Cordarone lowers the myocardial oxygen consumption of the resting anginal subject and puts a brake on the increase in that consumption as a result of effort.

It is therefore probable that Cordarone enables the anginal subject to produce a greater effort without bringing on the heart pain because it reduces the oxygen requirements of the cardiac muscle. Moreover, taking into account the fact that the cardiovascular disturbances appearing during an angina-producing effort reflect a hypersympathicotonic condition [488, 696, 1357, 1483, 1485, 1491] (the same applies during effort by a healthy subject, 293, 1545), both BARZIN and SOLVAY believe that their pathophysiological investigations make it possible, at least in part, to ascribe the clinical benefit derived by their patients from the treatment with Cordarone to the inhibiting properties which the medication possesses in respect of the orthosympathetic tonus, as evidenced in animals. Their view finds a further argument in the fact that BEKAERT [123] finds that, with a man undergoing Cordarone treatment, the tachycardia induced by the intravenous injection of adrenaline is sharply reduced as compared with that found prior to starting the treatment.

2.3.3. Master Type Effort Test

ROOKMAKER [1551] applied an effort test during which the ECG is recorded by remote control whilst climbing a flight of stairs [1552]. There was adopted as a criterion giving the most precise results, applicable in every case without exception, the appearance (or aggravation) of a drop in level in the S-T segment by 0.1 mV. This effort test is reported to give considerably more accurate information than the Master two step test [1552].

Clinical experimentation with Cordarone has been done under double-blind conditions to compare it with similar experimentation with a placebo. The investigation involved a group of 15 carefully selected patients with an anginal syndrome confirmed by the typical electrocardiographic deteriorations at rest and/or under effort and free from other major diseases. Each patient was previously given the effort test on three different occasions under identical conditions, all antianginal medication being suppressed for a certain length of time prior to this test. The average of the three results obtained in each case was taken as a ,,basic value" for reference purposes.

Each patient was then treated for 3 weeks with the placebo and Cordarone successively at a dose of 300 mg per day. At the end of each of the 3 week periods the patients were given a further effort test followed by a series of questions as to the development of their subjective symptomatology during the previous fortnight. In 9 cases out of 15, ROOKMAKER finds with Cordarone a reduction in the drop in level of the S-T segment of the ECG, together with a more rapid return to the resting values of the heart rate which had risen during the effort. In no case did he find any objective improvement with the placebo.

Struck by the fact that, with certain of their patients treated at the dosage of 600 mg of Cordarone, the disappearance of the anginal attacks went hand in hand with a considerable increase in the walking distance which could be covered, HUEBER and KOTZAUREK [868] also applied the Master effort test. By way of example, they quote the findings with several patients whose electrocardiogram during the check effort test showed a very considerable drop in level of the S-T segment and a negative T wave. These electrocardiographic signs were no longer in evidence during the same test applied after three months Cordarone treatment.

KNEBEL [1002] also used the Master effort test, but under different dosage conditions to those of the foregoing authors. He selected patients suffering from severe angina pectoris for whom the Master test, applied on several occasions without any medicinal treatment, showed up on the electrocardiogram (reconstituted on the basis of a vectocardiogram recorded from three orthogonal leads) highly positive signs of effort-induced myocardial ischaemia.

He administered 150 mg of Cordarone in the vein. He repeated the Master test during the 5—6 min following the injection. He found that the drop in level of the S-T segment was greatly reduced or disappeared altogether. In the view of the author, these facts reflect an improvement in cardiac muscle irrigation due to Cordarone, probably resulting from a coronary vaso-dilating effect. KNEBEL stresses the fact that, according to the haemodynamic studies which he made on other patients also treated with 150 mg of Cordarone injected into the vein, heart rate, cardiac output, systemic blood pressure and pulmonary arterial pressure do not change during the 20 min continuous observation following the injection.

2.4. Effects on the Pathological Electrocardiogram in Coronary Angina

Several authors have made a systematic check on the development of the electrocardiogram in the case of their patients treated with Cordarone. Their findings can be summed up by saying that in a relatively high percentage of cases, the resting-state ECG does not reflect the clinical benefit [100, 1776, 1927].

However, it is fairly usual to find a considerable improvement in the electrical indications which can undoubtedly be attributed to the effect of the medication and which goes hand in hand with the clinical benefit [100, 149, 868, 1927, 32a, 6c].

2.5. Anti-Arrhythmic Effects

Cordarone has a favourable effect on certain forms of cardiac arrhythmia. Clinical research into this effect is only in its early stages. Five investigations however are already available [1923, 1947, 1974, 198c, 320c]. These involved 218 patients with various types of arrhythmia conditions who, in the majority of cases, had already been treated with various other drugs (digitalis, quinidine, ajmaline, procainamide, propranolol, lidocaine, diphenylhydantoin) administered in succession or even in association without producing any satisfactory results. 180 of these 218 cases (i.e. 83%) were completely cured of their rhythm disorders or were improved to a marked degree. Table 15 shows the main points observed

Table 15

Type of arrhythmia	Number of cases treated	Results Good to excellent	Fair to nil
Supraventricular extrasystoles	17	15	2
Ventricular extrasystoles	66	49	17
Sinus tachycardia	8	8	0
Supraventricular paroxystic tachycardia	22	19	3
Ventricular paroxystic tachycardia	1	1	0
Paroxystic atrial flutter or fibrillation	49	44	5
Chronic atrial fibrillation or flutter	50	35	15
Wolf-Parkinson-White syndrome	2	2	0
Related arrhythmia	3	3	0

by these five clinicians in connection with the anti-arrhythmic effects of Cordarone.

In the view of these cardiologists, Cordarone is a worthy acquisition as a therapeutic aid in various cardiac rhythm disorders.

Other research going on at the moment will enable the clinical indications to be specified and also make it possible to assess the eventual advantages of Cordarone in those arrhythmic conditions which provide an added complication to the development of myocardial infarction over the first few days.

2.6. Clinical Tolerance and Side Effects

Fairly often there is found a reduction in heart rate as a result of Cordarone treatment. In the vast majority of cases, this slowing down does not exceed 10—15%. It is accompanied by no subjective or objective upsets. Generally speaking, the higher the basic heart rate, the more accentuated is the slowing effect on cardiac rhythm so much so that this effect is only very slight or even non-existent when initial heart rate is low [4e].

In certain cases the heart rate may drop below 50 beats/min, especially where treatment has been prolonged at high dosages, mainly in the case of very elderly subjects. This bradycardia may be accompanied by subjective disorders such as lipothymic tendences. It yields to a temporary suspension of the medication or to a reduction in the posology.

Cases of veritable bradycardia, where the decrease in cardiac rate exceeds 15%, represent some 0.6% of known cases to date. This slowing down of rhythm is accompanied on the electrocardiogram by an extension of the electrical systole, involving only the slow wave of the ventricular complex [517, 6c]. FRIART and RASSON [4e] found that the prolongation of the Q—T interval was due to lengthening of both the upward and downward curves of the T wave, the S—T segment remaining unaffected.

More often than not, the T wave undergoes a characteristic change but not for the worse [517, 1924, 6c], and in certain cases a U wave can be seen to emerge [517, 1924, 4e]. These changes merely reflect the impregnation of the myocardial muscle by the drug and the action of the drug upon the heart [4e]. All these changes are reversible [517]. Both atrio-ventricular conduction and ventricular conduction remain unaffected [517, 6c], to the extent that the presence of a branch block is not a contra-indication for administering Cordarone [517].

In view of the fact that Cordarone inhibits, without actually blocking, the haemodynamic manifestations which arise from stimulation of the adrenergic β-receptors, and that it is necessary to maintain the integrity of these latter for the physiological compensation which the body brings into play to maintain the cardiac functions [620], special attention has been paid during clinical investigations to the possibility of a cardio-depressive effect liable to aggravate pre-existing cardiac insufficiency. The intravenous injection of 150 mg does not alter cardiac output either in a normal man [1322] or in the anginal patient [1002]. Furthermore, one month's treatment at the daily dose of 600 mg does not lower cardiac output in an anginal patient, even where symptoms of a hyposystolic condition exist [100]. The absence of effect on cardiac output by prolonged oral treatment has been confirmed [41a]. Experience has shown that Cordarone does not set up any cardiac decompensation [517, 1520]. Over a survey of more than 10,000 cases, 11 angina subjects with compensated cardiac insufficiency displayed signs of cardiac insufficiency during treatment with Cordarone. Since these patients were not necessarily properly balanced by their digitalis and/or diuretic treatment, the clinicians who report these observations [868, 1113] conclude that the re-appearance of the clinical signs of decompensation cannot be ascribed to the administration of Cordarone. Adaptation of cardiotonic and/or diuretic treatment has in every case enabled the Cordarone treatment to be continued.

All the clinical investigations, including some under double-blind conditions [1939] stress the absence of potentialising effect by Cordarone on the synthetic anticoagulants [61, 29 b].

Cordarone does not involve any phenomena of dyspnoea [157].

It is frequent during treatment with Cordarone to find the appearance of corneal deposits. This is a very superficial pigmentation, localised at the corneal epithelium and perhaps at the Bowman membrane, but not going as far as the stroma which remains unaffected [518, 576, 1961], yellowish in colour and formed by a more or less dense fine dotted line arranged more often than not along the force lines of a magnetic field.

These corneal deposits can only be seen with a biomicroscope. They become localised electively in the lower outside half or third of the cornea, and more often outside the pupillary area; they are two-sided and often symmetrical. Their frequency and density depend on the dosage adopted [305]. They are reversible with the cessation of treatment [15 c, 80 c]. Their disappearance seems to depend on the duration of the treatment and may need 4—5 months or more in the case of prolonged treatment [65, 518, 576, 577, 1961].

In the vast majority of cases, these corneal deposits do not involve any subjective disorder. A few patients only complain of seeing coloured halos, which coincide in most cases with pre-pupillary localisation of the corneal deposits. It seems that these halos only occur in the case of patients who have been treated at a high dosage, continuously and over a long period. They are reversible with cessation of treatment.

Ophthalmologists who have found no impairment of the crystalline lens or of the retina [65, 518, 576, 577, 1961], even with patients treated for 2 years [42 a, 126 a], consider that this side effect is benign and can in no way give cause for halting treatment. At the very most it would seem advisable to reduce the posology for patients suffering from over-extensive deposits leading to the appearance of halos.

Great care should be taken before attributing to Cordarone any lack of visual acuity or any change in the electroretinogram noticed during treatment, for VERIN [126 a] stresses the fact that such anomalies were present prior to starting the treatment in over half of his patients.

The appearance of corneal deposits should perhaps be placed in relation to the slow transit and the storing up of Cordarone in the case of man [236]. The nature of these deposits has not yet been completely cleared up.

Micro-analyses by activation reveal an *iodine* content which would indicate that these corneal deposits are only formed of Cordarone or its iodinated metabolites in the proportion of approximately one part in 200. An analysis of human corneas with an electronic microscope indicates the presence of pigments which could be either melanines or lipofuscins [124 a].

Another side effect occurring during Cordarone therapy consists of melanodermatitis, which is localized on the face and seems to be promoted by sunlight. These cases are extremely rare, this pigmentation appearing only in patients who received very high doses during particularly long periods [334 c]. Such cutaneous manifestations do not appear with normal posology [334 c]. Histochemical studies have shown that this pigmentation was due to melanines and lipofuscins [334 c]. Photosensitization (erythema and itching) has also been reported on the body parts which are exposed to sun [6c]. Its incidence seems to be very low, only in 1% of cases.

Hepatic tolerance to prolonged treatments is satisfactory, since the hepatic functional tests are not upset [1458].

The true place of Cordarone in the treatment of coronary insufficiency can only be clearly defined once a very large number of cases have been treated and followed up over a sufficiently lenghty subsequent period. For the moment "it is a substance which has proved itself effective with animals and which, in the case of humans, seems to offer considerable interest" [1374].

Miscellaneous

Besides the antianginal medications which have been examined up to now, there are numerous other drugs whose pharmacological properties were considered as comprising a therapeutic potential for the subject suffering from angina pectoris.

We have felt it possible for the time being to group them under the heading "miscellaneous". They have been split up into three sections without being able to use as a basis for their grouping clearly defined norms or criteria. This subdivision is therefore of a necessarily rigid character which is accounted for neither by any sort of chemical affinity nor by any similarity in pharmacological properties, and even less so by a comparable quality of therapeutic effect. Despite its artificial character, this breakdown is based on characteristics which are outlined successively on pages 288 for section 1, 299 for section 2 and 307 for section 3.

Section no. 1

The present section considers various medications which are suggested for treating angina but which are too recent for their actual value to be assessed. Because of their recent appearance, they have for the most part only been investigated in a limited or preliminary way. They are dealt with in alphabetical order.

Adenylocrat

A preparation containing adenylic acids, a myocardial extract and crataegus (and containing 200 mg % adenosine and 20 mg % adenosine monophosphoric acids), Adenylocrat is said to be the medication par excellence for treating stenocardic pain attacks [200]. According to WILDE [339c], chronic treatment with Adenylocrat at doses ranging from 45 to 80 drops daily was successful in 452 of 488 patients, including cases with coronary hypoxia, coronary sclerosis and conduction disturbances. No side effects were observed. In 50 cases of coronary hypoxia who suffered in the same time from cardiac insufficiency, a combined treatment with Adenylocrat and Digoxin was effective in 47 cases. It must be pointed out that the available clinical reports devoted to Adenylocrat are based upon open trials, so that their results need to be checked by controlled double-blind investigations.

Aminocetone

An aminocetone answering to the formula

$$C_8H_{17}\!-\!\!\bigcirc\!\!-\!\!\underset{\underset{O}{\|}}{C}\!-\!CH_2\!-\!CH_2\!-\!N\!\!\bigcirc$$

and known as N-1113 has been investigated by KARPATI et al. [941, 942]. It has a

coronary dilating effect which is greater and of considerably longer duration than
that of prenylamine on a isolated cat's heart and *in situ*. This effect is said to be
of a musculotropic nature.

Anginin

$$CH_3-NH-\overset{\overset{\text{O}}{\|}}{C}-O-CH_2-\underset{N}{\bigcirc}-CH_2-O-\overset{\overset{\text{O}}{\|}}{C}-NH-CH_3$$

Anginin or pyridinol carbamate is an antagonist of bradykinine, with protective
effects as regards experimental atherosclerosis in rabbits. The first clinical trials
carried out in Japan [1741, 1742] claim a favourable effect in angina, and even the
opening up of occluded arteries in the case of atherosclerotic patients. It has been
shown, however, in a double-blind test that when administered at the daily dose
of 3×1500 mg to 30 angina patients it had no significant effect [1340]. In another
double blind cross-over study on 40 patients with angina pectoris, pyridinol carbamate given at the dose of 1 g orally three hours prior to MASTER two step
exercise decreased the incidence of exercise-induced angina [341c and 342c].
Thirty-three of the patients under placebo but only 17 under treatment developed
ischaemic ECG alterations. There was also a reduction in the adhesive platelet
counts. It is believed that pyridinol carbamate averts the exercise ECG changes
possibly by limiting acute mural oedema in vessels injured by exercise or by biochemical stress, notably adrenaline release or cholesterol deposition. Histoenzym-
atic studies in animals [238c] revealed that oedematous changes of arterial wall
induced by cholesterol or adrenaline are prevented by pyridinol carbamate,
which increased both glycolytic and hydrolytic enzyme activities. These histo-
enzymatic features suggest that the effect of the drug is characterised by healing
through the regeneration of smooth muscle in atheromatous lesions.

The effect of pyridinol carbamate was investigated in a controlled double-
blind cross-over clinical trial on 43 patients suffering from obliterans atherosclerosis with claudication [113a]. After a ten week treatment at the daily dose
of 1.5 g, claudication time was significantly prolonged. This effect could be due to
an anti-atherosclerotic action, but histological examinations are still required. In
another double-blind cross-over trial [14c], pyridinol carbamate administered at
the daily dose of 1.5 g for an average of 45 weeks in 180 male patients improved
intermittent claudication of obliterans atherosclerosis in 51% of cases. Pain
disappeared in 83% of cases.

Baralgin

A central antalgic, a myotropic and parasympathicolytic spasmolytic [1144],
Baralgin when administered intravenously is said to be capable of neutralising the
cardiac pain from infarct in 77% of cases, and the pain resulting from coronary
insufficiency in 95% of cases, the action appearing within a few minutes and able
to last for more than 12 hours [1898].

Baxacor

$$\underset{O-CH_2-CH_2-N(C_2H_5)_2}{\bigcirc\overset{\overset{\text{O}}{\|}}{C}-CH_2-CH_2-\bigcirc}$$

Baxacor (generic name: etafenon) is a diethylaminoethoxy-phenylpropio-
phenone. Its structure can thus be likened to that of Ildamen (see p. 196). It brings

19*

about a drop in coronary resistance in an isolated guinea-pig and rabbit heart, thus causing a considerable increase in the perfusion flow [1053] which is said not to be due to an increase in myocardial oxygen consumption.

Experimental investigation into it has recently been extended. With dogs, for instance [782], the intravenous administration of 0.1 mg/kg increases coronary arterial flow by 50%, but increasing the doses up to 5 mg/kg brings no proportionate increase and repeated doses seem to bring about a tolerance phenomenon. At the minimal coronary-active dose, etafenon does not alter either peripheral arterial flow or blood pressure or heart rate. The oxygen content of the coronary venous blood increases, despite the presence of a positive inotropic effect. Conversely, at higher doses, heart contraction is depressed.

KUKOVETZ [1055] confirms the coronary-dilating effect of etafenon on the isolated heart of guinea-pigs and rabbits, and shows that it depends on the dosages, 0.1 mg being necessary to double the coronary flow. He also observes, from the dosage of 0.02 mg upwards, a cardiac depression which he considers as being greater than in the case of papaverine, dose for dose. Finally he shows that at these doses, etafenon does not change the phosphorylasic activity of the heart.

Etafenon has no effect on the adrenergic system [782] and does not affect the activity of the β-receptors [782]. According to other authors, the drug does however exert a competitive antagonism vis-à-vis these receptors [1053].

Etafenon is quickly resorbed when orally administered to rats, guinea-pigs and dogs. It is said to concentrate electively in the cardiac and skeletal muscles [781].

On the basis of papers devoted to it up to now, Baxacor can thus be considered as a purely coronary-dilating substance whose action mechanism seems to be of the papaverine type since it antagonises the coronary constrictive effect of barium chloride [1055]. The pharmacological file on this substance is still far from complete, mainly because of the fact that its effect on myocardial oxygen consumption and cardiac output has not been studied, and its action on the contractile force of the myocardium, varying with dosages [782], has still to be clarified.

From the clinical viewpoint, the file on Baxacor is as yet still rudimentary. In the case of humans, it produces favourable changes in the electrocardiographic indications of ischaemia induced by the LEVY hypoxia test [1465]. It is said to be very effective in intravenous administration against the pain of angina pectoris, provided it is given in 3 min, failing which the pain quite unexpectedly becomes more acute. In oral treatment at 3×25 or 50 mg per day 1 hour before meals, it is said to keep the coronary insufficiency condition with angina under control [1465].

HOHL et al. [62a] strongly recommend this medication in cases of heart disease with coronary insufficiency, those which comprise a previous incidence of infarction, and those accompanied by functional angina pectoris, because in such cases they found a general improvement with the administration of a strong Baxacor tablet (the dose is not specified) three times a day over a period of from 3 to 6 weeks. Although their investigation involved a total of 523 cases, it is to be regretted that none of these patients were treated under double-blind conditions, since the percentage of good and very good effects is only in the region of 50% for each of the three groups, i.e. a frequency which is only 10% greater than that achieved with placebo-therapy.

The effect of Baxacor on lung function in guinea-pigs was investigated. A ten-minute exposure to an 8% solution administered by aerosol had no effect on respiration, in contrast with marked bronchospasm followed by collapse reported with propranolol [78a]. The changes in vital capacity and pneumometer values after intravenous injection of 10 mg Baxacor were investigated in 11 patients with chronic bronchial spasm. Results showed that bronchospasm was not intensified by Baxacor [78a].

Eucilat

Introduced very recently on the pharmaceutical market as a medication intended for the treatment of peripheral arteritis and angina pectoris, Eucilat (generic name: benfurodil) is a derivative of benzofuranne which answers to the following formula:

$$CH_3-CH \quad | \quad O-CO-(CH_2)_2-COOH$$

The results of pharmacological investigations not having yet been published, reference must be made to the concepts outlined in clinical reports. It would appear that Eucilat is primarily a peripheral vasodilator which also exerts its myolytic properties on the coronary circulation, the intravenous injection of 1 mg/kg bringing about a 35% increase in the coronary venous flow of an anaesthetised dog.

From the clinical viewpoint, we have up to now four reports involving anginal subjects. The first is that by NEEL [27b] covering 33 patients suffering from effort-induced and/or spontaneous anginal attacks. At the average daily dose of 4×50 mg tablets, the author reports 42% very good results and 21% good results. It can be considered that these are very moderate results if account is taken of the fact that the improvement criteria are not very severe, good and very good results corresponding respectively to 30 and 60% subjective improvement. Furthermore, the assessment could have been distorted by the fact that in the case of certain patients already treated with other antianginal medications Eucilat was added to the treatments already initiated.

The paper by FELIX et al. [10b] covers 22 coronary patients. The criteria for assessing efficacy are not clearly specified since this publication deals with a total of 109 patients, the great majority suffering from peripheral arteritis either alone or associated with an anginal syndrome. For this reason it is difficult to analyse the quality of the results of this report.

Ten cases are reported by MICHELETTI and RENAULT [25b]: a favourable result was obtained in 4 cases at the average daily dosage of 6—8 tablets. According to WAREMBOURG et al. [41b], a daily dosage of 3 tablets for an average of 1 month provides a favourable result in 19 out of 24 cases.

None of these clinical tests has the character of an absolutely controlled investigation in the sense in which this is at present understood. We shall therefore have to wait until double-blind tests have been carried out before being in a position to pronounce a substantiated opinion as to the true therapeutic value of this new medication for the treatment of angina.

It appears that arterial diseases of the limbs are the major indication for Eucilat [14b].

Griseofulvine

Griseofulvine increases coronary flow in dogs [1580] and causes stimulation of the myocardium, with an increase in heart rate and a drop in blood pressure [19]. It is said to have provided some clinical benefit for anginal subjects [415] but these observations have never had any therapeutic sequel.

Mederel

$$O\!\!\diagdown\!\!N-CH_2-\underset{\underset{\underset{O}{\overset{|}{C}}}{\overset{|}{O}}}{\overset{|}{CH}}\!\!-CH_2-O-CH_2-CH_2-CH\!\!\diagup^{\overset{CH_3}{}}_{\underset{CH_3}{}}$$

Offered to the medical profession in 1969 as an antianginal medication, Mederel or 730 C.E.R.M. (amoproxan) was perfected by Duchene-Marullaz and his colleagues [457]. From this animal experimentation, the following essential facts emerge. We have here a drug which increases coronary venous flow and the oxygen content of the coronary venous blood to an extent proportionate to the doses used, i.e. 2.5, 5 and 10 mg/kg administered intravenously to an anaesthetised dog. Heart rate is not altered, ventricular contraction force is slightly reduced, and blood pressure rises to a moderate extent. No information is given as to cardiac work nor the heart's oxygen requirements, so that as far as is known so far, Mederel can only be considered as a drug which increases myocardial irrigation, the more so since it has no effect on the adrenergic system.

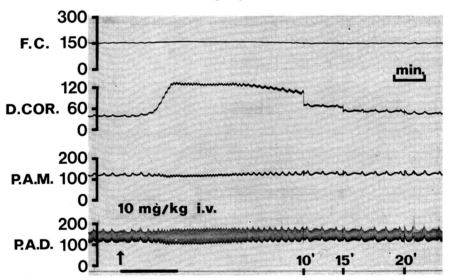

Fig. 54. Effect of amoproxan on heart rate, coronary arterial blood flow, and systemic blood pressure in the anaesthetized dog. From top to bottom: F.C.: Heart rate (beats/min). D.Cor.: Mean blood flow in the left circumflex coronary artery, measured with an electromagnetic probe (ml/min). P.A.M.: Mean blood pressure in the femoral artery (mm Hg). P.A.D.: Phasic blood pressure in the femoral artery (mm Hg). At signal mark: intravenous injection of amoproxan, 10 mg/kg. Parts of tracings recorded successively 10—15 and 20 min after injection

From our own experimental investigations with dogs, Mederel sharply increases coronary arterial blood flow at the intravenous dose of 10 mg/kg. There was a slight rise in heart rate, and the systemic blood pressure did not change significantly. The coronary effect disappeared after 20—30 min (Fig. 54).

Mederel also possesses minor anti-arrhythmic properties, far less potent than those of procainamide [457].

This substance is quickly resorbed by a healthy man after oral administration and only starts disappearing from the blood an hour after ingestion.

The first clinical investigation into Mederel was necessarily carried out by the non-controlled method [1432]. With some forty anginal patients, the average daily dosage of 500 mg administered for 1—2 months was effective in 72% of cases in the light of the purely subjective criteria of frequency, intensity and duration of pains. No information is given as to any reduction in nitroglycerin intake nor regarding any possible improvement in tolerance to the standard effort tests.

The antianginal effect of Mederel is said to be statistically better than that of the nitro derivatives, without however the nature of these being specified. The authors did not consider themselves in a position to assess the drug's effect on the electrocardiogram of the patients treated.

It was only possible to check for an anti-arrhythmic effect on twelve patients subject to extrasystoles whose nature is not specified. The effect of Mederel does not appear to be outstanding since it was non-existent in half the cases and doubtful in two others.

The efficacy of Mederel as an antianginal medication has been confirmed in three further clinical trials. HATT [17b] achieved 90% good and excellent results on 34 patients treated for an average of one month at a mean daily dosage of 750 mg for the first fortnight, subsequently reduced to 450 mg. CLOAREC and GROSGOGEAT [6b] report on a cross-section of 94 patients where Mederel administered for an average of one month at a daily dose of 450 mg achieved an excellent result in 77% of cases of effort-induced angina and in 79% of spontaneous angina cases. Electrocardiograph anomalies were improved in 25% of the cases. AUDIER and ARNOUX [2b] report 70% favourable results out of 48 cases treated at the average dosage of 600 mg for periods of from 2 weeks to 2 months. As stressed by HATT [17b], these investigations cannot be taken other than as guide-lines. The results submitted will need to be checked by carefully controlled tests under double-blind conditions.

Tolerance to Mederel would seem to be satisfactory [1432]. Gastrointestinal upsets have been reported in 12% of cases [1432]. No harmful effect on cardiac decompensation has been found.

It is obvious that these encouraging results obtained with an antianginal medication which only claims coronary dilating properties must be taken as merely preliminary and that the possible usefulness of this new drug can only be assessed after sufficient time has elapsed.

Mederel was withdrawn from the pharmaceutical market in mid-1970 because of the frequency and serious nature of undesirable cutaneous-mucosae manifestations.

Opticardon

A medication, not of an original character, associating pentaerythritol tetranitrate, ethaverine, theophylline, theobromine and hydroxyzine, Opticardon is said to have achieved 90% good to excellent results in 73 cases of coronary insufficiency [545]. The drug is said to increase cardiac efficiency in healthy humans [284c].

Pexid

Perhexiline maleate is 2-(2,2-dicyclohexylethyl)piperidine maleate. Also known as Pexid, it answers to the formula:

It is therefore chemically very similar to hexadylamine whose dilating properties as regards the systemic and coronary vessels, leading to an increase in the amount of oxygen made available to the myocardium, have been reported by Rowe et al. [1573].

The main pharmacological properties of perhexiline can be summed up as follows [22a, 63a]. In dogs, perhexiline dilates the coronary and femoral vascular beds: intravenous doses of 0.3 mg/kg upwards decrease arterial blood pressure and heart rate, and increase coronary flow. Atrio-ventricular conduction is depressed [153c]. Perhexiline blocks isoprenaline-induced tachycardia and is said to have a quinidine-like effect on membrane action potential [39a], but HUDAK et al. [153c] found that the substance produced no inhibition of the cardiovascular effects of isoprenaline in anaesthetised dogs and cats, and that there was no inhibition of adenosine deaminase. It also has broncho-dilating properties as regards dogs, healthy humans and asthmatic subjects [39a].

Rowe et al. [12d] showed that perhexiline decreases coronary vascular resistance, and increases coronary blood flow and coronary sinus blood oxygen content in the anaesthetised dog. These effects are long lasting following an intravenous infusion at the rate of 0.6 mg/kg/min, but very transient after a single intravenous injection at doses of 0.3—0.6 and 1.2 mg/kg. In man with proven coronary artery disease, a single intravenous injection of 40 or 60 mg reduces heart rate, left ventricular work, cardiac output, stroke volume and coronary sinus blood oxygen content; coronary blood flow was not significantly altered.

With humans, perhexiline counters effort-induced tachycardia [19a]. GRUPP et al. [130c] designed experiments in order to quantitate this observation in 12 normal subjects and to determine the time of onset and the duration of drug effect. A double-blind experiment in which 400 mg daily of perhexiline was compared with placebo resulted in a decrease of the exercise-induced tachycardia when drug was taken. The time of onset of drug action was not immediate. Maximum drug effect was not attained for at least five days, and there was evidence that the drug effects persist for at least that long after drug is withdrawn. The resting heart rate was not affected, an observation which tends to rule out β-receptor blockade as the mode of action. Taking also into consideration the results of experiments on animals, it is concluded that the effect of perhexiline is not due to β-adrenergic receptor blockade, ganglionic blockade, or cholinergic stimulation. The possible mechanism of action is postulated as a direct effect on the myocardium, which may interfere in a nonspecific manner with sympathetic activation.

Perhexiline has been tested on angina subjects. An initial clinical application involving 13 patients [841] with a daily dose of 300—400 mg showed a favourable effect, reflected in a reduction in the number of attacks and need for nitroglycerin, and in an increase in tolerance to effort. In a cross-over double-blind study of 10 patients with well-documented histories of angina pectoris, WINSOR [136a] found that the oral administration of perhexiline for 6 weeks at the daily dose of 4×100 mg significantly decreased the number of anginal attacks. While the resting heart rate was not altered, the exercise heart rate was slower during treatment than during placebo administration. Occasional evidence of ECG improvement was noted, as also similar evidence in respect of the exercise tolerance test.

Piridoxilate

Injected in a chloralosed dog at doses of 5 and 10 mg/kg i.v., piridoxilate or Glyo-6 considerably increases the oxygen content of the coronary venous blood, without changing either coronary venous flow or cardiac contraction force, or pulse rate or blood pressure. This effect is considered to reflect a drop in myocardial oxygen consumption [8b]. Piridoxilate sharply reduces the oxygen consumption of sections of rabbit myocardium measured with the Warburg apparatus [22b, 192c] and increases resistance time to anoxia in isolated guinea-pig auricles at concentrations ranging from 10^{-2} and 5.10^{-3} [8b, 12b] and in an isolated guinea-pig heart [12b]. It prolongs the survival time of mice subjected to anoxia [12b].

Administered to an anginal patient at the daily dose of 300 mg for from 3 to 8 weeks, piridoxilate reduces the frequency of pain attacks during an investigation which is not particularly convincing in view of its elementary character [623].

Polarising Solutions

Polarising solutions containing glucose, insulin and potassium cause the rapid disappearance in dogs of the electrocardiographic indications of experimental infarction [1767]. In anaesthetised dogs, the period of ventricular tachycardia induced by digitalis, which lasted for 3 hours in control animals, was significantly reduced to 85 minutes in 85% of dogs by large intravenous infusions of polarising solutions [201c].

The separate administration of potassium to coronary patients is said to have an antianginal effect and to bring about increased tolerance to exercise [752, 1769]. Polarising solutions themselves would appear to speed up the evolution of acute infarct in man and to be effective against pain [1768, 1770]. Since these conclusions were not accepted by other authors [565, 1211], FLETCHER et al. [566] carried out a double-blind test on 80 patients which resulted in negative findings.

An identical opinion is reached from another investigation [1430] carried out on 200 patients where polarising solutions did not alter the percentage of mortality or the incidence of forms of arrhythmia. The same goes for 256 patients treated over the two weeks following their acute infarct by the combined administration by mouth of potassium and glucose, and the subcutaneous injection of insulin [875]. Various parameters were studied by CUELLAR [72c] in 127 patients with myocardial infarction treated with polarising solutions and compared with those found in 137 similar patients receiving conventional therapy. No improvement of the clinical course has been observed.

In a multicentre controlled clinical trial of polarising solutions in the treatment of acute myocardial infarction involving 840 patients [256c], no significant benefit was shown to be derived from the regimen, the mortality rate at twenty eight days in the treated group (410 patients) being 23.9% and in the control group 25.3% (430 patients). The incidence of cardiac arrhythmias also was not significantly altered by the treatment. COTTERILL et al. [69c] reported on the same subject, with opposite conclusions. A random sample of 286 myocardial infarction cases were studied; 112 received polarising solutions treatment and 174 were controls. A highly significant difference was seen concerning death rate, since 19.5% of treated cases died whereas there were 46.5% of deaths in the control group. COTTERILL thinks that the failure of the abovementioned trial to show any advantage for the treatment could perhaps have been due to more intensive nursing and monitoring, which could have pre-empted any gain from polarising solutions.

Recently VEGA DIAZ and PEREZ CASAR [323c] showed that in 112 cases of myocardial infarction treated with polarising solutions, there was a shortening of the period of clinical evolution, and an improvement in the usual clinical features (hyperthermia, hypotension, shock, sedimentation rate, enzymatic alterations). Symptomatic benefit was especially seen in the cases in which electrocardiographic pathological pattern persisted. In view of these conflicting results, there would not appear therefore to be any advantage in using these polarising solutions in the treatment of acute myocardial infarction in the hope of exerting a favourable effect on its evolution as regards the appearance of complications, whether of shock, cardiac decompensation, arrhythmia or mortality.

Despite these unfavourable views, the supporters of this therapeutic attitude continue to advocate it in the treatment of acute myocardial infarction [115a].

The mode of action of this therapy being poorly understood, BAJUSZ [3b] carried out some experimental studies which indicate that certain K-salts, given alone or in combination with glucose and insulin, have a marked influence on the structural aspects of hereditary degenerative cardiomyopathy. As a result, it was observed that healing of the spontaneous focal myocardial lesions consistently found in an inbred strain of hamsters was significantly enhanced by treatment with K-aspartate or K-orotate. Insulin or combined glucose-insulin therapy similarly accelerated healing, but to a lesser extent, whilst K-salts and glucose-insulin potentialised each other's effect in this respect. Such treatments probably act through their ability to stimulate protein synthesis and/or by enhancing fibroblastic proliferation in the injured area. These observations do not allow of the conclusion that K-salts and K-containing "polarising" solutions act in a similar manner in human degenerative heart disease; they merely suggest this possibility.

In the opinion of OPIE [239c], increasing blood glucose concentrations may theoretically benefit the ischaemic myocardium by increasing the rate of anaerobic glycolysis, by reversing ion losses, by a direct membrane effect, by altering the extracellular volume, and by decreasing the circulating free fatty acid concentrations. Several of these actions may be enhanced by the simultaneous administration of insulin and potassium. Each of these aims seems desirable. But even if all these aims were achieved, we cannot be sure of undisputed therapeutic benefit to the ischaemic myocardium. We need even more basic work before the apparently attractive "glucose hypothesis" can be converted into a practical plan of treatment that can be recommended to the clinician without reservation. But, taking all these indications for glucose treatment together, we can conclude that the administration of glucose (or glucose, insulin and potassium) to patients with myocardial infarction remains an attractive field for therapeutic investigation, provided that suitable selection of patients is made.

Sandolanid

Sandolanid or acetyldigoxin is claimed to have proved of real benefit in 40 out of 56 anginal patients treated, bringing about improvement in the ECG and a reduction in the number, duration and intensity of angina attacks, and a decrease in nitroglycerin intake [1698]. On the other hand, WILLEMS [2001 bis] found no sign of improvement in the electrocardiograph indications of myocardial ischaemia in 12 cases of coronary insufficiency. DITTRICH [432] also obtained relief from precordial pain, going hand in hand with an increase in work capacity, in some twenty patients suffering from functional coronary insufficiency not accompanied by cardiac insufficiency. Nitro-Sandolanid contains 0.1 mg acetyldigoxin and 20 mg pentaerythrityl tetranitrate per tablet. It was given to 40 patients with chronic coronary insufficiency for at least 14 days, 3—6 tablets daily [134a]. The results were poor in severe insufficiency, but marked improvement was seen in patients with mild insufficiency. As the preparation was well tolerated, it was concluded that the drug is worth a trial in mild cases of coronary insufficiency.

According to JUNG [19b], a 2 week treatment at the daily dose of 3 tablets reduced the frequency of angina attacks in 41 out of 43 patients with chronic coronary insufficiency. 14 patients found their pains vanishing during the first week, and 24 during the second week. The ECG was improved in 19 cases. In a clinical trial published by TOKER [312c] and carried out on 30 patients receiving 3 tablets daily of Nitro-Sandolanid for 12 days, there was a distinct subjective improvement: 24 patients discontinued taking nitroglycerin, and only 4 showed ischaemic deterioration of the ECG during a bicycle ergometer exercise.

Surheme

Surheme or LA 1221 answers to the formula:

$$CH_3-(CH_2)_3$$
$$|$$
$$CH_3-(CH_2)_3-N-(CH_2)_2-NH-\overset{N}{\underset{O}{\|}}\text{-phenyl}$$

This is primarily a potent and long-lasting peripheral vasodilator, which increases coronary flow in an isolated rabbit heart and antagonises the coronary constricting effect on that organ of barium chloride and pituitrine [38b]. When administered intravenously to an anaesthetised dog at the dose of 10 mg/kg, Surheme increases the coronary venous flow whilst at the same time reducing cardiac output, work and rate [38b]. In the anaesthetised dog, Surheme increases blood flow in the femoral and carotid arteries. The effect is moderate and very transient by intravenous injection, moderate but more prolonged by oral administration, conspicuous and long lasting by intraarterial injection [5d].

Administered orally at an average daily dosage of 120—360 mg, Surheme is said to be effective as regards functional disorders in peripheral arteritis [37b]. The author of these clinical observations mentions in passing that he had obtained "very brilliant results" with some twenty patients suffering from angina pectoris [37b]. The lack of further information does not allow the quality of the therapeutic effects observed to be assessed.

It appears however that the main therapeutic indication for Surheme is peripheral arteriopathy, where significantly better results than those obtained with the placebo have been reported in a double blind study in which patients were randomly allocated to active drug or placebo treatment groups [40c].

Terodiline

$$\text{(diphenyl)}-CH-CH_2-CH-NH-C\overset{CH_3}{\underset{CH_3}{\overset{\diagup}{\diagdown}}}CH_3$$
$$|$$
$$CH_3$$

Terodiline (trade name Bicor) or 1-methyl-3,3-diphenyl-1-N-terbutyl-propylamine provides a marked increase in coronary blood flow through relaxation of smooth vascular muscle, resulting in decreased coronary vascular resistance [79a].

WIBELL [133a] demonstrated favourable effects on nitroglycerin intake and pain incidence in a double-blind cross-over study on 16 patients with coronary artery disease.

Terodiline was administered intravenously at a dosage of 50—100 mg to 10 patients who suffered anginal pain as a result of an exercise test [79a]. When the exercise test was repeated one hour after the injection, there was a drop in pulmonary capillary venous pressure, an effect which is considered as indicating improvement in left ventricular failure. There was also definite subjective improvement (no pain or reduced pain) in 4 out of the 10 patients. On the basis of these results, LECEROF and MALMBORG believe that terodiline should be tried as an adjunctive also in oral long-term therapy of angina pectoris.

Tromcardin

Tromcardin consists of equal parts of potassium and magnesium aspartate. According to WOELKE [137a] who treated 104 ischaemic heart disease patients by intravenous injections twice daily, angina disappeared in most cases after 2—3 injections. Side effects included only a warm sensation in the precordial region and transient pain at the injection site. Contra-indications are severe renal damage and atrio-ventricular conduction disturbances.

Tromcardin has been associated with pentaerythritol tetranitrate and methaqualon under the trade name of Steno-Tromcardin, and with Digoxin under the trade name of Digi-Tromcardin.

Vastarel

$$CH_3O-\text{⟨⟩}-CH_2-N\underset{}{\overset{}{\bigcirc}}NH$$
$$CH_3O \quad OCH_3$$

Vastarel (generic name: trimetazidine) is a moderate coronary vaso-dilating agent [528] with adrenolytic and noradrenolytic properties, which appears to exert its spasmolytic action rather more on the peripheral circulation, which entails a drop in venous return and a decrease in cardiac output. These effects would appear from a certain angle to be comparable to those of nitroglycerin [458]. There is a drop in blood pressure and also in stroke volume, cardiac output and cardiac work. Heart rate and myocardial metabolism are not altered [325c].

Some clinicians have tested Vastarel on angina pectoris subjects with no more than satisfactory results [919, 943, 1175]. Other clinical trials by WAREMBOURG [14d], JOUVE [7d], HERTAULT [6d], MEHROTRA [10d] and BRODBIN [1d] resulted at the utmost in satisfactory results. No double-blind well controlled investigation is available.

The period which elapses before its antianginal effect becomes apparent is said to be very long [274].

Vialibran

$$\text{⟨⟩}_2CH-N\underset{}{\overset{}{\bigcirc}}N-CH_2-\text{⟨⟩}\overset{O}{\underset{O}{\diagdown}}CH_2$$

Vialibran (generic name: medibazine) is a coronary dilating agent on an isolated heart [1085]. In the case of a chloralosed dog, it sharply increases the coronary venous flow and the oxygen content of coronary venous blood, whilst at the same time having no effect on heart rate, work or output nor on its oxygen consumption [1083, 1084].

Although several non-controlled clinical investigations report 60% favourable results with angina patients [285, 1433, 1957], this medication certainly does not provide any outstanding results, as witness a study by CANTOR [275] under double-blind conditions ending up with 4 patients improved out of ten treated.

Section no. 2

This second section deals with several medications which may be grouped into two categories:

a) those which, by their direct impact on the central nervous system, are likely to contribute, by reason of their sedative properties, to an improvement in the anxiety state specific to the sufferer from angina pectoris: morphine, the barbiturates, ethyl alcohol and Valium;

b) those which, by virtue of their dilator properties as regards the myocardial vessels, have been deemed worthy of clinical tests on angina subjects but whose therapeutic effect either has not been considered good or has been appreciably improved on by recent medications: the phenothiazines, diphenylhydantoin, the cinchona alkaloids, Daucarine, a-tocopherol, hexoestrol and adenosine and its derivatives.

Morphine

Opinions differ on the effect of morphine on coronary flow. KOUNTZ [1023] reported an increase in the perfused, resuscitated human heart but, because of the reduction in the amplitude of ventricular contraction, this could have been due merely to reduction in the extravascular support; ELEK and KATZ [484] demonstrated the occurrence of a direct coronary vasodilator effect in the fibrillating isolated heart of the dog, an effect which has been confirmed by KAVERINA [963]. However, VAN EGMOND [1918] saw no change in the flow in the isolated heart of the cat and WEGRIA et al. [1970] reported mostly reduction in blood pressure and coronary flow in the anaesthetized dog with average doses of 0.25—0.5 mg/kg given intravenously. Morphine given in similar dosage and by the same route did not alter the flow from the coronary venous sinus in the dog [917]. In the hands of DÖRNER and WICK [443], there was only a small and inconstant rise in arterial coronary flow in the dog, whether anaesthetized or not. MELVILLE [1269 p. 502] considers that, experimentally, small doses do not increase the coronary flow, which is only augmented by doses which cannot be attained in the intact organism.

Permanent use of morphine in angina is contra-indicated as, acting only on the pain without improving coronary efficiency, it may create a false sense of well-being which may lead the patient to undertake exertions for which his myocardium is not functionally suited [1594, 1619].

Barbiturates

By using a thermostromuhr in the unanaesthetized dog, ESSEX et al. [509] were able to record a considerable increase of coronary flow which persisted for almost 90 min after intravenous injection of pentobarbital, 15 mg/kg.

The clinical employment of barbiturates is only indicated to counteract the mental tension and anxiety which are an integral part of the anginal syndrome; they are particularly useful at the beginning of treatment. RUSSEK [1595] prefers meprobamate to them.

Ethyl Alcohol

Some angina pectoris patients derive benefit from the moderate use of alcohol. Although the sedative and central depressant action of alcohol, resulting in a raising of the threshold for pain, can explain such results, it has been suggested that they may also result from a coronary vasodilator action.

Ethyl alcohol has been sometimes stated to be practically devoid of activity on coronary vessels, or again to have good vasodilator properties. DIXON [433], on the isolated rabbit heart, and SULZER [1855], on a heart-lung preparation of the dog, failed to observe any significant increase in coronary flow, even with high concentrations. In the anaesthetized dog, the flow from the coronary venous sinus was unchanged [657, 1077] with a dose of 250 mg/kg given intravenously (corresponding to 40 mg per 100 ml in the blood), but it increased by 50% with 375 mg/kg (65 mg % in the blood), there being a simultaneous fall in arterial pressure, and by 120% with 500 mg/kg [1077].

The coronary arterial flow behaved in the same manner. Thus, according to these authors, the coronary flow increased with doses of alcohol which produced blood concentrations similar to those found in man after the ingestion of moderate quantities of alcohol (two or three cocktails). As there is a fall of blood pressure, it must be admitted that alcohol reduces the resistance of the coronary vessels but so far no experimental observations have made it possible to determine the factors responsible for this effect. Using the nitrous oxide method, SCHMITTHENNER et al. [1687] were unable, however, to confirm the increase of coronary flow found by the preceding authors, although the blood concentrations of alcohol were comparable.

In conscious dogs with implanted electromagnetic flow transducers, alcohol (1 g/kg intravenously) resulted in a significant decrease in coronary (41%) and peripheral (17%) vascular resistance, whereas heart rate, mean aortic pressure and cardiac output were not significantly changed [253c]. Both propranolol (1 mg/kg intravenously) and anaesthesia with pentobarbital (25 mg/kg intravenously) diminished the coronary and peripheral vasodilator effects. Results of this investigation suggest that in the conscious dog alcohol provokes a significant increase in coronary blood flow and a fall in coronary and peripheral vascular resistance. The coronary vasodilatation cannot be explained by excitement, since the characteristic cardiac acceleration and pressor effects of excitement did not occur. The possibility that the coronary vasodilatation may be the result of a central vasomotor depression, as has been proposed for the cutaneous vasodilatation seen after alcohol, must be considered.

EVANS and HOYLE [515] stated that half their anginal patients who benefited greatly from nitroglycerin reported an identical effect from the taking of alcohol. Although they, too, observed that in a number of their patients alcohol was capable of averting an attack of pain or could terminate one in the same way as, for example, nitroglycerin, RUSSEK et al. [1612, 1614] deny it had any coronary vasodilator effect as it never modified the electrocardiogram of myocardial ischaemia produced by standardized exercise: the therapeutic effect of alcohol was thus merely that of a rapidly acting sedative. Its use as a preventive in relation to anticipated exertion must be severely condemned as it can create a false feeling of perfect physical conditions which invites the coronary subject to engage in immoderate exertion when the pain-alarm no longer exists to limit this exertion; as the coronary flow is not increased by alcohol, there is a risk of infarct precipitation [1826].

The relevance of experimental investigations carried out in healthy anaesthetized dogs to the atherosclerotic coronary patient being open to question, CONWAY

[359] has studied the haemodynamic changes in patients with stable coronary heart disease after a drink of alcohol equivalent to 3 or 4 whiskies (0.5 g per kg). At rest, 45 min after this alcohol intake, blood pressure and cardiac output fell progressively, so that the calculated peripheral resistance did not alter.

No change occurred in the heart rate. Left ventricular work and myocardial oxygen uptake declined. All these changes occurred also during exercise, and no significant alteration was observed in the amount of work required to produce angina.

The conclusion was reached that alcohol was acting as a myocardial depressant. This opinion is shared by REGAN et al. [1513, 1514, 1515] chiefly because in young alcoholics without heart disease, alcohol intake prevents the normal increase in stroke volume when left end-diastolic ventricular pressure rises during an i.v. infusion of angiotensine. CONWAY's opinion is that it would seem prudent for patients with angina to take alcohol in moderation only. However, it seems that the acute haemodynamic effects of ethanol could be different in normal non-alcoholic human beings since, according to RIFF et al. [107a], there was a significant increase in cardiac output, due to an increase in heart rate without change in stroke volume 30 min after ingestion of whisky in such an amount that peak blood alcohol levels, reached within 30 min in the majority of subjects, ranged from 85 to 136 mg/100 ml. Blood pressure and left ventricular contractility remained unchanged, and there was no effect on the haemodynamic response to a given work-load.

MOHIUDDIN et al. [91a] measured left coronary artery flow in four male alcoholics receiving an i.v. infusion of 300 ml of 16% alcohol in normal saline. Mean blood alcohol level was 97.7 mg %. Alcohol failed to modify coronary flow but myocardial metabolism was profoundly altered as there was an increase in the myocardial lactate (66%) and glucose (290%) uptake and a decrease in pyruvate (17%) and palmitate (43%) uptake.

Following ingestion of alcohol, there were significant differences in left ventricular systolic time intervals between normal individuals and patients with coronary heart disease without heart failure [122c]. These differences were not related to heart rate or diastolic blood pressure but may be explained by a postulated lack of increase in stroke volume or in the contractility of the ischaemic myocardium or both.

Summarizing the present view about alcohol, GOULD stated recently that it has a depressant action on the heart and that it has no place in the therapy of angina pectoris, except as a sedative [15b].

Valium

Valium (diazepam) is employed in general practice as a psychotropic drug. It has in dogs some antiarrhythmic properties which are thought to merit further investigations in controlled clinical trials [297c]. Valium is used in angina to reduce anxiety, and its intravenous administration is recommended 5—10 min prior to cardioversion since it relieves undesirable psychic tension and apprehension. Valium develops also some effects on the coronary circulation in animals.

According to ABEL et al. [1a], Valium increased coronary blood flow when injected i.v. at doses of 0.1 up to 0.2 mg/kg in anaesthetized dogs on cardiopulmonary bypass. Since heart rate and aortic blood pressure (coronary head pressure) were maintained constant artificially, the rise in blood flow was considered to be a consequence of a decrease in coronary vascular resistance. In a second paper, ABEL et al. [1c] attempt to define the mechanism by which Valium produces the side-effects of coronary and systemic vasodilatation. No significant alteration in the vasodilatation produced by the drug was observed following either vagotomy or a-adrenoceptor blockade. Partial inhibition of the effect occurred after β-adrenoceptor blockade or catecholamine depletion (reserpine pretreatment). Nearly total inhibition was observed after small doses of atropine or ganglion-blocking agent (trimethaphan i.v. infusion). These results suggest that Valium may stimulate specifically vasodilating mechanisms, both adrenergic and cholinergic, at the post-ganglionic neurone, thereby causing active decrease in coronary vascular resistance.

Phenothiazines

Chlorpromazine

Chlorpromazine (Largactil) has powerful effects on the coronary circulation. In the isolated rabbit heart, the coronary outflow is increased by 60—100% with doses of 0.05—1.0 mg; this effect is, however, less powerful than that of promethazine [373]. The minimum active dose would appear to be 0.1 γ [254]. On the same preparation the coronary inflow increased very considerably; the effect increased with the dose, rising from 100% for a dose of 10 γ to 500 % for 500 γ [1271]. As there was only an insignificant reduction in the amplitude of the cardiac contractions, at any rate with low dosage, the authors are of the opinion that there was direct dilator action on the coronary vessels, an opinion which corroborates the observations of SZABO [1862] and of WITZLEB and BUDDE [2023], who, in the dog, were unable to establish any changes in cardiac metabolism during increase in the coronary flow. Nevertheless, the reduced extravascular pressure resulting from the marked reduction in the amplitude of the contractions was largely responsible for the enormous increase in the flow following large doses [1271].

In contrast with these reports, WIRTH et al. [2022] found that the coronary vasodilator effect of chlorpromazine on the perfused isolated guinea-pig's heart was only moderate and transient. Likewise, LONGSLET [1172] reported that chlorpromazine reduced coronary flow in the isolated rat heart for concentrations of 10^{-4} and 10^{-5}, a small and transient increase being noted for weaker strengths.

Given in therapeutic doses to the dog, chlorpromazine was incapable of increasing the collateral coronary flow, measured after acute occlusion of the anterior interventricular artery [1863]. Injected intravenously in a dose of 25 mg to normal man, it checked development of the electrocardiographic signs of hypoxia produced by inhalation of an atmosphere containing only 6% oxygen [1865].

Although the pharmacological effects of chlorpromazine on the coronary circulation might have been expected to have led to extensive research for an assessment of its usefulness in the prevention of anginal attacks, clinical investigations have hitherto been relatively few and have dealt with only very limited numbers of patients. FRIEDBERG [595] described a spectacular effect in an intractable case of angina which might have been a "tranquillizing" effect. SZABO et al. [1865] reported the observation of four patients, in two of whom the cardiac pains disappeared, the other two being very much improved; this therapeutic result was said to be due less to absolute improvement in the coronary flow than to reduction of cardiac metabolism, coupled with an action on the sensory paths for pain [1864]. On the other hand, COLE [349] was only able to observe temporary improvement in four patients with a daily dose of 40 mg, and this improvement could not be maintained although the dose was subsequently increased to 200 mg. WAX and DEGRAFF [1963] obtained no more effect with a daily dose of 75 mg than with a placebo.

The potential therapeutic importance of chlorpromazine in angina pectoris could be restricted, however, by the fact that it possesses powerful peripheral vasodilator properties. Its use has never been favoured.

Mepazine

Mepazine or Pacatal (N-methyl-piperidyl-3-methyl-phenothiazine), injected in dosage of 2—5 mg/kg intravenously, increased the coronary sinus flow by 50—80% in the cat; the heart rate fell, the amplitude of the contractions increased and the blood pressure fell by 25—30 mm Hg but returned to normal within 10—15 min [2041]. The reduction in the coronary flow produced by pituitrine yielded in 2—3 min to the intravenous injection of 5 mg/kg mepazine; given before pituitrine, mepazine prevented development of the spasm. Mepazine would appear to be more active than chlorpromazine [962]. Coronary vasodilatation was also observed in the isolated guinea-pig heart [1367], and the increase of coronary flow was not accompanied by changes in cardiac metabolism in the dog [2023].

Chloracizine

Following ZAKUSOV and KAVERINA [2038, 2040], chloracizine or 10 (β-diethylaminopropionyl)-2-chlorphenothiazine, which possesses potent coronary vasodilator effects, does not affect the systemic blood pressure level; coronary blood flow increased considerably without any change in the myocardial oxygen consumption. The drug was also found to be very effective in experimental myocardial infarction in contributing to the development of collateral circulation and the restoration of normal blood pressure and electrocardiogram [1295].

Chloracizine has been reported to improve almost 60% of the 140 anginous patients which have been treated, the drug having no beneficial effect on the pathological ECG [2039]. This study is unfortunately far from being convincing.

Diphenylhydantoin

Diphenylhydantoin, whose effects on myocardial excitability and automaticity have been recently reinvestigated by BIGGER et al. [31c] in the canine heart *in situ*, is used as an anti-arrhythmic drug. ZEFT et al. [345c] studied the effect of an intravenous injection of diphenylhydantoin sodium at a dose of 5 mg/kg on coronary haemodynamics in unanaesthetized dogs, with chronically implanted electromagnetic flow probes on the left circumflex coronary artery and proximal aorta. Coronary arterial flow increased by 36%, coronary vascular resistance falling by an average of 40%. The effect was very transient, blood flow returning to control levels in 3—5 min. At a dose of 10 mg/kg, myocardial blood flow rose by more than 100%. Conclusion has been reached that i.v. diphenylhydantoin in doses similar to those administered clinically to treat ventricular arrhythmias produces significant but transient coronary vasodilatation.

Cinchona Alkaloids

Whatever experimental method is employed, the effect of quinidine on the coronary circulation appears to depend on the dose: with low dosage, there was no change in the coronary flow in a heart-lung preparation of the dog [193] or in the perfused isolated heart of man [1023] or dog [484]; on the same preparations large doses increased the flow by a mechanism of direct coronary vasodilation [193, 484].

According to SZEKERES and LENARD [1867bis], the direction of quinidine's effect on the isolated rabbit heart, beating or fibrillating, depended on the temperature of the perfusion fluid: at 38°C it reduced coronary flow, but increased it powerfully at 26°C. In the dog the intravenous injection of 15 mg quinidine gluconate increased coronary flow and cardiac metabolism considerably and there was important reduction in the coronary vascular resistance and in myocardial efficiency [1576]; the tachycardia that was present was probably partly responsible for the increase of coronary flow.

According to MERCIER et al. [1283], quinidine produced an increase in the coronary outflow in the anaesthetized dog provided the systemic blood pressure did not fall; flow was reduced in case general hypotension occurred. In rats, quinidine sulfate (oral route) and dihydroquinidine gluconate (intraperitoneal injection) antagonized the coronary spasm provoked by pitressin [1294].

As clinical reports described good effects with quinidine in some cases of angina pectoris [584, 1469, 1532, 1533] and the use of quinine in angina had been suggested by BLACK [181] as long ago as 1795, RISEMAN et al. [1534] examined the effects in angina of five alkaloids of cinchona, namely, quinine, quinidine, cinchonine, cinchonidine and cinchamidine.

Using their own assessment technique (see p. 106), they were of the opinion that, with the exception of cinchonine which had little activity, these alkaloids yielded appreciable results, better than those with Peritrate and much superior to results with papaverine or khellin. The alkaloids of cinchona could be classed among the drugs most effective for the treatment of angina pectoris; quinine and quinidine were the most active of the four, and quinine appeared therapeutically superior in view of its general pharmacological activity as it was less toxic, particularly for the myocardium, and also cheaper. The quinoline nucleus was thought to be the fraction of the molecule primarily responsible for the therapeutic effect which corresponded, pharmacologically, to a coronary vasodilatation, which has been demonstrated mainly by HEDBOM [795] on the isolated mammalian heart.

RUSSEK's opinion [1594] is opposed to that of RISEMAN: as it failed to alter the electrocardiographic signs of the myocardial ischaemia of effort in the anginal patient, quinidine was not thought to be of any therapeutic importance in angina.

Despite the favourable results reported by RISEMAN, most authorities are of the opinion that quinidine should not be used as a daily prophylactic treatment in chronic coronary insufficiency [692 p. 723].

Daucarine

Dating from 1958, Daucarine, or alcoholic extract of carrot seeds, is a preparation which has been the subject of Soviet publications. The only references to this substance are abstracts which have appeared in various medical periodicals. According to ANGARSKAYA et al. [34] Daucarine causes a definite reduction in the tone of smooth muscle fibre in the animal. Administered to eighty-eight anginal patients by mouth in a daily dose of 60—100 mg for 1—3 weeks, it gave distinct improvement in 66% of cases, had a doubtful effect in 16%, and was ineffective in 18%. The improvement was particularly evident in the anginal cases with associated hypertension.

No side-effects developed.

Vitamin E (α-Tocopherol)

While the nutritional importance of vitamin E is now well established, its therapeutic value in coronary disease is still very controversial. LU, ALLMARK and GRAHAM [1183] failed to observe any coronary vasodilator effect (or any significant action on the myocardium) in the perfused isolated rabbit heart following large doses of α-tocopherol. In the first clinical trials, anginal patients were improved subjectively and objectively by 200—300 mg α-tocopherol daily, the reduction in the number of attacks of pain being associated with reduction in nitroglycerin requirements and improved exercise tolerance [1749]. Some later clinical investigations have not, however, been able to confirm these satisfactory results [69, 82, 1122, 1210, 1499]. The carefully controlled and double-blind observations of RINZLER et al. [1528] established definitely that vitamin E had no more beneficial action in angina pectoris than the placebo.

Nevertheless, VOGELSANG [328 c] reported recently the results of the use of α-tocopherol in degenerative cardiovascular disease over 24 years. The drug has been found beneficial in coronary insufficiency (coronary sclerosis or angina pectoris) at the daily dose of 400 international units. According to this investigator, an appropriate presentation should be used because enteric-coated tablets were found to be most effective since they only dissolve in the intestinal tract, whereas gelatin capsules are partially inactivated in the stomach. Listed contra-indications for the use of α-tocopherol are: hyperthyroidism, iron medication or simultaneous administration of laxatives containing mineral oil.

Hexoestrol

In addition to the male sex hormones, particularly testosterone propionate, the effect of which in angina was excellent according to some authors [1110] and nil according to others [1118], several derivatives of Stilbene and of hexoestrol have been tried in the treatment of angina pectoris; apart from the fact that the results obtained have always been very debatable, the undesirable repercussions of these drugs on the sex habitus restricts their employment very greatly.

In 1958, 4,4'-diethylaminoethoxyhexoestrol was recommended under the names of Coralgyl or Trimanyl "MG.345", as being free from oestrogen effects. Having coronary vasodilator properties in the isolated rabbit heart and no effect on peripheral vessels, this substance, which increased the coronary arterial flow only slightly in the dog [443], was given by BECKER [117] to fifty anginal patients with alleged very good results; the author also stated that the electrocardiographic changes associated with infarct disappeared in most cases after only 3—6 days of treatment; no side-effects and no changes in arterial pressure were observed.

According to BALATRE and MERLEN [77], the drug should be considered as one of the best antianginal medications although it was found to be just equal to methylchromone, which is now known as being devoid of value in the treatment of angina.

Adenosine and Related Substances

When added to the perfusate in an isolated guinea-pig heart, adenosine increased coronary flow proportionally to the concentration of the solution [1689].

Adenosine and adenylic acid (of muscle or yeast) increased the coronary venous outflow in a heart-lung preparation of the dog [451bis] and in the anaesthetized entire dog, where they were active in doses that produced no change in blood pressure [1967]; they were twenty times more powerful than sodium nitrite on the isolated rabbit heart [1966]. Adenine and guanosine have likewise been reported to be coronary vasodilators [1966].

Adenosine phosphoric acid increased the coronary flow in the unanaesthetized dog [509]. According to ECKSTEIN et al. [474], a product liberated by mechanical destruction of red cells, which is probably adenosine triphosphate (ATP) or adenosine diphosphate (ADP), is a powerful coronary vasodilator.

Examining more particularly the effects of ATP, FOLKOW [567] showed that this substance, when injected by the intracoronary route in the fibrillating heart of the dog *in situ*, increased the coronary flow markedly by a direct dilator effect on the smooth muscle fibre, and that the minimum active dose, calculated on the basis of equimolar concentrations, was ten times smaller than that of acetylcholine.

Comparing the activities of various adenosine derivatives on the arterial coronary flow of the dog heart *in situ*, WINBURY et al. [2016] calculated the respective activities of ATP, ADP, AMP and adenosine as 100, 95, 28 and 25, adenine being inactive. As these estimations were not in agreement with some earlier works, WOLF and BERNE [2028] took up this question again and made a comparative study of the action of a number of adenine nucleotides on the coronary inflow in the dog. Adenosine triphosphate and diphosphate had identical coronary vasodilator activities, whereas the monophosphate and adenosine itself had effects which were four times weaker (all the findings thus confirmed those of WINBURY). Inactive substances were adenine and the monophosphate, diphosphate and triphosphate of inosine, of guanosine and of cytidine; of the uridine phosphates, only the triphosphate had a coronary vasodilator effect, which was a fourth of that of ATP.

According to the same authors, ATP caused increase in the oxygen consumption of the myocardium, but the rise in coronary blood flow was greater than was necessary to meet the increased oxygen requirements. Its action on the coronary circulation can then be considered primary on the vessels, and not secondary to elevation of myocardial metabolism.

The adenosine-induced increment in myocardial blood flow is nonuniformly distributed within the left ventricular wall, the outer layers receiving a proportionately greater fraction of the flow augmentation than the inner layers [193c].

The effects of adenosine are transient as it is rapidly destroyed by a deaminase [35]. An analogue of adenosine, 2-chloroadenosine has vasodepressor effects which are much more powerful [332] as it is not inactivated by the adenosine deaminase [1889]. It has the pharmacological characteristics of adenosine but it is more active and its vasodilator effects are more sustained; at coronary level it is ten times more powerful than adenosine [1890]. As it is readily absorbed when administered by mouth, THORP and COBBIN [1890] thought that this substance might be useful in angina pectoris and in arterial hypertension.

N^6-[naphthyl-(1)]-methyl-adenosine, a recent adenosine derivative, developped in anaesthetized dogs and cats sustained coronarodilator properties, cardiac output being also increased in the same time while there was a small fall in blood pressure. In the conscious dog, its coronarodilator activity seemed to be five times higher than that of dipyridamole [890].

Thyroxine

Injected intravenously in a dose of 1 mg/kg in the unanaesthetized dog, thyroxine increased the coronary flow, as measured by means of a thermostromuhr, within 48 hr, the maximum of increase being reached after periods of from 48 to 96 hr in different dogs, whereafter the flow fell again progressively [508]. ESSEX et al.

[509] found thyroxine more active than nitrites, and the action was very prolonged. It could precipitate angina in man, and it thus affords a classical example of a powerful coronary vasodilator which cannot be used therapeutically on man as it greatly increases cardiac metabolism [2004 p. 370]. This traditional opinion would appear to be erroneous, according to RUSSEK [1597], as he has observed favourable effects in 80% of euthyroid coronary patients from daily administration of thyroid extract in combination with laevothyroxine and the vitamin B complex.

Section no. 3

In this last section, some medications will be briefly considered, which are used by the physician as peripheral vasodilators. All of them may improve the coronary circulation in animals under various experimental conditions. They have therefore been occasionally tested in anginous patients in order to define some possible therapeutic interest, but inconsistent and questionable effects resulted in discarding them for this nosologic indication.

Phenoxy-Isopropyl-Norsuprifen

Phenoxy-isopropyl-norsuprifen (Caa 40, Duvadilan, Vasodilan) is endowed with peripheral vasodilator properties [245], involving mainly the deep muscular arteries [930], which increase the blood flow in the limb muscles. The occurrence of coronary vasodilator effects has been demonstrated on the normal dog in an indirect manner, in that, when injected intravenously in a dose of 0.25—0.5 mg/kg, the drug counteracts development of the electrocardiographic signs of ischaemia produced by the injection of large doses of pituitrine [245]. The coronary flow of the fibrillating isolated rabbit heart is also increased [1326].

The use of Duvadilan in the treatment of the anginal syndrome appears to have yielded very favourable results [161, 753, 1326], but these clinical observations cannot carry conviction as the number of patients treated was excessively small or as the conclusions were based exclusively on subjective impressions supplied by the patients and were not subject to critical control [460].

Phenyl-Isobutyl-Norsuprifen

Phenyl-isobutyl-norsuprifen (Dilatropon, Dilatal, Dilatol, Arlidin) is very closely related to the preceding substance. The close relationship of the two chemical structures presages a certain degree of analogy in pharmacological effects. Tests demonstrated that this is so.

WIEMERS [1991] showed that, in man, the dog and the cat, Dilatropon produced a considerable fall in blood pressure which was neither histaminic, cholinergic nor sympatholytic in character, but was due purely to peripheral action.

In the coronary arteries, Dilatropon produced a marked increase of flow, probably due to direct dilatation of the vessels in the myocardium [1992]. Although this is the probable mode of action, it has not been strictly proved as the simultaneous increases in the cardiac output and heart rate were themselves capable of producing considerable change in the flow.

Identical effects have been observed in heart-lung preparations of the dog [684]. In the normal dog, Dilatropon prevented development of the electrocardiographic abnormalities of myocardial ischaemia produced by the coronary vasoconstrictor effects of pituitrine [245].

We have no knowledge of any clinical paper on the use of Dilatropon in angina pectoris.

Cyclospasmol

A peripheral vasodilator with musculotropic activity, Cyclospasmol (cyclandelate) increased the coronary flow in the isolated rabbit heart [160]; the force of the ventricular contractions was reduced at the same time. It is an antagonist of barium chloride.

In the cat, myocardial infarct produced by ligature of the anterior interventricular coronary artery disappeared earlier in Cyclospasmol-treated animals (20 mg daily) than in the controls [17].

Used mainly for treatment of arteritic conditions in the limbs [662, 822, 936, 1997], Cyclospasmol would appear to give good results in angina pectoris associated with arterial hypertension [94].

Vasculat

Vasculat which is derived from Sympatol is a peripheral vasodilator, intravenous administration of which to the dog, cat or rabbit induces a fall of blood pressure proportionate to the dose injected and of lasting character; the effect is produced on the muscle fibre itself [1912]. Accordingly, the clinical employment of Vasculat is primarily directed to the treatment of peripheral vascular disorders [202, 788].

Vasculat increased the coronary flow of the perfused isolated rabbit heart and stimulated the force and frequency of the cardiac contractions [1226]. As this change in the extracoronary support might have contributed to increase the outflow, the same authors also experimented with conditions in which there was practically no cardiac contraction (perfusion at low pressure): as the coronary flow was again increased in the apparent absence of any change in cardiac dynamics, they concluded that there was a direct dilator effect.

Vasculat is of very little further interest to clinicians for the treatment of angina pectoris, although BOUREL and LENOIR [202], after observing three cases of acute coronary insufficiency, express the view that it may have a favourable effect.

Reserpine

The coronary vasodilator properties of reserpine on the isolated heart of the rabbit and cat are of the papaverine type as it antagonizes the coronary vasoconstrictor action of pituitrine and barium chloride [1899, 1900]. These properties were abolished by an antihistaminic (Pyribenzamine), and adrenolytic (Regitine) and by vasoconstrictors (barium chloride, pituitrine).

Contrary to preceding observations, BULLE [254] reported the incidental finding that reserpine always reduced the coronary flow in the isolated rabbit heart, this effect being evident with doses of from 0.1 γ and being more pronounced with higher doses.

Confirming the observations of TRIPOD and MEIER [1899] we have shown that reserpine increased the coronary flow powerfully in the isolated rabbit heart [301].

According to VARMA et al. [1921], reserpine prevented the depression in S-T segment induced by the injection of picrotoxine into the lateral cerebral ventricle in the rabbit.

Clinically, LEWIS et al. [1131], using the double-blind technique and the daily report card of GREINER, showed that the alseroxylon fraction of Rauwolfia serpentina (Rauwiloid) reduced the frequency and severity of the attacks progressively and at the same time improved effort tolerance in fourteen of fifteen cases of angina pectoris; the effect was unusually prolonged. Raubasine has been reported to give promising results [1443]. RUSSEK [1594], on the other hand, found that reserpine had no therapeutic importance in this field as it did not prevent the electrocardiographic signs of myocardial ischaemia appearing in the angina patient in consequence of the performance of a standard exercise.

Padutin

Padutin which is an insulin-free pancreatic extract developped a coronary dilator effect which was double that of aminophylline on the isolated rabbit heart [486, 1379] and on the heart-lung preparation of the dog [1844]. According to GREENE [719], the fact that a considerable fall of blood pressure accompanied this increase in coronary flow proves that there is a direct effect, although of short duration. VAQUEZ et al. [1919] obtained remarkable results in about 20 angina patients with the insulin-free pancreatic extract prepared by GLEY and KISTHI-NIOS [672]. These observations were confirmed by WOLFFE et al. [2029].

FREY et al. [590, 591, 1044] have isolated from the urine of normal human subjects and animals a substance in pure form, the Frey hormone, which has pharmacological properties similar to those of insulin-free pancreatic extract and which is active in the angina syndrome [590, 591, 1107]. NUZUM and ELLIOT [1379] considered that insulin-free pancreatic extract and Frey hormone probably contain the same active principle (kallicrein). They obtained quite definitely beneficial effects with pancreatic extract in 70% of anginal patients as well as in cases of intermittent claudication.

Although some other clinical reports favoured the use of Padutin in the treatment of angina pectoris [514, 843], it must be admitted that, with the passage of time, the effects reported have become definitely less favourable in coronary diseases than in peripheral vessels disorders [1564]. Its employment is particularly indicated in disturbances of the arterial circulation in the extremities [1313] and in various pathological conditions of the peripheral arterial system in which hyperaemia brings clinical improvement [246, 589, 788, 789].

Recosen

Recosen is a total extract of fresh heart which, in the anaesthetized dog, has an augmentor effect on coronary flow which is probably due to vessel dilatation as the general blood pressure was not increased [184]. It is impossible, however, to exclude the possible intervention of changes in cardiac dynamics which undoubtedly occur, as the amplitude of contraction was increased in the isolated guinea-pig heart, perfused in the Langendorff method [1833] and in the papillary muscle [1178]. The coronary dilator effect is in no way specific, contrary to the opinion of STERN [1833], as the increase in coronary flow runs parallel with the increase in cardiac activity. On the isolated heart of the guinea-pig [357, 1621], rabbit and cat [357], Recosen reduces the resistance of the coronary vessels, and this effect cannot be due to adenosine or adenylic acid [1621], the coronary vasodilator properties of which are known [1966, 2028]. In the dog Recosen produces a transient increase of 50% in the coronary flow with a dose of 0.03 ml per g of heart in both denervated heart-lung preparation and the heart *in situ* with its nerves intact [2024]. In the normal dog Recosen cannot prevent development of the ischaemic electrocardiographic wave induced by pituitrine unless it has been administered in large doses intramuscularly for several days [1150].

Recosen has been used in the anginal syndrome by a number of clinicians [895, 1267, 1363, 1453, 1519, 1565, 1847, 1857] with favourable results which, however, do not carry conviction as the observations were not carefully controlled.

Cortunon

An aqueous extract preparation of mammalian liver [2054], Cortunon produced direct coronary vasodilator effects on the rabbit or dog heart, isolated or *in situ* [1180], which are due neither to the histamine nor to the choline which it contains [1181]. Some batches of the preparation may be three times as active as others [1182], and this probably explains the inconstancy of the results recorded in relation to the use of this preparation in clinical work on man [1646].

Heparin

The sodium salt of heparin increases the coronary flow in the anaesthetized dog slightly but the barium salt is inactive [658]. This observation suggested to its authors that the favourable results obtained in the course of anticoagulant treatment of acute cardiac infarction and in angina pectoris might be due primarily to improvement in the blood supply to the heart.

In the dog heparin definitely reduced the incidence of coronary thrombosis and myocardial infarct (seen at autopsy 24 hours after the experiment) caused by the intracoronary injection of sodium ricinoleate; it had a definitely prophylactic effect in relation to the parietal thrombus which is produced in the dog by ligature of a large left collateral branch of the anterior interventricular artery followed by subendocardial infiltration of the myocardium in the apical region with 2 ml sodium ricinoleate, this procedure being followed in heparinized animals merely by necrosis without thrombus [1771, 1772]. Also working with the dog but in a slightly different manner, AUDIER et al. [63] tied the same branch of the anterior interventricular coronary artery in animals in which the postoperative sequelae were observed clinically and electrocardiographically for a period of three weeks, after which the animals were killed and the part of the myocardium supplied by the ligatured artery was submitted to macroscopic and microscopic examination.

Two groups of animals were examined in parallel, one lot of controls which were untreated and one lot which received daily injections of heparin, 5 mg/kg, for 10 days after the operation. Clinically, there was no difference in the behaviour of the two groups but the late ischaemic electrocardiographic changes were more important and more frequent in the untreated group. The effect of heparin was more evident in the pathological aspect as the untreated dogs exhibited an extensive myocardial necrosis which was absent or very limited and circumscribed in the heparinized dogs. As the untreated animals showed few signs of thrombosis, the authors rejected the intervention of an anticoagulant effect, the results favouring a direct tissue action. On the other hand, when administered by continuous perfusion during the 24 hours following immediately after ligature of the anterior interventricular artery in the dog (102 experiments), heparin did not alter the extent of the infarct, as measured a week after occlusion of the artery [1540].

An interesting observation reported that, in the normal subject, heparin normalized the coronary blood flow when reduced by 20% during the hyperlipemic postprandial phase [1512].

Heparin is used frequently in clinical medicine in the treatment of the anginal syndrome, either alone or as complementary treatment. Heparin appears to improve the prognosis for patients who have developed myocardial infarct as a result of coronary atherosclerosis: (a) the frequency of myocardial infarction and of angina of effort was greater in the presence of high blood levels of low-density lipoproteins, and a single injection of heparin suppressed the anginal pain of effort for 3—10 days in almost 100% of patients treated [1199]; (b) the pains and the number of nitroglycerin tablets were spectacularly reduced in almost 100% of sixty anginal patients who received intravenous or intramuscular injections of 50—100 mg heparin twice weekly [704].

On the other hand, the employment of heparin in the treatment of angina did not justify itself in a number of investigations [162, 295, 750, 792, 1529, 1615, 1616, 1619] which showed that the drug was both ineffective against the subjective symptoms (number of attacks, nitroglycerin requirements) and also incapable of increasing exercise tolerance or preventing development of the electrocardiographic signs of ischaemia following performance of a standard exercise by angina patients. Having seen favourable effects in 50% of cases treated with, STEVENSON and WILSON [1838] think, however, that heparin should merit trial in patients in whom attacks are very frequent and easily produced by exertion.

Heparin seems to be indicated more in acute myocardial infarction as the prolonged treatment of 163 patients with large doses (200—300 mg daily) reduced mortality considerably in comparison with a control group and also a Dicoumarol-treated group [742].

As far as the acute pain of cardiac infarction is concerned, intravenous injection of heparin had no significant antalgic effect tested in a double-blind study [255].

A double-blind trial has been undertaken to evaluate the effect of small doses of heparin in the treatment of acute coronary occlusion. 103 patients were given 10,000 units heparin subcutaneously twice daily for 16 days and then once daily for 8 days while 109 patients were given corresponding volumes of placebo [120a]. Although death rate in both groups was not significantly different, thromboembolic complications occurred in 13.6% of the heparin group and in 25.7% of the placebo group, a statistically significant difference. The number of deaths due to such complications was 18 in the placebo group and 6 in the treated group, again a significant difference. In author's opinion, the promising result in prevention of thromboembolic complications indicates that the investigation should be continued.

Dicoumarol

In view of the concept that the favourable effects reported with Dicoumarol in coronary thrombosis cannot in all probability be explained solely by an anticoagulant effect, GILBERT and NALEFSKI [658] considered a coronary vasodilator effect possible: Dicoumarol in fact caused a considerable and prolonged increase of coronary venous flow in the heart *in situ* of the anaesthetized dog and in the isolated dog heart perfused at constant pressure; its action was greater and more prolonged than that of theobromine-sodium acetate. RUSKIN [1586] also thinks that Dicoumarol has a coronary vasodilator action, and this effect is for KRANTZ and CARR [1026] as important as the anticoagulant properties in the beneficial effects seen in the treatment of coronary thrombosis.

In view of the fact that the clinical investigations in which it was concluded that Dicoumarol had a remarkable effect on the anginal pain [115, 173, 1174, 1400, 1952] were based on excessively simple subjective methods, with no controls or sound scientific basis, GABRIELSEN and MYHRE [618] have re-examined this question by applying the Greiner method to ten anginal patients, treated for more than two years, or the equivalent of 8500 patient-days. They concluded that the Dicoumarol effect was not better than that of a placebo: neither the pain state nor the nitroglycerin requirements were changed. RUSSEK [1616, 1619] is of the same opinion.

Ilidar

RANDALL and SMITH [1494] observed increased flow in the isolated rabbit heart equal, dose for dose, to that produced by papaverine, an effect which they attribute, rather hastily, to direct coronary vasodilator action, as the drug produced marked change in both directions (reduction followed by increase) in the contractile force of the heart. In the anaesthetized dog the intracoronary injection of a large dose (1—30 mg) was followed by reduction in the coronary arterial resistance, which, as it was observed by direct measurement of the peripheral coronary pressure at the end of cardiac diastole, indicated direct dilatation of the coronary arterioles [413]. No clinical study has been made in anginous patients.

Priscol

Priscol increases the coronary flow in the perfused isolated heart of the dog and the cat, and it also increases the amplitude and frequency of the cardiac contractions; in the rabbit, on the other hand, its effect would appear to be exactly the reverse [16]. According to MEIER and MÜLLER [1264], the coronary flow in the isolated heart of the calf or rabbit is unchanged except with large doses, in which case it diminished. GOWDEY [702] found that the effect was uniformly constrictor in the rabbit, but in the cat it could be vasoconstrictor or vasodilator, depending on the animal.

In the anginal syndrome, RUSSEK [1616, 1619] has shown that the electrocardiographic abnormalities produced by exercise are uninfluenced or may even be influenced adversely by Priscol.

Hydergine

Hydergine is a mixture of equal parts of the methanesulphonates of three alkaloids of ergot, namely, dihydroergocornine, dihydroergocristine and dihydroergokryptine.

Although, as far as we know, Hydergine has never been demonstrated to have an augmentor effect on coronary flow, the various effects that it exercises on the heart should be favourable for the treatment of disturbances of the coronary circulation: (a) slowing in heart rate [1566, 1567] and reduction of systolic output [1669, 1671, 1850] resulting, along with the hypotensive effect, in reduction of the work of the heart; (b) reduction in the oxygen consumption of the myocardium. PICHUGIN [248c] has recently shown that in the anaesthetised cat, dihydroergotoxine at doses from 0.2 to 1 mg/kg by intravenous injection induces changes in coronary flow (sinusal outflow) which parallel the changes produced in the systemic blood pressure: during the hypertensive phase (first twenty minutes) the coronary flow increases by 42%. Then, with the onset of the fall in blood pressure, the flow decreased by 50%. In experiments where the blood pressure was maintained constant, the coronary flow was always reduced.

It is debatable whether these effects are associated with sympatholytic action on the tone of the coronary vessels, this being asserted only by those who consider that sympathetic nervous influences are vasoconstrictor for the coronary arteries, which is by no means certain.

SCHIMERT [1669] thinks that, although it has no true coronary vasodilator action, Hydergine does, by virtue of its various effects on the cardiovascular system, modify circulatory dynamics in such a way that what he terms the coronary reserve is improved.

Good results have been obtained with Hydergine in anginal patients, particularly those showing signs of cardiac erethism [1065, 1671, 1810, 1850, 1851]. KÜHNS [1052] considers that the effect is beneficial in 50% of patients, 7% showing restoration of a pathological electrocardiogram to normal.

Ronicol

We have found only one paper relating to the effect of Ronicol on the coronary arteries: the flow in a heart-lung preparation increased slightly [675]. From what we know of the general pharmacology of Ronicol in relation to that of nicotinic acid (of which Ronicol is an alcoholic derivative), namely that it possesses all the general actions of nicotinic acid, it can also be assumed that Ronicol should increase the coronary flow, as this effect has been described for nicotinic acid [916, 1390, 1648] and is accompanied in the isolated rabbit heart by definite increase in the amplitude of the cardiac contractions and a slight increase in their frequency [270]; the occurrence of these two latter phenomena make it impossible to attribute the increased coronary flow to a coronary vasodilator effect with certainty.

Nicotinic acid produces favourable changes in the electrocardiograms of anginal cases treated, which suggests improvement in the coronary circulation [119] and MELVILLE [1269, p. 500] mentions that the bi-weekly intravenous injection of 100—300 mg nicotinic acid for three weeks produced a beneficial effect on the clinical course of angina pectoris.

GOLDSBOROUGH [682] recorded good results in 60 cases of ischaemic heart disease with daily doses of 600 mg given by mouth. The fact that the drug lowered the plasma cholesterol levels suggests that the benefit observed in these cases cannot be entirely ascribed to vasodilatation in the heart muscle.

Ronicol does not appear to be useful in coronary affections, and RUSSEK et al. [1616, 1619] have demonstrated its inability to produce favourable changes in the electrical tracings of myocardial ischaemia produced by standardized exertion in anginal patients.

Poly-Methoxyphenol Derivatives

KARCZMAR et al. [939] described the coronary vasodilator properties of several substances derived from dimethoxyphenyl by the substitution of various alkyl groups on one of the two carbon atoms in the lateral chain; these compounds have also antiaccelerator activity in relation to the heart, but are devoid of sympathicolytic, adrenolytic and cholinergic properties. One of these derivatives, 3-dimethylamino-1,1,2-tris-(4-methoxyphenyl)-1-propene hydrochloride (Win 5494, Amotriphene, Myordil), had a coronary vasodilator activity two or three times that of papaverine. Both intracoronary and intravenous injections of Win 5494 dilated the coronary bed without increasing the forcefulness of heart contraction [192], but according to BROWN et al. [244] the contractile force of the heart increased by 20% for i.v. administration of 2 up to 16 mg/kg, heart rate being reduced respectively by 16 and 44%.

In dogs given sublethal doses of cardiac glycosides, Amotriphene was able to convert the digitalis cardiac arrhythmias to normal sinus rhythm [243, 244]. According to BOBB and GREEN [192], this substance would appear to possess the desirable traits of the nitrites and to be superior to aminophylline and papaverine as a coronary vasodilator.

In anginous patients, Amotriphene prevented the electrocardiographic signs of ischaemia appearing during a Master exercise test in only 16% of cases [1588]. According to HARRIS [784], the therapeutic subjective effect of the drug was convincing, an observation which has been confirmed in only 50% of cases by RUSKIN [1588].

The clinical effect of this drug has been studied in 13 patients with angina pectoris, using a double-blind technique [1637]: no significant differences were found between Win 5494 and the placebo; no significant change in either the consumption of nitroglycerin or in exercise tolerance tests followed administration of the drug in a dose of 25 mg four times daily.

Triparanol

An inhibitor of cholesterol biosynthesis which has been withdrawn from use, triparanol had an antianginal effect in a group of cases, most of whom had a "stable form" of angina pectoris which had not responded to a number of different medications [850]; during triparanol therapy there was in some cases a definite improvement in the ECG tracings in response to exercise.

Subsequently, considerable clinical improvement has been reported in some cases of angina [1024]. Tolerance to exercise increased [363]. Cardiac pain disappeared in severe angina after 2 months of treatment [1158]. In another clinical trial involving 18 anginous patients, half of whom experienced functional benefit when taking triparanol [767], high blood cholesterol level was reduced by the same proportion in the group of patients who were improved and in the group of cases for whom the medication was inactive. Such an observation suggested to the investigator that the occasional beneficial action of triparanol in angina could not be linked with the fall in blood cholesterol level but with other mechanisms, possibly coronary vasodilation. RUSSEK [1600], on the other hand, considers that, despite an important reduction in high cholesterol levels in almost all of the 40 cases treated, the administration of triparanol at the daily dose of 250 mg for 3—5 months did not involve any clinical improvement, the electrocardiographic tracings also being unchanged. There was no better tolerance to the Master test, even after one year of daily administration [1603, 1605].

Varia

1. 1-p-ethoxyphenyl-3-diethylamino-indane increases coronary flow in rabbit and in isolated guinea-pig heart, cardiac work being unchanged [265]. Blood pressure varies only slightly. Oxygen content in the coronary venous blood rises sharply. Coronary spasm induced by pituitrine and ergometrine was counteracted.

Since the central mechanisms of the haemodynamic regulation were not perturbed, BUSCH et al. [264, 265] consider that the substance has a special affinity for the coronary vessels. They also demonstrated that the compound modifies favourably the intramyocardial circulatory alterations (and the consecutive electrocardiographic disturbances) which arise, as an anaphylactic reaction, from the administration of a protein in the previously sensitized rabbit.

2. *Perflavon*, a salt of (β-dimethylaminoethoxy)-7 flavone and of (carboxymethyl)-7 theophylline, is a flavone derivative which increases coronary blood flow in dogs when injected intravenously at a dose of 1 mg/kg. The clinical symptomatology of angina pectoris was reported to be improved in 80% of cases [1871].

3. *Tromasedan* (dibazole), which is the benzyl-2-benzimidazole, is an antianginal drug of soviet origin that was found to increase venous coronary blood flow and myocardial oxygen consumption in animals [989].

4. *Dialicor*, which is the trade name for o-(β-diethylaminoethoxy) phenylpropiophenone hydrochloride, enhances considerably coronary blood flow in dogs and was said to yield good therapeutic results in angina [1793].

5. *Oxygen*. In cases of angina which had not been relieved by conventional medical therapy, hyperbaric oxygen improved several patients both clinically and electrocardiographically [111 c].

Carotid Sinus Nerve Stimulation

A very recent approach to the treatment of *severe* angina pectoris has been reached: carotid sinus nerve electrical activation by a chronically implanted stimulator.

It is well known that profound circulatory changes can be induced by carotid sinus nerve stimulation, which result in a decrease in myocardial oxygen consumption by reducing the four prime determinants of myocardial oxygen needs, namely heart rate, ventricular wall tension, myocardial contractility and arterial blood pressure.

Since angina pectoris results from an imbalance between the heart's oxygen needs and the oxygen supply, ideal therapy would be to restore the balance between supply and demand in as physiologic a manner as possible, by increasing oxygen delivery and by reducing oxygen demands. In practice, this is difficult to achieve, particularly in patients with diffuse, severe atherosclerosis.

With this understanding of the determinants of myocardial oxygen consumption and of the pathophysiological underlying cause of angina in mind, BRAUNWALD et al. [44 c] sought to relieve angina by lowering myocardial oxygen consumption through electrical stimulation of the carotid sinus nerves. They at first studied a group of dogs for periods up to one year and observed that they tolerated electrical stimulation of these nerves without significant deleterious side effects. Since the experimental results were promising, and as manual stimulation of the carotid sinuses can abolish attacks of angina [336 c], BRAUNWALD et al. were encouraged to apply this method clinically in patients with angina pectoris.

In a recent report, EPSTEIN et al. [94 c] summarized the therapeutic and physiologic effects of the use of a radiofrequency carotid sinus nerve stimulator, which are based on a clinical investigation involving 17 patients with severe angina. Only patients with incapacitating angina without overt evidence of cardiac failure and who were still severely limited despite intensive medical management (including long acting nitrates and propranolol) were considered as potential candidates. Furthermore, implantation of the stimulator was carried out only if several criteria were fulfilled i.e. presence of obvious vascular narrowing revealed by coronary angiography, determination of a level of bicycle exercise that reproducibly precipitated angina, increase of exercise capacity after either nitroglycerin or isosorbide dinitrate, and intact baroreceptor reflexes documented by the response to the Valsalva manoeuvre. EPSTEIN et al. reported that use of the stimulator produced appreciable symptomatic improvement in 13 of 17 patients: nearly all episodes of angina were terminated by activation of the stimulator, and prophylactic use (when the patient anticipates that a given activity may precipitate an anginal attack) increased intensity and duration of exercise that could be performed, even when the effect of electric stimulation was controlled in a double-blind fashion. After long-term use, exercise capacity was increased in many patients. According to the results of haemodynamic measurements which were recorded in the course of an exercises program with use of the implanted stimulator, EPSTEIN et al. concluded that the physiologic changes most probably responsible for relieving the angina are a reduction in sympathetic stimulation to the heart and arterial bed, thereby diminishing two major determinants of myocardial oxygen consumption, arterial pressure and, to a lesser extent, heart rate.

The demonstration of such symptomatic benefit has aroused renewed interest in the general circulatory effects of the stimulation of carotid sinus nerves and specifically in the mechanisms involved in the relief of ischaemic cardiac pain. It was at first considered that the relief of angina afforded by carotid sinus nerve stimulation resulted entirely from a reduction of myocardial oxygen requirements. But the possibility was also raised that coronary vasodilatation may occur. Although FALICOV et al. [95c] and FEIGL [98c] found some restriction of this vascular bed during electric nerve stimulation in anaesthetised dogs, SOLTI et al. observed a considerable increase in coronary blood flow [296c]. Furthermore, experiments carried out on conscious dogs in whom a carotid sinus nerve stimulator had been implanted showed that the coronary blood flow typically remained close to control levels, but it decreased in some dogs while in other cases it actually increased [321c, 322c]. Calculated coronary vascular resistance declined by an average of 22% [322c], a phenomenon which was shown to be mediated primarily by a reduction of sympathetic vasoconstrictor impulses to the coronary bed. Thus, the possibility that coronary vasodilatation occurs in man must also be considered [44c]. But the most interesting events found in both anaesthetised and conscious dogs during carotid sinus nerves electric activation were a significant decrease in myocardial contractility and in cardiac work, due to a reduction in heart rate and in arterial pressure [95c, 321c, 322c]. The findings in dog are thus consonant with the observations in man.

In the opinion of BRAUNWALD and associates, the early clinical results have been sufficiently encouraging to warrant continued trial of this new mode of therapy [44c, 50c, 89c, 156c], which has also been applied in FRANCE [166c, 313c].

The surgical procedure for implanting the electrodes and the receiving unit is described by BRAUNWALD et al. [44c].

A carotid sinus nerve stimulator has been constructed (Angistat CSNS Medtronic). The patient may activate the device prophylactically prior to activity known to precipitate an anginal attack or he may use it at the onset of an attack to gain immediate relief of pain.

It must be pointed out that the fitting of such a stimulator for therapeutic purposes implies a certain risk because of the fact that it calls for an operation under general anaesthetic. Because of this, it should be restricted to patients for whom all medical steps taken hitherto have not been successful in diminishing the frequency of angina pectoris attacks [87a]. The question of the relative merits of carotid sinus nerve stimulation versus implantation of the internal mammary artery into the ischaemic myocardium or of reconstructive coronary artery surgery in patients with refractory angina pectoris is not settled. However, it appears that the method of providing symptomatic relief of angina by carotid sinus nerve stimulation is preferable in older patients with advanced heart disease, in whom the risks of thoracotomy are particularly hazardous [87a]. The same surgical procedure has also been applied for the treatment of essential hypertension [289c].

To round off this survey devoted to the antianginal medications at present available, there is no doubt that since the beginning of this century specialised research workers dealing with this type of activity have been increasingly concerned with and have succeeded in developing drugs with a real capacity for bringing considerable benefit to those suffering from angina pectoris. It can be anticipated that even more substantial progress will be made in the next few years. With ever closer cooperation between various branches of activity, with special emphasis on synthetic chemistry, pharmacology and biochemistry, biologists should be able in the future to develop more effective antianginal medications, either by following the lines at present considered to be promising because of the success they have achieved or by the opening up of other lines of research as yet unforeseeable.

Of these latter, some may be pioneered by pathophysiologists, notably in the field of myocardial biochemistry. Indeed, although certain metabolic processes of the normal cardiac muscle are beginning to be properly understood, the same is far from true as regards the myocardium of the anginal subject. True, the clinical investigation of the various aspects of cardiac metabolism in patients suffering from atherosclerosis and coronary insufficiency has already been under way for several years past, but the results it has achieved still remain fragmentary. The paucity of such knowledge is primarily due to the fact that it only relates to cardiac musculature as a whole, whereas there is no doubt whatsoever that the metabolic processes of the anginal subject's myocardium vary from one area to another, as is the case with the healthy myocardium.

It has been shown for instance that in the normal heart the blood supply to the inner layers of the ventricular wall is not equal to that which irrigates the outer layers. Moreover blood vessels leading to both layers are not the same [121 c]. It was also demonstrated [149 c], that in the normal heart, myocardial tissue pressure exceeding arterial blood pressure throughout systole in the inner half of the left ventricular wall, the gradient in coronary resistance which results therefrom causes a corresponding gradient in nutrient blood flow, to the extent that this latter in the deepest regions of the ventricular musculature is only half that found in the superficial ones. This flow gradient in turn causes transmural gradients in tissue oxygen tension and cell metabolism. Circulation through the left ventricular wall involves three pathways: epicardial, endocardial and collateral. If, for the sake of simplicity, the collateral circulation is not taken into account in these considerations since the regulatory factors are the same in this system as in the endocardial region [10e], we can take as a basis the schematic drawing of the circulation through the thickness of the left ventricle proposed by WINBURY et al. [2013] on the grounds of known anatomical features and which shows that the epicardial and endocardial regions compete for the available blood flow because of the unique pattern of circulation. This results in underperfusion of the inner layers, which is evidenced not only by a lower nutrient circulation in the endocardium but also by a lower tissue oxygen tension: WINBURY et al. [11e] have effectively shown that a transmural gradient of oxygen tension exists through the wall of the left ventricle and that the deeper subendocardial layers are relatively ischaemic as compared to the subepicardial layers.

If to these data relating to the normal cardiac muscle there is added the fact that the cardiac necrosis which follows a coronary occlusion is far more extensive and severe in the sub-endocardiac part of the ventricular wall, it will be realised that metabolic deteriorations resulting from the disturbances brought about in the blood flow by the atherosclerotic lesions found in coronary subjects must differ widely from one area of the cardiac musculature to another.

There are also good evidences to postulate that there are inequalities of myocardial perfusion in coronary artery disease [273 c], but direct measurement of blood flow in individual arteries and collateral vessels are required to demonstrate the validity of this concept. It was shown recently that myocardial perfusion is heterogeneous in some patients with coronary artery disease and that reduced regional perfusion may be localized to discrete lesions of coronary vessels [52c]: in 9 subjects with normal coronary arteries, mean myocardial blood flows ranged between normal values; in some patients with angiographic narrowing of coronary artery branches, myocardial perfusion was also normal in regions distal to minimal lesions and in regions beyond occlusions which were well supplied with collateral vessels but, in other patients, significantly reduced myocardial irrigation was observed in areas of myocardial fibrosis or areas of myocardium distal to markedly constricted or occluded vessels which were without visible collateral circulation.

Furthermore, regional variations in myocardial performance exist in normal hearts as revealed by coronary cineangiography, using biplane filming [187c]. This has been shown by measuring the true spatial distances between coronary bifurcations (which provide a myriad of epicardial landmarks) on successive biplane cine frames, a procedure which allows the onset, extent and rate of epicardial segment shortening to be quantitated and compared in multiple areas of the heart. Such regional variations in myocardial performance are exaggerated in coronary heart disease, and the myocardial segments supplied by stenotic arteries have a delay in mechanical activation and show either systolic lengthening or marked reduction in both extent and rate of shortening.

Segmentary exploration of the cardiac muscle aimed at investigating metabolic deteriorations due to coronary atherosclerosis or to degenerative myocardial lesions is at present still handicapped by the difficulty of gathering in humans the "fractional" biological material necessary for such examinations. Any progress in this area is thus closely linked to the development of new investigation techniques, especially as regards methods and apparatus. Some attempts in this direction are now in progress both in animal and man. A technique for the study of *local* metabolic changes in coronary venous blood draining from a small area of ischaemic myocardium has been designed for acute experiments in dogs [240c]. Positive changes in values for local coronary venous blood lactate, pyruvate, lactate/pyruvate ratio, glucose, phosphate and potassium detected by local coronary venous sampling were not observed in coronary sinus blood samples. Clinical implications are that negative metabolic changes in blood samples obtained by presently available methods from the coronary venous system of patients with ischaemic heart disease in no way exclude gross local venous metabolic changes. In man, a method was devised to study regional myocardial perfusion by simultaneously measuring the clearance constants of Xe^{133} washout from multiple areas of myocardium with a multiple-crystal scintillation camera [52c]. The perfusion patterns so obtained were compared to the coronary vascular patterns observed in the same patients by angiography. In 25 subjects, Xe^{133} dissolved in saline was injected into the right and/or left coronary artery and counts/sec were recorded on magnetic tape from each of 294 NaI scintillation crystals viewing the precordium via a multichannel collimator. The slopes of the initial monoexponential segment of the isotope washout curves were calculated for each crystal by the method of least squares on an IBM 360/91 computer. Myocardial blood flow was also calculated assuming a partition coefficient of 0.72. Scintiphotographs showing isotope arrival and washout from different regions of myocardium were made by replaying the tape on an oscilloscope.

It is also vital that research workers should carry out parallel metabolic and clinical investigations in man, since a more thorough understanding of the metabolic deterioration underlying clinical manifestations should contribute to improved knowledge of the pathogenesis of ischaemic heart disease. It is only in the light of the data obtained by correlating clinical facts and biochemical observations that it will be easier to interpret the metabolic effects of antianginal medications, since the biochemical characteristics of the normal heart and of the diseased heart as known at present still fall far short of enabling us to say in what direction myocardial metabolism should be diverted if a therapeutic benefit is to be obtained [79 c, 410].

Even if this line of research, which would in fact tend towards the biochemical correction of the myocardial functional disturbances producing the anginal syndrome, were to lead to perfecting effective therapeutic media, it could still be held that these were rather more of a symptomatic than prophylactic character. This is why a special interest should be attached to research which is being developed in parallel and which aims at stabilising, diminishing and, even better, preventing the development of coronary atherosclerosis, the major initial cause of angina-producing coronary insufficiency. The therapeutic prospects offered by this research are certainly not immediate, but they are probably very real.

Pending the results of such diverse and probably promising developments in medicinal research, there is no doubt that effective means are even now within the reach of the medical practitioner. He has a wide choice of antianginal medications which, as shown by the facts outlined in this monograph, owe their therapeutic effect to highly diverse mechanisms. It is up to him to use them with the full knowledge of the facts, on rational grounds dictated primarily by the aetiology and symptomatology of each case taken individually, and also in the light of such side effects as these medications might entail. These undesirable effects should nevertheless be gauged in a critical light, and especially with an eye to the individual severity of the disease in question. Whilst bearing in mind the "primum non nocere" of Hippocrates, the doctor must appreciate that any therapeutic action which entails the use of active medications necessarily involves the hasard inherent in any effective form of treatment. Faced with the possible use of genuinely effective medications, any negative therapeutic attitude justifying itself by systematic fear of risk or by the practitioner's preoccupation with his own peace of mind is a medically indefensible abdication. It may also be prejudicial to the patient, since by reason of its unfavourable prognosis, angina pectoris jeopardises the patient's health in a chronically incapacitating manner, produces an especially uncomfortable social state dominated by constant apprehension, sometimes severely handicaps professional activity, and last but not least lays the subject open to cardiac episodes which are often irreducible and to the constant threat of sudden death which is always unpredictable.

Faced with an undoubted anginal syndrome, systematic therapeutic abstention as regards long term antianginal medication on the part of the practitioner can be considered as an attitude running contrary to the Hippocratic precept and to the moral responsibility of the doctor whose duty it is to see to the social rehabilitation of the patient suffering from angina pectoris. As things stand at present as regards the treatment of coronary insufficiency, the doctor can no longer be satisfied with applying a purely symptomatic treatment. As VASTESAEGER [1927] puts it: "L'angor coronarien typique ou atypique est de loin le symptome le plus fréquent en cardiologie. Il représente, pour celui qui en subit les premières atteintes, un choc moral d'autant plus grave que les profanes savent que l'évolution du mal coronarien est souvent inexorable et qu'elle peut mener vers une mort brutale ou douloureuse. Ces deux raisons font que le cardiologue se doit de consacrer au traitement de l'angor coronarien un effort maximal. Aussi ne peut-il se contenter, comme le voudraient certains désabusés, de prescrire de la nitroglycérine pour couper les crises douloureuses. Il importe en effet que le malade soit persuadé que son médecin essaye au moins de prévenir les sensations angoreuses et qu'il ne borne pas son action à un traitment palliatif et par trop manifestement symptomatique".

Table 16. *Main side effects in man of the most commonly used antianginal drugs*

Trade name	Generic name or common name or code number	Side effects
Adenylocrat	—	Specific data not available
Algocor	Benziodarone	See Amplivix
Aminal	Triethanolamine trinitrate (Trolnitrate phosphate)	See Metamine
Aminocardol	Theophylline ethylene diamine (Aminophylline)	Gastric discomfort, nausea, vomiting
Amplivix	Benziodarone	Gastrointestinal disturbances, diarrhoea. Potentiation of some anticoagulants
Anginine	Glyceryl trinitrate (Nitroglycerin)	See Trinitrin
Angitrit	Triethanolamine trinitrate (Trolnitrate phosphate)	See Metamine
Angoron	Amiodarone (L. 3428)	See Cordarone
Aptin	Alprenolol (H 56/28)	All side effects inherent to the β-blocking drugs (see Inderal)
Avlocardyl	Propranolol	See Inderal
Baralgin	—	Specific data not available
Baxacor	Etafenon	Specific data not available
Cardilate	Erythrityl tetranitrate	Severe pulsatile headache. Mild gastrointestinal disturbances
Cardiloid	Erythrityl tetranitrate	See Cardilate
Cardine	—	See Carduben
Cardivix	Benziodarone	See Amplivix
Carduben	—	Specific data not available
Carvasin	Isosorbide dinitrate	See Isordil
Cholegyl, Choledyl	Choline theophyllinate (Oxtriphylline)	Gastric discomfort. Nausea, vomiting
Clinium	Lidoflazine	Arrhythmias which may be severe. Flushing of the face. Gastro-intestinal disturbances. Headache, vertigo, tinnitus
Complamin	Oxypropyltheophylline nicotinate (Xanthinol nicotinate)	Specific data not available
Cordarone	Amiodarone (L. 3428)	Corneal deposits. Bradycardia principally with high dosage and prolonged treatment in elderly patients. Actinic dermatitis
Cordilox	Iproveratril, Verapamil	See Isoptin
Corontin	Prenylamine	See Hostaginan
Dociton	Propranolol	See Inderal
Duotrate	Pentaerythritol tetranitrate	See Peritrate
Eraldin	Practolol (ICI 50.172)	Bradycardia and cardiac insufficiency with overdosage. Occasionally: skin rashes, nausea, sleep disturbance, paraesthesia
Erinitrit	Sodium nitrite	Hypotension
Etrynit	Propatylnitrate	Headache. Postural hypotension
Eucilat	Benfurodil	Specific data not available
Gina	Propatylnitrate	See Etrynit

Table 16 continued

Trade name	Generic name or common name or code number	Side effects
Gubernal	Alprenolol (H 56/28)	See Aptin
Hostaginan	Prenylamine	Nausea, vomiting, diarrhoea. Flushing. Skin rashes
Ildamen	Oxyfedrine	Specific data not available
Inderal	Propranolol	Bradycardia, cardiac insufficiency, bronchospasm. Occasionally: gastrointestinal disturbances, tiredness and dizziness. Feelings of faintness or weakness associated with bradycardia and/or hypotension
INPEA	—	Specific data not available
Intensaine	Carbochromen, Chromonar	Arthralgia
Irrigor	Imolamine (LA 1211)	Somnolence, vertigo, lipothymia
Isoptin	Iproveratril, Verapamil	Cardiac insufficiency and arrhythmia following intravenous administration
Isordil	Isosorbide dinitrate	Throbbing vascular headaches (may be severe and persistent). Cutaneous vasodilation with flushing. Transient dizziness and weakness. Postural hypotension
Kellin	Khellin	Nausea which may be particularly troublesome. Insomnia, vertigo, weakness, fatigue, depression, anorexia, epigastric distress, constipation, vomiting
Maxitate	Mannitol hexanitrate	See Nitranitol
Mederel	Amoproxan (730 C.E.R.M.)	Withdrawn from use in 1970. Cutaneousmucosae manifestations with phlyctenae. Stomatitis, dysphagia. Optic neuritis
Metamine	Triethanolamine trinitrate (Trolnitrate phosphate)	Headache. Gastrointestinal disturbances. Transient episodes of dizziness and weakness
Myocardol	Pentaerythritol tetranitrate	See Peritrate
Nilatil	Itramin tosylate	Specific data not available
Nitranitol	Mannitol hexanitrate	Specific data not available
Nitretamin	Triethanolamine trinitrate (Trolnitrate phosphate)	See Metamine
Nitroglyn	Glyceryl trinitrate	Specific data not available
Nitrol	Glyceryl trinitrate	Headache
Nitropol	Glyceryl trinitrate	See Nitroglyn
Octyl nitrite	—	Throbbing vascular headaches. Flushing. Dizziness and weakness. Hypotension
Ortin	Triethanolamine trinitrate (Trolnitrate phosphate)	See Metamine
Pavabid	Papaverine	Nausea, gastric distress, anorexia, constipation, weakness, drowsiness, vertigo, sweating, headache
Pentafin	Pentaerythritol tetranitrate	See Peritrate
Pentanitrine	Pentaerythritol tetranitrate	See Peritrate
Pentritol	Pentaerythritol tetranitrate	See Peritrate

21*

Table 16 continued

Trade name	Generic name or common name or code number	Side effects
Peritrate	Pentaerythritol tetranitrate	Headache. Nausea. Gastrointestinal disturbances
Persantine	Dipyridamole	Gastrointestinal intolerance. Nausea, vomiting, diarrhoea. Headache, vertigo, dizziness
Pexid	Perhexiline	Specific data not available
Prenitron	Triethanolamine trinitrate (Trolnitrate phosphate)	See Metamine
Provismine	—	See Carduben
Quintrate	Pentaerythritol tetranitrate	See Peritrate
Recetan	Butidrine	All side effects inherent to the β-blocking drugs (see Inderal)
Reoxyl	Hexobendine, Hexabendin	See Ustimon
Retrangor	Benziodarone	See Amplivix
Sandolanid	—	Specific data not available
Segontin	Prenylamine	See Hostaginan
Sorbitrate	Isosorbide dinitrate	See Isordil
Sotalol	M.J. 1999	All side effects inherent to the β-blocking drugs (see Inderal)
Sursum	Iproclozide	Orthostatic hypotension. Liver damage. Potentiation of many medications in current use
Sustac	Glyceryl trinitrate	See Nitroglyn
Synadrin	Prenylamine	See Hostaginan
Tetranitrin	Erythrityl tetranitrate	See Cardilate
Tetranitrol	Erythrityl tetranitrate	See Cardilate
Trangorex	Amiodarone (L. 3428)	See Cordarone
Trasicor	Oxprenolol (Ciba 39089-Ba)	All side effects inherent to the β-blocking drugs (see Inderal)
Trinitrin	Glyceryl trinitrate (Nitroglycerin)	Headache. Cutaneous vasodilation with flushing. Skin rashes
Ustimon	Hexobendine, Hexabendin	None has been reported
Vaporol	Amyl nitrite	Headache
Vasangor	Propatylnitrate	See Etrynit
Vasodiatol	Pentaerythritol tetranitrate	See Peritrate
Vastarel	Trimetazidine	Specific data not available
Vialibran	Medibazine	Specific data not available
Vibeline	—	See Carduben
Visken	Pindolol (LB 46)	All side effects inherent to the β-blocking drugs (see Inderal)
Visnadin	—	See Carduben
Visnamine	—	See Carduben

References: 1. MEYLER, L. — Side effects of drugs. Excerpta Medica Foundation, 1966.
2. The MERCK Index, 8th Edition, 1968.
3. GOODMAN, L.S., GILMAN, A. — The pharmacological basis of therapeutics, 4th Edition. New-York: Macmillan Cy, 1970.

References

1. ABAZA, A., RUTLISBERGER, P.A.: Presse méd. **68**, 963 (1960).
2. ABERG, G., DZEDIN, T., LUNDHOLM, L., OLSSON, L., SVEDMYR, N.: Life Sci. **8**, 353 (1969).
3. ABLAD, B., BROGARD, M., Ek, L.: Acta Pharmacol. Toxicol. **25**, Suppl. 2, 9 (1967).
4. — JOHNSSON, G., NORRBY, A., SÖLVELL, L.: Acta Pharmacol. Toxicol. **25**, Suppl. 2, 85 (1967).
5. ABRAHAMSEN, A.M., KIIL, F.: Brit. med. J. **1**, 456 (1966).
6. ABRAMS, W.B., BECKER, M.C., LEWIS, D.W., KILLOUGH, J.H.: Amer. J. Cardiol. **5**, 634 (1960).
7. — LEWIS, D.W., SHOSHKES, M., ROTHFELD, E., BECKER, M.: Amine oxidase inhibitors in angina pectoris. Symposium International on "The Catecholamines in Cardiovascular Pathology". Burlington (Vermont), 23 Aug. 1959, Summary, p. 6.
8. ACETO, M.D., KINNARD, W.J., BUCKLEY, J.P.: Fed. Proc. **20**, 102 (1961).
9. — — — Fed. Proc. **22**, 304 (1962).
10. AELLIG, W.H., PRICHARD, B.N.C., RICHARDSON, G.A.: Brit. J. Pharmacol. **37**, 527 (1969).
11. AFONSO, S.: Amer. J. Physiol. **216**, 297 (1969).
12. — O'BRIEN, G.S.: Circulat. Res. **20**, 403 (1967).
13. — — CRUMPTON, C.W.: a) J. Lab. clin. Med. **68**, 852 (1966). b) Circulat. Res. **22**, 43 (1968).
14. AHLQUIST, R.P.: Amer. J. Physiol. **153**, 586 (1948).
15. — Ann. Rev. Pharmacol. **8**, 259 (1968).
16. — HUGGINS, R.A., WOODBURY, R.A.: J. Pharmacol. exp. Ther. **89**, 271 (1947).
17. AKKER, S. van den, BIJLSMA, U.G., VAN DONGEN, K., TEN THIJE, J.H.: Arzneimittel-Forsch. **7**, 15 (1957).
18. ALBERT, A.: J. Lancet **81**, 112 (1961).
19. ALDINGER, E.E.: Circulat. Res. **22**, 589 (1968).
20. ALGAN, O., KIENLE, H.: Med. Mschr. **21**, 232 (1967).
21. ALLANBY, K.D., COX, A.G.C., MACLEAN, K.S., PRICE, T.M.L., SOUTHWELL, N.: Lancet **1961 I**, 138.
22. ALLMARK, M.G., LU, F.C., CARMICHAEL, E., LAVALLEE, A.: Amer. Rev. Tuberc. **68**, 199 (1953).
23. ALTMAN, G.E., RISEMAN, J.E.F., KORETSKY, S.: Amer. J. med. Sci. **240**, 66 (1960).
24. ALTSCHULE, M.D.: Amer. Heart J. **27**, 322 (1944).
25. ALVARO, A.B., MacALPIN, R.N., KATTUS, A.A.: Circulation **36**, Suppl. 2, 51 (1967).
26. AMMERMANN, E.O.: Med. Welt **18**, 1498 (1967).
27. AMSTERDAM, E.A., GORLIN, R., WOLFSON, S.: J. Amer. med. Ass. **210**, 103 (1969).
28. — WOLFSON, S., GORLIN, R.: Ann. intern. Med. **68**, 1151 (1968).
29. — — — Amer. J. Cardiol. **23**, 104 (1969).
30. — — — Amer. J. Cardiol. **24**, 305 (1969).
31. ANDERSON, F.F., CAMERON, A.: J. Amer. pharm. Ass. **39**, 183 (1950).
32. — CRAVER, B.N.: J. Pharmacol. exp. Ther. **93**, 135 (1948).
33. ANDRUS, C.E.: Circulation **22**, 979 (1960).
34. ANGARSKAYA, M.A., KHADZHAI, Y.I., KOLESNIKOV, D.G., PROKOPENKO, A.P., DUBINSKY, A.A., SHUBOV, M.I.: Klin. Med. **36**, 29 (1958), abstract in Circulation **18**, 466 (1958).
35. ANGKAPINDU, A., STAFFORD, A., THORP, R.H.: Arch. int. Pharmacodyn. **119**, 194 (1959).
36. ANREP, G.V.: Medical Sciences **3**, 245 (1936).
37. — BARSOUM, G.S., KENAWY, M.R.: Gaz. Faculty Med. Cairo **2**, 1 (1947).
38. — — — J. Pharm. Pharmacol. **1**, 164 (1949).
39. — — — MISRAHY, G.: Brit. Heart J. **8**, 171 (1946).
40. — — — — Lancet **1947 I**, 557.
41. — — SCHÖNBERG, A.: J. Pharm. Pharmacol. **5**, 166 (1953).
42. — — TALAAT, M.: J. Physiol. (Lond.) **86**, 431 (1936).
43. — BLALOCK, A., HAMMOUDA, M.: J. Physiol. (Lond.) **67**, 87 (1929).
44. — HÄUSLER, H.: J. Physiol. (Lond.) **65**, 357 (1928).
45. — KENAWY, M.R., BARSOUM, G.S.: Amer. Heart J. **37**, 531 (1949).
46. ANTHONY, J.R., JICK, H., SPODICK, D.H.: Amer. Heart J. **77**, 598 (1969).
47. ANTONIO, A., ROCHA E SILVA, M.: Circulat. Res. **11**, 910 (1962).
48. APTHORP, G.H., CHAMBERLAIN, D.A., HAYWARD, G.W.: Brit. Heart J. **26**, 218 (1964).
49. Aptin: Leaflet ASTRA (Sweden), p. 24 and 28.
50. ARAVANIS, C., LUISADA, A.A.: Ann. intern. Med. **44**, 1111 (1956).

51. ARBORELIUS, M., LECEROF, H., MALM, A., MALMBORG, R.O.: Brit. Heart J. **30**, 407 (1968).
52. ARESKOG, N.H., ADOLFSSON, L.: Brit. med. J. **1969**II, 601.
53. ARMAND, P., PAECHT, A., LICHAH, E., BREMOND, C.: Gaz. Hôp. (Paris) **142**, 205 (1970).
54. ARMBRUST, C.A., LEVINE, S.A.: Amer. J. med. Sci. **220**, 127 (1950).
55. ARMITAGE, A.K., BOSWOOD, J., LARGE, B.J.: Brit. J. Pharmacol. **16**, 59 (1961).
56. ARONOW, W.S., KAPLAN, M.A.: a) New Engl. J. Med. **280**, 847 (1969); b) Ann. intern. Med. **70**, 1072 (1969).
57. ASCHENBECK, G.: Dtsch. med. J. **16**, 137 (1965).
58. ASKANAZY, S.: Dtsch. Arch. klin. Med. **56**, 209 (1895).
59. ASTROM, H.: Brit. Heart J. **30**, 44 (1968).
60. ATTERHÖG, J.H., PORJÉ, G.: Svenska Läk.-Tidn. **63**, 2071 (1966).
61. AUDIER, M., SERRADIMIGNI, A., POGGI, L., BORY, M., DIANE, P.: Arch. Méditerr. méd. **5**, 265 (1969).
62. — ARNOUX, E., GIRAUD, M.: Sem. Hôp. (Thérapeutique) **42**, 355 (1966).
63. — DEVIN, R., BONNEAU, H., RUF, G.: Presse méd. **62**, 803 (1954).
64. AYAD, H.: Lancet **1949**I, 305.
65. BABEL, J., STANGOS, N.: Arch. Ophthal. **30**, 197 (1970).
66. BACHAND, R.T., SOMANI, P., HARDMAN, H.T.: Clin. Res. **16**, 221 (1968).
67. BACQ, Z.M., CHEYMOL, J., DALLEMAGNE, M.J., HAZARD, R., LABARRE, J., REUSE, J.J., WELSCH, M.: Pharmacodynamie biochimique, Ed. Sciences et Lettres, Liège, 1961, p. 176.
68. BAEDER, D.H.: Fed. Proc. **20**, 103 (1961).
69. BAER, S., HEINE, W.I., GELFOND, D.B.: Amer. J. med. Sci. **215**, 542 (1948).
70. BAGOURI, M.M.: J. Pharm. Pharmacol. **1**, 177 (1949).
71. BAISSE, J.: Bull. Soc. chim. Fr. p. 769 (1949).
72. BAKER, J.B.E.: J. Physiol. (Lond.) **115**, 30P (1951).
73. BAKER, L.D., LESHIN, S.J., SHARMA, G.V.R.K., MESSER, J.V.: Amer. J. Cardiol. **23**, 104 (1969).
74. — MATHUR, V.S., LESHIN, S.J., MESSER, J.V.: Circulation **38**, Suppl. 6, 37 (1968).
75. BAKST, H., KISSIN, M., LEIBOWITZ, S., RINZLER, S.: Amer. Heart J. **36**, 527 (1948).
76. BALAGUER-VINTRO, I., OTER RODRIGUEZ, R., DUARTE MANTILLA, G., VILALTA BERNET, C.: An. Med. (Med.) **55**, 97 (1969).
77. BALATRE, P., MERLEN, J.F.: Thérapie **15**, 83 (1960).
78. — — GRANJEAN, L.: Presse méd. **57**, 1067 (1949).
79. BALCON, R., JEWITT, D.E., DAVIES, J.P.H., ORAM, S.: a) Amer. Heart J. **74**, 582 (1967); b) Lancet **1966**II, 917.
80. — MALOY, W.C., SOWTON, E.: Brit. med. J. **3**, 91 (1968).
81. BALDES, E.J., HERRICK, J.F.: Proc. Soc. exp. Biol. (N.Y.) **37**, 432 (1937).
82. BALL, K.P.: Lancet **1948**I, 116.
83. BANES, D.: J. pharm. Sci. **57**, 893 (1968).
84. BANKS, T., SHUGOLL, G.I.: J. Amer. med. Ass. **200**, 1031 (1967).
85. BANSE, H.J., ZAHNOW, W.: Münch. med. Wschr. **52**, 2036 (1958).
86. BARBARESI, F., BACUZZI, E., MANFREDI, M., STARCICH, R.: G. Clin. med. **47**, 849 (1966).
87. BARBI, G.L., TALLONE, G.: Clin. ter. **32**, 236 (1965).
88. BARGHEER, R., FIEGEL, G., SAITO, S., GUTTMANN, W.: Arzneimittel-Forsch. **17**, 288 (1967).
89. BAROLDI, G., MANTERO, O., SCOMOZONI, G.: Circulat. Res. **4**, 223 (1956).
90. BAROUSCH, R.: Wien. klin. Wschr. **79**, 856 (1967).
91. BARRERA, J.A., TURIELLA, R.G.: Pren. méd. argent. **47**, 111 (1959).
92. BARRETT, A.M.: J. Pharm. Pharmacol. **21**, 241 (1969).
93. — CROWTHER, A.F., DUNLOP, D., SHANKS, R.C., SMITH, L.H.: Arch. Pharmacol. exp. Path. **259**, 152 (1968).
94. BARRETT, C.T.: S. Afr. med. J. **26**, 734 (1952).
95. BARRY, A.J., DALY, J.W., PRUETT, E.D.R., STEINMETZ, J.R., BIRKHEAD, N.C., RODAHL, K.: Amer. J. Cardiol. **17**, 1 (1966).
96. BARSOUM, G.S., KENAWY, M.R.: Amer. Heart J. **47**, 297 (1954).
97. BARTELSTONE, H.J., SCHERLAG, B.J., CRANEFIELD, P.F., HOFFMAN, B.F.: Bull. N.Y. Acad. Med. **42**, 951 (1966).
98. BARTHEL, W., MARKWARDT, F.: Biochem. Pharmacol. **18**, 1899 (1969).
99. BARZIN, J.: Rev. méd. Liège **23**, 135 (1968).
100. — FRESON, A.: Brux.-méd. **49**, 105 (1969).
101. BASTENIE, P.A., VANHAELST, L., NEVE, P.: Lancet **1967**II, 1221.
102. BATEMAN, F.J.A.: Lancet **1967**II, 418.
103. BATLOUNI, M., BETOLAMI, V., DUPRAT, R.: Arqui. Brasil. Cardiol. **21**, 321 (1968).

104. BATTERMAN, R.C.: J. Amer. med. Ass. **157**, 1333 (1955).
105. — Ann. N.Y. Acad. Sci. **64**, 499 (1956).
106. — GROSSMAN, A.J., SCHWIMMER, J., BLACKMAN, A.L.: J. Amer. med. Ass. **157**, 234 (1955).
107. — MOURATOFF, C.J.: Calif. Med. **98**, 318 (1963).
108. BATTOCK, D.J., ALVAREZ, H., CHIDSEY, C.A.: Circulation **38**, Suppl. 6, 39 (1968).
109. — — — Circulation **39**, 157 (1969).
110. BAUDINE, A., CHAILLET, F., CHARLIER, R., HOSSLET, A.: Arch. int. Pharmacodyn. **169**, 469 (1967).
111. BAUE, A.: J. Amer. med. Ass. **208**, 849 (1969).
112. BAUMGARTEN, A.: Med. J. Aust. **49**, 429 (1962).
113. BAY, G., LARSEN, L.P., LORENTSEN, E., SIVERTSSEN, E.: Brit. med. J. **1967I**, 141.
114. BAYLEY, R.H., LA DUE, J.S., YORK, D.J.: Amer. Heart J. **27**, 657 (1944).
115. BEAUMONT, J.L., COBLENTZ, B., MAURICE, P., CHEVALIER, H., LENEGRE, J.: Sem. Hôp. Paris **28**, 1926 (1952).
116. BECK, C.S., LEIGHNINGER, D.S.: J. Amer. med. Ass. **156**, 1226 (1954).
117. BECKER, A.: Medizinische **52**, 2152 (1958).
118. BECKER, M.C.: J. Amer. med. Ass. **203**, 56 (1968).
119. BECKMAN, H.: Pharmacology in Clinical Practice, 1 vol., 839 pp. Philadelphia and London: Saunders and Co. 1954, p. 191.
120. BECKSCHÄFER, W.: Arzneimittel-Forsch. **18**, 1079 (1968).
121. BEECHER, H.K.: J. Amer. med. Ass. **158**, 399 (1955).
122. — J. Amer. med. Ass. **159**, 1602 (1955).
123. BEKAERT, J.: Personal communication 1968.
124. — AUBERT, P.: Ther. Umsch. **18**, 317 (1961).
125. — — Ther. Umsch. **28**, 326 (1966).
126. — DELTOUR, G., BROEKHUYSEN, J.: Arch. int. Pharmacodyn. **132**, 339 (1961).
127. BELL, H., AZARNOFF, D.L., DUNN, M.: Clin. Pharmacol. Ther. **9**, 40 (1968).
128. BELLIVEAU, R.E., COVINO, B.G.: Arch. int. Pharmacodyn. **180**, 341 (1969).
129. BEN, M., WARREN, M., DRINNON, V., SCOTT, C.: Angiology **11**, 62 (1960).
130. BENAIM, S., DIXON, M.F.: Brit. med. J. **5104**, 1069 (1958).
131. BENDA, L., DONEFF, D., LUJF, A., MOSER, K.: Wien. med. Wschr. **117**, 829 (1967).
132. BENDER, F., SCHMIDT, E.: Vth European Congress of Cardiology, Athenes, Sept. 1968, Abstracts p. 41.
133. BENFEY, B.G., GREEFF, K., HEEG, E.: Brit. J. Pharmacol. **30**, 23 (1967).
134. BENTHE, H.F., CHENPANICH, K.: Arch. Pharmacol. exp. Path. **255**, 3 (1966).
135. BERGEN, S.S., jr., VAN ITALLIE, T.B., SEBRELL, W.H.: Proc. Soc. exp. Biol. (N.Y.) **103**, 39 (1960).
136. BERKESY, L.: Ther. d. Gegenw. **73**, 55 (1932).
137. BERMAN, J.K., FIELDS, D.C., JUDY, H., MORI, V., PARKER, R.J.: Surgery **39**, 399 (1956).
138. BERNAL, P., ABITEBOUL, J.: Sem. thér. **44**, 2338 (1968).
139. BERNE, R.M.: Circulat. Res. **6**, 644 (1958).
140. — Amer. J. Physiol. **204**, 317 (1963).
141. — Physiol. Rev. **44**, 1 (1964).
142. — Circulat. Res. **14—15**, Suppl. 261 (1964).
143. — BLACKMON, J.R., GARDNER, T.H.: J. clin. Invest. **36**, 1101 (1957).
144. BERNSMEIER, A., RUDOLPH, W.: Münch. med. Wschr. **104**, 46 (1962).
145. BERNSTEIN, A., SOMON, F.: Vasc. Dis. **2**, 6 (1965).
146. BERNSTEIN, L., FRIESINGER, G.C., LICHTLEN, P.R., ROSS, R.S.: Circulation **33**, 107 (1966).
147. BERRY, J.W., CARNEY, R., LANKFORD, H.: Angiology **12**, 254 (1961).
148. BERTACCINI, G., IMPICCIATORE, M., VISIOLI, O., MALAGNINO, G.: Il Farmaco **23**, 183 (1968).
149. BERTEAU, P.: Rev. méd. Normande **11**, 215 (1969).
150. BEST, M.M., COE, W.S.: Circulation **2**, 344 (1950).
151. — — Amer. J. Med. **222**, 34 (1951).
152. — DUNCAN, CH.H.: Circulation **22**, 666 (1960).
153. BESTERMAN, E.M.M., FRIEDLANDER, D.H.: Postgrad. med. J. **41**, 526 (1965).
154. BETZ, E., BRAASCH, D., HENSEL, H.: Arzneimittel-Forsch. **11**, 333 (1961).
155. — SCHMAHL, F.W., HENSEL, H.: Arzneimittel-Forsch. **14**, 1319 (1964).
156. BEUMER, H.M.: Pharmacol. Clin. **1**, 172 (1969).
157. — Personal communication 1969.
158. BIANCHI, C., STARCICH, R., LUCCHELLI, P.E.: Vth European Congress of Cardiology. Athenes, Sept. 1968. Abstracts p. 46.
159. — LUCCHELLI, P.E., STARCICH, R.: Pharmacol. Clin. **1**, 161 (1969).

160. BIJLSMA, V.G., FUNCKE, A.B.H., TERSTEEGE, H.M., REKKER, R.F., ERNSTING, M.J.E., NAUTA, W.T.: Arch. int. Pharmacodyn. **105**, 145 (1956).
161. BILLIOTTET, J., FERRAND, J.: Sem. Hôp. Paris, thér. **8**, 834 (1958).
162. BINDER, M.J., KALMANSON, G.M., DRENICK, E.J., ROSOVE, L.: J. Amer. med. Ass. **151**, 967 (1953).
163. BINET, L., BURSTEIN, M.: C.R. Acad. Sci. (Paris) **221**, 197 (1945).
164. BING, R.J.: Circulation **32**, 620 (1965).
165. — BENNISH, A., BLUEMCHEN, G., COHEN, A., GALLAGHER, J.P., ZALESKI, E.J.: Circulation **29**, 833 (1964).
167. — COWAN, C., BOTTCHER, D., CORSINI, G., DANIELS, C.G.: J. Amer. med. Ass. **205**, 277 (1968).
168. BIÖRCK, G.: Amer. Heart J. **32**, 689 (1946).
169. — PANNIER, R.: Acta cardiol. (Brux.) **1**, 283 (1946).
170. BIRKETT, D.A., CHAMBERLAIN, D.A.: Brit. med. J. **1966 I**, 500.
171. BISIANI, M., FRESIA, P., GENOVESE, E., MORTARI, A.: Minerva med. **49**, 4231 (1958).
172. BITTAR, N., SOSA, J.A., CRONIN, R.F.P.: Circulation **34**, Suppl. 3, 57 (1966).
173. BJERLOV, H.: Nord. Med. **55**, 291 (1956).
174. BJÖRK, L., CULLHED, I., HALLEN, A.: Circulation **36**, 868 (1967).
175. BJÖRNTORP, P.: Acta med. scand. **182**, 285 (1967).
176. — Acta med. scand. **184**, 259 (1969).
177. — EK, L., OLSSON, S., SCHRÖDER, G.: Acta Pharmacol. Toxicol. **25**, Suppl. 2, 51 (1967).
178. BLACK, J.W., CROWTHER, A.F., SHANKS, R.G., SMITH, L.H., DORNHORST, A.C.: Lancet **1964 I**, 1080.
179. — DUNCAN, W.A.M., SHANKS, R.G.: Brit. J. Pharmacol. **25**, 577 (1965).
180. — STEPHENSON, J.S.: Lancet **1962 II**, 311.
181. BLACK, S.: Mem. Med. Soc. (Lond.) **4**, 261 (1795). Quoted by Riseman, ref. 1534.
182. BLACKBURN, C.H., BYRNE, L.J., CULLUM, V.A., FARMER, J.B., LEVY, G.P.: J. Pharm. Pharmacol. **21**, 488 (1969).
183. BLINKS, J.R.: Ann. N.Y. Acad. Sci. **139**, 673 (1967).
184. BLÖMER, H., SCHIMERT, G.: Schweiz. med. Wschr. **45**, 1108 (1951).
185. BLOOM, N.: Virginia med. Mth. **87**, 23 (1960).
186. BLOOMFIELD, D.A., SOWTON, E.: Circulat. Res. **21**, Suppl. 3, 243 (1967).
187. BLUMGART, H.L., FREEDBERG, A.S., KURLAND, G.S.: Circulation **1**, 1105 (1950).
188. — — — Circulation **16**, 110 (1957).
189. — RISEMAN, J.E.F., DAVIS, D., BERLIN, D.D.: Arch. intern. Med. **52**, 165 (1933).
190. — SCHLESINGER, M.J., ZOLL, P.M.: Arch. intern. Med. **68**, 181 (1941).
191. — ZOLL, P.M.: Circulation **20**, 301 (1960).
192. BOBB, J.R.R., GREEN, H.D.: Fed. Proc. **17**, 17 (1958).
193. BODO, R.: J. Physiol. (Lond.) **64**, 365 (1927).
194. BOEHM, G.: Münch. med. Wschr. **68**, 106 (1921).
195. BOERTH, R.C., COVELL, J.W., POOL, P.E., ROSS, J.: Circulat. Res. **24**, 725 (1969).
196. BÖHM, C., SCHLEPPER, M., WITZLEB, E.: Dtsch. med. Wschr. **85**, 1405 (1960).
197. BOHR, D.F.: Ann. N.Y. Acad. Sci. **139**, 799 (1967).
198. BOISSIER, J.R., SCHMITT, H., GIUDICELLI, J.J., VIARS, P.: Thérapie **23**, 1371 (1968).
199. BOLLINGER, A.: Dtsch. med. Wschr. **92**, 1399 (1967).
200. BOSSE, J.: Med. Mschr. **22**, 321 (1968).
201. BOTTI, G., VISIOLI, O., AMBANELLI, U.: Cardiologia **49**, Suppl., 45 (1966).
202. BOUREL, M., LENOIR, P.: Thérapie **14**, 523 (1959).
203. BOVET, D., BOVET-NITTI, F.: Arch. int. Pharmacodyn. **73**, 367 (1947).
204. BOYER, N.H.: J. Amer. med. Ass. **122**, 306 (1943).
205. — GREEN, H.D.: Amer. Heart J. **21**, 199 (1941).
206. BOYLES, C.M., SIEBER, H.A., ORGAIN, E.S.: J. Amer. med. Ass. **153**, 12 (1953).
207. BRAASCH, W., FLECK, D.: Arzneimittel-Forsch. **11**, 336 (1961).
208. BRACHFELD, N., BOZER, J., GORLIN, R.: Circulation **19**, 697 (1959).
209. — SCHEUER, J.: Amer. J. Physiol. **212**, 603 (1967).
210. BRÄNDSTRÖM, A., CORRODI, H., JUNGGREN, U., JÖNSSON, T.E.: Acta pharm. Suec. **3**, 303 (1966).
211. BRANDT, J.L., CACCESE, A., DOCK, W.: Amer. J. Med. **12**, 650 (1952).
212. BRAUNSTEINER, H., HERBST, M., SAILER, S., SANDHOFER, F.: Schweiz. med. Wschr. **98**, 828 (1968).
213. BRAUNWALD, E.: Amer. J. Cardiol. **18**, 303 (1966).
214. — COHEN, L.S.: Circulation **34**, Suppl. 3, 64 (1966).
215. — EPSTEIN, S.E., GLICK, G., WECHSLER, A.S., BRAUNWALD, N.: New Engl. J. Med. **277**, 1278 (1967).
216. BREDMOSE, P.: Ugeskr. Laeg. **124**, 941 (1962).

217. BRETSCHNEIDER, H.J.: Dtsch. med. Wschr. **86**, 1649 (1961).
218. — Angina Pectoris, Dietrich-Steinkopf **27**, 1962 (1961).
219. — Langenbecks Arch. klin. Chir. **298**, 774 (1961).
220. — Dtsch. med. J. **13**, 457 (1962).
221. — Kreislaufmessungen, 4e Colloque, Fribourg, Ed. Fleckenstein, München **4**, 104 (1963).
222. — Verh. dtsch. Ges. inn. Med. **69**, 583 (1963).
223. — Landarzt **41**, 845 (1965).
224. — Arzneimittel-Forsch. **16**, 189 (1966).
225. — Regensburg. Jb. ärztl. Fortbild. **15**, 1 (1967).
226. — EBERLEIN, H.J., KABUS, H.M., NELLE, G., REICHMANN, W.: Arzneimittel-Forsch. **13**, 255 (1963).
227. — FRANK, A., BERNARD, U., KOCHSIEK, K., SCHELER, F.: Arzneimittel-Forsch. **9**, 49 (1959).
228. BRICK, I., HUTCHINSON, K.J., McDEVITT, D.G., RODDIE, I.C., SHANKS, R.G.: Brit. J. Pharmacol. **34**, 127 (1968).
229. — RODDIE, I.C., SHANKS, R.G.: Arch. Pharmacol. exp. Path. **259**, 156 (1968).
230. BRIQUEMONT, F.: Brux. méd. **44**, 533 (1964).
231. BRODY, A.J.: J. Amer. med. Ass. **171**, 1195 (1959).
232. BROEKHUYSEN, J.: In press 1971.
233. — DELTOUR, G., GHISLAIN, M.: Arzneimittel-Forsch. **19**, 1850 (1969).
234. — — DELBRUYERE, M.: Biochem. Pharmacol. **16**, 2077 (1967).
235. — LARUEL, R., DEBRUCQ-LARUEL, A., DELTOUR, G.: Biochem. Pharmacol. **16**, 2069 (1967).
236. — — SION, R.: Arch. int. Pharmacodyn. **177**, 340 (1969).
237. BROFMAN, B.L.: J. Amer. med. Ass. **162**, 1603 (1956).
238. BROUSTET, P.: Personal Communication 1968.
239. — LAPORTE, G.: Personal Communication 1969.
240. BROWN, H.R., HOFFMAN, M.J., DE LALLA, V.: Circulation **1**, 132 (1950).
241. BROWN, J.H., RIGGILO, D.A.: Proc. Soc. exp. Biol. (N.Y.) **127**, 1158 (1968).
242. BROWN, M.G., RISEMAN, J.E.F.: J. Amer. med. Ass. **109**, 256 (1937).
243. BROWN, T.G., GREEN, T.J.: Fed. Proc. **18**, 372 (1959).
244. — — GREEN, R.L.: Amer. Heart J. **61**, 531 (1961).
245. BRÜCKE, F., HERTTING, G., LINDNER, A., LOUDON, M.: Wien. klin. Wschr. **68**, 183 (1956).
246. BRÜCKNEROVA, O.: Z. ges. inn. Med. **14**, 118 (1959).
247. BRUGGER, A., SALVA, J.A., SOPENA, M.: Thérapie **24**, 805 (1969).
248. BRUGMANS, J.: Personal communication 1969 and according to RUDOLPH, quoted by DE GEEST and PIESSENS (ref. 400).
249. BRUNNER, H., HEDWALL, P.R., MEIER, M.: Arzneimittel-Forsch. **18**, 164 (1968).
250. BRUNTON, T.L.: Lancet **1867 II**, 97.
251. BUCKLEY, J.P., ACETO, M.D.G., KINNARD, W.J.: Angiology **12**, 259 (1961).
252. BUISSON, P.: Sud méd. chir. **103**, 13950 (1968).
253. Bull. Soc. Int. Cardiologie **1/9**, 1 (1969).
254. BULLE, P.H.: Science **126**, 24 (1957).
255. BULPITT, C.J.: Brit. med. J. **3**, 279 (1967).
256. BUNAG, R.D., DOUGLAS, C.R., IMAI, S., BERNE, R.M.: Circulat. Res. **15**, 83 (1964).
257. BURCH, RAY (1948): Cited by MELVILLE (ref. 1269, p. 485).
258. BURCH, G.E., DE PASQUALE, N.P.: Amer. Heart J. **72**, 842 (1966).
259. BURCHELL, H.B., PRUITT, R.D., BARNES, A.R.: Amer. Heart J. **36**, 373 (1948).
260. BÜRGIN, D.: Schweiz. med. Wschr. **98**, 940 (1968).
261. BURGISON, R.M., LU, G.G., KRANTZ, J.C., jr.: Fed. Proc. **20**, 102 (1961).
262. BURKART, F., BAROLD, S., SOWTON, E.: Amer. J. Cardiol. **20**, 509 (1967).
263. BUSCH, E.: Arch. exp. Pathol. Pharmakol. **237**, 565 (1960).
264. — Biochem. Pharmacol. **8**, 134 (1961).
265. — Arch. int. Pharmacodyn. **135**, 257 (1962).
266. BUSSMANN, W.D., KRAYENBUEHL, H.P.: Helv. physiol. pharmacol. Acta **26**, 199 (1968).
267. — LOCHNER, W.: Arzneimittel-Forsch. **16**, 51 (1966).
268. BUYANOV, V.V.: Farmakol. i Toksikol. **30**, 30 (1967).
269. CAHEN, P., FINAS, C., FROMENT, R.: Lyon méd. **37**, 411 (1959).
270. CALDER, R.M.: Proc. Soc. exp. Biol. (N.Y.) **65**, 76 (1947).
271. CALLSEN, H.: Therapiewoche **17**, 2072 (1967).
272. CAMERON, A., CRAVER, B.N.: Proc. Soc. exp. Biol. (N.Y.) **74**, 271 (1950).
273. CAMPUS, S., FABRIS, F., RAPPELLI, A., MATHIS, I.: Bull. Soc. Ital. Biol. Sper. **43**, 304 (1967).
274. CANDAELE, G., VASTESAEGER, M.: Scalpel (Brux.) **8**, 133 (1969).
275. CANTOR, S.A.: Med. J. Aust. **2**, 983 (1967).

276. Cardoe, N.: Brit. J. clin. Pract. **22**, 299 (1968).
277. Carlsson, A., Hillarp, N.A., Waldeck, B.: Acta physiol. scand. **59**, Suppl. 215, 1 (1963).
278. Carson, R.P., Wilson, W.S., Nemiroff, M.J., Weber, W.J.: Amer. Heart J. **77**, 579 (1969).
279. Case, R.B., Brachfeld, N.: Amer. J. Cardiol. **9**, 425 (1962).
280. — Roven, R.B.: Progr. cardiovasc. Dis. **6**, 45 (1963).
281. — — Some considerations of coronary flow. In: Modern trends in diseases of coronary arteries and ischemic heart disease. Ed. C.K. Friedberg. New York: Grune and Stratton 1964, p. 45.
282. Castenholz, A.: Arzneimittel-Forsch. **18**, 1073 (1968).
283. Castro De, B., Parchi, C.: G. Clin. med. **41**, Fasc. 6 (1960).
284. Catecholamines and the heart. Lancet **1969 I**, 1200.
285. Catinat, J., Sauvan, R.: Presse méd. **74**, 1854 (1966).
286. Ceremuzynski, L., Staszewska-Barczak, J., Herbaczynska-Cedro, K.: Cardiovasc. Res. **3**, 190 (1969).
287. Cesarman, T.: Arch. Inst. Cardiol. Mex. **27**, 563 (1957).
288. — J. clin. exp. Psychopath. **19**, Suppl. 1, 169 (1958).
289. — Aterosclerosis y enfermedad coronaria, 1 vol. Mexico: Ed. Interamericana 1960, p. 377.
290. — Cazes, D.: Arch. Inst. Cardiol. Mex. **24**, 514 (1954).
291. — Chamberlain, D.A.: Amer. J. Cardiol. **18**, 321 (1966).
292. — Davis, W.G., Mason, D.F.J.: Lancet **1967 II**, 1257.
293. — Turner, P., Sneddon, J.M.: Lancet **1967 II**, 12.
294. Chamla, J.: Sem. thér. **44**, TH 406 (1968).
295. Chandler, H.L., Mann, G.V.: New Engl. J. Med. **249**, 1045 (1953).
296. Charlier, R.: Acta cardiol. (Brux.), Suppl. VII (1959).
297. — Arzneimittel-Forsch. **10**, 732 (1960).
298. — Aterosclerosis y enfermedad coronaria, 1 vol. Mexico: Ed. Interamericana 1960, p. 363.
299. — Ther. Umsch. **17**, 6 (1960).
300. — 3rd European Congress of Cardiology, Roma, Sept. 1960. Abstracts p. 1067.
301. — Vaso-dilatateurs coronariens, Paris: Ed. Gauthier Villars 1962.
302. — Proc. 3rd Asian Pacific Congress of Cardiology, Kyoto 1964, p. 731.
303. — 1966 and 1968, unpublished.
304. — Rev. méd. Liège **23**, 232—269—299 (1968).
305. — J. Suisse de Pharmacie **107**, 523 (1969).
306. — Brux.-méd. **49**, 543 (1969).
307. — Brux.-méd. **50**, 651 (1970).
308. — Brit. J. Pharmacol. **39**, 668 (1970).
309. — Baudine, A., Chaillet, F.: Arch. int. Physiol. **75**, 787 (1967).
310. — — — Deltour, G.: Acta cardiol. (Brux.) **22**, 323 (1967).
311. — — Delaunois, G., Bauthier, J.: 4th International Congress of Pharmacology, Basle 1969, Abstracts p. 257.
312. — — — Deltour, G.: Cardiologia **54**, 83 (1969).
313. — Deltour, G.: Méd. et Hyg. (Genève) **20**, 230 (1962).
313bis — — Vth European Congress of Cardiology, Athenes, Sept. 1968, Abstracts p. 81.
314. — — In: Médicaments et Métabolisme du Myocarde, Nancy: Ed. Lamarche and Royer, 1969, p. 291.
315. — — J. de Pharmacol. **1**, 175 (1970).
316. — — Baudine, A.: Arch. int. Physiol. **75**, 508 (1967).
317. — — — Chaillet, F.: Arzneimittel-Forsch. **18**, 1408 (1968).
318. — — Tondeur, R., Binon, F.: Arch. int. Pharmacodyn. **139**, 255 (1962).
319. — Hosslet, A., Baudine, A.: Arch. int. Pharmacodyn. **132**, 116 (1961).
320. Chatillon, J.: Méd. et Hyg. (Genève) **25**, 1212 (1967).
321. Chavez, I.: Aterosclerosis y enfermedad coronaria, 1 vol. Mexico: Ed. Interamericana 1960, p. 21.
322. Cherian, G., Brockington, I.M., Shah, P.M., Oakley, G.M., Goodwin, J.F.: Amer. Heart J. **73**, 140 (1967).
323. Chessin, M., Dubnick, B., Leeson, G., Scott, C.C.: Ann. N.Y. Acad. Sci. **80**, 597 (1959).
324. Chevalier, H., Simon, J.: Amer. Heart J. **58**, 120 (1959).
325. Chiche, P., Botteri, L., Derrida, J.: Sem. Hôp. Paris **43**, 1 (1967).
326. Chidsey, E.A., Braunwald, E.: Pharmacol. Rev. **18**, 685 (1966).
327. Christakis, G., Rinzler, S.H., Archer, M., Winslow, G., Jampel, S., Stephenson, J., Friedman, G., Fein, H., Kraus, A., James, G.: Amer. J. publ. Hlth **56**, 299 (1966).

328. CHRISTENSSON, B., KARLEFORS, T., WESTLING, H.: Brit. Heart J. **27**, 511 (1965).
329. CHRISTMAN, W.: Med. Welt (Berl.) **46**, 2559 (1968).
330. *Claims for Cordilox.* Drug. Ther. Bull. **5**, 85 (1967).
331. CLARK, L.C., JR., WOLF, R., GRANGER, D., TAYLOR, Z.: J. appl. Physiol. **6**, 189 (1953).
332. CLARKE, D.A., DAVOLL, J., PHILIPS, F.S., BROWN, G.B.: J. Pharmacol. exp. Ther. **106**, 291 (1952).
333. CLAUSEN, J., JORGENSEN, F.S., ROIN, J., FELSBY, M., NIELSEN, B.L., STRANGE, B.: Lancet **1966II**, 920.
334. CLAUSEN, J.P., LARSEN, O.A., TRAP-JENSEN, J.: Circulation **40**, 143 (1969).
335. CLOAREC, M.: Sem. Hôp. Thérapeut. **37**, 8, 753 (1961).
336. COBB, F., BACHE, R., EBERT, P., REMBERT, B., GREENFIELD, J.: Clin. Res. **17**, 58 (1969).
337. COBB, F.R., BACHE, R.J., EBERT, P.A., REMBERT, B.S., GREENFIELD, J.C.: Circulat. Res. **25**, 331 (1969).
338. CODE, C.F., EVANS, C.L., GREGORY, R.A.: J. Physiol. (Lond.) **92**, 344 (1938).
339. COHEN, A., GALLACHER, J.P., LUEBS, E.D., VARGA, Z., YAMANAKA, J., ZALESKI, E.J., BLUEMCHEN, C., BING, R.J.: Circulation **32**, 636 (1965).
340. COHEN, B.M.: Curr. ther. Res. **9**, 618 (1967).
341. COHEN, E.I.: Arch. Mal. Cœur **11**, 1048 (1957).
342. COHEN, L.S., BRAUNWALD, E.: Circulation **35**, 847 (1967).
343. — — Acquis. Nouv. Pathol. Cardio-vasc. **11**, 243 (1968).
344. — ELLIOTT, W.C., GORLIN, R.: Amer. J. Physiol. **206**, 997 (1964).
345. — — KLEIN, M.D., GORLIN, R.: Amer. J. Cardiol. **17**, 153 (1966).
346. — — ROLETT, E.L., GORLIN, R.: Circulation **31**, 409 (1965).
347. COLE, R.E., GOLDBERG, R.I.: Curr. ther. Res. **9**, 551 (1967).
348. COLE, S.L.: Dis. Chest **34**, 330 (1958).
349. — KAYE, H., GRIFFITH, G.C.: Circulation **15**, 405 (1957).
350. — — — J. Amer. med. Ass. **168**, 275 (1958).
351. Cold induced angina. Lancet **1969I**, 407.
352. CONDORELLI, L.: Vth European Congress of Cardiology. Athenes, Sept. 1968. Symposia p. 125.
353. CONN, J.J., KISSANE, R.W., KOONS, R.A., CLARK, T.E.: Ann. intern. Med. **36**, 1173; **38**, 23 (1952).
354. CONN, R.D., BRUCE, R.A.: Clin. Res. **15**, 92 (1967).
355. CONSTANTIN, B., ARDISSON, J.L., GASPARINI, J.J.: C.R. Soc. Biol. (Paris) **161**, 2227 (1967).
356. CONTRO, S., HARING, O.M., GOLDSTEIN, W.: Circulation **6**, 250 (1952).
357. CONWAY, C.M.: J. Pharm. Pharmacol. **11**, 477 (1959).
358. CONWAY, E.J., COOKE, R.: Biochem. J. **33**, 479 (1939).
359. CONWAY, N.: Amer. Heart J. **76**, 581 (1968).
360. — GUPTA, G.D., SOWTON, E.: Acta cardiol. (Brux.) **23**, 434 (1968).
361. — SEYMOUR, J., GELSON, A.: Brit. med. J. **2**, 213 (1968).
362. CORCONDILAS, A., ROUBELAKIS, G., IOANNIDIS, P., KOROXENIDIS, G., TSITOURIS, G., MICHAELIDES, G.: Vth European Congress of Cardiology. Athenes, Sept. 1968. Abstracts p. 92.
363. CORCORAN, A.C., ZIMMERMANN, H.A., CUTURELLI, R.: Progr. cardiovasc. Dis. **2**, 576 (1960).
364. *Cordilox up to date:* Drug and Therap. Bull. **7**, 19 (1969).
365. CORMAN, A., BREST, A.N.: Geriatrics **23**, 157 (1968).
366. COSBY, R.S., MAYO, M.: Amer. J. Cardiol. **3**, 444 (1959).
367. COSSIO, P.: Amer. Heart J. **56**, 113 (1958).
368. COTTET, J.: Thérapie **13**, 16 (1958).
369. — Path. et Biol. **7**, 2113 (1959).
370. — MATHIVAT, A., REDEL, J.: Presse méd. **62**, 939 (1954).
371. — VITTU, C.: Presse méd. **75**, 1355 (1967).
372. COULSHED, N.: Brit. Heart J. **22**, 79 (1960).
373. COURVOISIER, S., FOURNEL, J., DUCROT, R., KOLSKY, M., KOETSCHET, P.: Arch. int. Pharmacodyn. **92**, 305 (1953).
374. COVA, N., BREGANI, P.: Minerva cardioangiol. **8** (1960).
375. CRAVEN, P., PITT, B.: Circulation **38**, Suppl. 6, 61 (1968).
376. CRIOLLOS, R.L., AL-SHAMMA, A.M., ROE, B.B.: a) Circulation **37**, Suppl. 2, 27 (1968). b) Ann. Thorac. Surg. **4**, 151 (1967).
377. CUGURRA, F., ECHINARD-GARIN, P.: Arch. int. Pharmacodyn. **123**, 481 (1960).
378. CUMMING, G.R., CARR, W.: Canad. J. Physiol. Pharmacol. **44**, 465 (1966).
379. — — Canad. J. Physiol. Pharmacol. **45**, 813 (1967).
380. DAILHEU-GEOFFROY, P.: Quest méd. **3**, 319 (1950).

381. DAILHEU-GEOFFROY, P.: Clinique (Paris) **46**, 27 (1951).
382. — 3rd European Congress of Cardiology, Roma, Sept. 1960. Discussion of the Communication by CHARLIER (see ref. 300).
383. — Ouest méd. **19**, 185 (1966).
384. — NATAF, J.: Presse méd. **69**, 971 (1961).
385. — — Ther. Umsch. **19**, 483 (1962).
386. DALLE, X., MELTZER, L.E.: Acta cardiol. (Brux.) **22**, 247 (1967).
387. DAMATO, A.N., LAU, S.H., HELFANT, R.H., STEIN, E., BERKOWITZ, W.D., COHEN, S.I.: Circulation **39**, 287 (1969).
388. — — — — PATTON, R.D., SCHERLAG, B.J., BERKOWITZ, W.D.: Circulation **39**, 297 (1969).
389. — — PATTON, R.D., STEINER, C., BERKOWITZ, W.D.: Circulation **40**, 61 (1969).
390. DARBY, T.D., ALDINGER, E.E.: Circulat. Res. **8**, 100 (1960).
391. DAVIES, D.F., GROPPER, A.L., SCHRODER, H.A.: Circulation **3**, 543 (1951).
392. DAVIES, P., ORAM, S., CURWEN, M.P.: Brit. med. J. **1963 II**, 359.
393. DAVIS, J.A., WIESEL, B.H.: Amer. J. med. Sci. **230**, 259 (1955).
394. DAVIS, W.G., MACDONALD, D.C., MASON, D.F.J.: Brit. J. Pharmacol. **37**, 338 (1969).
395. DAWES, G.S.: J. Physiol. (Lond.) **99**, 224 (1941).
396. — MOTT, J.C., VANE, J.R.: J. Physiol. (Lond.) **121**, 72 (1953).
397. DAWSON, P.M.: Amer. J. Physiol. **50**, 443 (1920).
398. DAYTON, S., PEARCE, M.L.: Amer. J. Med. **46**, 751 (1969).
399. — — HASHIMOTO, S., DIXON, W.J., TOMIYASU, U.: Circulation **40**, Suppl. 2, 1 (1969).
400. DE GEEST, H., PIESSENS, J.: New Engl. J. Med. In press (1971).
401. DE GRAFF, A.C., LYON, A.F.: Amer. Heart J. **65**, 423 (1963).
402. DELAUNOIS, A.L.: Arch. int. Pharmacodyn. **134**, 245 (1961).
403. DELBARRE, F., AUSCHER, C., OLIVIER, J.L., ROSE, A.: Sem. Hôp. Paris **43**, 1128 (1967).
404. DELEIXHE, A., DELRÉE, G.: Rev. méd. Liège **24**, 377 (1969).
405. DELIUS, W.: Med. Klin. **62**, 1128 (1967).
406. DELTOUR, G.: Actualités pharmacol. **21**, 117 (1968).
407. — Circulatory Drugs. Ed. by A. BERTELLI. Amsterdam: North Holland Publ. Co. 1969, p. 71.
408. — BEKAERT, J., BROEKHUYSEN, J., CHARLIER, R.: Memorias del IV Congreso Mundial de Cardiologia, Mexico **5**, 141 (1962).
409. — BINON, F., TONDEUR, R., GOLDENBERG, C., HENAUX, F., SION, R., DERAY, E., CHARLIER, R.: Arch. int. Pharmacodyn. **139**, 247 (1962).
410. — BROEKHUYSEN, J.: In: Médicaments et Métabolisme du Myocarde. Nancy: Ed Lamarche and Royer 1969, p. 253.
411. — CHARLIER, R., BROEKHUYSEN, J.: Unpublished.
412. DEMEY, D., DERNIER, J., BLOCK, P., PAESMANS, M.: Brux.-méd. **50**, 639 (1970).
413. DENISON, A.B., BARDHANABAEDYA, S., GREEN, H.D.: Circulat. Res. **4**, 653 (1956).
414. — SPENCER, M.P., GREEN, H.D.: Circulat. Res. **3**, 39 (1955).
415. DE PASQUALE, N.P., BURKS, J.W., BURCH, G.E.: J. Amer. med. Ass. **184**, 421 (1963).
416. DE SCHAEPDRYVER, A.F., TASSON, J., LAMONT, H.: Europ. J. Pharmacol. **5**, 379 (1969).
417. DESHAYES, P., CARDINAEL, Y.: Rhumatologie **19**, 255 (1967).
418. DE SOLDATI, L.: IIIrd World Congress of Cardiology. Brussels 1958. Abstracts of Symposia, p. 517.
419. — NAVARRO-VIOLA, R., MEJIA, R.H.: Arch. Mal. Cœur **45**, 108 (1952).
420. DESRUELLES, J., DECALF, A., WAUCAMPT, J.J.: Mouvement thérapeutique (Lille) **11**, 3 (1966).
421. DETRY, R., LACHIEZE-REY, E., RAYMOND, J., PONT, M.: Lyon méd. **7**, 1 (1970).
422. DEUTICKE, B., GERLACH, E.: Arch. Pharmakol. exp. Path. **255**, 107 (1966).
423. DEWAR, H.A., GRIMSON, T.A.: Brit. Heart. J. **12**, 54 (1950).
424. — HORLER, A.R., NEWELL, D.J.: Brit. Heart J. **21**, 315 (1959).
425. — NEWELL, D.J.: Scot. med. J. **9**, 526 (1964).
426. D'HEER, H.: Belg. T. Geneesk. **23**, 1126 (1961).
427. DI CARLO, F.J., CREW, M.C., SKLOW, N.J., COUTINHO, C.B., NONKIN, P., SIMON, F., BERNSTEIN, A.: J. Pharmacol. exp. Ther. **153**, 254 (1966).
428. DIDISHEIM, J.C., UEBERSAX, R.: Méd. et Hyg. (Genève) **658**, 863 (1964).
429. DIETZ, A.J.: Biochem. Pharmacol. **16**, 2447 (1967).
430. DIGHIERO, J., HAZAN, J., AGUIRRE, C.V., RUDOLF, J.: Aterosclerosis y enfermedad coronaria, 1 vol. Mexico: Ed. Interamericana 1960, p. 387.
431. DIMOND, E.G., BENCHIMOL, A.: Brit. Heart J. **25**, 389 (1963).
432. DITTRICH, W.: Dtsch. med. Wschr. **94**, 1176 (1969).
433. DIXON, W.F.: J. Physiol. (Lond.) **35**, 346 (1907).
434. DOCK, W.: Med. Clin. N. Amer. **33**, 635 (1949).

435. DOHADWALLA, A.N., FREEDBERG, A.S., VAUGHAN WILLIAMS, E.M.: Brit. J. Pharmacol. **36**, 257 (1969).
436. DOLL, E., KEUL, J., BRECHTEL: Z. Kreisl.-Forsch. **55**, 1076 (1966).
437. DONATO, L., BARTOLOMEI, G., FEDERIGHI, G., TORREGGIANI, G.: Circulation **33**, 708 (1966).
438. — — GIORDANI, R.: Circulation **29**, 195 (1964).
439. DONNET, V., DUFLOT, J.C., JACQUIN, M., MURISASCO, A., FORNARIS, M.: C.R. Soc. Biol. (Paris) **161**, 2232 (1967).
440. — — — PEYROT, J., POMMIER DE SANTI, P.: C.R. Soc. Biol. (Paris) **161**, 2230 (1967).
441. DONOSO, E., COHN, L.J., NEWMAN, B.J., BLOOM, H.S., STEIN, W.G., FRIEDBERG, C.K.: Circulation **36**, 534 (1967).
442. DORNAUS, W.: Therapiewoche **17**, 784 (1967).
443. DÖRNER, J., WICK, E.: Arzneimittel-Forsch. **10**, 631 (1960).
444. DORNHORST, A.C.: Ann. N.Y. Acad. Sci. **139**, 968 (1967).
445. DOTREMONT, G., DE GEEST, H.: Acta clin. belg. **23**, 163 (1968).
446. DOTTI, F., PIVA, M., ONGARI, R.: Arzneimittel-Forsch. **18**, 1445 (1968).
447. DRESEL, P.E.: Canad. J. Biochem. **38**, 375 (1960).
448. DREWS, A.: Arzneimittel-Forsch. **18**, 1084 (1968).
449. DRILL, V.A.: Pharmacology in Medicine, 2nd ed., 1 vol. New York: McGraw-Hill 1958, 1243 pp.
450. DRISCOL, T.E., BERNE, R.M.: Proc. Soc. exp. Biol. (N.Y.) **96**, 505 (1957).
451. *Drugs for Angina:* Brit. med. J. **1969**II, 677.
451 bis DRURY, A.N., SZENT-GYORGYI, A.: J. Physiol. (Lond.) **68**, 213 (1929).
452. DRY, T.J.: Proc. Mayo Clin. **31**, 10 (1956).
453. DU BOIS, R.: Schweiz. med. Wschr. **98**, 1142 (1968).
454. DUCE, B.R., GARBERG, L., JOHANSSON, B.: Acta pharmacol. (Kbh.) **25**, Suppl. 2, 41 (1967).
455. DUCHENE-MARULLAZ, P., LAVARENNE, J.: Actualités pharmacol. **21**, 65 (1968).
456. — COSNIER, D., GRIMALD, J.: Thérapie **24**, 617 (1969).
457. — — Thérapie **24**, 665 (1969).
458. — LAVARENNE, J.: Actualités pharmacol. **21**, 65 (1968).
459. DUESEL, B.F., FAND, T.I.: Intern. Record Med. Gen. Pract. Clin. **167**, 245 (1954).
460. DULAC, J.F., MANY, P., PICARD, P.: Presse méd. **41**, 1546 (1959).
461. DUMKE, P.R., SCHMIDT, C.F.: Amer. J. Physiol. **138**, 421 (1943).
462. DUNGAN, K.W., LISH, P.M.: Fed. Proc. **23**, 124 (1964).
463. DUNLOP, D., SHANKS, R.G.: Brit. J. Pharmacol. **32**, 201 (1968).
464. DÜX, A., SCHAEDE, A.: Dtsch. med. Wschr. **94**, 1349 (1969).
465. DWYER, E.M., WIENER, L., COX, J.W.: Circulation **36**, Suppl. 2, 99 (1967).
466. DZIUBA, K.: Med. Welt (Berl.) **18**, 894 (1967).
467. EBERLEIN, H.J.: Arch. Kreisl.-Forsch. **50**, 18 (1966).
468. ECKENHOFF, J.E., HAFKENSCHIEL, J.H.: J. Pharmacol. exp. Ther. **91**, 362 (1947).
469. — — HARMEL, M.H., GOODALE, W.T., LUBIN, M., BING, R.J., KETY, S.S.: Amer. J. Physiol. **152**, 356 (1948).
470. — — LANDMESSER, C.M.: Amer. J. Physiol. **148**, 582 (1947).
471. — — — HARMEL, M.: Amer. J. Physiol. **149**, 634 (1947).
472. ECKSTEIN, R.W.: Circulat. Res. **2**, 460 (1954).
473. — Circulat. Res. **5**, 230 (1957).
474. — CHAMBLISS, J., DEMMING, J., WELLS, K.: Fed. Proc. **9**, 36 (1950).
475. — McEACHEN, J.A., DEMMING, J., NEWBERRY, W.B.: Science **113**, 385 (1951).
476. — NEWBERRY, W.B., McEACHEN, J.A., SMITH, G.: Circulation **4**, 534 (1951).
477. — — — — Circulation **4**, 534 (1951).
478. — STROUD, M., ECKEL, R., DOWLING, C.V., PRITCHARD, W.P.: Amer. J. Physiol. **163**, 539 (1950).
479. EDERY, H., LEWIS, G.P.: J. Physiol. (Lond.) **160**, 20P (1962).
480. EHRENBERGER, W.: Wien. Z. inn. Med. **41**, 323 (1960).
481. EHRLICH, J.C., SHINOHARA, Y.: Arch. Path. **78**, 432 (1964).
482. EISEL, K., KAISER, H.: Ther. d. Gegenw. **107**, 231 (1968).
483. EJRUP, B., KUMLIN, T.: Aktiebolaget Pharmacia **77**, 172 (1961).
484. ELEK, S.R., KATZ, L.N.: J. Pharmacol. exp. Ther. **75**, 178 (1942).
485. — — J. Amer. med. Ass. **120**, 434 (1942).
486. ELLIOT, A.H., NUZUM, F.R.: J. Pharmacol. exp. Ther. **43**, 463 (1931).
487. ELLIOT, E.C.: Canad. med. Ass. J. **85**, 469 (1961).
488. ELLIOTT, W.C., GORLIN, R.: Mod. Conc. cardiov. Dis. **35**, 111 (1966).
489. ELLIS, L.B., BLUMGART, H.L., HARKEN, D.E., SISE, H.S., STARE, F.J.: Circulation **17**, 945 (1958).

490. Ellis, L.B., Hancock, E.W.: J. Amer. med. Ass. **163**, 445 (1957).
491. Emele, J.F., Shanaman, J.E., Warren, M.R.: Fed. Proc. **18**, 387 (1959).
492. Endte, K.: Wien. med. Wschr. **41**, 792 (1959).
493. Enescu, V., Boszormenyi, E., Bernstein, H., Corday, E.: Animal and clinical pharmacologic techniques in drug evaluation. Vol. 2. Ed. by P.E. Siegler and J.H. Moyer. Chicago: Year Book Med. Publ. 1967, p. 444.
494. Engelhardt, A.: Arch. exp. Pathol. Pharmakol. **250**, 245 (1965).
495. Engelking, H.: Münch. med. Wschr. **110**, 289 (1968).
496. Enos, W.F.: J. Amer. med. Ass. **158**, 912 (1956).
497. — Holmes, R.H., Beyer, J.: J. Amer. med. Ass. **152**, 1090 (1953).
498. Enselme, J.: Brux.-méd. **42**, 1321 (1959).
499. Epstein, F.H.: Circulation **36**, 609 (1967).
500. Epstein, S.E., Beiser, G.D., Goldstein, R.E., Stampfer, M., Wechsler, A.S., Glick, G., Braunwald, E.: Circulation **40**, 269 (1969).
501. — — Stampfer, M., Glick, G., Wechsler, A.S., Goldstein, R.E., Cohen, L.S., Braunwald, N., Braunwald, E.: Circulation **38**, Suppl. 6, 72 (1968).
502. — Braunwald, E.: New Engl. J. Med. **275**, 1106 and 1175 (1966).
503. — — Ann. N.Y. Acad. Sci. **139**, 952 (1967).
504. — — Ann. intern. Med. **67**, 1333 (1967).
505. — Robinson, B.F., Kahler, R.L., Braunwald, E.: J. clin. Invest. **44**, 1745 (1965).
506. Eral, N.: Arzneimittel-Forsch. **18**, 1094 (1968).
507. Erbring, H., Uebel, H., Vogel, G.: Arzneimittel-Forsch. **17**, 283 (1967).
508. Essex, H.E., Herrick, J.F., Baldes, E.J., Mann, F.C.: Amer. J. Physiol. **117**, 271 (1936).
509. — Wegria, R., Herrick, J.F., Mann, F.C.: Amer. Heart J. **19**, 554 (1940).
510. Evans, A., Bourne, G.: Brit. Heart J. **3**, 69 (1941).
511. Evans, C.L.: Starling's Human Physiology, 11th edition. Philadelphia: Lea and Febiger 1952, p. 580.
512. — Starling, E.H.: J. Physiol. (Lond.) **46**, 413 (1913).
513. Evans, W.: Cardiology. New York: Hoeber 1949.
514. — Hoyle, C.: Quart. J. Med. **26**, 311 (1933).
515. — — Quart. J. Med. **3**, 105 (1934).
516. Facquet, J., Nivet, M.: Vth European Congress of Cardiology, Athenes, Sept. 1968, Abstracts p. 139.
517. — — Grosgogeat, Y., Alhomme, P., Vachon, J.: Thérapie **25**, 335 (1970).
518. — — Alhomme, P., Raharison, S., Grosgogeat, Y.: Presse méd. **77**, 725 (1969).
519. Faivre, G., Dodinot, B., Hua, G., Schmidt, C.: Ann. méd. Nancy **8**, 149 (1969).
520. — Gilgenkrantz, Lagarde, Vincent, Frenkiel: Arch. Mal. Cœur **51**, 68 (1958).
521. Fallen, E.L., Elliott, W.C., Gorlin, R.: Circulation **36**, 480 (1967).
522. Fam, W.M., McGregor, M.: Circulat. Res. **22**, 649 (1958).
523. — — Circulat. Res. **15**, 355 (1964).
524. — — Studies on myocardial oxygen tension. In: Cardiovascular and respiratory effects of hypoxia. Ed. by Hatcher. Basle: S. Karger 1966.
525. Farmer, J.B., Levy, G.P.: Brit. J. Pharmacol. **32**, 429P (1968).
526. — — Brit. J. Pharmacol. **34**, 116 (1968).
527. Farrehi, C., Perley, A., Ritzmann, L.W., Malinow, M.R., Judkins, M.R., Griswold, H.E.: Circulation **38**, Suppl. VI, 6 (1968).
528. Faucon, G., Duchene-Marullaz, P., Lavarenne, J., Schaff, G., Sagols, L., Collard, M.: C.R. Soc. Biol. (Paris) **158**, 314 (1964).
529. — Evreux, J.C., Kofman, J., Perrot, E.: C.R. Soc. Biol. (Paris) **162**, 945 (1968).
530. — — Lavarenne, J., Kofman, J., Perrot, E.: Thérapie **23**, 1123 (1968).
531. — Lavarenne, J., Kofman, J., Evreux, J.C.: Sem. Hôp. Paris **43**, 15 (1967).
532. Fauda, C., Candiani, C.: Minerva med. **50**, 1924 (1959).
533. Favaloro, R.G., Effler, D.B., Groves, L.K., Fergusson, D.J.G., Lozada, J.S.: Circulation **37**, 549 (1968).
534. Fellows, E.J., Killam, K.F., Toner, J.J., Dailey, R.A., Macko, E.: Fed. Proc. **9**, 271 (1950).
535. Fergusson, D.J., Shirey, E.K., Sheldon, W.C., Effler, D.B., Sones, F.M.: Circulation **37**, Suppl. 2, 24 (1968).
536. Ferrari, V., Finardi, G.: Minerva med. **46**, 1175 (1955).
537. Ferrero, C.: Ther. Umsch. **16**, 169 (1959).
538. — Arnold, E.F., Doret, J.P.: Cardiologia (Basel) **38**, 80 (1961).
539. Ferrini, R.: Arzneimittel-Forsch. **18**, 48 (1968).
540. — Miragoli, G., Croce, G.: Arzneimittel-Forsch. **18**, 829 (1968).

541. FERUGLIO, F.S., CAMPUS, S., PANDOLFO, G., DESSY, P., GAGNA, C., USLENGHI, E.: Boll. Soc. ital. Biol. sper. **43**, 313 (1967).
542. — — — — — — Boll. Soc. ital. Biol. sper. **43**, 315 (1967).
543. FIEGEL, G., BARGHEER, R., HEINDORF, M., KUKWA, D.: Med. Klin. **60**, 1044 (1965).
544. — KELLING, H.W., BARGHEER, R., KUKWA, D.: Med. Welt (Berl.) **17**, 976 (1963).
545. FIERLAFYN, E., QUERTON, M.: Brux.-méd. **48**, 845 (1968).
546. FIFE, R., HOWITT, G., STEVENSON, J.: Brit. med. J. **5174**, 692 (1960).
547. FISCH, S.: Amer. Heart J. **71**, 281 (1966).
548. — Amer. Heart J. **71**, 564 (1966).
549. — Amer. Heart J. **71**, 712 (1966).
550. — Amer. Heart J. **71**, 837 (1966).
551. — Amer. Heart J. **72**, 280 (1966).
552. — BOYLE, A., SPERBER, R., DEGRAFF, A.C.: 61st Annual Meeting of Amer. Therap. Soc., Miami Beach, 1960.
553. — DEGRAFF, A.C.: Dis. Chest **44**, 533 (1963).
554. FISCHER, E.K., FIEGEL, C.: Dtsch. med. J. **10**, 484 (1959).
555. FISCHER, K.: Med. Klin. **60**, 847 (1965).
556. FISHBEIN, M.: Angiology **11**, 53 (1960).
557. FITZGERALD, J.D.: Clin. Pharmacol. Ther. **10**, 292 (1969).
558. — BARRETT, A.M.: Lancet **1967 II**, 310.
559. — — Lancet **1967 II**, 509.
560. FLATTERY, K.V., SHUM, A., JOHNSON, G.E.: Arch. int. Pharmacodyn. **175**, 54 (1968).
561. FLECKENSTEIN, A., DÖRING, H.J., KAMMERMEIER, H.: Klin. Wschr. **46**, 343 (1968).
562. — KAMMERMEIER, H., DÖRING, H.J., FREUND, H.J.: Z. Kreisl.-Forsch. **56**, 839 (1967).
563. — TRITTHART, H., FLECKENSTEIN, B., HERBST, A., GRUEN, G.: Arch. ges. Physiol. **307**, R 25 (1969).
564. FLEMING, J., HAMER, J.: Brit. Heart J. **29**, 257 (1967).
565. FLETCHER, G.F., HURST, J.W., SCHLANT, R.C.: Circulation **34**, Suppl. 3, 102 (1966).
566. — — — Amer. Heart J. **75**, 319 (1968).
567. FOLKOW, B.: Acta physiol. scand. **17**, 311 (1949).
568. FOLLE, L.E., AVIADO, D.M.: J. Pharmacol. exp. Ther. **149**, 79 (1965).
569. FÖLSCH, E., BERNHARD, P.: Arzneimittel-Forsch. **19**, 308 (1969).
570. FOLTZ, E.L., PAGE, R.G., SHELDON, W.F., WONG, S.K., TUDDENHAM, W.J., WEISS, A.J.: Amer. J. Physiol. **162**, 521 (1950).
571. FORSBERG, S.A., JOHNSSON, G.: Acta pharmacol. (Kbh.) **25**, Suppl. 2, 75 (1967).
572. FOULDS, R., MAC KINNON, J.: Brit. med. J. **1960 II**, 835.
573. FOURNEAU, J.P.: Ann. pharm. franç. **11**, 685 (1953).
574. FOWLER, W.M., HUREVITZ, H.M., SMITH, F.M.: Arch. intern. Med. **56**, 1242 (1935).
575. FOX, R.H., GOLDSMITH, R., KIDD, D.J., LEWIS, G.P.: a) J. Physiol. (Lond.) **154**, 16 P (1960). b) J. Physiol. (Lond.) **157**, 589 (1961).
576. FRANCOIS, J.: Bull. Soc. belge Ophtal. **150**, 656 (1968).
577. — Docum. ophthal. (Den Haag) **27**, 235 (1969).
578. FRANCOIS-FRANCK, C.A.: C.R. Soc. Biol. (Paris) **55**, 1448 (1903).
579. FRANK, A., BRETSCHNEIDER, H.J., KANZOW, E., BERNARD, U.: Z. ges. exp. Med. **128**, 520 (1957).
580. FRANK, M.J., LEVINSON, G.E.: J. clin. Invest. **47**, 1615 (1968).
581. FRANKL, W.S., SOLOFF, L.A.: Amer. J. Cardiol. **22**, 266 (1968).
582. FRANKLIN, D.L.: Med. Elec. Biol. Eng. **3**, 27 (1965).
583. FREEDBERG, A.S.: Discussion of ref. 1600 in Progr. cardiovasc. Dis. **2**, 584 (1960).
584. — RISEMAN, J.E.F., SPIEGL, E.D.: Amer. Heart J. **22**, 494 (1941).
585. — SPIEGL, E.D., RISEMAN, J.E.F.: Amer. Heart J. **22**, 519 (1941).
586. — — — Amer. Heart J. **27**, 611 (1944).
587. FREMONT, R.E.: Curr. ther. Res. **9**, 235 (1967).
588. FRESIA, P., GENOVESE, E., MORTARI, A.: Minerva med. **49**, 4295 (1958).
589. FREY, E.K., HARTENBACH, W., SCHULTZ, F.: Münch. med. Wschr. **95**, 11 (1953).
590. — KRAUT, H.: Münch. med. Wschr. **75**, 763 (1928).
591. — — Arch. exp. Pathol. Pharmakol. **133**, 1 (1928).
592. FRICK, M.H., BALCON, R., CROSS, D., SOWTON, E.: Circulation **37**, 160 (1968).
593. — KATILA, M.: Circulation **37**, 192 (1968).
594. FRIEDBERG, C.K.: Canad. med. Ass. J. **68**, 95 (1953).
595. — Diseases of the Heart. Philadelphia: Saunders & Co. 1956.
596. — Discussion of ref. 1600 in Progr. cardiovasc. Dis. **2**, 583 (1960).
597. — Geriatrics **22**, 144 (1967).
598. — JAFFÉ, H.L., PORDY, L., CHESKY, K.: Circulation **26**, 1254 (1962).
599. FRIEDEN, J.: Amer. Heart J. **74**, 283 (1967).

600. FRIEDEMANN, M.: Schweiz. med. Wschr. **96**, 1656 (1966).
601. FRIEDMAN, J.J.: Amer. J. Physiol. **214**, 488 (1968).
602. FRIEND, D.G., O'HARE, J.P., LEVINE, H.D.: Amer. Heart J. **48**, 775 (1954).
603. FRIESE, G.: Münch. med. Wschr. **106**, 1084 (1964).
604. FRISCH, R.A., KAUFMAN, K.K., BEEZY, R., GARRY, M.W.: Amer. J. med. Sci. **224**, 304 (1952).
605. FRITZ, E.: Med. Klin. **59**, 1384 (1964).
606. FROHLICH, E.D., SCOTT, J.B.: Circulation **24**, 936 (1961).
607. — TARAZI, R.C., DUSTAN, H.P.: Arch. intern. Med. **123**, 1 (1969).
608. FRONĚK, A., GANZ, V.: Circulat. Res. **8**, 175 (1960).
609. — — 3rd European Congress of Cardiology, Roma, Sept. 1960, Pars Altera, p. 1069.
610. — — Cor et vasa (Praha) **2**, 120 (1961).
611. FRY, D.L., GRIGGS, D.M., GREENFIELD, J.G.: Circulat. Res. **14**, 73 (1964).
612. FUCCELLA, L.M., IMHOF, P.: Vth European Congress of Cardiology. Athenes, Sept. 1968. Abstracts p. 151.
613. FULLER, H.L., KASSEL, L.E.: J. Amer. med. Ass. **159**, 1708 (1955).
614. FULTON, W.F.M.: The coronary arteries. Arteriography, micro-anatomy, and pathogenesis of obliterative coronary artery disease. Springfield/Ill.: Ch. C. Thomas 1965.
615. FURBERG, C., JACOBSSON, K.A.: Acta med. scand. **181**, 729 (1967).
616. GAAL, P.G., KATTUS, A.A., ROSS, G.: Brit. J. Pharmacol. **26**, 713 (1966).
617. GABEL, L.P., WINBURY, M.M., ROWE, H., GRANDY, R.P.: J. Pharmacol. exp. Ther. **146**, 117 (1964).
618. GABRIELSEN, Z., MYHRE, J.R.: Circulation **17**, 348 (1958).
619. GADDUM, J.H., PEART, W.S., VOGT, M.: J. Physiol. (Lond.) **108**, 467 (1949).
620. GAFFNEY, T.E., BRAUNWALD, E.: Amer. J. Med. **34**, 320 (1963).
621. GAGLIANI, J., DE GRAFF, A.C., KUPPERMAN, H.S.: Intern. Record Med. Gen. Pract. Clin. **167**, 251 (1954).
622. GANDER, M., VERAGUT, U., KOHLER, R., LUTHY, E.: Cardiologia (Basel) **49**, 17 (1966).
623. GANELINA, I.E., DERYAGINA, G.P., KRIVORUCHENKO, I.V.: Sem. thér. **45**, 74 (1969).
624. GANZ, V., FRONĚK, A.: 3rd European Congress of Cardiology, Roma, Sept. 1960, Pars Altera, p. 707.
625. — — Cor et vasa (Praha) **2**, 107 (1961).
626. GARRONE, G., BOSSONEY, C.: Schweiz. med. Wschr. **86**, 417 (1956).
627. GARVEY, L., MELVILLE, K.I.: Pharmacologist **9**, 198 (1967).
628. — SHISTER, H.E., MELVILLE, K.I.: Canad. med. Ass. J. **98**, 113 (1968).
629. GAULT, J.E.: Med. J. Aust. **1**, 1066 (1969).
630. GAVEND, M., GAVEND, M.R., MERCIER, J.: C.R. Soc. Biol. (Paris) **154**, 2089 (1960).
631. GAZES, P.C., RICHARDSON, J.A., WOODS, E.F.: Circulation **19**, 657 (1959).
632. GEBHARDT, W., DRESSEL, J., STEIM, H., REINDELL, H.: Arzneimittel-Forsch. **11**, 962 (1961).
633. — REINDELL, H., KÖNIG, K., BÜCHNER, C.: Verh. dtsch. Ges. Kreisl.-Forsch. **31**, 99 (1965).
634. GELLER, H.M., BRANDFONBRENER, M., WIGGERS, C.J.: Circulat. Res. **1**, 152 (1953).
635. GENSINI, G.G., DI GIORGI, S., MURAD-NETTO, S., BLACK, A.: Angiology **13**, 550 (1962).
636. GENT, A.E., BROOK, C.G.D., FOLEY, T.H., MILLER, T.N.: Brit. med. J. **4**, 366 (1968).
637. GERARD, R., GRAS, A., BENYAMINE, R.: Sem. Hôp. Paris **43**, 44 (1967).
638. GERBAUX, A., LENEGRE, J.: Cardiologia **37**, Suppl. 2, 165 (1960).
639. — — Rev. Prat. (Paris) **31** bis, 107 (1962).
640. GERBAUX, J.O.: Revue du Rhumatisme **3**, 98 (1968).
641. GERBAUX, M.A.: Bull. Soc. méd. Paris **5**, 1 (1962).
642. GERHARD, W., SMEKAL, P.V., RENSCHLER, H.E., MUELLER, G.: Z. Kreisl.-Forsch. **57**, 876 (1968).
643. GERLACH, E., DEUTICKE, B.: Arzneimittel-Forsch. **13**, 48 (1963).
644. GEROLA, A., FEINBERG, H., KATZ, L.N.: Physiologist **1**, 31 (1957).
645. — — — Amer. J. Physiol. **196**, 394 (1959).
646. GERSMEYER, E.F., BEYER, E., LEICHT, E., SPITZBARTH, H.: Z. ges. exp. Med. **143**, 85 (1967).
647. — SPITZBARTH, H.: Med. Welt (Berl.) **13**, 764 (1967).
648. GERSTLAUER, E.: Med. Klin. **45**, 73 (1950).
649. GERSTNER, K.: Wien. med. Wschr. **115**, 1034 (1965).
650. GETTES, L.S., SURAWICZ: Amer. J. med. Sci. **254**, 257 (1967).
651. GIANELLY, R.E., GOLDMAN, R.H., TREISTER, B., HARRISON, D.C.: Ann. intern. Med. **67**, 1216 (1967).
652. — GRIFFIN, J.R., HARRISON, D.C.: Clin. Res. **15**, 118 (1967).
653. GIBSON, A.: J. Amer. med. Ass. **203**, 57 (1968).

654. GIBSON, D.G., BALCON, R., SOWTON, E.: Brit. med. J. 1968 III, 1961.
655. GIBSON, D., SOWTON, E.: Brit. med. J. 1968 I, 213.
656. GIESE, W., MÜLLER-MOHNSSEN, H.: Probleme der Coronardurchblutung. Berlin-Heidelberg-New York: Springer 1958, p. 159.
657. GILBERT, N.C., FENN, G.K.: Arch. intern. Med. 44, 118 (1929).
658. — NALEFSKI, L.A.: J. Lab. clin. Med. 34, 797 (1949).
659. GILLAM, P.M.S., PRICHARD, B.N.C.: Brit. med. J. 1965 II, 337.
660. — — Amer. J. Cardiol. 18, 366 (1966).
661. GILLE, H., RAUSCH, F.: Med. Welt (Berl.) 17, 715 (1966).
662. GILLOT, P.: Brux.-méd. 39, 1443 (1957).
663. — Acta cardiol. (Brux.) 14, 494 (1959).
664. — 3rd European Congress of Cardiology, Roma, Sept. 1960. Discussion of communication by CHARLIER (ref. 300).
665. — Brux.-méd. 50, 657 (1970).
666. GINN, W.M., ORGAIN, E.S.: J. Amer. med. Ass. 198, 1214 (1966).
667. GINSBERG, A.M., STOLAND, O.O.: J. Pharmacol. exp. Ther. 41, 195 (1931).
668. GIORDANO, G., TURRISI, E.: Clin. ter. 10, 670 (1956).
669. GIUDICELLI, J.-F., SCHMITT, H., BOISSIER, J.R.: J. Pharmacol. exp. Ther. 168, 116 (1969).
670. GLAVIANO, V.V.: Proc. Soc. exp. Biol. (N.Y.) 118, 1155 (1965).
671. GLEASON, W.L., BRAUNWALD, E.: J. clin. Invest. 41, 80 (1962).
672. GLEY, P., KISTHINIOS, N.: Presse méd. 37, 1279 (1929).
673. GLICK, G., PARMLEY, W.W., WECHSLER, A.S., SONNENBLICK, E.H.: Circulat. Res. 22, 789 (1968).
674. GODFRAIND, T., KABA, A., POLSTER, P.: Brit. J. Pharmacol. 28, 93 (1966).
675. GOKSEL, F.M.: Acta cardiol. (Brux.) 7, 630 (1952).
676. GOLD, H.: Amer. J. Med. 17, 722 (1954).
677. — KWIT, N.T., OTTO, H.: J. Amer. med. Ass. 108, 2173 (1937).
678. — TRAVELL, J., MODELL, W.: Amer. Heart J. 14, 284 (1937).
679. GOLDBERG, L.M.: Acta physiol. scand. 15, 173 (1948).
680. GOLDBERG, V.A.: Klin. Med. (Wien) 46, 100 (1968).
681. GOLDBERGER, E.: Amer. Heart J. 30, 60 (1945).
682. GOLDSBOROUGH, C.E.: Lancet 1960 II, 675.
683. GOLENHOFEN, K., HENSEL, H., HILDEBRANDT, G.: Durchblutungsmessung mit Wärmeleitelementen. Forschung und Klinik. Stuttgart: Georg Thieme 1963.
684. GOLLWITZER-MEIER, K., JUNGMANN, H.: Arch. exp. Pathol. Pharmakol. 214, 349 (1951).
685. — KRAMER, K., KRÜGER, E.: Pflügers Arch. ges. Physiol. 237, 639 (1936).
686. — KROETZ, C.: Klin. Wschr. 19, 580 (1940).
687. GOMEZ, C.G.R.: Angina de pecho, estudio preliminar de diez casos tratados con amiodarone. Tesis, Merida, Yucatan, Mexico. Imp. Massa, April 1969.
688. GOODALE, W.T., HACKEL, D.B.: Circulat. Res. 1, 502 (1953).
689. — — Circulat. Res. 1, 502 (1953).
690. — LUBIN, M., BANFIELD, W.G.: Amer. J. med. Sci. 214, 695 (1947).
691. — — ECKENHOFF, J.E., HAFKENSCHIEL, J.H., BANFIELD, W.G.: Amer. J. Physiol. 152, 340 (1948).
692. GOODMAN, L.S., GILMAN, A.: The Pharmacological Basis of Therapeutics, 1 vol., 2nd ed. New York: Macmillan 1955, 1831 pp.
693. GOODYER, A.V.N., HUVOS, A., ECKHARDT, W.F., OSTBERG, R.H.: Circulat. Res. 7, 432 (1959).
694. GORLIN, R.: Amer. J. Cardiol. 9, 419 (1962).
695. — Fed. Proc. 21, II, Suppl. 11, 93 (1962).
696. — Circulation 32, 138 (1965).
697. — J. Amer. med. Ass. 201, 27 (1967).
698. — BRACHFELD, N., McLEOD, C., BOPP, P.: Circulation 19, 705 (1959).
699. — — MESSER, J.V., TURNER, J.D.: Ann. intern. Med. 51, 698 (1959).
700. — COHEN, L.S., ELLIOTT, W.C., KLEIN, M.D., LANE, F.J.: Circulation 32, 361 (1965).
701. — TAYLOR, W.J.: J. Amer. med. Ass. 207, 907 (1969).
702. GOWDEY, C.W.: Brit. J. Pharmacol. 3, 254 (1948).
703. GRABNER, G., KAINDL, F., KRAUPP, O.: Arzneimittel-Forsch. 9, 45 (1959).
704. GRAHAM, D.M., LYON, T.P., GOFMAN, J.W., JONES, H.B., YANKLEY, A., SIMONTON, J., WHITE, S.: Circulation 4, 666 (1951).
705. GRAHAM, G.R.: J. Physiol. (Lond.) 128, 19 P (1955).
706. GRANATA, L., OLSSON, R.A., HUVOS, A., GREGG, D.E.: Circulat. Res. 16, 114 (1965).
707. GRANDJEAN, T.: Schweiz. med. Wschr. 97, 1559 (1968).
708. — RIVIER, J.L.: Brit. Heart J. 30, 50 (1968).

709. GRANT, R.H.E., KEELAN, P., KERNOHAN, R.J., LEONARD, J.C., NANCEKIEVILL, L., SINCLAIR, K.: Amer. J. Cardiol. **18**, 361 (1966).
710. — MCDEVITT, D.G., SHANKS, R.G.: Lancet **1968**I, 362.
711. GRAUMAN, S.J.: Amer. J. Cardiol. **3**, 544 (1959).
712. GRAY, W., RISEMAN, J.E.F., STEARNS, S.: New Engl. J. Med. **232**, 389 (1945).
713. GRAYSON, J., IRVINE, M., PARRATT, J.R.: Brit. J. Pharmacol. **30**, 488 (1967).
714. — — — Brit. J. Pharmacol. **37**, 523 P (1969).
715. — MENDEL, D.: Amer. J. Physiol. **200**, 968 (1961).
716. GREEFF, K., WAGNER, J.: Regensburg. Jb. ärztl. Fortbild. **15**, 28 (1967).
717. GREEN, H.D.: Publ. of Amer. Ass. Adv. Sci., Science Press **13**, 105 (1940).
718. — GREGG, D.E.: Amer. J. Physiol. **130**, 126 (1940).
719. GREENE, C.W.: J. Pharmacol. exp. Ther. **57**, 98 (1936).
720. GREGG, D.E.: Coronary Circulation in Health and Disease. Philadelphia: Lea & Febiger 1950.
721. — Ann. N.Y. Acad. Sci. **64**, 494 (1956).
722. — Circulation **27**, 1128 (1963).
723. — In: Oxygen in the animal organism. London: Pergamon Press 1964, p. 325.
724. — Int. Symp. on the coronary circulation and energetics of the myocardium, Milan 1966. Basle: S. Karger 1967, p. 54.
725. — ECKSTEIN, R.W.: Amer. J. Physiol. **132**, 781 (1941).
726. — FISHER, L.C.: Blood supply to the heart. In: Handbook of Physiology, Section 2: Circulation, 1963, **II**, chapter 44, 1517. Ed. by HAMILTON and Dow. Washington: American Physiological Society.
727. — GREEN, H.D.: Amer. J. Physiol. **130**, 114 (1940).
728. — KHOURI, E.M., RAYFORD, C.R.: Circulat. Res. **16**, 102 (1965).
729. — LONGINO, F.H., GREEN, P.A., CZERWONKA, L.J.: Circulation **3**, 89 (1951).
730. — PRITCHARD, W.H., ECKSTEIN, R.W., SHIPLEY, R.E., ROTTA, A., DINGLE, J., STEEGE, T.W., WEARN, J.T.: Amer. J. Physiol. **136**, 250 (1942).
731. — — SHIPLEY, R.E., WEARN, J.T.: Amer. J. Physiol. **139**, 726 (1943).
732. — SABISTON, D.C.: Circulation **13**, 916 (1956).
733. — SHIPLEY, R.E.: Amer. J. Physiol. **142**, 44 (1944).
734. — — Amer. J. Physiol. **151**, 13 (1947).
735. — — ECKSTEIN, R.W., ROTTA, A., WEARN, J.T.: Proc. Soc. exp. Biol. (N.Y.) **49**, 267 (1942).
736. GREGGIA, A., POGGIOLI, R.: Boll. Soc. ital. Biol. sper. **44**, 969 (1968).
737. GREIF, S., LIERTZER, V.: Ärztl. Forsch. **21**, 354 (1967).
738. GREINER, T., GOLD, H., CATTEL, M.K., TRAVELL, J., BAKST, H., RINZLER, S.H., BENJAMIN, Z.H., WARSHAW, L.J., BOBB, A.L., KWIT, N.T., MODELL, W., ROTHENDLER, H.H., MESSELOFF, C.R., KRAMER, M.L.: Amer. J. Med. **9**, 143 (1950).
739. GREMELS, H.: Arch. exp. Pathol. Pharmakol. **182**, 1 (1936).
740. GRIFFITH, G.C.: Aterosclerosis y enfermedad coronaria, 1 vol. Mexico: Ed. Interamericana 1960, p. 373.
741. — Circulation **22**, 1156 (1960).
742. — ZINN, W.J., ENGELBERG, H., DOOLEY, J.V., ANDERSON, R.: Circulation **18**, 728 (1958).
743. GRISWOLD, H.: Brit. med. J. **1969**II, 47.
744. GROBECKER, H., PALM, D., BAK, I.J., SCHMID, B.: Arch. Pharmakol. exp. Pathol. **263**, 215 (1969).
745. — — HOLTZ, P.: Arch. Pharmakol. exp. Path. **259**, 174 (1968).
746. — — — Arch. Pharmakol. exp. Path. **260**, 379 (1968).
747. GROSSMAN, A.J., BROOKS, A.M., BLACKMAN, A.L., SCHWIMMER, J., BATTERMAN, R.C.: Intern. Record Med. Gen. Pract. Clin. **167**, 263 (1954).
748. GRÜN, G., HAASTERT, H.P., DÖRING, H.J., KAMMERMEIER, H., FLECKENSTEIN, A.: Arzneimittel-Forsch. **18**, 381 (1968).
749. GRUND, G., WÜRZBACH, K.: Ärztl. Prax. **15**, 2490 (1963).
750. GRÜNER, A., HILDEN, T., RAASCHOU, F., VOGELIUS, H.: Amer. J. Med. **14**, 433 (1953).
751. GUADAGNO, L., GIANNELLI, G., GHIARA, F., GUADAGNO, P., ZUCCHELLI, G.P.: Minerva med. **58**, 3288 (1967).
752. GUBNER, R.S., BEHR, D.J.: Circulation **16**, 889 (1957).
753. GUILLEMAN, P.: Gaz. Hôp. (Paris) **25**, 909 (1958).
754. GUZMAN, F., BRAUN, C., LIM, R.K.S.: Arch. int. Pharmacodyn. **136**, 353 (1962).
755. HAAS, H.: Arzneimittel-Forsch. **14**, 461 (1964).
756. — Arzneimittel-Forsch. **18**, 89 (1968).
757. — BUSCH, E.: Arzneimittel-Forsch. **17**, 257 (1967).
758. — — Arzneimittel-Forsch. **18**, 401 (1968).
759. — HARTFELDER, G.: Arzneimittel-Forsch. **12**, 549 (1962).

760. HABERSANG, S., LEUSCHNER, F., VON SCHLICHTEGROLL, A.: Arzneimittel-Forsch. 17, 1478 (1967).
761. HAEFELY, W., HÜRLIMANN, A., THOENEN, H.: Angiologica 4, 203 (1967).
762. HAHN, N., FELIX, R., DRAZNIN, N., MEUSER, H.J., DÜX, A.: Arzneimittel-Forsch. 19, 300 (1969).
763. HAHN, R.A., PENDLETON, R.G., WARDELL, J.R.: J. Pharmacol. exp. Ther. 161, 111 (1968).
764. HAIGHT, C., FIGLEY, M.M., SLOAN, H., ELLSWORTH, W.J., MEYER, J.A., BERK, M.S., BOBLITT, D.E.: Circulation 18, 732 (1958).
765. HALE, G., DEXTER, D., JEFFERSON, K., LEATHAM, A.: Brit. Heart J. 28, 40 (1966).
766. HALMAGYI, M., HEMPEL, K.J., OCKENGA, T., RICHTER, G., WERNITSCH, W., ZEITLER, E.: Arzneimittel-Forsch. 17, 272 (1967).
767. HALPERIN, M.H.: Progr. cardiovasc. Dis. 2, 631 (1960).
768. HAMER, J., FLEMING, J.: Brit. Heart J. 29, 871 (1967).
769. — GRANDJEAN, T., MELENDEZ, L., SOWTON, G.E.: Brit. med. J. 1964 II, 720.
770. — SOWTON, E.: Brit. Heart J. 27, 892 (1965).
771. — — Amer. J. Cardiol. 18, 354 (1966).
772. HAMILTON, W.F., HIMMELSTEIN, A., NOBLE, R.P., REMINGTON, J.W., RICHARDS, D.W., WHEELER, N.C., WITHAM, A.L.: Amer. J. Physiol. 153, 309 (1948).
773. HAMM, J., RENSCHLER, H.E., ZACK, W.J.: Medizinische 3, 120 (1959).
774. HAMMERL, H., KLEIN, K., PICHLER, O.: Ärztl. Forsch. 13, 196 (1959).
775. — KRÄNZL, C., PICHLER, O., STUDLAR, M.: Arzneimittel-Forsch. 18, 309 (1968).
776. — SIEDEK, H.: Wien. klin. Wschr. 45, 788 (1961).
777. HANNA, C.: Arch. int. Pharmacodyn. 119, 305 (1959).
778. — PARKER, R.C.: Arch. int. Pharmacodyn. 126, 386 (1960).
779. — SHUTT, J.H.: Arch. exp. Pathol. Pharmakol. 220, 43 (1953).
780. HANSEN, A.T., HAXHOLDT, B.F., HUSFELDT, E., LASSEN, N.A., MUNCK, O., SORENSON, H.R., WINKLER, K.: Scand. J. clin. Lab. Invest. 8, 182 (1956).
781. HAPKE, H.-J., GIESE, W.: Arzneimittel-Forsch. 19, 1677 (1969).
782. — STERNER, W.: Arzneimittel-Forsch. 19, 1664 (1969).
783. HARLEY, B.J.S., DAVIES, R.O.: Canad. med. Ass. J. 99, 527 (1968).
784. HARRIS, R.: Amer. J. Cardiol. 4, 274 (1959).
785. HARRIS, W.S., SCHOENFELD, C.D., BROOKS, R.H., WEISSLER, A.M.: Amer. J. Cardiol. 17, 484 (1966).
786. HARRISON, D.C.: New Engl. J. Med. 280, 895 (1969).
787. HARRISON, J., TURNER, P.: Brit. J. Pharmacol. 36, 177 P (1969).
788. HARTENBACH, W.: Dtsch. med. Wschr. 31, 1061 (1953).
789. — Münch. med. Wschr. 16, 429 (1954).
790. HASHIMOTO, K., KUMAKURA, S., TANEMURA, I.: Arzneimittel-Forsch. 14, 1252 (1964).
791. HAUSNER, E., ESSEX, H.E., HERRICK, J.F., BALDES, E.J.: Amer. J. Physiol. 131, 43 (1940).
792. HAZARD, J.: Sem. Hôp. Paris 37, 2364 (1954).
793. HEATHCOTE, R.S.A.: J. Pharmacol. exp. Ther. 16, 327 (1921).
794. HEBB, A.R., GODWIN, T.F., GUNTON, R.W.: Canad. med. Ass. J. 98, 246 (1968).
795. HEDBOM, K.: Skand. Arch. Physiol. 8, 169 (1898).
796. HEFFERNAN, A., HICKEY, N., MULCAHY, R., FITZGERALD, O.: Acta cardiol. (Brux.) 24, 47 (1969).
797. HEFNER, L.L., FRIEDMAN, B., REEVES, T.J., EDDLEMAN, E.E., HARRISON, T.R.: 15, 111 (1957).
798. HEIM, F., WALTER, F.: Arzneimittel-Forsch. 18, 399 (1968).
799. HEIMANN, W., WILBRANDT, W.: Helv. Physiol. Acta 12, 230 (1954).
800. HEISTRACHER, P., KRAUPP, O., SPRING, G.: Arzneimittel-Forsch. 14, 1098 (1964).
801. — HELL, E., KRAUPP, O.: Arzneimittel-Forsch. 15, 146 (1964).
802. — KRAUPP, O., SCHIEFTHALER, T.: Arzneimittel-Forsch. 14, 1077 (1964).
803. HEJTMANCIK, M.R., FUTCH, E.D., HERRMANN, C.R.: Tex. St. J. Med. 49, 679 (1953).
804. HELBIG, J.: Münch. med. Wschr. 103, 100 (1961).
805. HELLEMS, H.K., ORD, J.W., TALMERS, F.N., CHRISTENSEN, R.C.: Circulation 16, 893 (1957).
806. HELLER, E.M.: Canad. med. Ass. J. 74, 197 (1956).
807. HELLERSTEIN, H.K., HIRSCH, E.Z., CUMLER, W., ALLEN, L., POLSTER, S., ZUCKER, N.: Reconditioning of the coronary patient. A preliminary report. In: Coronary Heart Disease, ed. by W. LIKOFF and J.H. MOYER. New York: Grune and Stratton 1963, p. 448.
808. — HORNSTEN, T.R.: J. Rehab. 32, 48 (1966).
809. HELLMAN, L., ZUMOFF, B., KESSLER, G., KARA, E., RUBIN, I.L., ROSENFELD, R.S.: Ann. intern. Med. 59, 477 (1963).

810. HENDERSON, F.G., SHIPLEY, R.E., CHEN, K.K.: J. Amer. pharm. Ass. **40**, 207 (1951).
811. HENKE, C., DUDIK, E., STEIM, H.: Arzneimittel-Forsch. **18**, 1103 (1968).
812. HENSALA, J.C., BURGISON, R.M., KRANTZ, J.C.: J. Pharmacol. exp. Ther. **131**, 261 (1961).
813. HENSEL, H.: Personal Communication 1965.
814. — HALLWACHS, H., SCHMIDT-MERTENS, H.H.: Arzneimittel-Forsch. **21**, 927 (1971).
815. — RUEF, J., GOLENHOFEN, K.: Pflügers Arch. ges. Physiol. **259**, 267 (1954).
816. HERD, J.A., HOLLENBERG, M., THORBURN, G.D., KOPALD, H.H., BARGER, A.C.: Amer. J. Physiol. **203**, 122 (1962).
817. HERMAN, M.V., ELLIOTT, W.C., GORLIN, R.: Circulation **35**, 834 (1967).
818. HERMANN, H., MORNEX, R.: Thérapie **15**, 993 (1960).
819. HERMANSEN, K.: Acta pharmacol. (Kbh.) **26**, 343 (1968).
820. — Brit. J. Pharmacol. **35**, 476 (1969).
821. HERREMAN, F.: Sem. Hôp. Paris **42**, 13 (1966).
822. HERSCHEL, J.G.: Geneesk. Gids **29**, 26 (1951).
823. HESS, H.: Therapiewoche **11**, 149 (1960).
824. HESS, M.H., BRIGGS, F.N., SHINEBOURNE, E., HAMER, J.: Nature (Lond.) **220**, 79 (1968).
825. HEUBNER, W., MANCKE, R.: In: Abderhalden's Handbuch der biologischen Arbeits-methoden. Berlin und Wien: Urban & Schwarzenberg 1935, Abt. V, Teil 8, p. 885.
826. HILGER, H.H., SCHAEDE, A., WAGNER, J., LOUVEN, B., WACKERBAUER, J., HELLWIG, H.: Z. Kreisl.-Forsch. **56**, 164 (1967).
827. — WAGNER, J., HELLWIG, H., LOUVEN, B., WACKERBAUER, J., SCHAEDE, A.: Z. Kreisl.-Forsch. **56**, 1192 (1967).
828. HILL, R.C., TURNER, P.: Brit. J. Pharmacol. **32**, 663 (1968).
829. — — Brit. J. Pharmacol. **36**, 368 (1969).
830. HILLESTAD, L., ANDERSEN, A.: Acta med. scand. **185**, 535 (1969).
831. — STORSTEIN, O.: Amer. Heart J. **77**, 137 (1969).
832. HILLS, E.A., DOWNES, E.M.: Lancet **1967** II, 1149.
833. HILTON, R., EICHHOLTZ, F.: J. Physiol. (Lond.) **59**, 413 (1925).
834. HILTON, S.M., LEWIS, G.P.: J. Physiol. (Lond.) **134**, 471 (1956).
835. — — Brit. med. Bull. **13**, 189 (1957).
836. HIMBERT, J.: Sem. Hôp. thér. **45**, 156 (1969).
837. HIRCHE, H.: Pflügers Arch. ges. Physiol. **288**, 162 (1966).
838. — SCHOLTHOLT, J.: Arzneimittel-Forsch. **15**, 1388 (1965).
839. HIRSCH, W.: Med. Klin. **61**, 1784 (1966).
840. — WOSCHEE, G.: Ther. d. Gegenw. **106**, 809 (1967).
841. HIRSHLEIFER, I.: Curr. ther. Res. **11**, 99 (1969).
842. HOBBS, L.F.: Angiology **11**, 86 (1960).
843. HOCHREIN, M., KELLER, C.J.: Arch. exp. Pathol. Pharmakol. **159**, 438 (1931).
844. HOCKERTS, T., BÖGELMANN, G.: Arzneimittel-Forsch. **9**, 47 (1959).
845. HOESCHEN, R.J., BOUSVAROS, G.A., KLASSEN, G.A., FAM, W.M., MCGREGOR, M.: Brit. Heart J. **28**, 221 (1966).
846. HOFBAUER, K.: Wien. med. Wschr. **116**, 1155 (1967).
847. HOFFMANN, P.: Med. Klin. **59**, 1387 (1964).
848. HOHENSTEIN, H.: Ther. d. Gegenw. **104**, 1242 (1965).
849. HOLDSWORTH, C.D., ATKINSON, M., GOLDIE, W.: Lancet **1961** II, 621.
850. HOLLANDER, W., CHOBANIAN, A.V., WILKINS, R.W.: J. Amer. med. Ass. **174**, 5 (1960).
851. — MADOFF, I.M., CHOBANIAN, A.V.: J. Pharmacol. exp. Ther. **139**, 53 (1963).
852. — WILKINS, R.W.: Symposium International "The catecholamines in cardiovascular pathology", Burlington, Aug. 23, 1959, Summary, p. 11.
853. — — In: Hypertension. Ed. by J.H. MOYER. Philadelphia: Saunders & Co. 1959, p. 399.
854. HOLLOSZY, J.O., SKINNER, J.S., BARRY, A.J., CURETON, T.K.: Amer. J. Cardiol. **14**, 761 (1964).
855. HOLMBERG, S.: Internat. Symp. on the coronary circulation and energetics of the myo-cardium. Milan 1966. Basle: S. Karger 1967, p. 268.
856. HOLZMANN, M.: Cardiologia **35**, 17 (1959).
857. HONIG, C.R., TENNEY, S.M., GABEL, P.V.: Amer. J. Med. **29**, 910 (1960).
858. HOOGERWERF, S.: Geneesk. Gids **33**, 368 (1955).
859. HORITA, A.: J. Pharmacol. exp. Ther. **122**, 176 (1958).
860. HORLICK, L.: Canad. med. Ass. J. **80**, 9 (1959).
861. HORWITZ, D., GOLDBERG, L.I., SJOERDSMA, A.: Circulation **24**, 959 (1961).
862. HOUTSMULLER, A.J.: Ned. T. Geneesk. **108**, 2211 (1964).
863. — Ned. T. Geneesk. **110**, 1325 (1966).
864. HOWARTH, S., MACMICHAEL, J.S., SHARPEY-SCHAFER, E.P.: Clin. Sci. **6**, 125 (1947).

865. HÜDEPOHL, M.: Münch. med. Wschr. 108, 2360 (1966).
866. HUEBER, E.F.: 3rd European Congress of Cardiology, Roma, Sept. 1960, Pars altera B, p. 1111.
867. — Wien. med. Wschr. 42, 961 (1967).
868. — KOTZAUREK, R.: Wien. med. Wschr. 118, 657 (1968).
869. — THALER, H.: Wien. klin. Wschr. 11, 187 (1957).
870. HUFF, J.W., GILFILLAN, J.L.: Proc. Soc. exp. Biol. (N.Y.) 103, 41 (1960).
871. HULTGREN, H.N., ROBERTSON, H.S., STEVENS, L.E.: J. Amer. med. Ass. 148, 465 (1952).
872. HUNSCHA, H., KALTENBACH, M., SCHELLHORN, W.: Therapiewoche 16, 1153 (1966).
873. HUNTER, F.E., KAHANA, S., FORD, L.: Fed. Proc. 12, 221 (1953).
874. HUPPERT, V.F., BOYD, L.J.: Bull. N.Y. med. Coll. 18, 58 (1956).
875. IISALO, E., KALLIO, V.: Curr. ther. Res. 11, 209 (1969).
876. IKEZONO, E., YASUDA, K., HATTORI, Y.: Anesthesiology 29, 199 (1968).
877. IKRAM, H., NIXON, P.G.F.: Lancet 1967 I, 336.
878. IRONS, G.V., GINN, W.N., ORGAIN, E.S.: Amer. J. Med. 43, 161 (1967).
879. ISAACS, J.H., WILBURNE, M., MILLS, H., KUHN, R.: J. Amer. med. Ass. 198, 1065 (1966).
880. ISHINOSE, Y.: Discussion of the communication by CHARLIER (ref. 313bis), Vth European Congress of Cardiology, Athenes, Sept. 1968.
881. IWAI, M., SASSA, K.: Arch. exp. Pathol. Pharmakol. 99, 215 (1923).
882. JABLONS, B., SCHILERO, A.J., SICAM, L., ESTRELLADO, T.: Intern. Amer. Congress of Cardiology, Havana, Cuba, Nov. 1956.
883. JACOB, M.I., BERNE, R.M.: a) Amer. J. Physiol. 198, 322 (1960). b) Proc. Soc. exp. Biol. (N.Y.) 107, 738 (1961).
884. JACOBI, H., LANGE, A., PFLEGER, K.: Arzneimittel-Forsch. 6, 41 (1956).
885. JACOBSSON, K.A., KOCH, G., LINDGREN, M., MICHAELSSON, G.: Acta med. scand. 180, 129 (1966).
886. JAGENEAU, A., BRUGMANS, J.: Quoted by BOSMANS et al. (ref. 39c).
887. — SCHAPER, W.: Arzneimittel-Forsch. 17, 582 (1967).
888. — — Nature (Lond.) 221, 184 (1969).
889. — VAN GERVEN, W.: Naunyn-Schmiedeberg's Arch. exp. Path. Pharmak. 265, 16 (1969).
890. JAHN, W.: Arzneimittel-Forsch. 19, 701 (1969).
891. Evaluation of a Coronary Vasodilator. Dipyridamole (Persantin). J. Amer. med. Ass. 188, 1141 (1964).
892. JAMES, T.N.: Circulation 32, 1020 (1965).
893. JAQUENOUD, P.: Ann. Anesth. Franç. 7, 3 (1966).
894. JARCHO, S.: Amer. J. Cardiol. 17, 879 (1966).
895. JASINSKI, B.: Cardiologia 23, 49 (1953).
896. JENKINS, C.D., ROSENMAN, R.H., ZYZANSKI, S.J.: Circulation 38, Suppl. VI, 11 (1968).
897. JEREMIAS, H.: Therapiewoche 16, 266 (1966).
898. JESCHKE, D., CAESAR, K., SCHOLLMEYER, P.: Med. Welt (Berl.) 1, 14 (1969).
899. JEWITT, D.E., MERCER, C.J., SHILLINGFORD, J.P.: Lancet 1969 II, 227.
900. JOERGENSEN, L., ROWSELL, H.C., HOVIG, T., GLYNN, M.F., MUSTARD, J.F.: Lab. Invest. 17, 616 (1967).
901. JOHNSEN, T.S.: Ugeskr. Læg. 124, 942 (1962).
902. JOHNSON, J.R., WIGGERS, C.J.: Amer. J. Physiol. 118, 38 (1937).
903. JOHNSON, P.C., SEVELIUS, G.: J. Amer. med. Ass. 173, 1231 (1960).
904. JOHNSSON, G.: Acta pharmacol. (Kbh.) 25, Suppl. 2, 63 (1967).
905. — NORRBY, A., SÖLVELL, L.: Acta pharmacol. (Kbh.) 25, Suppl. 2, 95 (1967).
906. JOLLIFFE, N.: Circulation 20, 109 (1959).
907. JOLLY, E.R.: Circulation 20, 1 (1959).
908. JONGEBREUR, G.: Arch. int. Pharmacodyn. 90, 384 (1952).
909. JORIS, H., SCHMETZ, J.: Rev. méd. Liège 16, 486 (1961).
910. JOSEPH, L.G., MANCINI, A.: Angiology 12, 264 (1961).
911. JOST, M., GASSER, P.: Cardiologia 38, 215 (1961).
912. JOURDAN, F., FAUCON, G.: Arch. Mal. Cœur 50, 748 (1957).
913. — — Thérapie 12, 927 (1957).
914. — — Arch. int Pharmacodyn. 116, 423 (1958).
915. — — Thérapie 13, 635 (1958).
916. — — Thérapie 14, 364 (1959).
917. — — Cardiologia 34, 376 (1959).
918. JOUVE, A.: Brux.-méd. 48, 23 (1968).
919. — GRAS, A., BENYAMINE, R.: Vie méd. 44, 115 (1963).
920. — MEDVEDOWSKY, J.L., BENYAMINE, R.: Annales de Cardiologie et d'Angéiologie 18, 65 (1969).

921. JUNEMANN, C.: Münch. med. Wschr. **101**, 340 (1959).
922. JUNKMANN, K.: Arch. exp. Pathol. Pharmakol. **195**, 175 (1940).
923. KABELA, E., MENDEZ, R.: Brit. J. Pharmacol. **26**, 473 (1966).
924. KADATZ, R.: Arzneimittel-Forsch. **9**, 39 (1959).
925. — In: Methods in drug evaluation. Ed. by P. MANTEGAZZA and F. PICCININI. Amsterdam: North Holland Publishers Co. 1966, p. 120.
926. — Arch. Kreisl.-Forsch. **58**, 263 (1969).
927. — Brux.-méd. **50**, 609 (1970).
928. — DIEDEREN, W.: Ärztl. Forsch. **21**, 51 (1967).
929. — PÖTZSCH, E.: 3rd European Congress of Cardiology, Roma, Sept. 1960, Pars Altera, p. 827.
930. KAINDL, F., PÄRTAN, J., POLSTERER, P.: Wien. klin. Wschr. **68**, 186 (1956).
931. KAISER, W., KLEPZIG, H.: Med. Welt (Berl.) **33**, 1786 (1968).
932. KALMANSON, F.M., DRENICK, E.J., BINDER, M.J., ROSOVE, L.: Arch. intern. Med, **95**, 819 (1955).
933. KALTENBACH, M., ZIMMERMANN, D.: Dtsch. med. Wschr. **93**, 25 (1968).
934. KANDZIORA, J.: Med. Welt (Berl.) **39**, 2314 (1967).
935. KANNEL, W.B., WIDMER, L.K., DAWBER, T.R.: Schweiz. med. Wschr. **95**, 18 (1965).
936. KAPPERT, A.: Schweiz. med. Wschr. **85**, 237 (1955).
937. — Zeitschr. für Therapie **3**, 82 (1965).
938. — Zeitschr. für Therapie **8**, 477 (1969).
939. KARCZMAR, A.G., BOURGAULT, P., ELPERN, B.: Proc. Soc. exp. Biol. (N.Y.) **98**, 114 (1958).
940. KARGES, O.: Med. Klin. **64**, 1280 (1969).
941. KARPATI, E., DOMOK, L., SZPORNY, L.: Arzneimittel-Forsch. **19**, 1011 (1969).
942. — SZPORNY, L., DOMOK, L., NADOR, K.: J. Pharm. Pharmacol. **20**, 735 (1968).
943. KARTUN, P.: Gaz. méd. Fr. **70**, 931 (1963).
944. KASSER, I.S., BRUCE, R.A.: Circulation **38**, Suppl. 6, 111 (1968).
945. KATORI, M., BERNE, R.M.: Circulat. Res. **19**, 420 (1966).
946. KATTUS, A.A.: Internat. Symp. on coronary circulation and energetics of the myocardium, Milan 1966. Basle: S. Karger 1967, p. 302.
947. — GREGG, D.E.: Circulat. Res. **7**, 628 (1959).
948. — MAC ALPIN, R.N.: Circulation **32**, Suppl. 2, 122 (1965).
949. KATZ, A., MESSIN, R.: Brux.-méd. **51**, 1815 (1961).
950. KATZ, A.M., KATZ, L.N., WILLIAMS, F.L.: Amer. J. Physiol. **180**, 392 (1955).
951. KATZ, G.: Arch. int. Pharmacodyn. **49**, 239 (1935).
952. KATZ, L.N.: Amer. Heart J. **10**, 322 (1935).
953. — Ann. N.Y. Acad. Sci. **64**, 505 (1956).
954. — JOCHIM, K., BOHNING, A.: Amer. J. Physiol. **122**, 236 (1938).
955. — — WEINSTEIN, W.: Amer. J. Physiol. **122**, 252 (1938).
956. — LINDNER, E.: Amer. J. Physiol. **124**, 155 (1938).
957. — — J. Amer. med. Ass. **113**, 2116 (1939).
958. — — WEINSTEIN, W., ABRAMSON, D.I., JOCHIM, K.: Arch. int. Pharmacodyn. **59**, 399 (1938).
959. — WEINSTEIN, W., JOCHIM, K.: Amer. J. Physiol. **113**, 76 (1935).
960. — WILLIAMS, F.L., LAURENT, D., BOLENE-WILLIAMS, C., FEINBERG, H.: Fed. Proc. **15**, 106 (1956).
961. KAUFMANN, H., BERGOGNE, C., PLESSIS, F.: Presse méd. **74**, 921 (1966).
962. KAVERINA, N.V.: Farmakol. i Toksikol. **21**, 39 (1958). Abstracted in Chem. Zentralbl. **46**, 13043 (1958).
963. — See ref. 2039, p. 93.
964. — VYSOTSKAYA, N.B., ROZONOV, Y.B., SHUGINA, T.M.: Bjul. Eksp. Biol. Med. **64**, 1310 (1968).
965. KEEFER, C.S., RESNIK, W.H.: Arch. intern. Med. **41**, 769 (1928).
966. KEELAN, P.: Brit. med. J. **1965 I**, 897.
967. KEMP, H.G., ELLIOTT, W.C., GORLIN, R.: Trans. Ass. Amer. Phys. **80**, 59 (1967).
968. KENAWY, M.R., BARSOUM, G.S.: Gaz. Faculty Med. Cairo **13**, 39 (1945).
969. KENNAMER, R., PRINZMETAL, M.: Amer. J. Cardiol. **3**, 542 (1959).
970. KERNOHAN, R.J.: Lancet **1967 II**, 716.
971. KERTES, K.: Gyogyszerészet **11**, 70 (1967).
972. KETY, S.S.: Amer. Heart J. **38**, 321 (1949).
973. — SCHMIDT, C.F.: Amer. J. Physiol. **143**, 53 (1945).
974. KEUL, J., DOLL, E., FRIEDEMANN, M., REINDELL, H.: Arzneimittel-Forsch. **17**, 1503 (1967).
975. — — — — Arzneimittel-Forsch. **18**, 78 (1968).

976. KEYS, A.: Aterosclerosis y enfermedad coronaria, 1 vol. Mexico: Ed. Interamericana 1960, p. 137.
977. KHOURI, E. M., GREGG, D. E.: J. appl. Physiol. **18**, 224 (1963).
978. — — LOWENSOHN, H. S.: Internat. Symp. on the coronary circulation and energetics of the myocardium, Milan 1966. Basle: S. Karger 1967, p. 250.
979. — — RAYFORD, C. R.: Circulat. Res. **17**, 427 (1965).
980. KIESE, M., LANGE, G.: Arch. exp. Pathol. Pharmakol. **231**, 149 (1957).
981. — — RESAG, K.: Z. ges. exp. Med. **132**, 426 (1960).
982. KIESEWETTER, E.: Wien. med. Wschr. **119**, 346 (1969).
983. KILLAM, K. F., FELLOWS, E. J.: Fed. Proc. **9**, 291 (1950).
984. KIMURA, E., USHIYAMA, K., YAMAZAKI, T., YOSHIDA, K., KOJIMA, N., KANIE, T.: Proceedings of the IIIrd Asian Pacific Congress of Cardiology, Kyoto **1**, 745 (1964).
985. KINNARD, W. J., VOGIN, E. E., ACETO, M. D., BUCKLEY, J. P.: Angiology **15**, 312 (1964).
986. KINSELLA, D., TROUP, W., McGREGOR, M.: Amer. Heart J. **63**, 146 (1962).
987. KIRCHHOFF, H. W., BURKHART, K., MEYER, J., GEBELEIN, H., HENZE, H.: Arzneimittel-Forsch. **19**, 64 (1969).
988. KISCH, B.: Exp. Med. Surg. **16**, 96 (1958).
989. KISIN, I. E.: Bjul. Eksp. Biol. Med. **12**, 61 (1959).
990. KLAKEG, C. H., PRUITT, R. D., BURCHELL, H. B.: Amer. Heart J. **49**, 614 (1955).
991. KLARWEIN, M., NITZ, R. E.: Arzneimittel-Forsch. **15**, 555 (1965).
992. KLEIBER, E. E.: Ann. intern. Med. **36**, 1179 (1952).
993. KLENSCH, H.: Z. Kreisl.-Forsch. **54**, 771 (1965).
994. — JUZNIC, G.: Z. Kreisl.-Forsch. **53**, 117 (1964).
995. — — Arzneimittel-Forsch. **14**, 982 (1964).
996. KLEVER, R.: Therapiewoche **18**, 838 (1968).
997. KLICH, R.: Therapiewoche **13**, 347 (1963).
998. KLIGGE, H.: a) Med. Klin. **59**, 1907 (1964). b) Münch. med. Wschr. **108**, 1169 (1966).
999. KLOCKE, F. J., KAISER, G. A., ROSS, J., BRAUNWALD, E.: Circulat. Res. **16**, 376 (1965).
1000. — — — — Amer. J. Physiol. **209**, 913 (1965).
1001. KLOSTER, J. H.: Ugeskr. Læg. **124**, 939 (1962).
1002. KNEBEL, R.: Personal Communication 1969.
1003. — OCKENGA, T.: Wien. klin. Wschr. **16**, 273 (1965).
1004. KNICK, B.: Arzneimittel-Forsch. **11**, 843 (1961).
1005. KNOCH, G.: Med. Klin. **58**, 1485 (1963).
1006. KNOCHE, H., SCHMITT, G.: Z. Zellforsch. **61**, 524 (1963).
1007. KNOEBEL, S. B., McHENRY, P. L., ROBERTS, D., STEIN, L.: Circulation **37**, 932 (1968).
1008. — — STEIN, L., SONEL, A.: Circulation **36**, 187 (1967).
1009. KOCH-WESER, J.: Fed. Proc. **25**, 2 (1966).
1010. KÖHLER, J. A., STERNITZKE, N.: Circulatory Drugs. Ed. by A. BERTELLI. Amsterdam: North Holland Publ. Co. 1969, p. 31.
1011. KÖHLER, W.: Medizinische **7**, 294 (1959).
1012. KOLIN, A.: Proc. Soc. exp. Biol. (N.Y.) **35**, 53 (1936).
1013. — Science **130**, 1088 (1959).
1014. — a) Proc. Soc. exp. Biol. (N.Y.) **35**, 53 (1936). b) Science **130**, 1088 (1959).
1015. — ARCHER, J. D., ROSS, G.: Circulat. Res. **21**, 889 (1967).
1016. — KADO, R. T.: Proc. nat. Acad. Sci. (Wash.) **45**, 1312 (1959).
1017. — ROSS, G., GROLLMAN, J. H., ARCHER, J.: Proc. nat. Acad. Sci. (Wash.) **59**, 808 (1968).
1018. KOLODZIG, S.: Therapiewoche **43**, 1479 (1966).
1019. KOROXENIDIS, G., TSITOURIS, G., PAPADOPOULOS, A., VASSILIKOS, C., CORCONDILAS, A., MICHAELIDES, G.: Vth European Congress of Cardiology, Athenes, Sept. 1968. Abstracts p. 209.
1020. KORY, R. C., TOWNES, A. S., MABE, R. E., DORRIS, E. R., MENEELY, G. R.: Amer. Heart J. **50**, 308 (1955).
1021. KOSS, F. W., BEISENHERZ, G., MAERKISCH, R.: Arzneimittel-Forsch. **12**, 1130 (1962).
1022. KOT, P. A., CROKE, R. P., PINKERSON, A. L.: Angiology **18**, 603 (1967).
1023. KOUNTZ, W. B.: J. Pharmacol. exp. Ther. **45**, 65 (1932).
1024. — Progr. cardiovasc. Dis. **2**, 541 (1960).
1025. — SMITH, J. R.: J. clin. Invest. **17**, 147 (1938).
1026. KRANTZ, J. C., CARR, C. J.: Pharmacologic Principles of Medical Practice. 1 vol, 1116 pp., 2nd ed., Baillière, Tindall & Cox, 1951, p. 824.
1027. — — BRYANT, H. H.: J. Pharmacol. exp. Ther. **102**, 16 (1951).
1028. — — FORMAN, S. E.: J. Pharmacol. exp. Ther. **64**, 302 (1938).
1029. — — — ELLIS, F. W.: J. Pharmacol. exp. Ther. **67**, 187 (1939).
1030. — — — — J. Pharmacol. exp. Ther. **67**, 191 (1939).
1031. KRASNIKOV, Y. A.: Ter Arkh. **39**, 84 (1967).

1032. KRASNOW, N., BARBAROSH, H.: Anesthesiology **29**, 814 (1968).
1033. — HOOD, W.B., ROLETT, E.L., YURCHAK, P.M.: Circulation **26**, 745 (1962).
1034. — ROLETT, E.L., YURCHAK, P.M., HOOD, W.B., GORLIN, R.: Amer. J. Med. **37**, 514 (1964).
1035. KRAUPP, W.E.: Arch. exp. Pathol. Pharmakol. **253**, 298 (1966).
1036. KRAUPP, O., GROSSMANN, W., STÜHLINGER, W., RABERGER, G.: Arzneimittel-Forsch. **18**, 1067 (1968).
1037. — HEISTRACHER, P., WOLNER, E., TUISL, E.: Arzneimittel-Forsch. **14**, 1086 (1964).
1038. — NELL, G., RABERGER, G., STÜHLINGER, W.: Arzneimittel-Forsch. **19**, 1691 (1969).
1039. — NIESSNER, H.: Arch. Pharmakol. exp. Path. **255**, 29 (1966).
1040. — — PLOSZCZANSKI, B., ADLER-KASTNER, L., SPRINGER, A., CHIRIKDJIAN, J.J.: Europ. J. Pharmacol. **1**, 140 (1967).
1041. — WOLNER, E.: Arch. exp. Pathol. Pharmakol. **253**, 57 (1966).
1042. — — ADLER-KASTNER, L., CHIRIKDJIAN, J.J., PLOSZCZANSKI, B., TUISL, E.: Arzneimittel-Forsch. **16**, 692 (1966).
1043. — — SUKO, J.: Arch. Pharmakol. exp. Path. **254**, 431 (1966).
1044. KRAUT, H., FREY, E.K., BAUER, E.: Z. phys. Chem. **175**, 97 (1928).
1045. KRAUTHEIM, J., SCHMID, E.: Arzneimittel-Forsch. **16**, 1500 (1966).
1046. KRUEGER, G.A.W.: Therapiewoche **19**, 169 (1969).
1047. KRUEGER, K.: Med. Klin. **62**, 1627 (1967).
1048. — Therapiewoche **18**, 1413 (1968).
1049. KÜBLER, W., BRETSCHNEIDER, H.J.: Pflügers Arch. ges. Physiol. **277**, 141 (1963).
1050. — — Pflügers Arch. ges. Physiol. **280**, 141 (1964).
1051. — — SPIECKERMANN, P.G.: Arzneimittel-Forsch. **19**, 185 (1969).
1052. KÜHNS, K.: Z. Kreisl.-Forsch. **41**, 721 (1952).
1053. KUKOVETZ, W.R.: Arzneimittel-Forsch. **14**, 1104 (1964).
1054. — Circulatory Drugs. Ed. by A. BERTELLI. Amsterdam: North Holland Publ. Co. 1969, p. 40.
1055. — Arzneimittel-Forsch. **19**, 1672 (1969).
1056. — FISCHER, G.: Arch. exp. Pathol. Pharmakol. **251**, 146 (1965).
1057. KUKWA, D.: Arzneimittel-Forsch. **17**, 290 (1967).
1058. KUNZE, K., LÜBBERS, D.W., RYBAK, B.: C.R. Acad. Sci. (Paris) **253**, 904 (1961).
1059. KURIYAMA, T.: Jap. Circulat. J. (Ni.) **24**, 1332 (1960).
1060. KURLAND, G.S., FREEDBERG, A.S.: Circulation **22**, 464 (1960).
1061. KUSCHKE, H.J.: Arch. int. Pharmacodyn. **106**, 100 (1956).
1062. — ECKMANN, F., IDRISS, H., BIECK, P.: Verh. dtsch. Ges. inn. Med. **70**, 191 (1964).
1063. KUTSCHA, W.: Med. Welt (Berl.) **28**, 1639 (1967).
1064. KUTSCHERA, W., PERGER, F.: Ars Med. **5**, 330 (1957).
1065. KUTZ-ECHAVE, R.: Cardiologia **20**, 129 (1952).
1066. KVAM, D.C., RIGGILO, D.A., LISH, P.M.: J. Pharmacol. exp. Ther. **149**, 183 (1965).
1067. LAFONTANT, R., FEINBERG, H., KATZ, L.N.: Circulation **22**, 774 (1960).
1068. LAMPRECHT, G., SCHMIDT-VOIGT, J.: Med. Klin. **61**, 18 (1966).
1069. Lancet: **1966 II**, 950.
1070. Lancet: **1966 II**, 1435.
1071. LANG, O.: Wien. klin. Wschr. **17**, 305 (1965).
1072. LANGE, G.: Biochem. Pharmacol. **8**, 136 (1961).
1073. — Arch. exp. Pathol. Pharmakol. **246**, 240 (1963).
1074. LANGENDORFF, O.: Pflügers Arch. ges. Physiol. **61**, 291 (1895).
1075. LARSEN, V.: Acta pharmacol. (Kbh.) **4**, 1 (1948).
1076. LASAGNA, L.: Cited by BATTERMAN (ref. 105), p. 503.
1077. LASKER, N., SHERROD, T.R., KILLAM, K.F.: J. Pharmacol. exp. Ther. **113**, 414 (1955).
1078. LASSEN, N.A., LINDBJERG, J., MUNCK, O.: Lancet **1964 I**, 686.
1079. LASZLO, B., LASZLO, K.: Wien. klin. Wschr. **79**, 875, (1967).
1080. LAU, S.H., COHEN, S.I., STEIN, E., HAFT, J.I., KINNEY, M.J., YOUNG, M.W., HELFANT, R.H., DAMATO, A.N.: Circulation **38**, 711 (1968).
1081. — DAMATO, A.N., BERKOWITZ, W.D., PATTON, R.D.: Circulation **40**, 71 (1969).
1082. — HAFT, J.I., COHEN, S.I., HELFANT, R.H., YOUNG, M.W., DAMATO, A.N.: Circulation **36**, Suppl. 2, 169 (1967).
1083. LAUBIE, M., LE DOUAREC, J.C., SCHMITT, H.: Arch. int. Pharmacodyn. **151**, 313 (1964).
1084. — SCHMITT, H.: Arch. int. Pharmacodyn. **155**, 1 (1965).
1085. — — Thérapie **20**, 519 (1965).
1086. — — PELTIER, J., DROUILLAT, M.: Arch. int. Pharmacodyn. **159**, 206 (1966).
1087. — — REMY, C.: Thérapie **21**, 203 (1966).
1088. LAUBRY, C., SOULIE, P., LAUBRY, P.: Arch. Mal. Cœur **30**, 265 (1937).
1089. LAUENROTH, G.: Med. Klin. **55**, 1434 (1960).

1090. LAUSTELA, E., TALA, P.: Arzneimittel-Forsch. **17**, 1125 (1967).
1091. LEDWICH, J.R.: Canad. med. Ass. J. **98**, 988 (1968).
1092. LEEPER, R.D., MEAD, A.W., MONEY, W.L., RAWSON, R.W.: Clin. Pharmacol. Ther. **2**, 13 (1961).
1093. LEHAN, P.H., OLDEWURTEL, H.A., WEISSE, A.B., ELLIOTT, M.S., REGAN, T.J.: Circulation **33**, Suppl. 3, 154 (1966).
1094. LEIBETSEDER, F.: Wien. klin. Wschr. **43**, 839 (1965).
1095. LEIGHNINGER, D.S., RUEGER, R., BECK, C.: Amer. J. Cardiol. **3**, 638 (1959).
1096. LEITCH, J.L., HALEY, T.J.: J. Amer. pharm. Ass. **41**, 512 (1952).
1097. LEKIEFFRE, J.: Mouvement thérapeutique **9**, 5 (1964).
1098. LEKOS, D., IOANNIDIS, P., CORCONDILAS, A., HADJIGEORGE, C., MARNEZOS, E., KOROXENIDIS, G., MICHAELIDES, G.: Vth European Congress of Cardiology. Athenes, Sept. 1968. Abstracts p. 218.
1099. LEMBERG, L., CASTELLANOS, A., ARCEBAL, A.G.: Ann. intern. Med. **70**, 1078 (1969).
1100. LENEGRE, J.: Cah. méd. de France **8**, 381 (1963).
1101. — Thérapie **22**, 141 (1967).
1102. LEPESCHKIN, E.: Circulation **22**, 986 (1960).
1103. LEQUIME, J., CLEEMPOEL, H., VAN THIEL, E.: 5th World Congress of Cardiology, New-Delhi Nov. 1966, Ed. Acta Cardiologica, Symposia p. 53.
1104. LEROY, G.V.: J. Amer. med. Ass. **116**, 921 (1941).
1105. — FENN, G.K., GILBERT, N.C.: Amer. Heart J. **23**, 637 (1942).
1106. — SPEER, J.H.: J. Pharmacol. exp. Ther. **69**, 45 (1940).
1107. LESCHKE, E.: Münch. med. Wschr. **77**, 1167 (1930).
1108. LESLIE, A., SCOTT, W.S., MULINOS, M.G.: Proc. Soc. exp. Biol. (N.Y.) **41**, 652 (1939).
1109. LESLIE, R.E.: West. Med. **2**, 56 (1961).
1110. LESSER, M.A.: J. clin. Endocr. **6**, 549 (1946).
1111. LETAC, B., CANNON, R., HOOD, W.B., LOWN, B.: Proc. Soc. exp. Biol. (N.Y.) **127**, 63 (1968).
1112. LEUSEN, I.R., ESSEX, H.E.: Amer. J. Physiol. **172**, 226 (1953).
1113. LEUTENEGGER, A., LUTHY, E.: Schweiz. med. Wschr. **98**, 2020 (1968).
1114. LEVEY, G.S., EPSTEIN, S.E.: Circulat. Res. **24**, 151 (1969).
1115. LEVINE, J.H., NEILL, W.A., WAGMAN, R.J., KRASNOW, N., GORLIN, R.: J. clin. Invest. **41**, 1050 (1962).
1116. — WAGMAN, R.J.: Amer. J. Cardiol. **9**, 372 (1962).
1117. LEVINE, S.A.: Clinical Heart Disease, 3rd ed. Philadelphia: Saunders & Co. 1945, p. 77.
1118. — LIKOFF, W.B.: New Engl. J. Med. **229**, 770 (1943).
1119. LEVITT, B., RAINES, A., MOROS, D., STANDAERT, F.G.: Europ. J. Pharmacol. **6**, 217 (1969).
1120. LEVY, B., AHLQUIST, R.P.: J. Pharmacol. exp. Ther. **133**, 202 (1961).
1121. — WILKENFELD, B.E.: Europ. J. Pharmacol. **5**, 227 (1969).
1122. LEVY, H., BOAS, E.P.: Ann. intern. Med, **28**, 1117 (1948).
1123. LEVY, J.V.: Europ. J. Pharmacol. **2**, 250 (1968).
1124. — Arch. int. Physiol. Biochim. **75**, 381 (1967).
1125. — RICHARDS, V.: J. Pharmacol. exp. Ther. **150**, 361 (1965).
1126. LEVY, R.L., BARACH, A.L., BRUENN, H.G.: Amer. Heart J. **15**, 187 (1938).
1127. — BRUENN, H.G., RUSSEL, N.G.: Amer. J. med. Sci. **197**, 241 (1939).
1128. — — WILLIAMS, N.E.: Amer. Heart J. **19**, 639 (1940).
1129. — WILLIAMS, N.E., BRUENN, H.G., CARR, H.A.: Amer. Heart J. **21**, 634 (1941).
1130. LEW, H.T., MARCH, H.W.: Clin. Res. **15**, 94 (1967).
1131. LEWIS, B.I., LUBIN, R.I., JANUARY, L.E., WILD, J.B.: Circulation **14**, 227 (1956).
1132. LEWIS, C.M., BRINK, A.J.: Amer. J. Cardiol. **21**, 846 (1968).
1133. LEWIS, G.P.: Biochem. Pharmacol. **10**, 29 (1962).
1134. LEWIS, T.: Arch. intern. Med. **49**, 713 (1932).
1135. LIBERMANN, D., DENIS, J.-C.: Bull. Soc. Chim. biol. (Paris) 1961, p. 1952.
1136. LICHTLEN, P., BAUMANN, P.C.: Praxis **58**, 135 (1969).
1137. LIEBOW, J.M., SEASOHN, P.O.: J. chron. Dis. **17**, 609 (1964).
1138. LIESICKE, J.: Dtsch. med. J. **18**, 526 (1967).
1139. LIKOFF, W., SEGAL, B.L., KASPARIAN, H.: New Engl. J. Med. **276**, 1063 (1967).
1140. LILL, G.: Therapiewoche **18**, 1816 (1968).
1141. LIM, H.F., DREIFUS, L.S., RABBINO, M.D.: Circulation **36**, Suppl. 2, 172 (1967).
1142. LINDER, E.: Acta physiol. scand. **68**, Suppl. 272, 5 (1966).
1143. — SEEMAN, T.: Angiologica **4**, 225 (1967).
1144. LINDNER, E.: Arzneimittel-Forsch. **6**, 124 (1956).
1145. — Arzneimittel-Forsch. **10**, 569 (1960).
1146. — Arzneimittel-Forsch. **10**, 573 (1960).

1147. LINDNER, E.: Arzneimittel-Forsch. **19**, 15 (1969).
1148. — Circulatory Drugs. Ed. by A. BERTELLI. Amsterdam: North Holland Publ. Co. 1969, p. 11.
1149. — KATZ, L.N.: J. Pharmacol. exp. Ther. **72**, 306 (1941).
1150. LINDNER, A., LOUDON, M., WERNER, G.: Schweiz. med. Wschr. **83**, 360 (1953).
1151. LINHART, J.W., BRAUNWALD, E., ROSS, J.: J. clin. Invest. **44**, 883 (1965).
1152. — HILDNER, F.J., BAROLD, S.S., SAMET, P.: Amer. J. Cardiol. **21**, 109 (1968).
1153. — — — — Ann. intern. Med. **70**, 1079 (1969).
1154. — — — — Amer. J. Cardiol. **23**, 379 (1969).
1155. LINKO, E., RUOSTEENOJA, R., SIITONEN, L.: Amer. Heart J. **75**, 139 (1968).
1156. — SIITONEN, L., RUOSTEENOJA, R.: Acta med. scand. **181**, 547 (1967).
1157. LINQUETTE, M., LUEZ, G., BEGHIN, B.: Sem. Hôp. Paris **43**, 35 (1967).
1158. LISAN, P.: Progr. cardiovasc. Dis. **2**, 618 (1960).
1159. LISH, P.M., WEIKEL, J.H., DUNGAN, K.W.: J. Pharmacol. exp. Ther. **149**, 161 (1965).
1160. LITTMANN, D., RODMAN, M.H.: Circulation **3**, 875 (1951).
1161. LITVAK, J., SIDERIDES, L.E., VINEBERG, A.M.: Amer. Heart J. **53**, 505 (1957).
1162. LOCHNER, W.: Proc. IIIrd Asian-Pacific Congress of Cardiology, Kyoto **1**, 661 (1964).
1163. — Personal Communication 1969.
1164. — HIRCHE, H.: Arzneimittel-Forsch. **13**, 251 (1963).
1165. — MERCKER, H., NASSERI, M.: Arch. exp. Pathol. Pharmakol. **236**, 365 (1959).
1166. — — SCHÜRMEYER, E.: Arch. exp. Pathol. Pharmakol. **227**, 373 (1956).
1167. — NASSERI, M.: Arzneimittel-Forsch. **10**, 636 (1960).
1168. — — Pflügers Arch. ges. Physiol. **271**, 405 (1960).
1169. — PARRATT, J.R.: Brit. J. Pharmacol. **26**, 17 (1966).
1170. LOGUE, B.: Circulation **22**, 1151 (1960).
1171. LOMBARDO, T.A., ROSE, L., TAESCHLER, M., TULUY, S., BING, R.J.: Circulation **7**, 71 (1953).
1172. LONGSLET, A.: Acta pharmacol. (Kbh.) **27**, 183 (1969).
1173. LOOS, H.: Ärztl. Prax. **11**, 503 (1964).
1174. LOPES, E.C., MOLENAAR, M.G.: Ned. T. Geneesk. **96**, 999 (1952).
1175. LOPEZ SALGADO, A.: Pren. méd. argent. **50**, 1470 (1963).
1176. LORD, C.O., KATZ, R.L., EAKINS, K.E.: Anesthesiology **29**, 288 (1968).
1177. LORDICK, H.: Dtsch. med. J. **19**, 435 (1968).
1178. LOUBATIERES, A., SASSINE, A.: Arch. int. Pharmacodyn. **95**, 246 (1953).
1179. LOVE, W.D., BURCH, G.E.: J. clin. Invest. **36**, 468 (1957).
1180. LU, F.C.: Rev. canad. Biol. **9**, 219 (1950).
1181. — Rev. canad. Biol. **10**, 42 (1951).
1182. — ALLMARK, M.G., CARMICHAEL, E.J., MacMILLAN, D.B., LAVALLEE, A.: J. Pharm. Pharmacol. **5**, 94 (1953).
1183. — — GRAHAM, W.D.: Canad. J. Biochem. **33**, 21 (1955).
1184. — MELVILLE, K.I.: J. Pharmacol. exp. Ther. **99**, 277 (1950).
1185. LUBAWSKI, I., WALE, J.: Europ. J. Pharmacol. **6**, 345 (1969).
1186. LUCCHESI, B.R.: J. Pharmacol. exp . Ther. **145**, 286 (1964).
1187. — Circulat. Res. **22**, 777 (1968).
1188. — IWAMI, T.: J. Pharmacol. exp. Ther. **162**, 49 (1968).
1189. — WHITSITT, L.S., BROWN, N.L.: Canad. J. Physiol. Pharmacol. **44**, 543 (1966).
1190. — — STICKNEY, J.L.: Ann. N.Y. Acad. Sci. **139**, 940 (1967).
1191. LUDUENA, F.P., MILLER, E., WILT, W.A.: J. Amer. pharm. Ass. **44**, 363 (1955).
1192. LUEBS, E.D., COHEN, A., ZALESKI, E.J., BING, R.J.: Amer. J. Cardiol. **17**, 535 (1966).
1193. LUJF, A., MOSER, K.: Wien. klin. Wschr. **79**, 343 (1967).
1194. — — Wien. klin. Wschr. **80**, 15 (1968).
1195. — — SCHWARZMEIER, J.: Inn. Mediz. **48**, 289 (1967).
1196. LUMB, G.D., SINGLETARY, H.P., HARDY, L.B.: Angiology **13**, 463 (1962).
1197. LYDTIN, H.: Dtsch. med. Wschr. **92**, 401 (1967).
1198. — KUSUS, T., DIETZE, G., SCHNELLE, K.: Arzneimittel-Forsch. **17**, 1456 (1967).
1199. LYON, T.P., GOFMAN, J.W., JONES, H.B., LINDGREN, F.T., GRAHAM, D.M.: (1951) Quoted by STEVENSON and WILSON (ref. 1838).
1200. MAASSEN, J.H.: Med. Klin. **58**, 1269 (1963).
1201. MAC DONALD, A.G., MC NEILL, R.S.: Brit. J. Anaesth. **40**, 508 (1968).
1202. MACHT, D.I.: Arch. intern. Med. **17**, 786 (1916).
1203. MACK, R.E., NOLTING, D.D., HOGANCAMP, C.E., BING, R.J.: Amer. J. Physiol. **197**, 1175 (1959).
1204. MACKINNON, J., ANDERSON, D.E., HOWITT, G.: Brit. med. J. **5168**, 243 (1960).
1205. MACREZ, C., BERNARD-BRUNEL, J., MARNETTE-LEBREQUIER, H.: Sem. Hôp. Paris **43**, 30 (1967).

1206. MADEIRA, R.G., DU MESNIL DE ROCHEMONT, W., GADD, C.W., STOCK, T.B., BING, R.J.: Amer. J. Cardiol. **19**, 686 (1967).
1207. MAGGI, G.C., BANNO, S.: Cardiologia (Basel) **47**, 247 (1965).
1208. — CANDIANI, C., FAUDA, C., ROMEO, D.: 3rd European Congress of Cardiology, Roma, Sept. 1960, Pars Altera, p. 1081.
1209. MAHAIM, I., ROTHBERGER, C.J.: Helv. med. Acta **2**, 687 (1936).
1210. MAKINSON, D.H., OLESKY, S., STONE, R.V.: Lancet **1948I**, 102.
1211. MALACH, M.: Amer. J. Cardiol. **19**, 141 (1967).
1212. MALININ, T., STOKES, J.R., HARDY, L.B., LUMB, G.: Johns Hopk. med. J. **122**, 102 (1968).
1213. MALMBORG, R.O.: Acta med. scand. **426** (Suppl.), 177 (1965).
1214. MALMSTRÖM, G.: Acta med. scand. Suppl. 195, 1—103 (1947).
1215. MALOY, W.C., SOWTON, E., BALCON, R.: Circulation **38**, Suppl. 6, 132 (1968).
1216. MANN, H.: J. Mt. Sinai Hosp. **23**, 279 (1956).
1217. MARCHETTI, G., MERLO, L., NOSEDA, V.: Pflügers Arch. ges. Physiol. **298**, 200 (1968).
1218. — — — Arzneimittel-Forsch. **18**, 43 (1968).
1219. MARCUS, E., KATZ, L.N., PICK, R., STAMLER, J.: Acta cardiol. (Brux.) **13**, 190 (1958).
1220. MARION, J., NAVARRANNE, P., ROUX, M., BUYCK, J., FRITZ, A., LEMOIGNE, P., LONGUET, D.: Sem. Hôp. (Thérap.) **40**, 560 (1964).
1221. MARKOFF, N.: Praxis **48**, 49 (1959).
1222. MARKWALDER, J., STARLING, E.H.: J. Physiol. (Lond.) **47**, 275 (1913—1914).
1223. MARMO, E., COSCIA, L., AULISIO, G.A.: Clin. ter. **39**, 137 (1966).
1224. — — — Angiologica **4**, 256 (1967).
1225. — MATERA, A., D'AVANZO, F.B.: Clin. ter. **45**, 327 (1968).
1226. MARSH, D.F., HERRING, D.A.: Arch. int. Pharmacodyn. **78**, 489 (1949).
1227. MASSEL, H.M.: J. Lab. clin. Med. **24**, 380 (1939).
1228. MASTER, A.M.: Amer. Heart J. **56**, 570 (1958).
1229. — DONOSO, E., ROSENFELD, I.: Circulation **20**, 738 (1959).
1230. — FIELD, L.E., DONOSO, E.: N.Y. St. J. Med. **57**, 1051 (1957).
1231. — FRIEDMAN, R., DACK, S.: Amer. Heart J. **24**, 777 (1942).
1232. — JAFFE, H.L., DACK, S.: Amer. J. med. Sci. **197**, 774 (1939).
1233. — NUZIE, S., BROWN, R.C., PARKER, R.C.: Amer. J. med. Sci. **207**, 435 (1944).
1234. — OPPENHEIMER, E.T.: Amer. J. med. Sci. **177**, 223 (1929).
1235. — ROSENFELD, I.: J. Amer. med. Ass. **172**, 265 (1960).
1236. — — DONOSO, E.: Advanc. Cardiol. **2**, 243 (1959).
1237. MATHISEN, H.S., HOLEN, N.: Nord. Med. **67**, 10 (1962).
1238. MATHIVAT, A., COTTET, J.: Bull. Mém. Soc. Méd. Hôp. Paris **30—31**, 1030 (1953).
1239. MATLOFF, J.M., WOLFSON, S., GORLIN, R., HARKEN, D.E.: Circulation **37**, Suppl. 2, 133 (1968).
1240. MAUTZ, F.R., GREGG, D.E.: Proc. Soc. exp. Biol. (N.Y.) **36**, 797 (1937).
1241. MAXWELL, G.M.: Arch. int. Pharmacodyn. **173**, 226 (1968).
1242. — CRUMPTON, C.W., ROWE, G.G., WHITE, D.H., CASTILLO, C.A.: J. Lab. clin. Med. **54**, 88 (1959).
1243. — WHITE, D.H., CRUMPTON, C.W., ROWE, G.G., CASTILLO, C.A.: Circulation **18**, 757 (1958).
1244. McALPIN, R.N., KATTUS, A.A., WINFIELD, M.E.: Circulation **31**, 869 (1965).
1245. McCALLISTER, B.D., YIPINTSOI, T., HALLERMANN, F.J., WALLACE, R.B., FRYE, R.L.: Circulation **37**, 921 (1968).
1246. McCLISH, A., ANDREW, D., NOISAN, A., MORIN, Y.: Canad. med. Ass. J. **98**, 113 (1968).
1247. — — — — Canad. med. Ass. J. **99**, 388 (1968).
1248. McDONALD, D.A.: Ann. Rev. Physiol. **30**, 525 (1968).
1249. McEACHERN, C.G., SMITH, F.H., MANNING, G.W.: Amer. Heart J. **21**, 25 (1941).
1250. McGREGOR, M.: Ann. intern. Med. **56**, 669 (1962).
1251. — Intern. Encyclopedia of Pharmacology and Therapeutics, Section 6, Vol. II. New York and London: Pergamon Press 1966, p. 377.
1252. — FAM, W.H.: Bull. N.Y. Acad. Med. **42**, 940 (1966).
1253. — PALMER, W.H.: Coronary Heart Disease. Ed. by W. LIKOFF and J.H. MOYER. New York: Grune and Stratton 1963, p. 178.
1254. McHENRY, P.L., KNOEBEL, S.B.: J. appl. Physiol. **22**, 495 (1967).
1255. McINERNY, T.K., GILMOUR, D.P., BLINKS, J.R.: Fed. Proc. **24**, 712 (1965).
1256. McINNES, L., PARRATT, J.R.: Brit. J. Pharmacol. **37**, 272 (1969).
1257. McKENNA, D.H., AFONSO, S., JARAMILLO, C.V., CRUMPTON, C.W., ROWE, G.G.: Arch. int. Pharmacodyn. **162**, 275 (1966).
1258. — CORLISS, R.J., SIALER, S., ZARNSTORFF, W.C., CRUMPTON, C.W., ROWE, G.G.: Circulat. Res. **19**, 520 (1966).

1259. Medical World News, 1966.
1260. MEDVEDOWSKY, J.L.: Presse méd. **73**, 2605 (1965).
1261. MEESMANN, W., BACHMANN, G.W.: Dtsch. med. Wschr. **91**, 1260 (1966).
1262. — — Arzneimittel-Forsch. **16**, 501 (1966).
1263. MEESTER, W.D., HARDMAN, H.F., BARBORIAK, J.J.: J. Pharmacol. exp. Ther. **150**, 34 (1965).
1264. MEIER, R., MULLER, R.: Schweiz. med. Wschr. **69**, 1271 (1939).
1265. MELIKOGLU, S.: Therapiewoche **18**, 201 (1968).
1266. MELLEN, H.S., GOLDBERG, H.S., FRIEDMAN, H.F.: New Engl. J. Med. **276**, 989 (1967).
1267. MELON, J.M.: Gaz. Hôp. (Paris) **19**, 715 (1955).
1268. MELVILLE, K.I.: J. Pharmacol. exp. Ther. **64**, 86 (1938).
1269. — Pharmacology in Medicine (Editor V.A. DRILL), 2nd ed. New York: McGraw-Hill 1958, chapter 9, section. 32, p. 482.
1270. — BENFEY, B.G.: Canad. J. Physiol. Pharmacol. **43**, 339 (1965).
1271. — DRAPEAU, J.V.: Arch. int. Pharmacodyn. **115**, 306 (1958).
1272. — GARVEY, H.L., GILLIS, R.A.: Pharmacologist **8**, 174 (1966).
1273. — KOROL, B.: XXth International Congress Physiol. Sciences, Brussels 1956, Abstracts of Communications, p. 635.
1274. — LU, F.C.: J. Pharmacol. exp. Ther. **99**, 286 (1950).
1275. — — Canad. med. Ass. J. **65**, 11 (1951).
1276. — MAZURKIEWICZ, I.: J. Pharmacol. exp. Ther. **118**, 249 (1956).
1277. — SHISTER, H.E., HUQ, S.: Canad. med. Ass. J. **90**, 761 (1964).
1278. MENDEL, D., WINTERTON, M.: Brit. med. J. **1963**II, 358.
1279. MENDEZ, R., ACEVES, J., PULIDO, P.: Aterosclerosis y enfermedad coronaria, 1 vol. Mexico: Ed. Interamericana 1960, p. 395.
1280. — KABELA, E.: Lancet **1966**I, 907.
1281. MENGE, H.G., KADATZ, R.: Arzneimittel-Forsch. **9**, 476 (1959).
1282. MERCIER, F., JOUVE, A., GAVEND, M., GAVEND, M.R., GERIN, J., MERCIER, J.: C.R. Soc. Biol. (Paris) **152**, 1556 (1958).
1283. MERCIER, J., GAVEND, M., GAVEND, M.R., MERCIER, F.: Arch. int. Pharmacodyn. **122**, 394 (1959).
1284. MERCKER, H., LOCHNER, W., GERSTENBERG, E.: Arch. exp. Pathol. Pharmakol. **232**, 459 (1958).
1285. MERIEL, P., BOULARD, C., GALINIER, F., BOUNHOURE, J., GAVALDA, J., BOUNHOURE, F.: Sem. Hôp. Paris **41**, 1039 (1965).
1286. MERLEN, J.F.: Thérapie **6**, 223 (1951).
1287. MESSER, J.V., LEVINE, H.J., WAGMAN, R.J., GORLIN, R.: Circulation **28**, 404 (1963).
1288. — NEILL, W.A.: Amer. J. Cardiol. **9**, 384 (1962).
1289. MESSERICH, J.: Med. Welt (Berl.) **36**, 1904 (1966).
1290. MESSIN, R., DENOLIN, H., DEGRÉ, S.: Arch. Mal. Cœur **58**, 305 (1965).
1291. MESSINA, B., GROSSI, F., GRASSI, M., SPADA, S., MESSINI, R.: Circulatory Drugs. Ed. by A. BERTELLI. Amsterdam: North Holland Publ. Co. 1969, p. 124.
1292. MEWISSEN, A.: Rev. méd. Liège **17**, 43 (1962).
1293. MEYER, J.M., CORRELL, H.L., PETERS, B.J., LINDERT, M.C.F.: Amer. Practit. **3**, 379 (1952).
1294. MEZZASALMA, G., MORPURGO, M.: Mal. cardiovasc. **1**, 399 (1960).
1295. MIAZDRIKOVA, A.A.: Biochem. Pharmacol. **8**, 136 (1961).
1296. MICHEL, D.: Med. Klin. **55**, 1428 (1960).
1297. MICHEL, R., DELTOUR, G.: Biochem. Pharmacol. **17**, 2481 (1968).
1298. MIGNAULT, J. DE L.: Canad. med. Ass. J. **95**, 1252 (1966).
1299. MILLOT, J., PATRUX, A.M.: Gaz. méd. Fr. **22**, 1 (1965).
1300. MINZ, B., THUILLIER, J.: C.R. Soc. Biol. (Paris) **153**, 962 (1959).
1301. MITCHELL, J.R.A.: Brit. med. J. **1**, 791 (1961).
1302. MIURA, M., TOMINAGA, S., HASHIMOTO, K.: Arzneimittel-Forsch. **17**, 976 (1967).
1303. MIZGALA, H.F., DAVIS, R.O., KHAN, A.S.: Canad. med. Ass. J. **98**, 114 (1968).
1304. — KHAN, A.S., DAVIS, R.O.: Canad. med. Ass. J. **100**, 756 (1969).
1305. MODELL, W.: Drugs of Choice. St. Louis: C.V. Mosby Co. 1958.
1306. — Drugs of Choice. St. Louis: C.V. Mosby Co. 1966, p. 407.
1307. — Drugs of Choice 1968—1969. St. Louis: C.V. Mosby Co. 1967.
1308. MOE, G.K., VISSCHER, M.B.: Heart and Circulation, A. A. A. Sci. Public. **13**, 100(1940).
1309. MOIR, T.W.: Circulat. Res. **19**, 695 (1966).
1310. MOKOTOFF, R., KATZ, L.N.: Amer. Heart J. **30**, 215 (1945).
1311. MOLINO, N., BELLUARDO, C.: Thérapie **21**, 1191 (1966).
1312. MOLL, A., PETZEL, H.: Z. Kreisl.-Forsch. **56**, 46 (1967).
1313. MOLLY, W.: Ther. d. Gegenw. **93**, 10 (1954).

1314. MONIZ DE BETTENCOURT, J., CORREIA RALHA, A., PERES GOMES, F., PRISTA MONTEIRO, H.: Presse méd. **64**, 1468 (1956).
1315. — PRISTA MONTEIRO, H.: Med. contemp. **11**, 521 (1955).
1316. MONROE, R.G., FRENCH, G.N.: Circulat. Res. **9**, 362 (1961).
1317. MORALES-ANGUILERA, A., VAUGHAN-WILLIAMS, E.M.: Brit. J. Pharmacol. **24**, 319 (1965).
1318. — — Brit. J. Pharmacol. **24**, 332 (1965).
1319. MORAN, N.C.: Ann. N.Y. Acad. Sci. **139**, 649 (1967).
1320. — PERKINS, M.E.: J. Pharmacol. exp. Ther. **124**, 223 (1958).
1321. MORAWITZ, P., ZAHN, A.: Zbl. Physiol. **26**, 465 (1912).
1322. MORET, P.R., BOUFAS, D., FOURNET, P.C.: Schweiz. med. Wschr. **99**, 1090 (1969).
1323. MOSER, K., LUJF, A.: Wien. klin. Wschr. **79**, 349 (1967).
1324. — — Arzneimittel-Forsch. **19**, 305 (1969).
1325. MOUQUIN, M., MACREZ, C.: Presse méd. **68**, 257 (1960).
1326. — MILOVANOVICH, J.B., SAUVAN, R., VONTHRON, A., GROSGOGEAT, Y.: Presse méd. **67**, 715 (1959).
1327. MÜLLER, J., STRASSBURG, K.H.: Therapiewoche **19**, 871 (1962).
1328. MÜLLER, O., RORVIK, K.: Brit. Heart J. **20**, 302 (1958).
1329. MURMANN, W., SACCANI-GUELFI, M., GAMBA, A.: Boll. chim. farm. **105**, 292 (1966).
1330. MURPHY, F.M., BARBER, J.M.: 3rd European Congress of Cardiology, Roma, Sept. 1960, Pars Altera, p. 121.
1331. — — Cardiologia **37**, Suppl. 2, 117 (1960).
1332. — — KILPATRICK, S.J.: Lancet **1961I**, 139.
1333. MURRAY, J.F., ESCOBAR, E., JONES, N.L., RAPAPORT, E.: Amer. Heart J. **72**, 38 (1966).
1334. MURRELL, W.: Lancet **1879I**, 80.
1335. NAJMI, M., GRIGGS, D.M., KASPARIAN, H., NOVACK, P.: Circulation **35**, 46 (1967).
1336. NAKANO, J., KUSAKARI, T.: Amer. J. Physiol. **210**, 833 (1966).
1337. NAKHJAVAN, F.K., SHEDROVILZKY, H., GOLDBERG, H.: Circulation **38**, 777 (1968).
1338. — SON, R., GOLDBERG, H.: Cardiovasc. Res. **2**, 226 (1968).
1339. NALEFSKI, L.A., RUDY, W.B., GILBERT, N.C.: Circulation **5**, 851 (1952).
1340. NASH, D.T.: J. clin. Pharmacol. **8**, 259 (1968).
1341. NAUGHTON, J., BALKE, B.: Amer. J. med. Sci. **247**, 286 (1964).
1342. NAYLER, W.G.: Circulat. Res. **20**, Suppl. 3, 213 (1967).
1343. — Vth European Congress of Cardiology. Athenes, Sept. 1968. Abstracts p. 253.
1344. — CHAN, J., LOWE, T.E.: Med. J. Aust. **1**, 1128 (1968).
1345. — CHIPPERFIELD, D., LOWE, T.E.: Cardiovasc. Res. **3**, 30 (1969).
1346. — McINNES, I., CARSON, V., SWANN, J., LOWE, T.E.: Amer. Heart J. **77**, 246 (1969).
1347. — — SWANN, J.B., CARSON, V., LOWE, T.E.: Amer. Heart J. **73**, 207 (1967).
1348. — — — PRICE, J.M., CARSON, V., RACE, D., LOWE, T.E.: J. Pharmacol. exp. Ther. **161**, 247 (1968).
1349. — — — RACE, D., CARSON, V., LOWE, T.E.: Amer. Heart J. **75**, 83 (1968).
1350. — — — — LOWE, T.E.: Cardiovasc. Res. **2**, 371 (1968).
1351. — PRICE, J.M., LOWE, T.E.: Cardiovasc. Res. **1**, 63 (1967).
1352. — STONE, J., CARSON, V., McINNES, I., MACK, V., LOWE, T.E.: J. Pharmacol. exp. Ther. **165**, 225 (1969).
1353. NEEDLEMAN, P., HUNTER, F.E.: Mol. Pharmacol. **2**, 134 (1966).
1354. NEILL, W.A.: Amer. J. Cardiol. **22**, 507 (1968).
1355. — LEVINE, H.J., WAGMAN, R.J., GORLIN, R.: Circulat. Res. **12**, 163 (1963).
1356. NEILSON, G.H., SELDON, W.A.: Med. J. Aust. **1**, 856 (1969).
1357. NESTEL, P.J., VERGHESE, A., LOVELL, R.H.: Amer. Heart J. **73**, 227 (1967).
1358. NEUMANN, H.: Ärztl. Prax. **11**, 678 (1959).
1359. NEUMANN, M., LUISADA, A.: Amer. J. med. Sci. **251**, 552 (1966).
1360. NEWHOUSE, M.T., McGREGOR, M.: Amer. J. Cardiol. **16**, 234 (1965).
1361. NICKERSON, M.: Circulat. Res. **14**, Suppl. 2, 130 (1964).
1362. NICKERSON, E.: Ann. N.Y. Acad. Sci. **139**, 571 (1967).
1363. NIDEGGER, J.C.: Rev. méd. Suisse rom. **74**, 414 (1954).
1364. NIEDERGERKE, R.: J. Physiol. (Lond.) **134**, 569 (1956).
1365. NIELSEN, K.C., OWMAN, C.: Life Sci. **5**, 1611 (1966).
1366. — — Experientia (Basel) **23**, 203 (1967).
1367. NIESCHULZ, O., POPENDIKER, K., SACK, K.H.: Arzneimittel-Forsch. **4**, 232 (1954).
1368. NIESSNER, H., CHIRIKDJIAN, J.J.: Arzneimittel-Forsch. **19**, 62 (1969).
1369. NITZ, R.E., PÖTZSCH, E.: Arzneimittel-Forsch. **13**, 243 (1963).
1370. — RESAG, K.: Sem. Hôp. Paris **43**, 8 (1967).
1371. — — Ars Medici **23**, 645 (1968).
1372. — SCHRAVEN, E., TROTTNOW, D.: Experientia (Basel) **24**, 334 (1968).
1373. NIVET, M.: Sem. thér. **44**, TH 551 (1968).

1374. NIVET, M.: Documentation interne du Département Médical de la S.A. Labaz.
1375. NORDENFELT, I., PERSSON, S., REDFORS, A.: Acta med. scand. **184**, 465 (1969).
1376. — WESTLING, H.: Acta med. scand. **182**, Suppl. 472, 81 (1967).
1377. NORRIS, R.M., CAUGHEY, D.E., SCOTT, P.J.: Brit. med. J. **1968**II, 398.
1378. Nos Artères (Bruxelles) 1968, No. 25.
1379. NUZUM, F.R., ELLIOT, A.H.: Arch. intern. Med. **49**, 1007 (1932).
1380. NYLIN, G., DE FAZIO, V., MARSICO, F.: Cardiologia (Basel) **17**, 191 (1950).
1381. OBIANWU, H.: Acta pharmacol. (Kbh.) **25**, 127 (1967).
1382. — Acta pharmacol. (Kbh.) **25**, 141 (1967).
1383. OBLATH, R.W.: Communication to the American Therap. Soc., 60th Annual Congress, Atlantic City, N. J., June 6, 1959.
1384. O'BRIEN, K.P., HIGGS, L.M., GLANCY, D.L., EPSTEIN, S.E.: Circulation **39**, 735 (1969).
1385. OGAWA, K., GUDBJARNASON, S.: Arch. int. Pharmacodyn. **172**, 172 (1968).
1386. — — BING, R.J.: J. Pharmacol. exp. Ther. **155**, 449 (1967).
1387. OLIVER, M.F.: Brit. med. J. **5129**, 1107 (1959).
1388. — Circulation **36**, 337 (1967).
1389. — Bull. N.Y. Acad. Med. **44**, 1021 (1968).
1390. OLLEON, J.: Valeur comparée de quelques médications coronarodilatatrices (étude expérimentale). Ed. A. REY. Thèse de Lyon: 1957, p. 133.
1391. OLSON, R.E.: Circulation **22**, 453 (1960).
1392. OLSSON, R.A., GREGG, D.E.: In: GREGG, KHOURI and RAYFORD. Circulat. Res. **16**, 102 (1965).
1393. — — Amer. J. Physiol. **208**, 231 (1965).
1394. OPIE, L.H., THOMAS, M.: J. Physiol. (Lond.) **202**, 23 P (1969).
1395. ORAM, S., SOWTON, E.: Brit. med. J. **5269**, 1745 (1961).
1396. OSCHAROFF, G.: Angiology **15**, 505 (1964).
1397. OSHER, H.L., KATZ, K.H., WAGNER, D.J.: New Engl. J. Med. **244**, 315 (1951).
1398. OSHER, W.J.: Amer. J. Physiol. **172**, 403 (1953).
1399. OVERKAMP, H.: Med. Klin. **55**, 1423 (1960).
1400. OWREN, P.A.: Schweiz. med. Wschr. **84**, 822 (1954).
1401. PAGE, I.H.: Aterosclerosis y enfermedad coronaria, 1 vol. Mexico: Ed. Interamericana 1960, p. 381.
1402. — SCHNECKLOTH, R.E.: Circulation **20**, 1075 (1959).
1403. — STAMLER, J.: Mod. Conc. cardiov. Dis. **37**, 119 and 125 (1968).
1404. PAGET, G.E.: Brit. med. J. **1963**II, 1266.
1405. PAL, J.: Dtsch. med. Wschr. **39**, 2068 (1913).
1406. PALEY, H.W., McDONALD, I.G., PETERS, F.W.: Circulation **31**, Suppl. 2, 167 (1965).
1407. PALIARD, P., PERROT, E.: Sem. Hôp. Paris **43**, 39 (1967).
1408. PALMER, D.W.: New Engl. J. Med. **276**, 989 (1967).
1409. PALMER, J.A., RAMSEY, C.G.: Canad. med. Ass. J. **65**, 17 (1951).
1410. PALMER, J.H.: Canad. med. Ass. J. **65**, 207 (1951).
1411. PAPP, G., SZEKERES, L., SZMOLENSZKY, T.: Acta physiol. Acad. Sci. hung. **32**, 365 (1967).
1412. PAPP, J.G., VAUGHAN-WILLIAMS, E.M.: Brit. J. Pharmacol. **36**, 178 P (1969) and **37**, 391 (1969).
1413. PARADE, G.W., MELIKOGLU, S., OHLER, T., TING, K.: Therapiewoche **18**, 47 (1968).
1414. PARKER, J.O., CHIONG, M.A., WEST, R.O., CASE, R.B.: Circulation **40**, 113 (1969).
1415. — DI GIORGI, S., WEST, R.O.: Amer. J. Cardiol. **17**, 470 (1966).
1416. — LEDWICH, J.R., WEST, R.O., CASE, R.B.: Circulation **39**, 745 (1969).
1417. — WEST, R.O., CASE, R.B., CHIONG, M.A.: Circulation **40**, 97 (1969).
1418. — — DI GIORGI, S.: Circulation **36**, 734 (1967).
1419. PARRATT, J.R.: Brit. J. Pharmacol. **22**, 34 (1964).
1420. — Lancet **1967**I, 955.
1421. — Progr. med. Chem. **6**, 11 (1969).
1422. — Cardiovasc. Res. **3**, 306 (1969).
1423. — GRAYSON, J.: Experientia (Basel) **19**, 161 (1963).
1424. — — Lancet **1966**I, 338.
1425. — WADSWORTH, R.M.: Brit. J. Pharmacol. **37**, 357 (1969).
1426. — Brit. J. Pharmacol. **37**, 524 P (1969).
1427. PARRY, E.H.O., WELLS, P.G.: Brit. med. J. **5165**, 26 (1960).
1428. PEEL, A.A., BLUM, K., LANCASTER, W.M., DALL, J.L., CHALMERS, G.L.: Scot. med. J. **6**, 403 (1961).
1429. PENTECOST, B.L., AUSTEN, W.G.: Amer. Heart J. **72**, 790 (1966).
1430. — MAYNE, N.M.C., LAMB, P.: Lancet **1968**I, 946.
1431. PERLMAN, A.: Angiology **3**, 16 (1952).
1432. PERNOD, J., KERMAREC, J.: Thérapie **24**, 675 (1969).

1433. Perrin, A., Pairard, J.: Lyon méd. **215**, 1743 (1966).
1434. Pescador, T.: Personal Communication 1968.
1435. Petzel, H., Moll, A.: Med. Welt (Berl.) **52**, 2852 (1966).
1436. Pfeiffer, H.: Klin. Wschr. **28**, 304 (1950).
1437. Pfleger, K., Schöndorf, H.: Arzneimittel-Forsch. **19**, 97 (1969).
1438. Phear, D.N.: Brit. med. J. **1968 II**, 740.
1439. Phear, D., Walker, W.C.: Brit. med. J. **5204**, 995 (1960).
1440. Pichler, E., Strauss, A.: Wien. klin. Wschr. **80**, 61 (1968).
1441. Pieper, H.P.: J. appl. Physiol. **19**, 1199 (1964).
1442. Pieri, J., Casalonga, L., Dejouhannet, S.: Sem. Hôp. Paris **42**, 5 (1966).
1443. — Wahl, M., Casalonga, J.: Presse méd. **66**, 1523 (1958).
1444. Pilkington, T.R.E., Purves, M.J.: Brit. med. J. **5165**, 38 (1960).
1445. Pinto, S.L., Telles, E.: Vth European Congress of Cardiology, Athenes, Sept. 1968, Abstracts p. 327.
1446. Pippig, L., Schneider, K.W.: Arzneimittel-Forsch. **15**, 1008 (1965).
1447. Pitt, A., Friesinger, G.C., Ross, R.S.: Cardiovasc. Res. **3**, 100 (1969).
1448. Pitt, B.: Int. Symp. on the Coronary Circulation and Energetics of the Myocardium, Milan 1966. Basle: S. Karger 1967, p. 89.
1449. — Elliot, E.C., Gregg, D.E.: Circulat. Res. **21**, 75 (1967).
1450. — Fortuin, N., Dagenais, G., Friesinger, G.C., Hodges, M.: Circulation **38**, Suppl. 6, 157 (1968).
1451. Pitt, W.A., Cox, A.R.: Amer. Heart J. **76**, 242 (1968).
1452. Piva, M., Ongari, R.: Arzneimittel-Forsch. **18**, 179 (1968).
1453. Plavsic, C.: Acta cardiol. (Brux.) **8**, 35 (1953).
1454. Pletscher, A.: Experientia (Basel) **14**, 73 (1958).
1455. — Gey, K.F., Burkard, W.P.: 3rd European Congress of Cardiology, Roma, Sept. 1960, Pars Altera, p. 1093.
1456. — — Pellmont, B.: Aterosclerosis y enfermedad coronaria, 1 vol. Mexico: Ed. Interamericana 1960, p. 391.
1457. — Pellmont, B.: J. clin. exp. Psychopath. **19**, 163 (1958).
1458. Plomteux, G., Heusghem, C., Ernould, H., Vandeghen, N.: a) Europ. J. Pharmacol. **8**, 369 (1969). b) Thérapie **24**, 973 (1969).
1459. Plotz, H.: Amer. J. med. Sci. **239**, 194 (1960).
1460. Plotz, M.: N.Y. St. J. Med. **52**, 16 (1952).
1461. Popovich, N.R., Roberts, F.F., Crislip, R.L., Menges, H.: Circulat. Res. **4**, 727 (1956).
1462. Popper, H.: J. Amer. med. Ass. **168**, 2235 (1959).
1463. Porter, W.T.: Amer. J. Physiol. **1**, 511 (1898).
1464. Powell, C.E., Slater, I.H.: J. Pharmacol. exp. Ther. **122**, 480 (1958).
1465. Praschl, E., Kubicek, F.: Med. Klin. **63**, 460 (1968).
1466. Prichard, B.N.C.: Brit. J. Pharmacol. **41**, 408 P (1971).
1467. — Gillam, P.M.S.: Brit. med. J. **1964 II**, 725.
1468. Proger, S.H., Ayman, D.: Amer. J. med. Sci. **184**, 480 (1932).
1469. — Minnich, W.R., Magendants, H.: Amer. Heart J. **10**, 511 (1935).
1470. Proudfit, W.L., Shirey, E.K., Sones, F.M.: Circulation **33**, 901 (1966).
1471. — — — Circulation **36**, 54 (1967).
1472. Provenza, V., Scherlis, S.: Circulation **20**, 35 (1959).
1473. — — Circulat. Res. **7**, 318 (1959).
1474. Pruitt, R.D., Burchell, H.B., Barnes, A.R.: J. Amer. med. Ass. **128**, 839 (1945).
1475. Puri, P.S., Ogawa, K., Robin, E., Martinez, M.A., Ribeilima, J., Bing, R.J.: Circulation **34**, Suppl. III, 192 (1966).
1476. Pyörälä, K., Ikkma, E., Siltanen, P.: Acta med. scand. **173**, 385 (1963).
1477. Queneau, P.: Rev. med. Lyon **16**, 753 (1967).
1478. Raab, W.: Ann. intern. Med. **14**, 688 (1940).
1479. — J. clin. Endocrinol. **1**, 977 (1941).
1480. — J. Amer. med. Ass. **128**, 249 (1945).
1481. — Ann. N.Y. Acad. Sci. **64**, 528 (1956).
1482. — Advances of Cardiology, vol. 1. Basle: S. Karger 1956, p. 65.
1483. — Amer. J. Cardiol. **9**, 576 (1962).
1484. — Jap. Circulat. J. (Ni.) **29**, 113 (1965).
1485. — Amer. Heart J. **72**, 538 (1966).
1486. — Cardiologia (Basel) **52**, 305 (1968).
1487. — Medical World News **10**, 7, 39 (1969).
1488. — Gigee, W.: Circulation **3**, 553 (1955).
1489. — Humphreys, R.J.: J. Pharmacol. exp. Ther. **89**, 64 (1947).
1490. — Lepeschkin, E.: Circulation **1**, 733 (1950).

1491. RAAB, W., VAN LITH, P., LEPESCHKIN, E., HERRLICH, H.C.: Amer. J. Cardiol. **9**, 455 (1962).
1492. RABKIN, R., STABLES, D.P., LEVIN, N.W., SUZMAN, M.M.: Amer. J. Cardiol. **18**, 370 (1966).
1493. RAHN, K.H., OCKENGA, T.: Klin. Wschr. **45**, 1087 (1967).
1494. RANDALL, L.O., SMITH, T.H.: J. Pharmacol. exp. Ther. **103**, 10 (1951).
1495. RAPER, C., WALE, J.: Europ. J. Pharmacol. **4**, 1 (1969).
1496. RATSCHOW, M., SCHOOP, W.: Med. Klin. **55**, 1421 (1960).
1497. — — Med. Klin. **55**, 1436 (1960).
1498. RAVERA, M.: Minerva med. **59**, 4561 (1968).
1499. RAVIN, I.B., KATZ, K.H.: New Engl. J. Med. **240**, 331 (1949).
1500. REALE, A.: Circulation **36**, 933 (1967).
1501. — Amer. J. Cardiol. **21**, 113 (1968).
1502. — D'INTINO, S., VESTRI, A.: Lancet **1968 I**, 52.
1503. — GIOFFRE, P.A., MOTOLESE, M., IMHOF, P.: Vth European Congress of Cardiology, Athenes, Sept. 1968, Abstracts p. 291.
1504. REES, J.R., REDDING, V.J.: Proc. roy. Soc. Med. **59**, Suppl., 30 (1966).
1505. — — Cardiovasc. Res. **1**, 169 (1967).
1506. — — Cardiovasc. Res. **1**, 179 (1967).
1507. — — Cardiovasc. Res. **2**, 43 (1968).
1508. — — Circulat. Res. **25**, 161 (1969).
1509. — — Amer. Heart J. **78**, 224 (1969).
1510. — — ASHFIELD, R., GIBSON, D., GAVEY, C.J.: Brit. Heart J. **28**, 374 (1966).
1511. REEVES, T.J., HEFNER, L.L., JONES, W.B., GOGHLAN, C., PRIETO, G., CARROLL, J.: Amer Heart J. **60**, 745 (1960).
1512. REGAN, T.J., BINAK, K., GORDON, S., DEFAZIO, V., HELLEMS, H.K.: Circulation **23**, 55 (1961).
1513. — KOROXENIDIS, G., MOSCHOS, C.B., OLDEWURTEL, H.A., LEHAN, P.H., HELLEMS, H.K.: J. clin. Invest. **45**, 270 (1966).
1514. — WEISSE, A.B., MOSCHOS, C.B., LESNIAK, L.J., NADINI, M., HELLEMS, H.K.: Trans. Ass. Amer. Phys. **78**, 282 (1965).
1515. — — OLDEWURTEL, H.A., HELLEMS, H.K.: J. clin. Invest. **43**, 1289 (1964).
1516. REGELSON, W., HOFFMEISTER, F.S., WILKENS, H.: Ann. N.Y. Acad. Sci. **80**, 981 (1959).
1517. REIN, H.: Z. Biol. **87**, 394 (1927).
1518. RENKIN, E.M.: Fed. Proc. **24**, 1092 (1965).
1519. REY, C., PATTANI, F.: Acta cardiol. (Brux.) **9**, 221 (1954).
1520. REYMOND, C.: Thérapie **25**, 323 (1970).
1521. RICHARDSON, A.T.: Proc. roy. Soc. Med. **62**, 872 (1969).
1522. RICHARDSON, A.W., DENISON, A.B., GREEN, H.D.: Circulation **5**, 430 (1952).
1523. RICHARDSON, J.A.: Modern trends in diseases of coronary arteries and ischemic heart disease. Ed. by C.K. FRIEDBERG. New York: Grune & Stratton 1964, p. 56.
1524. — WOODS, E.F.: The Catecholamines in Cardiovascular Pathology. Burlington, Aug. 23, 1959, Abstracts p. 17.
1525. RICHET, G., COTTET, J., AMIEL, C., LEROUX-ROBERT, C., PODEVIN, R.: Presse méd. **74**, 1247 (1966).
1526. RINZLER, S.H.: Amer. J. Med. **5**, 736 (1948).
1527. — Bull. N.Y. Acad. Med. **44**, 936 (1968).
1528. — BAKST, H., BENJAMIN, Z.H., BOBB, A.L., TRAVELL, J.: Circulation **1**, 288 (1950).
1529. — TRAVELL, J., BAKST, H., BENJAMIN, Z.H., ROSENTHAL, R.L., ROSENFELD, S., HIRSCH, B.B.: Amer. J. Med. **14**, 438 (1953).
1530. RISEMAN, J.E.F.: Circulation **14**, 422 (1956).
1531. — ALTMAN, G.E., KORETSKY, S.: Circulation **17**, 22 (1958).
1532. — BROWN, M.G.: Arch. intern. Med. **60**, 100 (1937).
1533. — — New Engl. J. Med. **229**, 670 (1943).
1534. — STEINBERG, L.A., ALTMAN, G.E.: Circulation **10**, 809 (1954).
1535. — STERN, B.: Amer. J. med. Sci. **188**, 646 (1934).
1536. — WALLER, J.V., BROWN, M.G.: Amer. Heart J. **19**, 683 (1940).
1537. RIVIER, J.L.: Schweiz. med. Wschr. **97**, 1564 (1968).
1538. — REYMOND, C., GRANDJEAN, T.: Ther. Umsch. **25**, 58 (1968).
1539. ROBBINS, S.L., SOLOMON, M., BENNETT, A.: Circulation **33**, 733 (1966).
1540. ROBERG, N.B., REQUARTH, W.H.: Circulation **1**, 1193 (1950).
1541. ROBERTS, J.T.: Circulation **16**, 929 (1957).
1542. ROBERTS, L.N., MASON, G.P., VILLANUEVA, M.P., BABACAN, B.C.: Canad. med. Ass. J. **98**, 113 (1968).
1543. ROBIN, E., COWAN, C., PURI, P., GANGULY, S., DE BOYRIE, E., MARTINEZ, M., STOCK, T., BING, R.J.: Circulation **36**, 175 (1967).

1544. ROBINSON, B.F.: Circulation **35**, 1073 (1967).
1545. — EPSTEIN, S.E., BEISER, G.D., BRAUNWALD, E.: Circulat. Res. **19**, 400 (1966).
1546. ROBINSON, C.R.: Clin. Med. **74**, 47 (1967).
1547. ROCHET, J., VASTESAEGER, M.M.: Scalpel (Brux.) **119**, 267 (1966).
1548. RODBARD, S., GRAHAM, G.R., WILLIAMS, F.: J. appl. Physiol. **6**, 311 (1953).
1549. RODRIGUES-PEREIRA, E., VIANA, A.P.: Arzneimittel-Forsch. **18**, 175 (1968).
1550. ROJAS, G.S.: Sem. méd. Méx. **54**, 262 (1967).
1551. ROOKMAKER, W.A.: In press 1971.
1552. — Enkele toepassingen van telemetrie in de cardiologie. Rotterdam: Wyt 1969.
1553. ROSENBERG, H.N., MICHELSON, A.L.: Amer. J. med. Sci. **230**, 254 (1955).
1554. ROSENBLUM, R., FRIEDEN, J., DELMAN, A.J.: Clin. Res. **15**, 220 (1967).
1555. — — — BERKOWITZ, W.D.: Circulation **36**, Suppl. 2, 226 (1967).
1556. ROSENFELD, I., DONOSO, E., MASTER, A.M.: Proc. Soc. exp. Biol. (N.Y.) **103**, 320 (1960).
1557. ROSENMAN, R.H., FISHMAN, A.P., KAPLAN, S.R., LEVIN, H.G., KATZ, L.N.: J. Amer. med. Ass. **143**, 160 (1950).
1558. — — KATZ, L.N.: A preliminary report on the use of khellin in angina pectoris and bronchial asthma. Program of the 22nd Scientific Sessions of the American Heart Assoc. (abstract), 1949, p. 43.
1559. ROSS, G., JORGENSEN, C.R.: J. Pharmacol. exp. Ther. **158**, 504 (1967).
1560. — — Amer. Heart J. **76**, 74 (1968).
1561. ROSS, R.S.: Circulation **27**, 107 (1963).
1562. — UEDA, K., LICHTLEN, P.R., REES, J.R.: Circulat. Res. **15**, 28 (1964).
1563. ROSSI, B.: Angiology **6**, 59 (1955).
1564. RÖTH, G.: Medizinische **25**, 852 (1953).
1565. ROTH, O.: Schweiz. med. Wschr. **80**, 206 (1950).
1566. ROTHLIN, E.: Helv. physiol. pharmacol. Acta **2**, C 48 (1944).
1567. — Bull. Acad. Suisse Sci. Méd. **2**, 249 (1946—1947).
1568. ROUGHGARDEN, J.W., NEWMAN, E.V.: Amer. J. Med. **41**, 935 (1966).
1569. ROWE, G.G.: Med. Clin. N. Amer. **46**, 1421 (1962).
1570. — Amer. Heart J. **68**, 691 (1964).
1571. — Clin. Pharmacol. Ther. **7**, 547 (1966).
1572. — Ann. Rev. Pharmacol. **8**, 95 (1968).
1573. — AFONSO, S., BOAKE, W.C., CASTILLO, C.A., LUGO, J.E., CRUMPTON, C.W.: Proc. Soc. exp. Biol. (N.Y.) **112**, 545 (1963).
1574. — CASTILLO, C.A., AFONSO, S., CRUMPTON, C.W.: Amer. Heart J. **67**, 457 (1964).
1575. — CHELIUS, C.J., AFONSO, S., GURTNER, H.P., CRUMPTON, C.W.: J. clin. Invest. **40**, 1217 (1961).
1576. — EMANUEL, D.A., MAXWELL, G.M., BROWN, J.F., CASTILLO, C., SCHUSTER, B., MURPHY, Q.R., CRUMPTON, C.W.: J. clin. Invest. **36**, 844 (1957).
1577. — TERRY, W., STENLUND, R.R., THOMSEN, J.H., QUERIMIT, A.S.: Arch. int. Pharmacodyn. **178**, 99 (1969).
1578. — THOMSEN, J.H., STENLUND, R.R., McKENNA, D.H., SIALER, S., CORLISS, R.J.: Circulation **39**, 139 (1969).
1579. ROWLANDS, D.J., HOWITT, G., MARKMAN, P.: Brit. med. J. **1965 I**, 891.
1580. RUBIN, A.A.: J. Amer. med. Ass. **185**, 971 (1963).
1581. RUBIO, R., BERNE, R.M.: Fed. Proc. **26**, 772 (1967).
1582. RUDOLPH, W., BERNSMEIER, A., HENSELMANN, L., BAEDEKER, W.D., HOFMANN, H.: Klin. Wschr. **42**, 667 (1964).
1583. — MEIXNER, L., KUNZIG, H.J.: Klin. Wschr. **45**, 333 (1967).
1584. RUSHMER, R.F.: Cardiovascular dynamics, 2nd ed. Philadelphia: Saunders Co. 1961, p. 443.
1585. — Handbook of Physiology. Ed. by W.F. HAMILTON and P. Dow, vol. 1, sect. 2. Baltimore: Williams and Wilkins 1962, p. 533.
1586. RUSKIN, A.: Physiological Cardiology. 1 vol., 370 pp., American Lecture Series. Springfield, Illinois: Ch. C. Thomas 1953, p. 140.
1587. — Fed. Proc. **20**, 102 (1961).
1588. — Circulation **23**, 681 (1961).
1589. RUSSEK, H.I.: J. Amer. med. Ass. **157**, 751 (1955).
1590. — J. Amer. med. Ass. **158**, 216 (1955).
1591. — Ann. N.Y. Acad. Sci. **64**, 533 (1956).
1592. — Circulation **18**, 774 (1958).
1593. — Circulation **18**, 774 (1958).
1594. — IIIrd World Congress of Cardiology, Brussels, Demonstration. Sept. 1958.
1595. — Amer. J. Cardiol. **3**, 547 (1959).
1596. — J. Amer. med. Ass. **171**, 503 (1959).

1597. RUSSEK, H.I.: Circulation 20, 761 (1959).
1598. — Amer. J. med. Sci. 239, 187 (1960).
1599. — Angiology 11, 76 (1960).
1600. — Progr. cardiovasc. Dis. 2, 578 (1960).
1601. — Progr. cardiovasc. Dis. 2, 582 (1960).
1602. — J. Kans. Cy Sthw. Clin. Soc. 36, 14 (1960).
1603. — Circulation 24, 1027 (1961).
1604. — Circulation 24, 1027 (1961).
1605. — Circulation 24, 1028 (1961).
1606. — Angiology 12, 239 (1961).
1607. — Amer. J. med. Sci. 254, 406 (1967).
1608. — Angiology 18, 15 (1967).
1609. — J. Amer. med. Ass. 204, 528 (1968).
1610. — Amer. J. Cardiol. 21, 44 (1968).
1611. — Geriatrics 24, 81 (1969).
1612. — NAEGELE, C.F., REGAN, F.D.: J. Amer. med. Ass. 143, 355 (1950).
1613. — REGAN, F.D., ANDERSON, W.H., DOERNER, A.A., NAEGELE, C.F.: N.Y. St. J. Med.
       52, 437 (1952).
1614. — SMITH, R.H., BAUM, W.S., NAEGELE, C.F., REGAN, F.D.: Circulation 1, 700 (1950).
1615. — URBACH, K.F., DOERNER, A.A.: J. Amer. med. Ass. 149, 1008 (1952).
1616. — — ZOHMAN, B.L.: J. Amer. med. Ass. 153, 207 (1953).
1617. — ZOHMAN, B.L.: J. Amer. med. Ass. 158, 1017 (1955).
1618. — ZOHMAN, B.L.: Circulation 38, Suppl. 6, 168 (1968).
1619. — DORSET, V.J.: Amer. J. med. Sci. 229, 46 (1955).
1620. — DRUMM, A.E., WEINGARTEN, W., DORSET, V.J.: Circulation 12, 169 (1955).
1621. RYSER, H., WILBRANDT, W.: Arch. int. Pharmacodyn. 96, 131 (1953).
1622. SAAMELI, K.: Helv. physiol. pharmacol. Acta 25, CR 219 (1967).
1623. — Helv. physiol. pharmacol. Acta 25, CR 432 (1967).
1624. SABISTON, D.C.: Internat. Symp. on Coronary Circulation and Energetics of the Myo-
       cardium. Milan 1966. Basle: S. Karger 1967, p. 280.
1625. SACHS, B.A.: Amer. Heart J. 75, 707 (1968).
1626. SAGALL, E.L., KURLAND, G.S., RISEMAN, J.E.F.: New Engl. J. Med. 235, 650 (1946).
1627. SAHM, F.: Med. Klin. 55, 1426 (1960).
1628. SAKAI, S., SANEYOSHI, S.: Arch. exp. Pathol. Pharmakol. 78, 331 (1915).
1629. SALANS, A.H., SILBER, E.H., KATZ, L.N.: Cited by SILBER and KATZ (ref. 1752).
1630. SALAZAR, A.E.: Circulat. Res. 9, 1351 (1961).
1631. SALLE, J., NAU, P.: Thérapie 13, 86 (1958).
1632. SAMAAN, K.: Quart. J. Pharm. 5, 6 (1932).
1633. — Quart. J. Pharm. 5, 183 (1932).
1634. — HOSSEIN, A.M., FAHIM, I.: J. Pharm. Pharmacol. 1, 538 (1949).
1635. SAMBHI, M.P., ZIMMERMAN, H.A.: Arch. intern. Med. 101, 974 (1958).
1636. SANDERS, K.: Lancet 7100, 432 (1959).
1637. SANDLER, G.: Amer. Heart J. 59, 718 (1960).
1638. — Brit. med. J. 1961 I, 792.
1639. — Brit. med. J. 1961 II, 1741.
1640. — CLAYTON, G.A.: Brit. med. J. 1967 IV, 268.
1641. — — THORNICROFT, S.G.: Brit. med. J. 1968 III, 224.
1642. — PATNEY, L.N., LAWSON, C.W.: Postgrad. med. J. 40, 217 (1964).
1643. SAPIENZA, P.L.: Clin. Med. 75, 30 (1968).
1644. SARNOFF, S.J., BRAUNWALD, E., WELCH, G.H., CASE, R.B., STAINSBY, W.N., MACRUZ,
       R.: Amer. J. Physiol. 192, 148 (1958).
1645. — CASE, R.B., MACRUZ, R.: Circulat. Res. 6, 522 (1958).
1646. SAULNIER, R.: Quoted by LU et al. (ref. 1182).
1647. SBAR, S., SCHLANT, C.: J. Amer. med. Ass. 201, 865 (1967).
1648. SCAFFIDI, V., D'AGOSTINO, L.: Quoted by CALDER (ref. 270). Riv. Pat. sper. 22, 437
       (1939).
1649. SCALES, B., McINTOSH, D.A.D.: J. Pharmacol. exp. Ther. 160, 261 (1968).
1650. SCARBOROUGH, W.R.: Progr. cardiovasc. Dis. 2, 263 (1959).
1651. — MASON, R.E., DAVIS, F.W., SINGEWALD, M.L., BAKER, B.M., LORE, S.A.: Amer.
       Heart J. 44, 645 (1952).
1652. SCEBAT, L., BENSAID, J., SOZUTEK, Y., LEFEVRE, M., RENAIS, J.: Sem. thér. 44, 686
       (1968).
1653. — MAURICE, M.: Personal Communication 1968.
1654. SCHACHTER, R.J., KIMURA, E.T., NOWARRA, G.M., MESTERN, J.: Intern. Record Med.
       Gen. Pract. Clin. 167, 248 (1954).

1655. SCHAEFER, L.E.: Ann. N.Y. Acad. Sci. **148**, 925 (1968).
1656. SCHAEFER, N., STAUCH, M.: Med. Klin. **64**, 1037 (1969).
1657. SCHAPER, W.K.A.: The Collateral Circulation in the Canine Coronary System. These Univ. Louvain (1967).
1658. — SCHAPER, J., XHONNEUX, R., VANDESTEENE, R.: Cardiovasc. Res. **3**, 315 (1969).
1659. — XHONNEUX, R., JAGENEAU, A.H.M.: Arch. exp. Pathol. Pharmakol. **252**, 1 (1965).
1660. — — — JANSSEN, P.A.J.: J. Pharmacol. exp. Ther. **152**, 265 (1966).
1661. SCHAUMANN, W., BODEM, R., BARTSCH, W.: Arch. Pharmacol. exp. Path. **255**, 328 (1966).
1662. SCHELLING, J.L., LASAGNA, L.: Clin. Pharmacol. Ther. **8**, 256 (1967).
1663. SCHERBEL, A.L.: Amer. J. Cardiol. **6**, 1125 (1960).
1664. SCHERF, D., SCHAFFER, A.I.: Amer. Heart J. **43**, 927 (1952).
1665. SCHERLAG, B.J., LAU, S.H., HELFANT, R.H., BERKOWITZ, W.D., STEIN, E., DAMATO, A.N.: Circulation **39**, 13 (1969).
1666. SCHERLIS, S., PROVENZA, D.V.: Circulation **18**, 777 (1958).
1667. SCHEUER, J.: Amer. J. Cardiol. **19**, 385 (1967).
1668. SCHILLING, F.J., BECKER, W.H., CHRISTAKIS, G.: Circulation **34**, Suppl. III, 28 (1966).
1669. SCHIMERT, G.: Schweiz. med. Wschr. **25**, 598 (1951).
1670. — SCHWALB, H.: Arzneimittel-Forsch. **21**, 465 (1971).
1671. — ZICKGRAF, H.: Klin. Wschr. **27**, 59 (1948).
1672. SCHLEPPER, M., WITZLEB, E.: Arzneimittel-Forsch. **12**, 559 (1962).
1673. SCHLESINGER, M.J.: J. Lab. clin. Invest. **6**, 1 (1957).
1674. — ZOLL, P.M.: Arch. Path. **32**, 178 (1941).
1675. SCHLUGER, J., McGINN, J.T., HENNESSY, D.J.: Amer. J. med. Sci. **233**, 296 (1957).
1676. SCHMALL, F.W., BETZ, E.: Arzneimittel-Forsch. **14**, 1159 (1964).
1677. SCHMID, E., KRAUTHEIM, J., WEIST, F.: Circulatory Drugs. Ed. by A. BERTELLI. Amsterdam: North Holland Publ. Co. 1969, p. 83.
1678. SCHMID, J.R., HANNA, C.: Pharmacologist **9**, 187 (1967).
1679. SCHMIDT, H.D., SCHMIER, J.: Arzneimittel-Forsch. **16**, 1058 (1966).
1680. — — Arzneimittel-Forsch. **17**, 861 (1967).
1681. SCHMIDT, L.: Klin. Wschr. **36**, 127 (1958).
1682. — ENGELHORN, R.: Arch. exp. Pathol. Pharmakol. **218**, 115 (1953).
1683. SCHMIDT-VOIGT, J.: Fortschr. Med. **84**, 23 (1966).
1684. SCHMITT, G.: Med. Welt (Berl.) **18**, 2943 (1967).
1685. — JUNGE-HÜLSING, G., WAGNER, H., HAUSS, W.H.: Arzneimittel-Forsch. **17**, 1500 (1967).
1686. — KNOCHE, H.: Verh. dtsch. Ges. Kreisl.-Forsch. **30**, 283 (1964).
1687. SCHMITTHENNER, J.E., HAFKENSCHIEL, J.H., FORTE, I., WILLIAMS, A.J., RIEGEL, C.: Circulation **18**, 778 (1958).
1688. SCHMUTZ, J., LAUENER, H., HIRT, R., SANZ, M.: Helv. chim. Acta **34**, 767 (1951).
1689. SCHOENDORF, H., RUMMEL, W., PFLEGER, K.: Experientia (Basel) **25**, 44 (1969).
1690. SCHOENMAKERS, J.: Probleme der Coronardurchblutung. Stuttgart: G. Thieme 1958, p. 133.
1691. SCHOEPKE, H.G., DARBY, T.D., BRONDYK, H.D.: Pharmacologist **8**, 204 (1966).
1692. SCHOFIELD, B.M., WALKER, J.M.: J. Physiol. (Lond.) **122**, 489 (1953).
1693. SCHOLIMEYER, P.J., JESCHKE, D.: Klin. Wschr. **47**, 42 (1969).
1694. SCHOLTHOLT, J., BUSSMANN, W.D., LOCHNER, W.: Pflügers Arch. ges. Physiol. **285**, 274 (1965).
1695. SCHÖNE, H.H., LINDNER, E.: Arzneimittel-Forsch. **10**, 583 (1960).
1696. — — Klin. Wschr. **40**, 1196 (1962).
1697. SCHRAVEN, E., NITZ, R.E.: Arzneimittel-Forsch. **18**, 396 (1968).
1698. SCHURGER, R.: Med. Welt (Berl.) **1**, 58 (1968).
1699. SCHWALB, H.: Med. Klin. **63**, 81 (1968).
1700. SCHWALBE, J.: Arzneimittel-Forsch. **18**, 1107 (1968).
1701. SCHWARTZ, W.: Clin. Med. **74**, 61 (1967).
1702. SCHWEITZER, F.: Prakt. Arzt. (Wien) **219**, 558 (1965).
1703. SCHWEIZER, W.: Cardiologia (Basel) **33**, 40 (1958).
1704. — BURKART, F., CREUX, G., WIDMER, L.K.: Schweiz. med. Wschr. **98**, 869 (1968).
1705. — VON PLANTA, P.: Schweiz. med. Wschr. **88**, 882 (1958).
1706. SCOTT, J.C.: Circulat. Res. **9**, 906 (1961).
1707. — Animal and Clinical Pharmacologic Techniques in Drug Evaluation. Ed. by NODINE and SIEGLER. Chicago: Year Book Medical Publications 1964, p. 176.
1708. SCOTT, R.C., IGLAUER, A., GREEN, R.S., KAUFMAN, J.W., BERMAN, B., McGUIRE, J.: Circulation **3**, 80 (1951).
1709. — SEIWERT, V.J.: Ann. intern. Med. **36**, 1190 (1952).
1710. — — FOWLER, N.O., McGUIRE, J.: Circulation **6**, 125 (1952).

1711. SCOTT, W.S., LESLIE, A., MULINOS, M.G.: Amer. Heart J. **19**, 719 (1940).
1712. SCRIABINE, A., McSHANE, W.K.: J. New Drugs **5**, 143 (1965).
1713. SEGAL, R.L., SILVER, S., YOHALEM, S.B., NEWBURGER, R.A.: Amer. J. Cardiol. **1**, 671 (1958).
1714. SEKIYA, A., VAUGHAN-WILLIAMS, E.M.: Brit. J. Pharmacol. **21**, 473 (1963).
1715. SELYE, H.: a) Amer. Heart J. **77**, 653 (1969). b) J. Amer. med. Ass. **206**, 103 (1968).
1716. — Méd. et Hyg. (Genève) **27**, 669 (1969).
1717. SELZER, A., SUDRANN, R.B.: Circulat. Res. **6**, 485 (1958).
1718. SEMMLER, F.: Ther. d. Gegenw. **106**, 673 (1967).
1719. SETNIKAR, I.: Farmaco, Ed. sci. **11**, 750 (1956).
1720. — MURMANN, W., RAVASI, M.T.: Arch. int. Pharmacodyn. **131**, 187 (1961).
1721. — RAVASI, M.T.: Arch. int. Pharmacodyn. **124**, 116 (1960).
1722. — ZANOLINI, T.: Farmaco, Ed. sci. **11**, 855 (1956).
1723. SEVELIUS, G., JOHNSON, P.C.: J. Lab. clin. Med. **54**, 669 (1959).
1724. SHANKS, R.G.: Brit. J. Pharmacol. **26**, 322 (1966).
1725. — Amer. J. Cardiol. **18**, 308 (1966).
1726. — Methods in Drug Evaluation. Ed. by P. MANTEGAZZA and F. PICCININI. Amsterdam: North Holland Publishers Co. 1966, p. 183.
1727. — Brit. J. Pharmacol. **29**, 204 (1967).
1728. — Lancet **1967**II, 560.
1729. — DUNLOP, D.: Cardiovasc. Res. **1**, 34 (1967).
1730. — WOOD, T.M., DORNHORST, A.C., CLARK, M.L.: Nature (Lond.) **212**, 88 (1966).
1731. SHAPIRO, A.: J. Amer. med. Ass. **203**, 57 (1968).
1732. SHAPIRO, A.K.: The Psychological Basis of Medical Practice. Ed. by LIEF, LIEF and LIEF. New York: Harper and Row 1963, p. 163.
1733. SHAPIRO, S.: Angiology **10**, 126 (1959).
1734. — Angiology **12**, 53 (1961).
1735. SHARMA, P.L.: Brit. J. Anaesth. **41**, 481 (1969).
1736. SHEFFIELD, L.T., HOLT, J.H., REEVES, T.J.: Circulation **32**, 622 (1965).
1737. — REEVES, T.J.: Mod. Conc. cardiov. Dis. **34**, 1 (1965).
1738. SHEN, Y., QUIROZ, A.C., BURCH, G.E., DEPASQUALE, N.P.: Amer. Heart J. **73**, 669 (1967).
1739. SHERBER, D.A., GELB, I.J.: Circulation **22**, 809 (1960).
1740. — — Angiology **12**, 244 (1961).
1741. SHIMAMOTO, T., MAEZAWA, H., YAMAZAKE, H., ATSUMZ, T., FUGITA, T., ISHIOKA, T., SUNAGA, T.: Amer. Heart J. **71**, 297 (1966).
1742. — NUMANO, F., FUGITA, T.: Amer. Heart J. **71**, 216 (1966).
1743. SHINEBOURNE, E., FLEMING, J., HAMER, J.: Lancet **1967**II, 1217.
1744. — — — Cardiovasc. Res. **2**, 379 (1968).
1745. — WHITE, R., HAMER, J.: Circulat. Res. **24**, 835 (1969).
1746. SHIPLEY, R.E., GREGG, D.E., WEARN, J.T.: Amer. J. Physiol. **136**, 263 (1942).
1747. — WILSON, C.: Proc. Soc. exp. Biol. (N.Y.) **78**, 724 (1951).
1748. SHOSHKES, M., ROTHFELD, E.L., BECKER, M.C., FINKELSTEIN, A., SMITH, C.C., WACHTEL, F.W.: Circulation **20**, 17 (1959).
1749. SHUTE, W., SHUTE, E., VOGELSANG, A.: Med. Rec. **160**, 91 (1947).
1750. SICUTERI, F., FANCIULLACCI, M., DELBIANCO, P.L.: Med. Pharmacol. exp. **15**, 73 (1966).
1751. SIESS, M.: Arzneimittel-Forsch. **12**, 683 (1962).
1752. SILBER, E.H., KATZ, L.N.: J. Amer. med. Ass. **153**, 1075 (1953).
1753. SILVA MALTEZ, J., DE SOUSA BORGES, A.: J. Méd. (Pôrto) **46**, 609 (1961).
1754. SIMAAN, J., FAWAZ, G.: Cardiovasc. Res. **2**, 68 (1968).
1755. SIMON, A.J., DOLGIN, M., SOLWAY, A.J.L., HIRSCHMANN, J., KATZ, L.N.: J. Lab. clin. Med. **34**, 992 (1949).
1756. SKINNER, M.S., LEIBESKIND, R.S., PHILLIPS, H.L., HARRISON, T.R.: Amer. Heart J. **61**, 250 (1961).
1757. SLOMAN, G., PITT, A., HIRSCH, E.Z., DONALDSON, A.: Med. J. Aust. **1**, 4 (1965).
1758. — STANNARD, M.: Brit. med. J. **1967**IV, 508.
1759. SMITH, F.M.: Arch. intern. Med. **28**, 836 (1921).
1760. — MILLER, G.H., GRABER, V.C.: J. clin. Invest. **2**, 157 (1925).
1761. SMITH, M.H., GORLIN, R.: Circulation **14**, 1002 (1956).
1762. SMITH, W.G.: Lancet **1967**I, 165.
1763. SMULYAN, H., EICH, R.H.: J. Lab. clin. Med. **71**, 378 (1968).
1764. SNOW, P.J.D.: Lancet **1965**II, 551.
1765. — Amer. J. Cardiol. **18**, 458 (1966).
1766. — ANDERSON, D.E.: Brit. Heart J. **21**, 323 (1959).

1767. Sodi-Pallares, D., Bisteni, A., Medrano, G.A., De Micheli, A., Ponce de Leon, J., Calva, E., Fishleder, B.L., Testelli, M.R., Miller, B.L.: Electrolytes and Cardiovascular Diseases. Basle: S. Karger 1966, 2, 198.
1768. — — — Testelli, M.R., De Micheli, A.: Dis. Chest. 43, 424 (1963).
1769. — Fishleder, B.L., Cisneros, F., Vizcaino, M., Bisteni, A., Medrano, G.A., Polansky, B.J., De Micheli, A.: Canad. med. Ass. J. 83, 243 (1960).
1770. — Testelli, M.R., Fishleder, B.L., Bisteni, A., Medrano, G.A., Friedland, C., De Micheli, A.: Amer. J. Cardiol. 9, 166 (1962).
1771. Solandt, D.Y., Best, C.H.: Lancet 1938II, 130.
1772. — Nassim, R., Best, C.H.: Lancet 1939II, 592.
1773. Soloff, L.A., Gimenez, J.L., Winters, W.L.: Amer. J. med. Sci. 243, 783 (1962).
1774. Solvay, H., Van Schepdael, J.: Electrodiagnostic-thérapie 5, 153 (1968).
1775. — — Electrodiagnostic-Thérapie, 6, 137 (1969).
1776. — — Arch. Mal. Cœur 12, 1700 (1969).
1777. Somani, P.: Pharmacologist 9, 249 (1967).
1778. — Amer. Heart J. 77, 63 (1969).
1779. — Bachand, R.T.: Europ. J. Pharmacol. 7, 239 (1969).
1780. — — Hardman, H.F.: Clin. Res. 16, 249 (1968).
1781. — — — Laddu, A.R.: Europ. J. Pharmacol. 8, 1 (1969).
1782. — Fleming, J.G., Chan, G.K., Lum, B.K.B.: J. Pharmacol. exp. Ther. 151, 32 (1966).
1783. — Lum, B.K.B.: J. Pharmacol. exp. Ther. 147, 194 (1965).
1784. — — J. Pharmacol. exp. Ther. 152, 235 (1966).
1785. — Watson, D.L.: J. Pharmacol. exp. Ther. 164, 317 (1968).
1786. Somerville, W.: Brit. med. J. 1969III, 46.
1787. — Proc. roy. Soc. Med. 62, 871 (1969).
1788. Sones, F.M., Shirey, E.K.: Mod. Conc. cardiov. Dis. 31, 735 (1962).
1789. Sonnenblick, E.H., Braunwald, E., Williams, J.F., Glick, G.: J. clin. Invest. 44, 2051 (1965).
1790. — Ross, J., Braunwald, E.: Amer. J. Cardiol. 22, 328 (1968).
1791. — — Covell, J.W., Kaiser, G.A., Braunwald, E.: Amer. J. Physiol. 209, 919 (1965).
1792. Sonntag, A.C.: Annual Reports in Medicinal Chemistry. Ed. by C.K. Cain. New York: Academic Press 1968, p. 71.
1793. Sorrentino, L., Di Rosa, M.: Méd. et Hyg. (Genève) 541, 232 (1962).
1794. — — Di Paco, G.F., Tauro, C.S.: Gazz. med. ital. 118, 3 (1959).
1795. Sosa, J.A., McGregor, M.: Canad. med. Ass. J. 89, 248 (1963).
1796. Soskin, S., Priest, W.S., Schultz, W.J.: Amer. J. Physiol. 108, 107 (1934).
1797. Soulie, P., Chiche, P., Carlotti, J., Baillet, J.: Presse méd. 62, 40, 847 (1954).
1798. Sowton, E., Balcon, R., Cross, D., Frick, M.H.: Cardiovasc. Res. 1, 301 (1967).
1799. — — — — Brit. med. J. 1968I, 215.
1800. — Hamer, J.: Amer. J. Cardiol. 18, 317 (1966).
1801. — Oram, S.: Brit. med. J. 1961I, 794.
1802. Spain, D.M., Bradess, V,A.: Amer. J. med. Sci. 240, 701 (1960).
1803. — Nathan, D.J.: J. Amer. med. Ass. 177, 683 (1961).
1804. Speckmann, K., Klensch, H., Maetzel, F.K., Meyer, J.D.: Dtsch. med. Wschr. 92, 1493 (1967).
1805. Spencer, F.C.: Acquis. Nouv. Pathol. Cardiovasc. 11, 397 (1969).
1806. Spier, C.: Clin. Med. 76, 23 (1969).
1807. Spitzbarth, H.: Arzneimittel-Forsch. 9, 59 (1959).
1808. Sprague, H.B.: Circulation 23, 648 (1961).
1809. — White, P.D.: Med. Clin. N. Amer. 16, 895 (1933).
1810. Spühler, O.: Schweiz. med. Wschr. 76, 1259 (1946).
1811. — Schweiz. med. Wschr. 79, 518 (1949).
1812. Srivastava, S.C., Dewar, H.A., Newell, D.J.: Brit. med. J. 1964II, 724.
1813. Stafford, A.: Brit. J. Pharmacol. 28, 218 (1966).
1814. — Nature (Lond.) 214, 390 (1967).
1815. Stampfer, E.: Wien. klin. Wschr. 81, 288 (1969).
1816. Stampfer, M., Epstein, S.E., Beiser, G.D., Goldstein, R.E., Braunwald, E.: Circulation 38, Suppl. 6, 188 (1968).
1817. Stanton, H.C.: Fed. Proc. 23, 124 (1964).
1818. — Kirchgessner, T., Parmenter, K.: J. Pharmacol. exp. Ther. 149, 174 (1965).
1819. Starcich, R.: Minerva med. 47, 887 (1956).
1820. — Ambanelli, V.: G. Clin. med. 40, 2 (1959).
1821. Starey, F.: Therapiewoche 19, 323 (1969).
1822. Starfinger, W.: Therapiewoche 17, 235 (1967).

1823. STARR, I., GAMBLE, C.J., MARGOLIES, A., DONAL, J.S., JOSEPH, N., ENGLE, E.: J. clin. Invest. **16**, 799 (1937).
1824. — PEDERSEN, E., CORBASCIO, A.N.: Circulation **12**, 588 (1955).
1825. STAUCH, M., SCHAIRER, K.: Z. Kreisl.-Forsch. **58**, 586 (1969).
1826. STEARNS, S., RISEMAN, J.E.F., GRAY, W.: New Engl. J. Med. **234**, 578 (1946).
1827. STEHLE, R.L.: J. Pharmacol. exp. Ther. **46**, 471 (1932).
1828. STEIN, P.D., BROOKS, H.L., MATSON, J.L., HYLAND, J.W.: Clin. Res. **15**, 223 (1967).
1829. — — — — Cardiovasc. Res. **2**, 63 (1968).
1830. STEINBERG, F., JENSEN, J.: J. Lab. clin. Med. **30**, 769 (1945).
1831. STEINER, C., WIT, A.L., DAMATO, A.N.: Circulat. Res. **24**, 167 (1969).
1832. STEPHEN, S.A.: Amer. J. Cardiol. **18**, 463 (1966).
1833. STERN, P.: Z. Kreisl.-Forsch. **40**, 726 (1951).
1834. STERN, S.: Amer. Heart J. **74**, 170 (1967).
1835. STERNE, J., HIRSCH, C.: 4th European Congress of Cardiology, Praha, 1964.
1836. — — Thérapie **20**, 89 (1965).
1837. STERNITZKE, N., KOEHLER, J.A., LANG, E.: Med. Welt (Berl.) **36**, 1910 (1966).
1838. STEVENSON, F.H., WILSON, D.G.: Lancet **1954I**, 1319.
1839. STEWART, H.J., HORGER, E.L., SORENSON, C.W.: Amer. Heart J. **36**, 161 (1948).
1840. — JACK, N.B.: Amer. Heart J. **20**, 205 (1940).
1841. STOCK, J.P.P., DALE, N.: Brit. med. J. **1963II**, 1230.
1842. STOCK, T.B., WENDT, V.E., HAYDEN, R.O., BRUCE, T.A., BING, R.J.: Med. Clin. N. Amer. **46**, 1497 (1962).
1843. STOKER, J.B.: Brit. J. clin. Pract. **22**, 384 (1968).
1844. STOLAND, O.O., GINSBERG, A.M., LOY, D.L., HIEBERT, P.E.: J. Pharmacol. exp. Ther. **51**, 387 (1934).
1845. STORCK, U.: Med. Welt (Berl.) **52**, 2926 (1965).
1846. STORMAN, H.: Arzneimittel-Forsch. **16**, 705 (1966).
1847. STORTI, R.: Minerva med. **79**, 605 (1952).
1848. STRAESSLE, B., BURCKHARDT, D.: Schweiz. med. Wschr. **95**, 667 (1965).
1849. STRAUSAK, A., COTTIER, P., SCHMID, A.: Cardiologia (Basel) **34**, 138 (1959).
1850. STRAUSS, L.H.: Cardiologia (Basel) **25**, 1 (1954).
1851. STRÖDER, U.: Cardiologia (Basel) **19**, 127 (1951).
1852. SUETTINGER, H.: Therapiewoche **17**, 1362 (1967).
1853. SULLIVAN, F.J., BENDER, A.D., HORVATH, S.M.: Arch. int. Pharmacodyn. **147**, 229 (1964).
1854. SULLIVAN, J.M., GORLIN, R.: Circulat. Res. **21**, 919 (1967).
1855. SULZER, R.: Heart **11**, 141 (1924).
1856. SUN, S.C., BURCH, G.E., DEPASQUALE, N.P.: Amer. Heaert J. **74**, 340 (1967).
1857. SURIYONG, R., VANNOTTI, A.: Schweiz. med. Wschr. **80**, 208 (1950).
1858. SUTTON, D.C., LUETH, H.C.: Arch. intern. Med. **45**, 827 (1930).
1859. SWANSON, L.W.: J. Lab. clin. Med. **30**, 376 (1945).
1860. Symposium on the Diagnosis of Thoracic Pain. Proc. Mayo Clin. **31**, 1 (1956).
1861. Sympsoium on evaluation of serum lipoprotein and cholesterol measurements as predictors of clinical complications of atherosclerosis. Circulation **14**, 691 (1956).
1862. SZABO, G.: Acta med. Acad. Sci. hung. **13**, 289 (1959).
1863. — MAGYAR, S., SOLTI, F.: Z. Kreisl.-Forsch. **47**, 971 (1958).
1864. — SOLTI, F., MAGYAR, S.: Z. Kreisl.-Forsch. **47**, 24 (1958).
1865. — — REV, J., REFI, Z., MEGYESI, K.: Z. Kreisl.-Forsch. **46**, 197 (1957).
1866. SZATMARY, J.: Wien. klin. Wschr. **16**, 282 (1965).
1867. SZEKELY, P., JACKSON, F., WYNNE, N.A., VOHRA, J.K., BATSON, G.A., DOW, W.I.M.: Amer. J. Cardiol. **18**, 426 (1966).
1867 bis. SZEKERES, L., LENARD, G.: Experientia (Basel) **14**, 338 (1958).
1868. — PAPP, J.G., FISCHER, E.: Europ. J. Pharmacol. **2**, 1 (1967).
1869. SZENTIVANYI, M., JUHASZ-NAGY, A., DEBRECENI, L.: Experientia (Basel) **22**, 171 (1966).
1870. — — — Acta physiol. Acad. Sci. hung. **31**, 9 (1967).
1871. SZIRMAI, E.: Hippokrates (Stuttg.) **32**, 491 (1961).
1872. TALLEY, R.W., BEARD, O.W., DOHERTY, J.E.: Amer. Heart J. **44**, 866 (1952).
1873. TARTARA, A., CORBETTA, F.: Folia cardiol. (Milano) **15**, 539 (1956).
1874. TATIBOUET, L.: In press 1971.
1875. TAYLOR, H.L., HENSCHEL, A., BROZEK, J., KEYS, A.: J. appl. Physiol. **2**, 223 (1944).
1876. TAYLOR, S.H., MACDONALD, H.R., ROBINSON, M.C., SAPRU, R.P.: Brit. Heart J. **29**, 352 (1967).
1877. TEOTINO, U.M., POLO FRIZ, L., STEIS, G., DELLA BELLA, D.: Farmaco, Ed. Sci. **17**, 252 (1962).
1878. The National Diet-Heart-Study. Final report. Circulation **37**, Suppl. 1, (1968).

1879. THIELE, K., GROSS, A., POSSELT, K., SCHULER, W.: Bull. chimie Thérap. **5**, 366 (1967).
1880. — KOBERSTEIN, E., NONNENMACHER, G.: Arzneimittel-Forsch. **18**, 1255 (1968).
1881. — POSSELT, K., VON BEBENBURG, W.: Arzneimittel-Forsch. **18**, 1263 (1968).
1882. — SCHIMASSEK, U., VON SCHLICHTEGROLL, A.: Arzneimittel-Forsch. **16**, 1064 (1966).
1883. THIEMER, K., STADLER, R.: Arzneimittel-Forsch. **16**, 1502 (1966).
1884. — — VON SCHLICHTEGROLL, A.: Arzneimittel-Forsch. **18**, 388 (1968).
1885. THIERFELDER, J.: Therapiewoche **13**, 695 (1963).
1886. THOMAS, C.B.: Circulation **20**, 25 (1959).
1887. THOMPSON, R.H., LETLEY, E.: Lancet **1967**II, 1149.
1888. THOMSEN, J.H., STENLUND, R.R., CORLISS, R.J., SIALER, S., ROWE, G.G.: a) Fed. Proc.
       26, 772 (1967). b) Arch. int. Pharmacodyn. **172**, 15 (1968).
1889. THORP, R.H.: Arch. int. Pharmacodyn. **120**, 130 (1959).
1890. — COBBIN, L.B.: Arch. int. Pharmacodyn. **118**, 95 (1959).
1891. TILSNER, V.: Med. Klin. **64**, 1120 (1969).
1892. *Today's Drugs:* Verapamil. Brit. med. J. **1968**I, 230.
1893. TODESCO, S., PERMUTTI, B.: Cuore e Circol. **47**, 169 (1963).
1894. TORRES, E.C., BRANDI, G.: Canad. J. Physiol. Pharmacol. **47**, 421 (1969).
1895. TOWERS, M.K., WOOD, P.: Brit. med. J. **5104**, 1067 (1958).
1896. TRANCHESI, J.: Aterosclerosis y enfermedad coronaria, 1 vol. Mexico: Interamericana
       1960, p. 173.
1897. Treatment of myocardial ischaemia. Brit. med. J. **1967**IV, 249.
1898. TRIMBORN, H.: Münch. med. Wschr. **110**, 615 (1968).
1899. TRIPOD, J., MEIER, R.: Arch. int. Pharmacodyn. **97**, 251 (1954).
1900. — — Arch. int. Pharmacodyn. **99**, 104 (1954).
1901. TRUITT, E.B.: J. Amer. pharm. Ass. **44**, 382 (1955).
1902. TSCHIRDEWAHN, B., KLEPZIG, H.: Dtsch. med. Wschr. **88**, 1702 (1963).
1903. — KNORPP, K., HEINRICH, F., SCHUETTERLE, G.: Dtsch. med. Wschr. **92**, 2204 (1967).
1904. TÜRKER, R.K., KAYAALP, S.O.: Experientia (Basel) **23**, 647 (1967).
1905. — — ÖZER, A.: Arzneimittel-Forsch. **18**, 1209 (1968).
1906. TURPEINEN, O., MIETTINEN, M., KARVONEN, M.J., ROINE, P., PEKKARINEN, M., LEH-
       TOSUO, E.J., ALIVIRTA, P.: Amer. J. clin. Nutr. **21**, 255 (1968).
1907. UHLENBROOCK, K., SCHWEER, M.: Arzneimittel-Forsch. **9**, 229 (1959).
1908. — — Arzneimittel-Forsch. **10**, 293 (1960).
1909. — SPEHN, W.: Münch. med. Wschr. **96**, 339 (1954).
1910. UHLMANN, F., NOBILE, F.: Arch. exp. Pathol. Pharmakol. **192**, 189 (1938).
1911. ULRYCH, M., FROHLICH, E.D., DUSTAN, H.P., PAGE, I.H.: Circulation **37**, 411 (1968).
1912. UNNA, K.: Arch. exp. Pathol. Pharmakol. **213**, 207 (1951).
1913. Unsaturated fats and coronary heart disease. Lancet **1968**II, 901.
1914. URSCHEL, C.W.: Amer. J. Physiol. **212**, 1497 (1967).
1915. VALORI, C., THOMAS, M., SHILLINGFORD, J.P.: Amer. J. Cardiol. **20**, 605 (1967).
1916. VAN DE BERG, L.: Acta chir. belg. **67**, 433 (1968).
1917. VANE, J.R.: J. Physiol. (Lond.) **121**, 97 (1953).
1918. VAN EGMOND, A.A.J.: Arch. exp. Pathol. Pharmakol. **65**, 197 (1911).
1919. VAQUEZ, H., GIROUX, R., KISTHINIOS, N.: Presse méd. **37**, 1277 (1929).
1920. VARKONYI, G.: Therapiewoche **16**, 191 (1966).
1921. VARMA, D.R., SHARE, N.N., MELVILLE, K.I.: Biochem. Pharmacol. **8**, 135 (1961).
1922. VARNAUSKAS, E., BERGMAN, H., HOUK, P., BJÖRNTORP, P.: Lancet **1966**II, 8.
1923. VASTESAEGER, M., GILLOT, P.H., VAN DER STRAETEN, P.: Brux.-méd. **51**, 99 (1971).
1924. — Personal Communication 1969.
1925. — BLOCK, P.: Ars Medici **25**, 1733 (1970).
1926. — CHARLIER, R., LELOUP, A.: Presse méd. **70**, 2050 (1962).
1927. — GILLOT, P., RASSON, G.: Acta cardiol. (Brux.) **22**, 483 (1967).
1928. — RASSON, G.: Ars Medici **22**, 399 (1967).
1929. — ROCHET, J., LELOUP, A.: Sem. Hôp. Paris (Thérapeutique) **37**, 937 (1961).
1930. — — GILLOT, P.: Personal Communication 1963.
1931. VAUGHAN WILLIAMS, E.M.: Amer. J. Cardiol. **18**, 399 (1966).
1932. — Int. Symp. on the coronary circulation and energetics of the myocardium. Basle:
       S. Karger 1967, p. 118.
1933. — Advanc. Cardiol. **4**, 275 (1970).
1934. — SINGH, B.N.: Brit. J. Pharmacol. **39**, 657 (1970).
1935. VECCHI, G.P., MARRAMA, P.: Folia cardiol. (Milano) **15**, 419 (1956).
1936. VERA, L.B. DE, CORDAY, E., GOLD, H.: Circulation **16**, 946 (1957).
1937. VERCRUYSSEN, J., CEYSSENS, W.: Revue Médicale de Louvain **1**, 11 (1962).
1938. VERHAEGHE, L.K.: Arzneimittel-Forsch. **19**, 1842 (1969).
1939. VERSTRAETE, M., VERMYLEN, J., CLAEYS, H.: Arch. int. Pharmacodyn. **176**, 33 (1968).

1940. VETTORI, G., ERLE, G., MAGARAGGIA, L., BAU, G.: Vth European Congress of Cardiology. Athenes, Sept. 1968. Abstracts p. 369.
1941. VINEBERG, A.M.: Canad. med. Ass. J. 55, 117 (1946).
1942. — CHARI, R.S., PIFARRE, R., MERCIER, C.: Canad. med. Ass. J. 87, 336 (1962).
1943. — MAHANTI, B., LITVAK, J.: Surgery 47, 765 (1960).
1944. VISIOLI, O., DALLAVALLE, L., BIANCHI, G., BOTTI, G., MALAGNINO, G.: Minerva cardio-angiol. 14, 613 (1966).
1945. — — BOTTI, G.: Folia cardiol. (Milano) 24, 417 (1965).
1946. Vital Statistics of the United States 2, Section 1, 8 (1961).
1947. VONK, J.T.C.: In Press 1971.
1948. VON OETTINGEN, W.F., DONAHUE, D.D., LAWTON, A.H., MONACO, A.R., YAGODA, H., VALAER, P.J.: Public Health Service Bulletin, 1944, N° 282, U.S. Public Health Service.
1949. VON PLANTA, W.: Personal Communication 1969.
1950. VORIDIS, E., ANTONIADIS, G., MARINAKIS, P., PAPAZOGLOU, N., PETRITIS, J.: Vth European Congress of Cardiology. Athenes, Sept. 1968. Abstracts p. 370.
1951. WAAL, H.J.: N.Z. med. J. 67, 291 (1968).
1952. WAALER, B.A.: Acta med. scand. 157, 289 (1957).
1953. WAGMAN, R.J., LEVINE, H.J., MESSER, J.V., NEILL, W.A., KRASNOW, N., GORLIN, R.: Amer. J. Cardiol. 9, 439 (1962).
1954. WAGNER, J., GREEFF, K., HEEG, E., PEREIRA, E.: Arch. exp. Pathol. Pharmakol. 253, 92 (1966).
1955. WALLACW, A.G., SCHAAL, S.F., SUGIMOTO, T., ROZEAR, M., ALEXANDER, J.A.: Bull. N.Y. Acad. Med. 43, 1119 (1967).
1956. WARBASSE, J.R., HAWLEY, R.R., GILLILAN, R.E.: Circulation 35, Suppl. 2, 263 (1967).
1957. WAREMBOURG, H.: Lille méd. 11, 619 (1966).
1958. — BERTRAND, M.: Lille méd. 9, 1138 (1967).
1959. — DELOMEZ, M.: Lille méd. 10, 545 (1965).
1960. — JAILLARD, J.: Lille méd. 14, 224 (1969).
1961. WATILLON, M., LAVERGNE, G., WEEKERS, J.F.: Bull. Soc. belge Ophtal. 150, 715 (1968).
1962. WATT, D.A.: Brit. med. J. 1967 IV, 744.
1963. WAX, D.S., DEGRAFF, A.C.: J. Amer. Geriat. Soc. 4, 151 (1956).
1964. WAYNE, E.J., LAPLACE, L.B.: Clin. Sci. 1, 103 (1933).
1965. WEARN, J.T.: J. exp. Med. 47, 293 (1928).
1966. WEDD, A.M.: J. Pharmacol. exp. Ther. 41, 355 (1931).
1967. — DRURY, A.N.: J. Pharmacol. exp. Ther. 50, 157 (1934).
1968. WEGRIA, R., ESSEX, H.E., HERRICK, J.F., MANN, F.C.: Amer. Heart J. 20, 557 (1940).
1969. — NICKERSON, J.L., CASE, R.B., HOLLAND, J.F.: Amer. J. Med. 10, 414 (1951).
1970. — WARD, H.P., FRANK, C.W., DREYFUSS, F., BROWN, E.M., HUTCHINSON, D.L.: Cited by WEGRIA (ref. 1969).
1971. WEINER, M.: J. Amer. med. Ass. 203, 57 (1968).
1972. WEISS, S., WILKINS, R.W., HAYNES, F.W.: J. clin. Invest. 16, 73 (1937).
1973. WEITZMAN, D.: Brit. med. J. 4851, 1409 (1953).
1974. WELLENS, H.J.: In press 1971.
1975. WELTI, J.J., FACQUET, J.: Sem. Hôp. Paris 35, 8, 697 (1959).
1976. WENDT, V.E., SUNDERMEYER, J.F., DEN BAKKER, P.B., BING, R.J.: Amer. J. Cardiol. 9, 449 (1962).
1977. WEST, J.W., BELLET, S., MANZOLI, U.C., MÜLLER, O.F.: Circulat. Res. 10, 35 (1962).
1978. — GUZMAN, S.V., BELLET, S.: Circulat. Res. 6, 389 (1958).
1979. — KOBAYASHI, T., ANDERSON, F.S.: Circulat. Res. 10, 722 (1962).
1980. — — GUZMAN, S.V.: Circulat. Res. 6, 383 (1958).
1981. WETTE, K.: Münch. med. Wschr. 22, 1238 (1966).
1982. WHALEN, R.E., MORRIS, J.J., BEHAR, V.S., THOMPSON, H.K., McINTOSH, H.D.: Clin. Res. 14, 265 (1966).
1983. WHITE, J.C.: Circulation 16, 644 (1957).
1984. — GARREY, W.E., ATKINS, J.A.: Arch. Surg. 26, 765 (1933).
1985. WHITE, P.D.: IIIrd World Congress of Cardiology, Brussels, 1958, Formal lectures, p. 43.
1986. — Aterosclerosis y enfermedad coronaria, 1 vol. Mexico: Interamericana 1960, p. 1.
1987. — Aterosclerosis y enfermedad coronaria, 1 vol. Mexico: Interamericana 1960, p. 339.
1988. WHITE, R., SHINEBOURNE, E.: Cardiovasc. Res. 3, 245 (1969).
1989. WHITSITT, L.S., LUCCHESI, B.R.: Circulat. Res. 21, 305 (1967).
1990. — — Circulat. Res. 23, 585 (1968).
1991. WIEMERS, K.: Arch. exp. Pathol. Pharmakol. 213, 283 (1951).
1992. — Arch. exp. Pathol. Pharmakol. 213, 314 (1951).
1993. WIENER, L., DWYER, E.M., COX, J.W.: Circulation 38, Suppl. 6, 206 (1968); 39, 623 (1969).
1994. — — — Circulation 38, 240 (1968).

1995. WIGGERS, C.J.: Circulat. Res. **2**, 271 (1954).
1996. — GREEN, H.D.: Amer. Heart J. **11**, 527 (1936).
1997. WIJK, T.W. VAN: Angiology **4**, 103 (1953).
1998. WILDE, W.: Therapiewoche **16**, 761 (1966).
1999. WILHELM, M., HEDWALL, P., MEIER, M.: Experientia (Basel) **23**, 651 (1967).
2000. WILKINS, R.W., HAYNES, F.W., WEISS, S.: J. clin. Invest. **16**, 85 (1937).
2001. WILKINSON, J.C.M.: Lancet **1967**II, 617.
2001bis. WILLEMS, D.: Med. Welt (Berl.) **13**, 719 (1969).
2002. WILLIAMS, J.F., GLICK, G., BRAUNWALD, E.: Circulation **32**, 767 (1965).
2003. WILLIAMS, N.E., CARR, H.A., BRUENN, H.G., LEVY, R.L.: Amer. Heart J. **22**, 252 (1941).
2004. WILSON, A., SCHILD, H.O.: Clark's Applied Pharmacology, 8th ed., 1 vol. Philadelphia and New York: Blakiston 1952, 691 pp.
2005. WILSON, D.F., TURNER, A.S.: N.Z. med. J. **66**, 682 (1967).
2006. — WATSON, O.F., PEEL, J.S., TURNER, A.S.: Brit. med. J. **1969**II, 155.
2007. WINBURY, M.M.: Advanc. Pharmacology **3**, 1 (1964).
2008. — Problems in laboratory evaluation of antianginal agents. Amsterdam: North Holland Publishers Co. 1967, p. 26.
2009. — Personal Communication 1968.
2010. — Internat. Encyclopedia of Pharmacology and Therapeutics. New York-London: Pergamon Press 1970, Section 78, Chapter 2.
2011. — GABEL, L.P.: Amer. J. Physiol. **212**, 1062 (1967).
2012. — — GRANDY, R.P.: Pharmacologist **4**, 180 (1962).
2013. — HOWE, B.B., HEFNER, M.A.: J. Pharmacol. exp. Ther. **168**, 70 (1969).
2014. — KISSIL, D., LOSADA, M.: Isotopes in Experimental Pharmacology. Ed. by L.J. ROTH. Chicago: University Press 1965, p. 229.
2015. — MICHIELS, P.M., HAMBOURGER, W.E., STOCKFISCH, W.J., COOK, D.L.: J. Pharmacol. exp. Ther. **99**, 343 (1950).
2016. — PAPIERSKI, D.H., HEMMER, M.L., HAMBOURGER, W.E.: J. Pharmacol. exp. Ther. **109**, 255 (1953).
2017. — PENSINGER, R.R.: Pharmacologist **8**, 222 (1966).
2018. WINDER, C.V., THOMAS, R.W., KAMM, O.: J. Pharmacol. exp. Ther. **100**, 482 (1950).
2019. WINEGRAD, S., SHANES, A.M.: J. gen. Physiol. **45**, 371 (1962).
2020. WINSOR, T., HUMPHREYS, P.: Angiology **3**, 1 (1952).
2021. — SCOTT, C.C.: Amer. Heart J. **49**, 414 (1955).
2022. WIRTH, W., GÖSSWALD, R., VATER, W.: Arch. int. Pharmacodyn. **123**, 78 (1959).
2023. WITZLEB, E., BUDDE, H.: Arch. int. Pharmacodyn. **104**, 33 (1955).
2024. — GOLLWITZER-MEIER, K., DONAT, K.: Klin. Wschr. **32**, 297 (1954).
2025. WOLF, H.: Wien. med. Wschr. **21**, 357 (1961).
2026. WOLF, S.: Pharmacol. Rev. **11**, 689 (1959).
2027. WOLFF, H.G., HARDY, J.D., GOODELL, H.: J. clin. Invest. **19**, 659 (1940).
2028. WOLFF, M.M., BERNE, R.M.: Circulat. Res. **4**, 343 (1956).
2029. WOLFFE, J.B., FINDLAY, D., DESSEN, E.: Ann. intern. Med. **5**, 625 (1931).
2030. — SHUBIN, H.: Clin. Med. **6**, 1563 (1959).
2031. WOLFSON, S., AMSTERDAM, E.A., GORLIN, R.: Circulation **36**, Suppl. 2, 274 (1967).
2032. — HEINLE, R.A., HERMAN, M.V., KEMP, H.G., SULLIVAN, J.M., GORLIN, R.: Amer. J. Cardiol. **18**, 345 (1966).
2033. — — KEMP, H.G., GORLIN, R.: Clin. Res. **14**, 265 (1966).
2034. WOLKERSTORFER, H.: Wien. klin. Wschr. **51**, 1012 (1965).
2035. WOLLHEIM, E.: Vth European Congress of Cardiology, Athenes, Sept. 1968, Symposia p. 41.
2036. WOODS, E.F., RICHARDSON, J.A., RICHARDSON, A.K., BOZEMAN, R.F.: J. Pharmacol. exp. Ther. **116**, 351 (1956).
2037. YURCHAK, P.M., ROLETT, E.L., COHEN, L.S., GORLIN, R.: Circulation **30**, 180 (1964).
2038. ZAKUSOV, V.V.: XXIst Internat. Congress Physiol. Sciences, Buenos-Aires, August 9—15, 1959. Abstractions of Communications, p. 299.
2039. — Novie dannie po farmakologii koronarnogo krovoobrachtenia. Moscow T. Agourskaia 1960, 1 vol., 287 pages.
2040. — KAVERINA, N.V.: Quoted in ref. 2039, p. 7.
2041. — — Sovjetsk. Med. **10**, 3 (1956) (Abstract).
2042. ZALESKI, E.J., COHEN, A., BING, R.J.: Animal and clinical pharmacologic techniques in drug evaluation, vol. 2. Ed. by P.E. SIEGLER and J.H. MOYER. Chicago: Year Book Med. Publ. 1967, p. 471.
2043. ZBINDEN, G.: Amer. Heart J. **60**, 450 (1960).
2044. ZEFT, H.J., PATTERSON, S.D., ORGAIN, E.S.: Ann. intern. Med. **70**, 1082 (1969).

2045. ZELLER, E.A., BARSKY, J.: Proc. Soc. exp. Biol. (N.Y.) **81**, 459 (1952).
2046. — — BERMAN, E.R.: J. biol. Chem. **214**, 267 (1955).
2047. — — FOUTS, J.R., KIRCHHEIMER, W.F., VAN ORDEN, L.S.: Experientia (Basel) **8**, 349 (1952).
2048. ZELVELDER, W.G.: Europ. J. Clin. Pharmacol. **3**, 158 (1971).
2049. ZIMMER, V.: Med. Welt (Berl.) **17**, 2806 (1966).
2050. ZIMMERMANN, W.: Arzneimittel-Forsch. **18**, 1112 (1968).
2051. ZION, M.M., BRADLOW, B.A.: S. Afr. med. J. **35**, 11 (1961).
2052. ZOLL, P.M., NORMAN, L.R., CASSIN, S.: Circulation **6**, 832 (1952).
2053. ZUBERBUHLER, R.C., BOHR, D.F.: Circulat. Res. **16**, 431 (1965).
2054. ZUELZER, G.: Med. Klin. **15**, 555 (1928).

Additional references (series a)

1a. ABEL, R.M., REIS, R.L., STAROSCIK, R.N.: Brit. J. Pharmacol. **38**, 620 (1970).
2a. AFONSO, S., O'BRIEN, G.S., CRUMPTON, C.W.: J. Lab. clin. Med. **74**, 844 (1969).
3a. AMEUR, M., HESSEL, F., LAVAL, G.: J. Méd. Nord et Est **6**, 88 (1969).
4a. ARESKOG, N.H., ADOLFSSON, L., RASMUSON, T.: Scand. J. clin. Lab. Invest. **24**, Suppl. 110, 114 (1969).
5a. ARONOW, W.S., SWANSON, A.J.: Clin. Res. **17**, 227 (1969).
6a. — — Ann. intern. Med. **71**, 599 (1969).
7a. — — Clin. Res. **17**, 227 (1969).
8a. AUBERT, A., NYBERG, G., SLAASTAD, R., TJELDFLAAT, L.: Brit. med. J. **1970 I**, 203.
9a. BECKER, L., FORTUIN, N.J., PITT, B.: Circulation **40**, Suppl. 3, 41 (1969).
10a. BENDER, F., SIEGER, W., DOTTERWEICH, K.: Ärztl. Forsch. **23**, 359 (1969).
11a. BERKOWITZ, W.D., WIT, A.L., LAU, S.H., STEINER, C., DAMATO, A.N.: Circulation **40**, 855 (1969).
12a. BITTAR, N., PAULY, T.J.: Clin. Res. **17**, 510 (1969).
13a. BLINKS, J.R.: Ann. N.Y. Acad. Sci. **139**, 673 (1967).
14a. BOSSE, J.A., SCHAUM, E.: Arch. exp. Pathol. Pharmakol. **264**, 221 (1969).
15a. BRAUNWALD, E., COVELL, J.W., MAROKO, P.R., ROSS, J.: Circulation **39—40**, Suppl. 4, 220 (1969).
16a. BRICHARD, G., ZIMMERMANN, P.E.: Lancet **1970 I**, 425.
17a. BROOKS, H.L., BANAS, J.S., DALEN, J.E., DEXTER, L.: Clin. Res. **17**, 231 (1969).
18a. — — MEISTER, S., SZUCS, M., DALEN, J., DEXTER, L.: Circulation **40**, Suppl. 3, 51 (1969).
19a. BUNDE, C.A., GRUPP, I.L., GRUPP, G.: Fed. Proc. **28**, 672 (1969).
20a. CAMPION, B., FRYE, R., ZITNIK, R.: Clin. Res. **17**, 233 (1969).
21a. CANTWELL, J.D., FLETCHER, G.F.: J. Amer. med. Ass. **210**, 130 (1969).
22a. CHO, Y.W., MATSUO, S., AVIADO, D.M.: Fed. Proc. **28**, 671 (1969).
23a. CHOU, C.C., RADAWSKI, D., GAZITUA, S., SCOTT, J.B.: J. Lab. clin. Med. **74**, 862 (1969).
24a. COBB, F.R., BACHE, R.J., EBERT, P.A., REMBERT, J.C., GREENFIELD, J.C.: Circulat. Res. **25**, 331 (1969).
25a. COHEN, L.S., VASTAGH, G.F., McLAUGHLIN, E., MITCHELL, J.H.: Circulation **40**, Suppl. 3, 60 (1969).
26a. COLLIER, J.G., DORNHORST, A.C.: Nature (Lond.) **223**, 1283 (1969).
27a. COWAN, C., DURAN, P.V.M., CORSINI, G., GOLDSCHLAGER, N., BING, R.J.: Amer. J. Cardiol. **24**, 154 (1969).
28a. — RIVAL, J., MATHES, P., BING, R.: Clin. Res. **17**, 235 (1969).
29a. COX, J.L., McLAUGHLIN, V.W., FLOWERS, N.C., MORAN, L.G.: Amer. Heart J. **76**, 650 (1968).
30a. DAMATO, A.N., LAU, S.H.: Circulation **40**, 527 (1969).
31a. DAVIES, R.O., MIZGALA, H.F., KHAN, A.S.: Clin. Res. **17**, 635 (1969).
32a. DENIS, B., GRUNWALD, D., RIVAL, M.A., MALLION, J.M., AVEZOU, F., LANNEY, E., MARTIN-NOEL, P.: Grenoble Médico-Chirurgical **9**, 35 (1970).
33a. DICARLO, F.J., MELGAR, M.D.: Amer. Chem. Soc., Abstract papers **158**, Biol. 335 (1969).
34a. DIEWITZ, M., LANGE, B.M.: Med. Klin. **64**, 1699 (1969).
35a. DOLL, E., KEUL, J.: Dtsch. med. Wschr. **94**, 2563 (1969).
36a. DOLLERY, C.T., PATERSON, J.W., CONOLLY, M.E.: Clin. Pharmacol. Ther. **10**, 765 (1969).
37a. ELLIOTT, W.C., STONE, J.M.: Acquis. Nouv. Pathol. Cardiovasc. **12**, 95 (1969).
38a. ENTMAN, M.L., LEVEY, G.S., EPSTEIN, S.E.: Circulat. Res. **25**, 429 (1969).
39a. FEINSILVER, O., AVIADO, D.M., CHO, Y.W.: Clin. Res. **17**, 414 (1969).
40a. FLECKENSTEIN, A., TRITTHART, H., FLECKENSTEIN, B., HERBST, A., GRUEN, G.: Arch. exp. Pathol. Pharmakol. **264**, 227 (1969).
41a. FOUCAULT, J.F., OLIVIER, J.: Gaz. méd. Fr. **9**, 1 (1970).

42a. FRANCOIS, J.: Docum. ophtal. (Den Haag) **27**, 235 (1969).
43a. FRICK, M.H.: Circulation **40**, 433 (1969).
44a. FROER, K.L., KOENIG, E., GRUENBERG, G.: Med. Klin. **64**, 1663 (1969).
45a. GARVEY, H.L., MELVILLE, K.I.: Canad. J. Physiol. Pharmacol. **47**, 675 (1969).
46a. GATTENLOEHNER, W., SCHNEIDER, K.W., ROST, R.: Med. Welt (Berl.) **42**, 2298 (1969).
47a. GENT, G., DAVIS, T.C., MCDONALD, A.: Brit. med. J. **1970**I, 533.
48a. GIANELLY, R.E., TREISTER, B.L., HARRISON, D.C.: Amer. J. Cardiol. **24**, 161 (1969).
49a. GIBSON, D., SOWTON, E.: Acquis. Nouv. Pathol. Cardiovasc. **12**, 19 (1969).
50a. GILL, E.: Dtsch. med. J. **20**, 553 (1969).
51a. GLANCY, D.L., HIGGS, L.M., O'BRIEN, K.P., EPSTEIN, S.E.: Circulation **40**, Suppl. 3, 89 (1969).
52a. GOLDBARG, A.N., MORAN, J.F., BUTTERFIELD, T.K., BERMUDEZ, G.A., NEMICKAS, R., CHILDERS, R.W.: Clin. Res. **17**, 242 (1969).
53a. — — — NEMICKAS, R., BERMUDEZ, G.A.: Circulation **40**, 847 (1969).
54a. GOLDSTEIN, R.E., BEISER, G.D., REDWOOD, D.R., ROSING, D.R., STAMPFER, M., EPSTEIN, S.E.: Circulation **40**, Suppl. 3, 92 (1969).
55a. — — — — — — Clin. Res. **17**, 579 (1969).
56a. GREEFF, K., GREVEN, G.: Arzneimittel-Forsch. **19**, 1763 (1969).
57a. GUTGESELL, H.P., TEMTE, J.V., MURPHY, Q.R.: J. Pharmacol. exp. Ther. **170**, 281 (1969).
58a. HARDEL, M., BAJOLET, A., GUERIN, R., GERARD, J., ELAERTS, J.: Ann. méd. Reims **6**, 161 (1969).
59a. HEDWORTH-WHITTY, R.B., HOUSLEY, E., ABRAHAM, A.S.: Cardiovasc. Res. **3**, 496 (1969).
60a. HELFANT, R.H., FORRESTER, J.S., HAMPTON, J.R., HAFT, J.I., GORLIN, R., KEMP, H.G.: Circulation **40**, Suppl. 3, 104 (1969).
61a. HOFFBRAND, B.I., FORSYTH, R.P.: Cardiovasc. Res. **3**, 426 (1969).
62a. HOHL, O., BERNHARDT, D., KENTSCHKE, G.E., METZGER, R.: Therapiewoche **19**, 1653 (1969).
63a. HUDAK, W.J., KUHN, W.L., LEWIS, R.E.: Fed. Proc. **28**, 671 (1969).
64a. IMHOF, P.R., BLATTER, K., FUCCELLA, L.M., TURRI, M.: J. appl. Physiol. **27**, 366 (1969).
65a. JUCHEMS, R., WERTZ, U.: Münch. med. Wschr. **111**, 2567 (1969).
66a. JURY, G.P.M.: Contribution à l'étude clinique de l'action de l'amiodarone sur l'angor coronarien. Imp. Conty, Clermont Ferrand, 1969.
67a. KABELA, E., JALIFE, J., PEON, C., CROS, L., MENDEZ, R.: Arch. int. Pharmacodyn. **181**, 328 (1969).
68a. KASTOR, J.A., DESANCTIS, R.W., LEINBACH, R.C., HARTHORNE, J.W., WOLFSON, I.N.: Circulation **40**, 535 (1969).
69a. KEROES, J., ECKER, R.R., RAPAPORT, E.: Circulat. Res. **25**, 557 (1969).
70a. KIRSCH, U., AUTENRIETH, G.: Arzneimittel-Forsch. **19**, 1826 (1969).
71a. KOFI EKUE, J.M., LOWE, D.C., SHANKS, R.G.: Brit. J. Pharmacol. **38**, 546 (1970).
72a. KRACKE, R.: Therapiewoche **19**, 2273 (1969).
73a. KUKOVETZ, W.R., JUAN, H., POECH, G.: Arch. exp. Pathol. Pharmakol. **264**, 262 (1969).
74a. — POECH, G.: Arzneimittel-Forsch. **19**, 1562 (1969).
75a. LADDU, A.R., SOMANI, P.: J. Pharmacol. exp. Ther. **170**, 79 (1969).
76a. LANDS, A.M., LUDUENA, F.P., BUZZO, H.J.: Life Sci. **6**, 2241 (1967).
77a. LANG, E., KÖHLER, J.A.: Arzneimittel-Forsch. **19**, 1870 (1969).
78a. LANGER, I.: Dtsch. med. J. **20**, 552 (1969).
79a. LECEROF, H., MALMBORG, R.O.: Acta med. scand. **186**, 231 (1969).
80a. LEDER, O., DOERING, H.J., REINDELL, A., FLECKENSTEIN, A.: Arch. ges. Physiol. **312**, R 9 (1969).
81a. LESBRE, J.P., CALAZEL, P., MERIEL, P., GUIRAUD, R., BRU, A.: Sem. Hôp. (Thérapeutique) **45**, 999 (1969).
82a. LINHART, J.W., HILDNER, F.J., BAROLD, S.S., LISTER, J.W., SAMET, P.: Circulation **40**, 483 (1969).
83a. LORENZ, D., DELL, H.D.: Arch. exp. Pathol. Pharmakol. **264**, 272 (1969).
84a. LOHMOELLER, G., LYDTIN, H.: Med. Klin. **64**, 2015 (1969).
85a. LUND LARSEN, G., SIVERTSSEN, E.: Acta med. scand. **186**, 187 (1969).
86a. MASON, D.T., BRAUNWALD, E.: Circulation **32**, 755 (1965).
87a. — SPANN, J.F., ZELIS, R., AMSTERDAM, E.A.: New Engl. J. Med. **281**, 1225 (1969).
88a. MASTERS, T.N., GLAVIANO, V.V.: J. Pharmacol. exp. Ther. **167**, 187 (1969).
89a. MIZGALA, H.F., KHAN, A.S., DAVIES, R.O.: Circulation **40**, Suppl. 3, 148 (1969).
90a. — — — Clin. Res. **17**, 637 (1969).
91a. MOHIUDDIN, S., TASKAR, P.K., MORIN, Y.: Clin. Res. **17**, 638 (1969).
92a. NIESSNER, H., LUJF, A., MOSER, K.: Z. ges. exp. Med. **151**, 163 (1969).

93a. PALMER, K.N.V., HAMILTON, W.F.D., LEGGE, J.S., DIAMENT, M.L.: Lancet 1969 II, 1092.
94a. PARKER, J.O., WEST, R.O., LEDWICH, J.R., DI GIORGI, S.: Circulation 40, 453 (1969).
95a. PARRATT, J.R., WADSWORTH, R.M.: Brit. J. Pharmacol. 38, 554 (1970).
96a. PFLEGER, K., NIEDERAU, D., VOLKMER, I.: Arch. Pharmakol. 265, 118 (1969).
97a. PITT, B., GREEN, L., SUGISHITA, Y.: Cardiovasc. Res. 4, 89 (1970).
98a. — MASON, J., CONTI, C.R., COLMAN, R.W.: Clin. Res. 17, 456 (1969).
99a. PROCTOR, J.D., ALLEN, F.J., WASSERMAN, A.J.: Pharmacologist 10, 221 (1968).
100a. — — — Arch. int. Pharmacodyn. 181, 363 (1969).
101a. PYFER, H.R., DOANE, B.L.: J. Amer. med. Ass. 210, 101 (1969).
102a. RABERGER, G., NELL, G., STUEHLINGER, W., KRAUPP, O.: Arch. exp. Pathol. Pharmakol. 264, 296 (1969).
103a. RAFF, W.K., DRECHSEL, U., SCHOLTHOLT, J., LOCHNER, W.: Arch. ges. Physiol. 312, R 21 (1969).
104a. RAPER, C., WALE, J.: Europ. J. Pharmacol. 8, 47 (1969).
105a. RESNEKOV, L.: J. Amer. med. Ass. 210, 126 (1969).
106a. RICE, A.J., FERGUSON, R.K., DELLE, M., WILSON, W.R.: a) Clin. Res. 17, 517 (1969). b) Clin. Pharmacol. Ther. 11, 567 (1970).
107a. RIFF, D.P., JAIN, A.C., DOYLE, J.T.: Amer. Heart J. 78, 592 (1969).
108a. ROSENBLUM, R., DELMAN, A.J.: Amer. Heart J. 79, 134 (1970).
109a. RUBIO, R., BERNE, R.M.: Circulat. Res. 25, 407 (1969).
110a. SANER, R.P.: Schweiz. med. Wschr. 100, 174 (1970).
111a. SCHAPER, W., JAGENEAU, A.: Circulation 40, Suppl. 3, 178 (1969).
112a. SHARMA, G.V.R.K., POMPOSIELLO, J.C., INAMDAR, A.N., MESSER, J.V.: Clin. Res. 17, 583 (1969).
113a. SHIMAMOTO, T.: Amer. Heart J. 79, 5 (1970).
114a. SINGH, B.M.: Lancet 1970 I, 563.
115a. SODI PALLARES, D., BISTENI, A., MEDRANO, G.A., CISNEROS, F., PONCE DE LEON, J.: Amer. J. Cardiol. 24, 607 (1969).
116a. SOMANI, P., LADDU, A.R.: Clin. Res. 17, 264 (1969).
117a. — — J. Pharmacol. exp. Ther. 170, 72 (1969).
118a. — — HARDMAN, H.F.: Life Sci. 8, 1151 (1969).
119a. SPIECKERMANN, P.G., HELLBERG, K., KETTLER, D., REPLOH, H.D., STRAUER, B.: Arch. ges. Physiol. 312, R 15 (1969).
120a. STEFFENSEN, K.A.: Acta med. scand. 186, 519 (1969).
121a. SUMMERS, D.N., RICHMOND, S., WECHSLER, B.M.: Circulation 40, Suppl. 3, 198 (1969).
122a. SVEDMYR, N., JAKOBSSON, B., MALMBERG, R.: Europ. J. Pharmacol. 8, 79 (1969).
123a. TEODORINI, S., SERBAN, M.: Rev. Roum. med. Int. 6, 337 (1969).
124a. TOUSSAINT, D., POHL, S.: Bull. Soc. belge Ophtal. 153, 675 (1969).
125a. TRITTHART, H., FLECKENSTEIN, A., FLECKENSTEIN, B., HERBST, A., KRAUSE, H.: Arch. exp. Pathol. Pharmakol. 264, 317 (1969).
126a. VERIN, M.P.: Bull. Soc. Ophtal. Fr. 70, 573 (1970).
127a. VOGEL, J.H.K., CHIDSEY, C.A.: Amer. J. Cardiol. 24, 198 (1969).
128a. WALE, J., PUN, L.-Q., RAND, M.J.: Europ. J. Pharmacol. 8, 25 (1969).
129a. WAREMBOURG, H., JAILLARD, J.: Sem. Hôp. Paris 45, 3055 (1969).
130a. WASSERMAN, A.J., PROCTOR, J.D., ALLEN, F.J., KEMP, V.E.: J. clin. Pharmacol. 10, 37 (1970).
131a. WEISSE, A.B., DIFLUMERI, A.A., REGAN, T.J.: Circulation 40, Suppl. 3, 214 (1969).
132a. — REGAN, T.J.: Acquis. Nouv. Pathol. Cardiovasc. 12, 83 (1969).
133a. WIBELL, L.: Acta Soc. Med. upsalien 73, 75 (1968).
134a. WICK, T.: Med. Welt (Berl.) 42, 2327 (1969).
135a. WILSON, A.G., BROOKE, O.G., LLOYD, H.J., ROBINSON, B.F.: Brit. med. J. 1969 IV, 399.
136a. WINSOR, T.: Clin. Pharmacol. Ther. 11, 85 (1970).
137a. WOELKE, F.: Ther. d. Gegenwart 108, 1586 (1969).
138a. WOLFSON, S., GORLIN, R.: Circulation 40, 501 (1969).
139a. YU, D.H., GLUCKMAN, M.I.: J. Pharmacol. exp. Ther. 170, 37 (1969).
140a. ZELIS, R., MASON, D.T.: Circulation 40, Suppl. 3, 221 (1969).
141a. ZSOTER, T.T., BEANLANDS, D.S.: Arch. intern. Med. 124, 584 (1969).

Additional references (series b)

1b. AISNER, M.: New Engl. J. Med. 282, 746 (1970).
2b. AUDIER, M., ARNOUX, E.: Arch. médit. de Médecine 2, 97 (1969).
3b. BAJUSZ, E.: Arzneimittel-Forsch. 19, 1830 (1969).
4b. BOUCEK, R.J., TAKESHITA, R., BRADY, A.H.: Anat. Rec. 153, 243 (1965).

5b. BUSSMANN, W.D., RAUH, M., KRAYENBUEHL, H.P.: Amer. Heart J. **79**, 347 (1970).
6b. CLOAREC, M., GROSGOGEAT, Y.: Vie méd. **7**, 1043 (1970).
7b. DAVIS, L.D., TEMTE, J.V.: Circulat. Res. **22**, 661 (1968).
8b. DUCHENE-MARULLAZ, P., COSNIER, D., PERRIERE, J.P., HACHE, J.: C.R. Soc. Biol. (Paris) **162**, 438 (1968).
9b. DWYER, E.M., WIENER, L., COX, J.W.: Circulation **38**, 250 (1968).
10b. FELIX, H., DuBOUREAU, L.H., SABY, G.: Vie méd. **4**, 1193 (1970).
11b. FLAMM, M.D., HARRISON, D.C., HANCOCK, E.W.: Circulation **38**, 846 (1968).
12b. FOURNEAU, J.P., DAVY, M., CLEMENT, M., LAMARCHE, M.: J. Pharmacol. (Paris) **1**, 149 (1970).
13b. FREIS, E.D.: Circulation **41**, 3 (1970).
14b. FRIEH, P., IMBERT, D.: Lyon méd. p. 687 (1970).
15b. GOULD, L.: Amer. Heart J. **79**, 422 (1970).
16b. HAAS, H.: Arzneimittel-Forsch. **20**, 501 (1970).
17b. HATT, P.Y.: Sem. Hôp. (Thérapeutique) **46**, 13 (1970).
18b. IGLOE, M.C.: J. Amer. Geriat. Soc. **18**, 233 (1970).
19b. JUNG, A.: Ther. d. Gegenwart **109**, 237 (1970).
20b. KANNEL, W.B., LEBAUER, E.J., DAWBER, T.R., McNAMARA, P.M.: Circulation **35**, 734 (1967).
21b. KOLASSA, N., PFLEGER, K., RUMMEL, W.: Europ. J. Pharmacol. **9**, 265 (1970).
22b. LAMARCHE, M., MARIGNAC, B.: Ann. méd. Nancy **8**, 343 (1969).
23b. LEVY, J.V.: Proc. Soc. exp. Biol. (N.Y.) **133**, 114 (1970).
24b. — Brit. J. Pharmacol. **38**, 743 (1970).
25b. MICHELETTI, J., RENAULT, B.: Information thérapeutique **4**, 5 (1966).
26b. MIYAHARA, M., IIMURA, O., YOKOYAMA, M., HOSHIKAWA, K.: Tohoju J. exp. Med. **97**, 95 (1969).
27b. NEEL, J.L.: Gaz. méd. Fr. **77**, 845 (1970).
28b. OLSSON, R.A.: Circulat. Res. **26**, 301 (1970).
29b. PERROT, J., LAVANDIER, G., GUYOT, J.C.: Cardiologue **20**, 173 (1970).
30b. PFLEGER, K., VOLKMER, I., KOLASSA, N.: Arzneimittel-Forsch. **19**, 1972 (1969).
31b. PIESSENS, J., KESTELOOT, H., DE GEEST, H.: Arzneimittel-Forsch. **20**, 355 (1970).
32b. PITT, B., GREGG, D.E.: Circulat. Res. **22**, 753 (1968).
33b. SCHMID, J.R., HANNA, C.: J. Pharmacol. exp. Ther. **156**, 331 (1967).
34b. SCHMITT, G., HAUSS, W.H.: Arzneimittel-Forsch. **17**, 959 (1967).
35b. SINGH, B.N., VAUGHAN-WILLIAMS, E.M.: Brit. J. Pharmacol. **38**, 749 (1970).
36b. SPACH, M.O., KANY, R., IMBS, J.L., SCHWARTZ, J.: C.R. Soc. Biol. (Paris) **163**, 1950 (1969).
37b. STERNE, J.: Thérapie **24**, 745 (1969).
38b. — PELE, M.F., HIRSCH, C.: Thérapie **24**, 735 (1969).
39b. TAKENAKA, T., TACHIKAWA, S.: Arzneimittel-Forsch. **20**, 351 (1970).
40b. VOEMEL, H.J.: Therapiewoche **19**, 2578 (1969).
41b. WAREMBOURG, H., LEKIEFFRE, J., POMMIER, M.: Lille méd. **13**, 1032 (1968).

Additional references (series c)

1c. ABEL, R.M., REIS, R.L., STAROSCIK, R.N.: Brit. J. Pharmacol. **39**, 261 (1970).
2c. ACHESON, J., DANTA, G., HUTCHINSON, E.C.: Brit. med. J. **1969I**, 614.
3c. ADAM, M., MITCHEL, B.F., LAMBERT, C.J.: Circulation **41**, Suppl. 2, 73 (1970).
4c. AELLIG, W.H., PRICHARD, B.N.C.: Brit. J. Pharmacol. **39**, 193 P (1970).
5c. AFONSO, S.: Circulat. Res. **26**, 743 (1970).
6c. ALIX, B., JURY, G., COURTADON, M., MAILLOT, S., JALLUT, H.: Méd. prat. **399**, 45 (1970).
7c. ANDERSON, T.W.: Lancet **1970II**, 753
8c. ANGELAKOS, E.T., KING, M.P., UZGIRIS, I.: Cardiovasc. Research, VIth World Congress of Cardiology, London, Sept. 1970, Abstracts p. 64.
9c. ARAVANIS, C., MICHAELIDES, G.: Acta cardiol. (Brux.) **25**, 501 (1970).
10c. ARFORS, K.E., HINT, H.C., DHALL, D.P., MATHESON, N.A.: Brit. med. J. **1968IV**, 430.
11c. ARONOW, W.S., CHESLUK, H.M.: a) Circulation **41**, 869 (1970). b) Clin. Res. **18**, 112 (1970).
12c. — — Circulation **42**, 61 (1970).
13c. ATKINS, J.M., BLOMQVIST, G., COHEN, L.S.: Clin. Res. **18**, 21 (1970).
14c. ATSUMI, T., MOTOMIYA, T., ISOKANE, N., SHIMAMOTO, T.: Cardiovasc. Research, VIth World Congress of Cardiology, London, Sept. 1970, Abstracts p. 67.
15c. BABEL, J., STANGOS, N., FERRERO, C.: a) Thérapie **25**, 331 (1970). b) Arch. Ophtal. **30**, 197 (1970).
16c. BAROLDI, G.: Acta cardiol. (Brux.), Suppl. 13, 17 (1969).

17c. BARRILLON, A., HIMBERT, J., FAYARD, J.M., LENEGRE, J.: Thérapie **25**, 349 (1970).
18c. BARTSCH, W., KNOPF, K.W.: Arzneimittel-Forsch. **20**, 1140 (1970).
19c. BAUER, G.E., MICHELL, G.: Med. J. Aust. **1**, 170 (1970).
20c. BENDER, F., DIEKMANN, L., HILGENBERG, F., DOTTERWEICH, K.: Cardiovasc. Research, VIth World Congress of Cardiology, London, Sept. 1970, Abstracts p. 76.
21c. BENDER, S.R.: Clin. Med. **77**, 33 (1970).
22c. BENICHOUX, R., MARCHAL, C., ROYER, R.: In: Médicaments et Métabolisme du Myocarde. Nancy: Lamarche and Royer 1969, p. 45.
23c. BENNETT, M.A., PENTECOST, B.L.: Circulation **41**, 981 (1970).
24c. BENSAID, J., CASTAN, R., SOZUTEK, Y., SCEBAT, L., LENEGRE, J.: Arch. Mal. Cœur **62**, 1404 (1969).
25c. — SOZUTEK, Y., CASTAN, R., SCEBAT, L., LENEGRE, J.: Acta cardiol. (Brux.) **25**, 378 (1970).
26c. BERNE, R.M., RUBIO, R.: Amer. J. Cardiol. **24**, 776 (1969).
27c. — — Circulation **40**, Suppl. 4, 240 (1969).
28c. BERNECKER, C., ROETSCHER, I.: Lancet **1970 II**, 662.
29c. BERNSTEIN, L., HAWKER, R., CATCHLOVE, B.: Cardiovasc. Research, VIth World Congress of Cardiology, London, Sept. 1970, Abstracts p. 80.
30c. Beta-Receptor Antagonists: Lancet **I**, 1380 (1970).
31c. BIGGER, J.T., WEINBERG, D.I., KOVALIK, A.T.W., HARRIS, P.D., CRANEFIELD, P.C., HOFFMAN, B.F.: Circulat. Res. **26**, 1 (1970).
32c. BJORNTORP, P., WALLENTIN, I.: Cardiovasc. Research, VIth World Congress of Cardiology, London, Sept. 1970, Abstracts p. 86.
33c. BLÜMCHEN, G., LANDRY, F., SCHLOSSER, V.: Arzneimittel-Forsch. **20**, 1067 (1970).
34c. BOGAERT, M.G., HERMAN, A.G., DE SCHAEPDRYVER, A.F.: Europ. J. Pharmacol. **12**, 215 (1970).
35c. — ROSSEEL, M.T., DE SCHAEPDRYVER, A.F.: Brux.-méd. **50**, 567 (1970).
36c. — — — Europ. J. Pharmacol. **12**, 224 (1970).
37c. BOISSIER, J.R., GIUDICELLI, J.F., MOUILLE, P.: C.R. Soc. Biol. (Paris) **164**, 255 (1970).
38c. BORRONI, G.: Clin. ter. **53**, 247 (1970).
39c. BOSMANS, P., VERCRUYSSEN, J., CLERCKX, A., VERSELDER, R., VAN HOORICKX, G., BRUGMANS, J., SCHUERMANS, V.: Acta cardiol. (Brux.) **25**, 429 (1970).
40c. BOUVRAIN, Y., ROUDY, G., MARINEAUD, J.-P.: Presse méd. **78**, 977 (1970).
41c. BRAASCH, W., BUCHHOLD, R.: Arzneimittel-Forsch. **20**, 808 (1970).
42c. BRAUNWALD, E.: Physiologist **12**, 65 (1969).
43c. — FRYE, R.L., AYGEN, M.M.: J. clin. Invest. **39**, 1874 (1960).
44c. — VATNER, S.F., BRAUNWALD, N.S., SOBEL, B.E.: Calif. Med. **112**, 41 (1970).
45c. BRAY, C.L., DINDA, P., OJO, S.A., RIDING, W.D., SETHNA, D.S.: Cardiovasc. Research, VIth World Congress of Cardiology, London, Sept. 1970, Abstracts p. 91.
46c. BRISTOW, J.D., VAN ZEE, B.E., JUDKINS, M.P.: Circulation **42**, 219 (1970).
47c. BRISTOW, M., GREEN, R.D.: Europ. J. Pharmacol. **12**, 120 (1970).
48c. BROEKHUYSEN, J., CHARLIER, R.: In Press (1971).
49c. BROOKS, H., BANAS, J., MEISTER, S., SZUCS, M., DALEN, J., DEXTER, L.: Circulation **42**, 99 (1970).
50c. BROTSLOW, J., ALEXANDER, M., GAINES, M., McALLISTER, E.: Nursing Clinics of North America **4**, 143 (1969).
51c. BROWSE, N.L., HALL, J.H.: Lancet **1969 II**, 718.
52c. CANNON, P.J., DELL, R.B., DWYER, E.M.: Cardiovasc. Research, VIth World Congress of Cardiology, London, Sept. 1970, Abstracts p. 98.
53c. CAPPELEN, C.: Cardiovasc. Research, VIth World Congress of Cardiology, London, Sept. 1970, Abstracts p. 47.
54c. CARDENAS, M., NADAL, B., SANZ, G., BRENES, C.: Cardiovasc. Research, VIth World Congress of Cardiology, London, Sept. 1970, Abstracts p. 99.
55c. CARLIER, J.: Rev. méd. Liège **25**, 620 (1970).
56c. CASE, R.B., NASSER, M.G., CRAMPTON, R.S.: Amer. J. Cardiol. **24**, 766 (1969).
57c. CASTILLO, C.A.: Cardiovasc. Research, VIth World Congress of Cardiology, London, Sept. 1970, Abstracts p. 101.
58c. — CASTELLANOS, A.: Circulation **42**, 271 (1970).
59c. CHAPMAN, D.W., PETERSON, P.K., MORRIS, G.C., HOWELL, J., LISTON BEAZLEY, H., WINTERS, L.: Cardiovasc. Research, VIth World Congress of Cardiology, London, Sept. 1970, Abstracts p. 103.
60c. CHITI, E.: Clin. ter. **53**, 315 (1970).
61c. CLARK, J.P., KILMORE, M.A., VICTOR, M., TERRY, W.H., ORCUTT, J.A.: Pharmacologist **12**, 284 (1970).

62c. CLAUSEN, J.P., TRAP-JENSEN, J.: Circulation **42**, 611 (1970).
63c. — — Cardiovasc. Research, VIth World Congress of Cardiology, London, Sept. 1970, Abstracts p. 106.
64c. COHEN, B.M.: Clin. Med. **77**, 25 (1970).
65c. COLTART, D.J.: Brit. J. Pharmacol. **40**, 147 P (1970).
66c. — MELDRUM, S.J.: Brit. J. Pharmacol. **40**, 148 P (1970).
67c. CONTI, C.R., PITT, B., GUNDEL, W.D.: Circulation **40**, Suppl. 3, 61 (1969).
68c. CROSS, D.F.: Amer. J. Cardiol. **26**, 217 (1970).
69c. COTTERILL, J.A., HUGHES, J.P., JONES, R., PAULLEY, J.W., ROBERTSON, P.D.: Lancet **1970I**, 1176.
70c. COWAN, M., FRIEDMAN, J., FEIGL, E., WALDHAUSEN, J.A.: Clin. Res. **18**, 301 (1970).
71c. CRONIN, R.F., EDELSTEIN, M., ROSE, C.: Cardiovasc. Research, VIth World Congress of Cardiology, London, Sept. 1970, Abstracts p. 112.
72c. CUELLAR, A., MEDRANO, G., ARRIAGA, J., HERNANDEZ, A.: Cardiovasc. Research, VIth World Congress of Cardiology, London, Sept. 1970, Abstracts p. 113.
73c. CUNDEY, P.E., LEET, C.J., FIELD, D.E., FRANK, M.J.: Clin. Res. **18**, 22 (1970).
74c. DAGENAIS, G.R., PITT, B., MASON, R.E., FRIESINGER, G.C., ROSS, R.S.: Amer. J. Cardiol. **25**, 90 (1970).
75c. DAMATO, A.N.: Cardiovasc. Research, VIth World Congress of Cardiology, London, Sept. 1970, Abstracts p. 33.
76c. DART, C.H., SCOTT, S., FISH, R., TAKARO, T.: Circulation **41**, Suppl. 2, 64 (1970).
77c. DE CARO, L., BALDRIGHI, V., BALDRIGHI, G., GORINI, M.: Cardiovasc. Research, VIth World Congress of Cardiology, London, Sept. 1970, Abstracts p. 118.
78c. DELAUNOIS, G., BAUTHIER, J., CHARLIER, R.: Arch. int. Pharmacodyn. **187**, 265 (1970).
79c. DELTOUR, G.: Thérapie **25**, 293 (1970).
80c. DEODATI, F., BEC, P., CUQ, G., VERGNES, R.: Rev. méd. Toulouse **6**, 211 (1970).
81c. DETRY, J.M.R., PIETTE, F., BRASSEUR, L.A.: Circulation **42**, 593 (1970).
82c. DIDISHEIM, P.: Thrombos. Diathes. haemorrh. (Stuttg.) **20**, 257 (1968).
83c. DI MATTEO, J., VACHERON, A., LAFONT, H., KELLERSHOHN, C., DE VERNEJOUL, P., MESTAN, J.: Cardiovasc. Research, VIth World Congress of Cardiology, London, Sept. 1970, Abstracts p. 123.
84c. DREBINGER, K.: Herz-Kreislauf **2**, 358 (1970).
85c. DRIMAL, J., AVIADO, D.M.: Pharmacologist **12**, 212 (1970).
86c. DUCE, B.R., GARBERG, L., SMITH, E.R.: Brit. J. Pharmacol. **39**, 809 (1970).
87c. ELIASSON, R., BYGDEMAN, S.: Scand. J. clin. Lab. Invest. **24**, 145 (1969).
88c. ELKELES, R.S., HAMPTON, J.R., HONOUR, A.J., MITCHELL, J.R.A.: Lancet **1968II**, 751.
89c. ELLIOTT, W.C., KING, R.D., ROSS, E., McHENRY, P.L.: J. Indiana med. Ass. **62**, 176 (1969).
90c. EMMONS, P.R., HARRISON, M.J.G., HONOUR, A.J., MITCHELL, J.R.A.: Lancet **1965II**, 603.
91c. ENRIGHT, L.P., HANNAH, H. III., REIS, R.L.: Circulat. Res. **26**, 307 (1970).
92c. ENSON, Y., BRISCOE, W.A., POLANYI, M.L., COURNAND, A.: J. appl. Physiol. **17**, 552 (1962).
93c. — JAMESON, A.G., COURNAND, A.: Circulation **29**, 499 (1964).
94c. EPSTEIN, S.E., BEISER, G.D., GOLDSTEIN, R.E., REDWOOD, D., ROSING, D.R., GLICK, G., WECHSLER, A.S., STAMPFER, M., COHEN, L.S., REIS, R.L., BRAUNWALD, N.S., BRAUNWALD, E.: New Engl. J. Med. **280**, 971 (1969).
95c. FALICOV, R.E., RESNEKOV, L., KOCANDRLE, V., KING, S., KITTLE, C.F.: Circulation **41**, Suppl. 2, 172 (1970).
96c. FALSETTI, H.L., MATES, R.E., GRANT, C., GREENE, D.G., BUNNELL, I.L.: Circulat. Res. **26**, 71 (1970).
97c. FAVALORO, R.G.: Cardiovasc. Research, VIth World Congress of Cardiology, London, Sept. 1970, Abstracts p. 42.
98c. FEIGL, E.O.: Circulat. Res. **23**, 223 (1968).
99c. FERMOSO, J., FOURCADE, A., ETCHEVERRY, J., GOBBEE, R.: Cardiovasc. Research, VIth World Congress of Cardiology, London, Sept. 1970, Abstracts p. 136.
100c. FERRINI, R., MIRAGOLI, G., CROCE, G.: Arzneimittel-Forsch. **20**, 1074 (1970).
101c. FREEDBERG, A.S., PAPP, J.G., VAUGHAN WILLIAMS, E.M.: J. Physiol. (Lond.) **207**, 357 (1970).
102c. FRICK, M.H., KATILA, M., VALTONEN, E.: Cardiovasc. Research, VIth World Congress of Cardiology, London, Sept. 1970, Abstracts p. 30.
103c. FRIEDBERG, C.K.: Cardiovasc. Research, VIth World Congress of Cardiology, London, Sept. 1970, Abstracts p. 42.
104c. FROMENT, R.: Acta cardiol. (Brux.) Suppl. 13, 210 (1969).
105c. FULTON, W.F.M.: Acta cardiol. (Brux.) Suppl. 13, 38 (1969).

106c. GAMBLE, W.J., HUGENHOLTZ, P.G., MONROE, R.G., POLANYI, M., NADAS, A.S.: Circulation **31**, 328 (1965).
107c. GAUTIER, J.C., DEROUESNE, C., HELD, T., LHERMITTE, F.: Presse méd. **78**, 1775 (1970).
108c. GAZAIX, M., ALZEARI, J.B.: Nice Médical **8**, 69 (1970).
109c. GENT, A.E., BROOK, C.G.D., FOLEY, T.H., MILLER, T.N.: Brit. med. J. **1968IV**, 366.
110c. GEORGE, C.F., NAGLE, R.E., PENTECOST, B.L.: Brit. med. J. **1970II**, 402.
111c. GERARD, R., FREDENUCCI, P., DEMART, F., JOUVE, A., APPAIX, A.: Cardiovasc. Research, VIth World Congress of Cardiology, London, Sept. 1970, Abstracts p. 146.
112c. GETTES, L.S., YOSHONIS, K.F.: Circulation **41**, 689 (1970).
113c. GIANELLY, R.E., HARRISON, D.C.: Geriatrics **25**, 120 (1970).
114c. GIUSTI, C.: Minerva med. **61**, 2063 (1970).
115c. GOLDBARG, A., MORAN, J.F., RESNEKOV, L.: Amer. J. Cardiol. **26**, 84 (1970).
116c. GOLDREYER, B.N., BIGGER, J.T.: Circulation **40**, Suppl. 3, 92 (1969).
117c. — — Circulation **41**, 935 (1970).
118c. GOLDSTEIN, R.E., BEISER, G.D., REDWOOD, D.R., ROSING, D.R., EPSTEIN, S.E.: Clin. Res. **18**, 307 (1970).
119c. GOMOLL, A.W.: Pharmacologist **12**, 213 (1970).
120c. GOODMAN, L.S., GILMAN, A.: The Pharmacological Basis of Therapeutics, 4th Edition. New York: Macmillan Co. 1970, p. 754.
121c. GORLIN, R.: Brit. Heart J. **33**, suppl., 9 (1971).
122c. GOULD, L., JAYNAL, F., ZAHIR, M., GOMPRECHT, R.F.: Clin. Res. **18**, 309 (1970).
123c. GRANATA, L., CARAFFA BRAGA, E., CEVESE, A., DATA, P.G.: Boll. Soc. ital. Biol. sper. **46**, 170 (1970).
124c. GREEN, G.E., STERTZER, S.H., GORDON, R.B., TICE, D.A.: Circulation **41**, Suppl. 2, 79 (1970).
125c. GREENBERG, B.H., McCALLISTER, B.D., FRYE, R.L., WALLACE, R.B.: Amer. J. Cardiol. **26**, 135 (1970).
126c. GREGG, D.E.: Acta cardiol. (Brux.) Suppl. 13, 1 (1969).
127c. — Acta cardiol. (Brux.) Suppl. 13, 114 (1969).
128c. — KHOURI, E.M., PASYK, S.: Cardiovasc. Research, VIth World Congress of Cardiology, London, Sept. 1970, Abstracts p. 155.
129c. GRIFFITH, G.C.: Amer. J. Cardiol. **25**, 730 (1970).
130c. GRUPP, I.L., BUNDE, C.A., GRUPP, G.: J. clin. Pharmacol. **10**, 312 (1970).
131c. GURTNER, H.P., DOLDER, M., KAUFMANN, M.: Cardiovasc. Research, VIth World Congress of Cardiology, London, Sept. 1970, Abstracts p. 156.
132c. HAAS, H.: Brux.-méd. **50**, 665 (1970).
133c. — GOKEL, M.: Arzneimittel-Forsch. **20**, 647 (1970).
134c. HABERSANG, S.: Arch. Pharmakol. **266**, 344 (1970).
135c. HAHN, N., FELIX, R., DUEX, A., DRAZNIN, N.: Europ. J. Physiol. **316**, R 18 (1970).
136c. HAMER, J., FLEMING, J.: Cardiovasc. Research, VIth World Congress of Cardiology, London, Sept. 1970, Abstracts p. 159.
137c. HAMM, J., HUNEKOHL, E., SCHMIDT, A.: Klin. Wschr. **48**, 457 (1970).
138c. HAMPTON, J.R.: J. Atheroscler. Res. **7**, 729 (1967).
139c. — HARRISON, M.J.G., HONOUR, A.J., MITCHELL, J.R.A.: Cardiovasc. Res. **1**, 101 (1967).
140c. — KEMP, H.G., GORLIN, R.: Cardiovasc. Research, VIth World Congress of Cardiology, London, Sept. 1970, Abstracts p. 160.
141c. HEDWORTH-WHITTY, R.B., HOUSLEY, E., ABRAHAM, A.S.: Cardiovasc. Res. **4**, 301 (1970).
142c. HEHENKAMP, G.: Med. Mschr. **24**, 313 (1970).
143c. HEIMBECKER, R.O.: Cardiovasc. Research, VIth World Congress of Cardiology, London, Sept. 1970, Abstracts p. 42.
144c. HELFANT, R.H., FORRESTER, J.S., HAMPTON, J.R., HAFT, J.I., KEMP, H.G., GORLIN, R.: Circulation **42**, 601 (1970).
145c. HELLERSTEIN, H.K.: Cardiovasc. Research, VIth World Congress of Cardiology, London, Sept. 1970, Abstracts p. 163.
146c. HERXHEIMER, H., LANGER, I.: Klin. Wschr. **22**, 1149 (1967).
147c. HICKIE, J.B.: Med. J. Aust. **2**, 268 (1970).
148c. HILGER, H.H.: Brux.-méd. **50**, 557 (1970).
149c. HONIG, C.R., KIRK, E.S., MYERS, W.W.: International Symposium on the Coronary Circulation and Energetics of the Myocardium. Milan 1966. Basle: S. Karger 1967, p. 31.
150c. HORWITZ, L.D., GORLIN, R., TAYLOR, J., KEMP, H.G.: Clin. Res. **18**, 312 (1970).
151c. HÖSEMANN, R., DIEKMANN, L., HILGENBERG, F.: Herz-Kreislauf **2**, 333 (1970).
152c. HOUDAS, Y., BERTRAND, M., KETELERS, J.Y.: In: Médicaments et Métabolisme du Myocarde. Nancy: Lamarche and Royer 1969, p. 77.

153c. HUDAK, W.J., LEWIS, R.E., KUHN, W.L.: J. Pharmacol. exp. Ther. 173, 371 (1970).
154c. HUGENHOLTZ, P.G., ELLISON, R.C., URSCHEL, C.W., MIRSKY, I., SONNENBLICK, E.H.: Circulation 41, 191 (1970).
155c. — GAMBLE, W.J., MONROE, R.G., POLANYI, M.: Circulation 31, 344 (1965).
156c. HYMAN, A.L., PEARCE, C.W., BARNES, G.E.: J. La med. Soc. 120, 386 (1968).
157c. IZBICKI, M.: Praxis 37, 1293 (1970).
158c. JAFFE, H.L.: N.Y. St. J. Med. 70, 1766 (1970).
159c. JAMES, T.N.: Circulation 42, 189 (1970).
160c. — BEAR, E.S., FRINK, R.J., LANG, K.F., TOMLINSON, J.C.: J. Lab. clin. Med. 76, 240 (1970).
161c. JANKE, J., FLECKENSTEIN, A., JAEDICKE, W.: Europ. J. Physiol. 316, R 10 (1970).
162c. JEWITT, D.E., BURGESS, P.A., SHILLINGFORD, J.P.: Cardiovasc. Res. 4, 188 (1970).
163c. — HUBNER, P., MAURER, B., MILLS, C., SHILLINGFORD, J.: Cardiovasc. Research, VIth World Congress of Cardiology, London, Sept. 1970, Abstracts p. 176.
164c. JOHNSON, W.D., FLEMMA, R.J., LEPLEY, D.: Amer. J. Cardiol. 25, 105 (1970).
165c. JOUVE, A., BENYAMINE, R., MALFROY, P.: Acta cardiol. (Brux.) Suppl. 13, 224 (1969).
166c. — TORRESANI, J., CHEVALIER-CHOLAT, A.M.: Thérapie 25, 267 (1970).
167c. KAISER, G.C., BARNER, H.B., JELLINEK, M., MUDD, G., HANLON, C.R.: Circulation 41, Suppl. 2, 49 (1970).
168c. KALMANSON, D., VEYRAT, C., CHICHE, P., DERAI, C., NOVIKOFF, N.: Cardiovasc. Research, VIth World Congress of Cardiology, London, Sept. 1970, Abstracts p. 47.
169c. KALTENBACH, M., BECKER, H.J., GRAEF, F., HUNSCHA, H.: Med. Klin. 65, 494 (1970).
170c. KARPPINEN, K.: Acta med. scand. 187, Suppl. 506, 7 (1970).
171c. KAVERINA, N.V., BENDIKOV, E.A., ROZONOV, Y.B.: Byull. éksp. Biol. Med. 68, 1373 (1969).
172c. KAZEMI, H., PARSONS, E.F., VALENCA, L.M., STRIEDER, D.J.: Circulation 41, 1025 (1970).
173c. KELLIHER, G.J., BUCKLEY, J.P.: J. pharm. Sci. 59, 1276 (1970).
174c. KEMP, H.G., MANCHESTER, J.H., AMSTERDAM, E.A., TAYLOR, W.J., GORLIN, R.: Circulation 41, Suppl. 2, 55 (1970).
175c. KERBER, R.E., GIANELLY, R.E., GOLDMAN, R.H.: Clin. Res. 18, 115 (1970).
176c. — GOLDMAN, R.H., ALDERMAN, E.L., HARRISON, D.C.: Pharmacologist 12, 233 (1970).
177c. KERR, J.W., PATEL, K.R.: Lancet 1970 II, 777.
178c. KEULEN, U.W.: Cardiovasc. Research, VIth World Congress of Cardiology, London, Sept. 1970, Abstracts p. 185.
179c. KHAJA, F., PARKER, J.O., LEDWICH, R.J., WEST, R.O., ARMSTRONG, P.W.: Amer. J. Cardiol. 26, 107 (1970).
180c. KINCAID-SMITH, P.: Lancet 1969 II, 920.
181c. KLOCKE, F.J., WITTENBERG, S.M., GREENE, D.G., BUNNELL, I.L., FALSETTI, H.L.: Cardiovasc. Research, VIth World Congress of Cardiology, London, Sept. 1970, Abstracts p. 188. See also Amer. J. Cardiol. 23, 548 (1969).
182c. KNOEBEL, S.B., ELLIOTT, W.C., ROSS, E., McHENRY, P.L.: Cardiovasc. Res. 4, 306 (1970).
183c. KOEHLER, M.: Z. Kreisl.-Forsch. 59, 708 (1970).
184c. KOFI EKUE, J.M., SHANKS, R.G., ZAIDI, S.A.: Brit. J. Pharmacol. 39, 184 P (1970).
185c. KOLASSA, N., TRAM, M., PFLEGER, K.: Arch. Pharmakol. 266, 373 (1970).
186c. KOLIN, A.: Cardiovasc. Research, VIth World Congress of Cardiology, London, Sept. 1970, Abstracts p. 46.
187c. KONG, Y., MORRIS, J.J.: Cardiovasc. Research, VIth World Congress of Cardiology, London, Sept. 1970, Abstracts p. 190.
188c. KOPITAR, Z.: Arzneimittel-Forsch. 20, 253 (1970).
189c. KRUG, A., KRUG, C., DHARAMADHACH, A.: Z. Kreisl.-Forsch. 59, 487 (1970).
190c. KUBLER, W., SPIECKERMANN, P.G., BRETSCHNEIDER, H.J.: J. molec. Cell. Cardiol. 1, 23 (1970).
191c. KUKOVETZ, W.R., PÖCH, G.: Brux.-méd. 50, 589 (1970).
192c. LAMARCHE, M., ROYER, R.: In: Médicaments et Métabolisme du Myocarde. Nancy: Lamarche and Royer 1969, p. 351.
193c. LAMMERANT, J., BECSEI, I., MERTENS-STRIJTHAGEN, J., DE SCHRYVER, C.: Arch. int. Pharmacodyn. 186, 166 (1970).
194c. LANG, E., KÖHLER, J.A.: Arzneimittel-Forsch. 19, 1870 (1969).
195c. LANGER, I.: J. Physiol. (Lond.) 190, 41 P (1967).
196c. LARAIA, P.J., CRAIG, R.J., REDDY, W.J.: Amer. J. Cardiol. 21, 107 (1968).
197c. LAVY, S., STERN, S.: Arch. int. Pharmacodyn. 184, 257 (1970).
198c. LEFERINK, B.H.G., TAN, H.S.: In press 1971.
199c. LENKE, D.: Arzneimittel-Forsch. 20, 655 (1970).

200c. LESBRE, J.P., RUMEAU, M., MERIEL, P.: Rev. méd. Toulouse **6**, 253 (1970).
201c. LEVINSON, R.S., MCILDUFF, J.B., REGAN, T.J.: Amer. Heart J. **80**, 70 (1970).
202c. LEVY, B., WASSERMAN, M.: Brit. J. Pharmacol. **39**, 139 (1970).
203c. LICHTLEN, P., ALBERT, H.: Z. Kreisl.-Forsch. **59**, 193 (1970).
204c. — — MOCCETTI, T.: Thérapie **25**, 403 (1970).
205c. — — — Cardiovasc. Research, VIth World Congress of Cardiology, London, Sept. 1970, Abstracts p. 199.
206c. — — SPIEGEL, M.: Z. Kreisl.-Forsch. **59**, 207 (1970).
207c. LIVESLEY, B., CATLEY, P.F., ORAM, S.: Cardiovasc. Research, VIth World Congress of Cardiology, London, Sept. 1970, Abstracts p. 202.
208c. LUCCHESI, B.R., HODGEMAR, R.J.: Pharmacologist **12**, 213 (1970).
209c. MACLEOD, C.A., HIRSCH, E.Z., SCHWARTZ, H.: Cardiovasc. Research, VIth World Congress of Cardiology, London, Sept. 1970, Abstracts p. 207.
210c. MADAN, B.R., MISHRA, S.N., KHANNA, V.K.: Arch. int. Pharmacodyn. **182**, 121 (1969).
211c. MALINDZAK, G.S., GREEN, H.D., STAGG, P.L.: J. appl. Physiol. **29**, 17 (1970).
212c. MARCHETTI, G.: Acta cardiol. (Brux.) Suppl. 13, 188 (1969).
213c. MARCHIORO, T., FELDMAN, A., OWENS, J.C., SWAN, H.: Circulat. Res. **9**, 541 (1961).
214c. MASIRONI, R.: Bull. Wld Hlth Org. **42**, 103 (1970).
215c. MASON, D.T.: Amer. J. Cardiol. **23**, 516 (1969).
216c. MASSUMI, R.A.: Circulation **42**, 287 (1970).
217c. MCCALLISTER, B.D., RICHMOND, D.R., SALTUPS, A., HALLERMANN, F.J., WALLACE, R.B., FRYE, R.L.: Circulation **42**, 471 (1970).
218c. MCCREDIE, R.M.: Cardiovasc. Research, VIth World Congress of Cardiology, London, Sept. 1970, Abstracts p. 206.
219c. MCNEILL, R.S.: Lancet **1964 II**, 1102.
220c. MERLEN, J.F., FLAMENT, G.: Brux.-méd. **50**, 571 (1970).
221c. MICHEL, D.: Cardiovasc. Research, VIth World Congress of Cardiology, London, Sept. 1970, Abstracts p. 218.
222c. MILLS, C.J.: Cardiovasc. Research, VIth World Congress of Cardiology, London, Sept. 1970, Abstracts p. 46.
223c. MITCHELL, J.R.A., EMMONS, P.R., HARRISON, M.J.G., HONOUR, A.J.: Nature (Lond.) **208**, 255 (1965).
224c. Mixed reception for myocardial revascularization. J. Amer. med. Ass. **213**, 616 (1970).
225c. MIYAHARA, M.: Acta cardiol. (Brux.), Suppl. 13, 174 (1969).
226c. MODELL, W.: Clin. Pharmacol. Ther. **3**, 97 (1962).
227c. MORGENSTERN, C., ARNOLD, G., HOELJES, U., LOCHNER, W.: Europ. J. Physiol. **315**, 173 (1970).
228c. MOSS, A.J., JOHNSON, J., SENTMAN, J.: Cardiovasc. Res. **4**, 441 (1970).
229c. MUSTARD, J.F., PACKHAM, M.A.: Pharmacol. Rev. **22**, 97 (1970).
230c. NARULA, O.S., SAMET, P.: Circulation **41**, 947 (1970).
231c. NEWELL, D.J., and clinical collaborators: Brit. Heart J. **32**, 16 (1970).
232c. NICKERSON, M.: Vasodilator drugs. In: The pharmacological basis of therapeutics. Ed. by GOODMAN and GILMAN. New York: Macmillan Co. 1965, p. 748.
233c. NIESSNER, H., LUJF, A., MOSER, K.: Intern. J. clin. Pharmacol. Ther. Toxicol. **3**, 277 (1970).
234c. NIMURA, Y., MOCHIZUKI, S., MATSUO, H., KITABATAKE, A., KATO, K., ABE, H.: Cardiovasc. Research, VIth World Congress of Cardiology, London, Sept. 1970, Abstracts p. 234.
235c. Nitroglycerine in Angina. Brit. med. J. **1970 III**, 239.
236c. NORDOY, A., RODSET, J.M.: Acta med. scand. **188**, 133 (1970).
237c. NOTT, M.W.: Brit. J. Pharmacol. **39**, 287 (1970).
238c. NUMANO, F., TAKENOBU, M., KATSU, K., SHIMAMOTO, T.: Cardiovasc. Research, VIth World Congress of Cardiology, London, Sept. 1970, Abstracts p. 236.
239c. OPIE, L.H.: J. molec. cell. Cardiol. **1**, 107 (1970).
240c. OWEN, P., THOMAS, M., YOUNG, V., OPIE, L.: Amer. J. Cardiol. **25**, 562 (1970).
241c. PAGE, I.H., BERRETTONI, J.N., BUTKUS, A., SONES, F.M.: Circulation **42**, 625 (1970).
242c. PARKER, J.O., CASE, R.B., KHAJA, F., LEDWICH, J.R., ARMSTRONG, P.W.: Circulation **41**, 593 (1970).
243c. — CHIONG, M.A., WEST, R.O., CASE, R.B.: Circulation **42**, 205 (1970).
244c. PARRATT, J.R.: In: Médicaments et Métabolisme du Myocarde. Nancy: Lamarche and Royer 1969, p. 265.
245c. — Acta cardiol. (Brux.), Suppl. 13, 191 (1969).
246c. — WADSWORTH, R.M.: Brit. J. Pharmacol. **39**, 296 (1970).
247c. PHILIP, R.B.: Thrombos. Diathes. haemorrh. (Stuttg.) **23**, 129 (1970).
248c. PICHUGIN, V.V.: Byull. éksp. Biol. Med. **69**, 58 (1970).

249c. PIETTE, F., DETRY, J.M., BRASSEUR, L.: Louvain Médical **89**, 149 (1970).
250c. PITT, A., ANDERSON, S.T.: Med. J. Aust. **1**, 1089 (1970).
251c. PITT, B., BECKER, L., ZARET, B., FORTUIN, N.J.: Cardiovasc. Research, VIth World Congress of Cardiology, London, Sept. 1970, Abstracts p. 250.
252c. — CRAVEN, P.: Cardiovasc. Res. **4**, 176 (1970).
253c. — SUGISHITA, Y., GREEN, H.L., FRIESINGER, G.C.: Amer. J. Physiol. **219**, 175 (1970).
254c. POMPOSIELLO, J.C., BAKER, L.D., SNOW, J.A., SHARMA, G.V., MESSER, J.V.: Cardiovasc. Research, VIth World Congress of Cardiology, London, Sept. 1970, Abstracts p. 252.
255c. POTANIN, C., HUNT, D., SHEFFIELD, L.T.: Circulation **42**, 199 (1970).
256c. Potassium, glucose, and insulin treatment for acute myocardial infarction. Lancet **1968II**, 1355.
257c. PRICHARD, B.N.C., GILLAM, P.M.S.: Ann. intern. Med. **68**, 1160 (1968).
258c. — — Brit. med. J. **1969I**, 7.
259c. PUECH, P., GROLLEAU, R., LATOUR, H.: Cardiovasc. Research, VIth World Congress of Cardiology, London, Sept. 1970, Abstracts p. 33.
260c. PURI, P.S., BING, R.J.: Dis. Chest **55**, 235 (1969).
261c. RABERGER, G., KRAUPP, O.: Brux.-méd. **50**, 645 (1970).
262c. — — Arch. Pharmakol. **266**, 430 (1970).
263c. — — STUEHLINGER, W., NELL, G., CHIRIKDJIAN, J.J.: Europ. J. Physiol. **317**, 20 (1970).
264c. RACKLEY, C.E., DEAR, H.D., BAXLEY, W.A., JONES, W.B., DODGE, H.T.: Circulation **41**, 605 (1970).
265c. RAFF, W.K., DRECHSEL, U., SCHOLTHOLT, J., LOCHNER, W.: Pflügers Arch. **317**, 336 (1970).
266c. REDWOOD, D.R., ROSING, D.R., GOLDSTEIN, R.E., BEISER, G.D., EPSTEIN, S.E.: Cardiovasc. Research, VIth World Congress of Cardiology, London, Sept. 1970, Abstracts p. 259.
267c. REES, J.R.: Brit. Heart J. **32**, 137 (1970).
268c. RENAUD, S., KUBA, K., GOULET, C., LEMIRE, Y., ALLARD, C.: Circulat. Res. **26**, 553 (1970).
269c. RIVIER, J.L., NISSIOTIS, E., JAEGER, M.: Thérapie **25**, 245 (1970).
270c. RODBARD, S., WILLIAMS, C.B., RODBARD, D.: Circulat. Res. **14**, 139 (1964).
271c. — WILLIAMS, F., WILLIAMS, C.B.: Amer. Heart J. **57**, 348 (1959).
272c. ROSS, G., JORGENSEN, C.R.: Cardiovasc. Res. **4**, 148 (1970).
273c. ROWE, G.G.: Circulation **42**, 193 (1970).
274c. RUDOLPH, W., MARKO, I.: Arzneimittel-Forsch. **20**, 1054 (1970).
275c. — — Arzneimittel-Forsch. **20**, 1190 (1970).
276c. — — BAUBKUS, H., MULLER-SEYDLITZ, P., GADOMSKI, M., POSSE, P., GULDE, M., JETSCHGO, G.: Arzneimittel-Forsch. **20**, 637 (1970).
277c. RUSSEK, H.I.: Cardiovasc. Research, VIth World Congress of Cardiology, London, Sept. 1970, Abstracts p. 270.
278c. SALWAN, F.A., LEIGHNINGER, D.S., BECK, C.S.: Dis. Chest **53**, 197 (1968).
279c. SANDLER, G.: Brux.-méd. **50**, 669 (1970).
280c. — CLAYTON, G.A.: Brit. med. J. **1970II**, 399.
281c. SANER, R.: Thérapie **25**, 393 (1970).
282c. SCHAPER, W., JAGENEAU, A., XHONNEUX, R.: Brux.-méd. **50**, 635 (1970).
283c. — XHONNEUX, R., JAGENEAU, A., VANDESTEENE, R., SCHAPER, J.: Acta cardiol. (Brux.), Suppl. 13, 74 (1969).
284c. SCHIRMER, R., HAMACHER, J.: Arch. Pharmakol. **266**, 440 (1970).
285c. SCHMIDT, H.D., SCHMIER, J.: Acta cardiol. (Brux.), Suppl. 13, 68 (1969).
286c. SCHMIER, J., KADEN, F., SCHMIDT, H.D.: Brux.-méd. **50**, 617 (1970).
287c. SCHNELLBACHER, K., REINDELL, H., ROSKAMM, H., REINDELL, A.: Herz-Kreislauf **2**, 364 (1970).
288c. SCHUILENBURG, R.M., DURRER, D.: Circulation **41**, 967 (1970).
289c. SCHWARTZ, S.I., GRIFFITH, L.S.C., NEISTADT, A., HAGFORS, N.: Amer. J. Surg. **114**, 5 (1967).
290c. SEALEY, B.J., LILJEDAHL, J., NYBERG, G., ABLAD, B.: Cardiovasc. Research, VIth World Congress of Cardiology, London, Sept. 1970, Abstracts p. 281.
291c. SETTI, L., RAZZABONI, G.: Boll. Soc. ital. Biol. sper. **45**, 1191 (1969).
292c. SINGER, D.H., LAZZARA, R., HOFFMAN, B.F.: The Myocardial Cell. Ed. by BRILLER and CONN. Philadelphia: University of Pennsylvania Press 1966, p. 98.
293c. SINGH, B.N., VAUGHAN WILLIAMS, E.M.: Brit. J. Pharmacol. **39**, 675 (1970).
294c. SINGH, R., RANIERI, A.J., VEST, H.R., BOWERS, D.L., DAMMANN, J.F.: Amer. J. Cardiol. **25**, 579 (1970).

295c. SNOW, J.A., OLSSON, R.A.: Clin. Res. **18**, 331 (1970).
296c. SOLTI, F., SZABO, Z., FEDINA, L., RENYI-VAMOS, F., SARAI, K.: Cardiovasc. Research, VIth World Congress of Cardiology, London, Sept. 1970, Abstracts p. 290.
297c. SPRACKLEN, F.H., CHAMBERS, R.J., SCHRIRE, V.: Cardiovasc. Research, VIth World Congress of Cardiology, London, Sept. 1970, Abstracts p. 295.
298c. STEINBERG, D.: Circulation **41**, 723 (1970).
299c. STERNITZKE, N., MEYTHALER, M.: Brux.-méd. **50**, 583 (1970).
300c. — — Z. Kreisl.-Forsch. **59**, 153 (1970).
301c. STORSTEIN-SPILKER, L.: Cardiovasc. Research, VIth World Congress of Cardiology, London, Sept. 1970, Abstracts p. 298.
302c. STRAUER, B.E., TAUCHERT, M., COTT, L., KOCHSIEK, K., BRETSCHNEIDER, H.J.: Cardiovasc. Research, VIth World Congress of Cardiology, London, Sept. 1970, Abstracts p. 300.
303c. STRAUSS, H.C., BIGGER, J.T., HOFFMAN, B.F.: Circulat. Res. **26**, 661 (1970).
304c. STROBBIA, R., MANZONI, A., ZOTTO U DAL: Minerva med. **61**, 3507 (1970).
305c. STRONG, J.P., RICHARDS, M.L., McGILL, H.C., EGGEN, D.A., McMURRY, M.T.: J. Atheroscler. Res. **10**, 283 (1969).
306c. SULLIVAN, J.M., HARKEN, D.E., GORLIN, R.: New Engl. J. Med. **279**, 576 (1968).
307c. — — — Circulation **39**, Suppl. 1, 149 (1969).
308c. SVEDMYR, N., ANDERSSON, R., EKSTROM-JODAL, B., HOLMBERG, S., HAGGENDAL, E., MALMBERG, R.: In: Médicaments et Métabolisme du Myocarde. Nancy: Lamarche and Royer 1969, p. 211.
309c. — MALMBERG, R., HAGGENDAL, E.: Pharmacol. Clin. **2**, 82 (1970).
310c. SZENTIVANYI, M., KUNOS, G.: In: Médicaments et Métabolisme du Myocarde. Nancy: Lamarche and Royer 1969, p. 535.
311c. THOMPSON, M.E., LEON, D.F., SHAVER, J.A., McDONALD, R.H.: Pharmacologist **12**, 213 (1970).
312c. TOKER, Y.: Münch. med. Wschr. **112**, 809 (1970).
313c. TORRESANI, J., CHEVALIER CHOLAT, A.M., COURBIER, R., HEUILLET, G., JOUVE, A.: Cardiovasc. Research, VIth World Congress of Cardiology, London, Sept. 1970, Abstracts p. 308.
314c. TOUBES, D.B., FERGUSON, R.K., RICE, A.J., AOKI, V.S., FUNK, D.C., WILSON, W.R.: Clin. Res. **18**, 345 (1970).
315c. TREMBLAY, G.M., DE CHAMPLAIN, J.A., NADEAU, R.A.: Cardiovasc. Research, VIth World Congress of Cardiology, London, Sept. 1970, Abstracts p. 309.
316c. TUNA, N., AMPLATZ, K.: Cardiovasc. Research, VIth World Congress of Cardiology, London, Sept. 1970, Abstracts p. 312.
317c. TURNER, P.: Brit. J. Pharmacol. **40**, 146 P (1970).
318c. VAN BELLE, H.: Europ. J. Pharmacol. **10**, 290 (1970).
319c. — Europ. J. Pharmacol. **11**, 241 (1970).
320c. VAN SCHEPDAEL, J., SOLVAY, H.: Presse méd. **78**, 1849 (1970).
321c. VATNER, S.F., FRANKLIN, D.C., VAN CITTERS, R.L., BRAUNWALD, E.: Clin. Res. **17**, 269 (1969).
322c. — — — — Circulat. Res. **27**, 11 (1970).
323c. VEGA DIAZ, F., PEREZ CASAR, F.: Cardiovasc. Research, VIth World Congress of Cardiology, London, Sept. 1970, Abstracts p. 318.
324c. VESTER, J.W., SUNDER, J.H., AARONS, J.H., DANOWSKI, T.S.: Clin. Pharmacol. Ther. **11**, 689 (1970).
325c. VIGNE, J.: Brux.-méd. **50**, 601 (1970).
326c. VINEBERG, A.: Cardiovasc. Research, VIth World Congress of Cardiology, London, Sept. 1970, Abstracts p. 42.
327c. — VELENA, S., LONG, J.: Cardiovasc. Research, VIth World Congress of Cardiology, London, Sept. 1970, Abstracts p. 319.
328c. VOGELSANG, A.: Angiology **21**, 275 (1970).
329c. VOHRA, J.K., DOWLING, J.T., SLOMAN, G.: Med. J. Aust. **2**, 228 (1970).
330c. VYDEN, J.K., CARVALHO, M., BOSZORMENYI, F., LANG, T., BERNSTEIN, H., CORDAY, E.: Amer. J. Cardiol. **25**, 53 (1970).
331c. WAGNER, H.R., GAMBLE, W.J., ALBERS, W.H., HUGENHOLTZ, P.G.: Circulation **37**, 694 (1968).
332c. WALE, J.: Europ. J. Pharmacol. **9**, 387 (1970).
333c. WALKER, J.A., FRIEDBERG, H.D., JOHNSON, W.D., FLEMMA, R.J., LEPLEY, D.: Cardiovasc. Research, VIth World Congress of Cardiology, London, Sept. 1970, Abstracts p. 321.
334c. WANET, J., ACHTEN, G., BARCHEWITZ, G., MESTDAGH, C., VASTESAEGER, M.: Ann. Derm. Syph. Paris **98**, 131 (1971).

335c. WAREMBOURG, H., HOUDAS, Y., BERTRAND, M.E., KETELERS, J.Y.: In: Médicaments et Métabolisme du myocarde. Nancy: Lamarche and Royer 1969, p. 203.
336c. WASSERMANN, S.: Wien. klin. Wschr. 41, 1514 (1928).
337c. WATT, D.A.L., LIVINGSTONE, W.R., MACKAY, R.K.S., OBINECHE, E.N.: Brit. Heart J. 32, 453 (1970).
338c. WIENER, L., KASPARIAN, H.: Cardiovasc. Research, VIth World Congress of Cardiology, London, Sept. 1970, Abstracts p. 324.
339c. WILDE, W.: Med. Mschr. 24, 177 (1970).
340c. WIRZ, P., SCHONBECK, M., MEHMEL, H., KRAYENBUHL, H.P., RUTISHAUSER, W.: Cardiovasc. Research, VIth World Congress of Cardiology, London, Sept. 1970, Abstracts p. 326.
341c. YAMAZAKI, H., KOBAYASHI, I.: a) Cardiovasc. Research, VIth World Congress of Cardiology, London, Sept. 1970, Abstracts p. 328; b) Amer. Heart J. 79, 640 (1970).
342c. — SANO, T., ODAKURA, T., TAKEUCHI, K., SHIMAMOTO, T.: Amer. Heart J. 79, 640 (1970).
343c. YIGITBASI, O., NALBANTGIL, I.: Praxis 59, 1218 (1970).
344c. ZACHARIAS, F.J.: Brit. med. J. 1969I, 712.
345c. ZEFT, H.J., CURRY, C.L., REMBERT, J.C., GREENFIELD, J.C.: Clin. Res. 18, 72 (1970).

Additional references (series d)

1d. BRODBIN, P., O'CONNOR, C.A.: Brit. J. clin. Pract. 22, 395 (1968).
2d. CLOAREC, M.: Thérapeutique 46, 921 (1970).
3d. CONTI, C.R., PITT, B., GUNDEL, W.D., FRIESINGER, G.C., ROSS, R.S.: Circulation 42, 815 (1970).
4d. Etude clinique de 405 cas traités au trinitrate d'ettriol. Ars Medici 25, 1399 (1970).
5d. FONTAINE, J.L., FONTAINE, R.: Thérapie 25, 961 (1970).
6d. HERTAULT, J.: Médecine pratique 2, 44 (1967).
7d. JOUVE, A., GRAS, A., BENYAMINE, R.: Vie méd. 44, 115 (1963).
8d. KAPLAN, H.R., ROBSON, R.D.: J. Pharmacol. exp. Ther. 175, 168 (1970).
9d. LADDU, A.R., SOMANI, P.: Pharmacologist 12, 307 (1970).
10d. MEHROTRA, T.N., BASSADONE, E.T.: Brit. J. clin. Pract. 21, 11 (1967).
11d. ROBSON, R.D., KAPLAN, H.R.: J. Pharmacol. exp. Ther. 175, 157 (1970).
12d. ROWE, G.G., SPRING, D.A., AFONSO, S.: Arch. int. Pharmacodyn. 187, 377 (1970).
13d. SHEVDE, S., SPILKER, B.A.: Brit. J. Pharmacol. 38, 448P (1970).
14d. WAREMBOURG, H., BERTRAND, M.: Lille méd. 8, 965 (1963).
15d. WETTENGEL, R., FABEL, H.: Dtsch. med. Wschr. 95, 1816 (1970).

Additional references (series e)

1e. ADAM, K.R., BOYLES, S., SCHOLFIELD, P.C.: Brit. J. Pharmacol. 40, 534 (1970).
2e. CARLIER, J.: Rev. méd. Liège 25, 797 (1970).
3e. DWYER, E.M.: Circulation 42, 1111 (1970).
4e. FRIART, J., RASSON, G.: Arzneimittel-Forsch. Sept. 1971 (In press).
5e. HAKKINEN, P., RELANDER, A., OKA, M.: Scand. J. clin. Lab. Invest. 25, Suppl. 113, 40 (1970).
6e. KUKOVETZ, W.R., PÖCH, G.: Naunyn-Schmiedeberg's Arch. exp. Path. Pharmak. 267, 189 (1970).
7e. LUCCHESI, B.R., HODGEMAN, R.J.: J. Pharmacol. Exp. Therap. 176, 200 (1971).
8e. Oxprenolol and Practolol: new beta blockers: Drug and Therap. Bull. 9, 1 (1971).
8e (bis). PETTA, J.M., ZACCHEO, V.I.: J. Pharmacol. Exp. Therap. 176, 328 (1971).
9e. SOMANI, P., LADDU, A.R., HARDMAN, H.F.: J. Pharmacol. Exp. Therap. 175, 577 (1970).
9e (bis). VAN CAUWENBERGE, H.: Rev. méd. Liége, 26, 221 (1971).
10e. WINBURY, M.M.: Circulation Research, 28, Suppl. 1, 140 (1971).
11e. — HOWE, B.B., WEISS, H.R.: J. Pharmacol. Exp. Therap. 176, 184 (1971).

Author Index

The numbers in *italics* shown in square brackets are the numbers of the references in the bibliography. Page numbers in *italics* refer to the bibliography.

Aarons, J. H., see Vester, J. W. [324c], 16, *370*

Abaza, A., Rutlisberger, P. A. [1], 162, *323*

Abe, H., see Nimura, Y. [234c], 78, *368*

Abel, R. M., Reis, R. L., Staroscfk, R. N. [1a, 1c], 301, *360, 363*

Aberg, G., Dzedin, T., Lundholm, L., Olsson, L., Svedmyr, N. [2], 249, 250, 251, *323*

Abiteboul, J., see Bernal, P. [138], 279, 280, *325*

Ablad, B., Brogard, M., Ek, L. [3], 216, 230, 231, 234, *323*

— Johnsson, G., Norrby, A., Sölvell, L. [4], 207, 232, *323*

— see Sealey, B. J. [290c], 233, *369*

Abraham, A. S., see Hedworth-Whitty, R. B. [59a, 141c], 57, 79, *361, 366*

Abrahamsen, A. M., Kiil, F. [5], 136, 143, *323*

Abrams, W. B., Becker, M. C., Lewis, D. W., Killough, J. H. [6], 163, *323*

— Lewis, D. W., Shoshkes, M., Rothfeld, E., Becker, M. [7], 163, *323*

Abramson, D. I., see Katz, L. N. [958], 66, 67, 121, 145, *340*

Aceto, M. D., Kinnard, W. J., Buckley, J. P. [8, 9], 146, *323*

— see Kinnard, W. J. [985], 149, *341*

Aceto, M. D. G., see Buckley, J. P. [251], 146, *327*

Aceves, J., see Mendez, R. [1279], 161, *346*

Acheson, J., Danta, G., Hutchinson, E. C. [2c], 51, *363*

Achten, G., see Wanet, J. [334c], 287, *370*

Adam, K. R., Boyles, S., Scholfield, P. C. [1e], 239, 240, *371*

Adam, M., Mitchel, B. F., Lambert, C. J. [3c], 12, *363*

Adler-Kastner, L., see Kraupp, O. [1040, 1042], 192, 194, *342*

Adolfsson, L., see Areskog, N. H. [52, 4a], 233, 240, 241, *324, 360*

Aellig, W. H., Prichard, B. N. C. [4c], 236, *363*

— — Richardson, G. A. [10], 227, 241, 252, *323*

Afonso, S. [11, 5c], 186, 202, *323, 363*

— O'Brien, G. S. [12], 185, *323*

— — Crumpton, C. W. [13, 2a], 186, 201, 202, *323, 360*

— see McKenna, D. H. [1257], 4, *345*

— see Rowe, G. G. [1573 to 1575, 12d], 81, 140, 294, *351, 371*

Aguirre, C. V., see Dighiero, J. [430], 163, *330*

Ahlquist, R. P. [14, 15], 173, 175, 205, *323*

— Huggins, R. A., Woodbury, R. A. [16], 312, *323*

— see Levy, B. [1120], 175, *343*

Aisner, M. [1b], 20, *362*

Akker, S. van den, Bijlsma, U. G., Van Dongen, K., Ten Thije, J. H. [17], 308, *323*

Albers, W. H., see Wagner, H. R. [331c], 91, *370*

Albert, A. [18], 147, *323*

Albert, H., see Lichtlen, P. [203c, 204c, 205c, 206c], 214, 247, *368*

Alderman, E. L., see Kerber, R. E. [176c], 233, *367*

Aldinger, E. E. [19], 291, *323*

— see Darby, T. D. [390], 129, *330*

Alexander, J. A., see Wallacw, A. G. [1955], *358*

Alexander, M., see Brotslow, J. [50c], 316, *364*

Algan, O., Kienle, H. [20], 188, *323*

Alhomme, P., see Facquet, J. [517, 518], 280, 286, 287, *332*

Alivirta, P., see Turpeinen, O. [1906], 14, *357*

Alix, B., Jury, G., Courtadon, M., Maillot, S., Jallut, H. [6c], 279, 286, 288, *363*

Allanby, K. D., Cox, A. G. C., Maclean, K. S., Price, T. M. L., Southwell, N. [21], 163, *323*

Allard, C., see Renaud, S. [268c], 50, *369*

Allen, F. J., see Proctor, J. P. [99a, 100a], 230, 231, 233, *362*

— see Wasserman, A. J. [130a], 230, 233, 235, *362*

Allen, L., see Hellerstein, H. K. [807], 10, *337*

Allmark, M. G., Lu, F. C., Carmichael, E., Lavallee, A. [22], 161, *323*

— see Lu, F. C. [1182, 1183] 72, 151, 158, 305, 310, *344*

Al-Shamma, A. M., see Criollos, R. L. [376], 10, *329*

Altman, G. E., Riseman, J. E. F., Koretsky, S. [23], 140, *323*

— see Riseman, J. E. F. [1531, 1534], 106, 108, 135, 137, 138, 139, 140, 142, 143, 146, 304, *350*

Altschule, M. D. [24], 20, *323*

Alvarez, H., see Battock, D. J. [108, 109], 213, 214, *325*

Alvaro, A. B., MacAlpin, R. N., Kattus, A. A. [25], 214, *323*

Alzeari, J. B., see Gazaix, M. [108c], 279, *366*

Ambanelli, U., see Botti, G. [201], 253, *326*

Ambanelli, V., see Starcich, R. [1820], 36, *355*

Ameur, M., Hessel, F., Laval, G. [3a], 279, *360*

Amiel, C., see Richet, G. [1525] 172, *350*

Ammermann, E. O. [26], 142, *323*

Amplatz, K., see Tuna, N. [316c], 96, *370*

Amsterdam, E. A., Gorlin, R., Wolfson, S. [27], 212, *323*
— Wolfson, S., Gorlin, R. [28, 29, 30], 114, 212, 215, *323*
— see Kemp, H. G. [174c], 12, *367*
— see Mason, D. T. [87a], 39, 130, *361*
— see Wolfson, S. [2031], 212, *359*

Andersen, A., see Hillestad, L. [830], 235, *338*

Anderson, D. E., see Mackinnon, J. [1204], 163, *344*
— see Snow, P. J. D. [1766], 162, *354*

Anderson, F. F., Cameron, A. [31], 66, *323*
— Craver, B. N. [32], 66, *323*

Anderson, F. S., see West, J. W. [1979], 89, *358*

Anderson, R., see Griffith, G. C. [742], 311, *336*

Anderson, S. T., see Pitt, A. [250c], 227, *369*

Anderson, T. W. [7c], 7, *363*

Anderson, W. H., see Russek, H. I. [1613], 104, 158, *352*

Andersson, R., see Svedmyr, N. [308c], 211, 251, *370*

Andrew, D., see McClish, A. [1246, 1247], 221, *345*

Andrus, C. E. [33], 96, *323*

Angarskaya, M. A., Khadzhai, Y. I., Kolesnikov, D. G., Prokopenko, A. P., Dubinsky, A. A., Shubov, M. I. [34], 304, *323*

Angelakos, E. T., King, M. P., Uzgiris, I. [8c], 63, *363*

Angkapindu, A., Stafford, A., Thorp, R. H. [35], 306, *323*

Anthony, J. R., Jick, H., Spodick, D. G. [46], *323*

Antoniadis, G., see Voridis, E. [1950], 226, *358*

Antonio, A., Rocha e Silva, M. [47], 63, *323*

Anrep, G. V. [36], 55, *323*
— Barsoum, G. S., Kenawy, M. R. [37, 38], 157, *323*
— — — Misrahy, G. [39, 40], 157, 158, *323*
— — Schönberg, A. [41], 160, *323*
— — Talaat, M. [42], 60, *323*
— Blalock, A., Hammouda, M. [43], 68, *323*
— Häusler, H. [44], 55, *323*
— Kenawy, M. R., Barsoum, G. S. [45], 67, 157, 158, 159, *323*

Aoki, V. S., see Toubes, D. B. [314c], 252, *370*

Appaix, A., see Gerard, R. [111c], 315, *366*

Apthorp, G. H., Chamberlain, D. A., Hayward, G. W. [48], 275, *323*

Aptin [49], 234, *323*

Aravanis, C., Luisada, A. A. [50], 155, *323*
— Michaelides, G. [9c], *363*

Arborelius, M., Lecerof, H., Malm, A., Malmborg, R. O. [51], 131, *324*

Arcebal, A. G., see Lemberg, L. [1099], 221, *343*

Archer, J., see Kolin, A. [1017], 78, *341*

Archer, J. D., see Kolin, A. [1015], 4, 78, *341*

Archer, M., see Christakis, G. [327], 14, *328*

Ardisson, J. L., see Constantin, B. [355], *329*

Areskog, N. H., Adolfsson, L. [52], 240, 241, *324*
— — Rasmuson, T. [4a], 233, *360*

Arfors, K. E., Hint, H. C., Dhall, D. P., Matheson, N. A. [10c], 51, *363*

Armand, P., Paecht, A., Lichah, E., Bremond, C. [53], 279, *324*

Armitage, A. K., Boswood, J., Large, B. J. [55], 156, *324*

Armbrust, C. A., Levine, S. A. [54], 158, *324*

Armstrong, P. W., see Khaja, F. [179c], 31, 32, *367*
— see Parker, J. O. [242c], 131, 133, *368*

Arnold, E. F., see Ferrero, C. [538], 129, *332*

Arnold, G., see Morgenstern, C. [227c], 207, *368*

Arnoux, E., see Audier, M. [62, 2b], 140, 164, 293, *324, 362*

Aronow, W. S., Chesluck, H. M. [11c, 12c], 5, 110, 147, 148, *363*
— Kaplan, M. A. [56], 110, 213, *324*
— Swanson, A. J. [5a—7a], 16, *360*

Arriaga, J., see Cuellar, A. [72c], 295, *365*

Aschenbeck, G. [57], 190, *324*

Ashfield, R., see Rees, J. R. [1510], 123, 125, *350*

Askanazy, S. [58], 152, *324*

Astrom, H. [59], 211, *324*

Atkins, J. A., see White, J. C. [1984], 19, *358*

Atkins, J. M., Blomqvist, G., Cohen, L. S. [13c], 252, *363*

Atkinson, M., see Holdsworth, C. D. [849], 163, *338*

Atsumi, T., Motomiya, T., Isokane, N., Shimamoto, T. [14c], 289, *363*

Atsumz, T., see Shimamoto, T. [1741], 289, *354*

Atterhög, J. H., Porjé, G. [60], 179, *324*

Aubert, A., Nyberg, G., Slaastad, R., Tjeldflaat, L. [8a], 233, *360*

Aubert, P., see Bekaert, J. [124, 125], 169, 170, 171, 172, *325*

Audier, M., Arnoux, E. [2b], 293, *362*
— — Giraud, M. [62], 140, 164, *324*
— Devin, R., Bonneau, H., Ruf, G. [63], 310, *324*
— Serradimigni, A., Poggi, L., Bory, M., Diane, P. [61], 279, 287, *324*

Aulisio, G. A., see Marmo, E. [1223, 1224], 208, 245, 250, *345*

Auscher, C., see Delbarre, F. [403], 172, *330*

Austen, W. G., see Pentecost, B. L. [1429], 217, *348*

Autenrieth, G., see Kirsch, U. [70a], 198, *361*

Avezou, F., see Denis, B. [32a], 279, *360*

Aviado, D. M., see Cho, Y. W. [22a], 294, *360*
— see Drimal, J. [85c], 222, *365*
— see Feinsilver, O. [39a], 294, *360*
— see Folle, L. E. [568], 214, *333*

Ayad, H. [64], 158, *324*

Aygen, M. M., see Braunwald, E. [43c], 33, *364*

Ayman, D., see Proger, S. H. [1468], 137, *349*

Azarnoff, D. L., see Bell, H. [127], 190, *325*

Babacan, B. C., see Roberts, L. N. [1542], 187, *350*

Babel, J., Stangos, N. [65], 287, *324*
— — Ferrero, C. [15c], 287, *363*

Bachand, R. T., Somani, P., Hardman, H. T. [66], 127, *324*
— see Somani, P. [1779—1781] 134, 249, 251, *355*

Bache, R., see Cobb, F. [336], 208, *329*

Bache, R. J., see Cobb, F. R. [337, 24a], 208, *329, 360*

Bachmann, G. W., see Meesmann, W. [1261, 1262], 45, 53, 86, 182, 183, *346*

Bacq, Z. M., Cheymol, J., Dallemagne, M. J., Hazard, R., Labarre, J., Reuse, J. J., Welsch, M. [67], 173, *324*

Bacuzzi, E., see Barbaresi, F. [86], 248, 249, *324*

Baedeker, W. D., see Rudolph, W. [1582], 186, 187, *351*

Baeder, D. H. [68], 146, 147, *324*

Baer, S., Heine, W. I., Gelfond, D. B. [69], 305, *324*

Bagouri, M. M. [70], 158, 159, *324*

Baillet, J., see Soulie, P. [1797], 160, *355*

Baisse, J. [71], 156, *324*

Bajolet, A., see Hardel, M. [58a], 279, *361*

Bajusz, E. [3b], 296, *362*

Bak, I. J., see Grobecker, H. [744], 166, *336*

Baker, B. M., see Scarborough, W. R. [1651], 95, *352*

Baker, J. B. E. [72], 66, *324*

Baker, L. D., Leshin, S. J., Sharma, G. V. R. K., Messer, J. V. [73], 26, *324*

— Mathur, V. S., Leshin, S. J., Messer, J. V. [74], *324*

— see Pomposiello, J. C. [254c] *369*

Bakst, H., Kissin, M., Leibowitz, S., Rinzler, S. [75], 112, 155, *324*

— see Greiner, T. [738], 110, 111, 112, 113, 116, 158, 308, *336*

— see Rinzler, S. H. [1528, 1529], 305, 311, *350*

Balaguer-Vintro, I., Oter Rodriguez, R., Duarte Mantilla, G., Vilalta Bernet, C. [76], 279, 280, *324*

Balatre, P., Merlen, J. F. [77], 305, *324*

— — Granjean, L. [78], 141, *324*

Balcon, R., Jewitt, D. E., Davies, J. P. H., Oram, S. [79], 217, 218, 221, *324*

— Maloy, W. C., Sowton, E. [80], 99, 100, *324*

— see Frick, M. H. [592], 4, 30, 34, 93, 100, 109, 128, 130, 133, *333*

— see Gibson, D. G. [654], 243, *335*

— see Maloy, W. C. [1215], 100, *345*

Balcon, R., see Sowton, E. [1798, 1799], 4, 93, 100, 128, 240, *355*

Baldes, E. J., Herrick, J. F. [81], 76, *324*

— see Essex, H. E. [508], 120, 306, *332*

— see Hausner, E. [791], 55, *337*

Baldrighi, G., see De Caro, L. [77c], 247, *365*

Baldrighi, V., see De Caro, L. [77c], 247, *365*

Balke, B., see Naughton, J. [1341], 10, *347*

Ball, K. P. [82], 305, *324*

Banas, J., see Brooks, H. [49c], 252, *364*

Banas, J. S., see Brooks, H. L. [17a, 18a], 249, 251, *360*

Banes, D. [83], 137, *324*

Banfield, W. G., see Goodale, W. T. [690, 691], 79, *335*

Banks, T., Shugoll, G. I. [84], 48, *324*

Banno, S., see Maggi, G. C. [1207], 138, *345*

Banse, H. J., Zahnow, W. [85], 156, *324*

Barach, A. L., see Levy, R. L. [1126], 106, *343*

Barbaresi, F., Bacuzzi, E., Manfredi, M., Starcich, R. [86], 248, 249, *324*

Barbarosh, H., see Krasnow, N. [1032], 221, *342*

Barber, J. M., see Murphy, F. M. [1330—1332], 163, *347*

Barbi, G. L., Tallone, G. [87], 253, *324*

Barboriak, J. J., see Meester, W. D. [1263], 248, *346*

Barchewitz, G., see Wanet, J. [334c], 287, *370*

Bardhanabaedya, S., see Denison, A. B. [413], 312, *330*

Barger, A. C., see Herd, J. A. [816], 83, *338*

Bargheer, R., Fiegel, G., Saito, S., Guttmann, W. [88], 159, *324*

— see Fiegel, G. [543, 544], 163, 190, *333*

Barner, H. B., see Kaiser, G. C. [167c], 11, *367*

Barnes, A. R., see Burchell, H. B. [259], 96, *327*

— see Pruitt, R. D. [1474], 96, *349*

Barnes, G. E., see Hyman, A. L. [156c], 316, *367*

Barold, S., see Burkart, F. [262], 109, *327*

Barold, S. S., see Linhart, J. W. [1152—1154, 82a], 3, 11, 34, 126, 130, *344, 361*

Baroldi, G. [16c], 53, *363*

— Mantero, O., Scomozoni, G. [89], 53, *324*

Barousch, R. [90], 179, *324*

Barrera, J. A., Turiella, R. G. [91], 162, *324*

Barrett, A. M. [92], 215, *324*

— Crowther, A. F., Dunlop, D., Shanks, R. C., Smith, L. H. [93], 235, 236, 242, *324*

— see Fitzgerald, J. D. [558, 559], 172, 173, 174, 177, 178, *333*

Barrett, C. T. [94], 308, *324*

Barrillon, A., Himbert, J., Fayard, J. M., Lenegre, J. [17c], 163, *364*

Barry, A. J., Daly, J. W., Pruett, E. D. R., Steinmetz, J. R., Birkhead, N. C., Rodahl, K. [95], 10, *324*

— see Holloszy, J. O. [854], 10, *338*

Barsky, J., see Zeller, E. A. [2045—2047], 160, *360*

Barsoum, G. S., Kenawy, M. R. [96], 158, *324*

— see Anrep, G. V. [37—42, 45], 60, 67, 157, 158, 159, 160, *323*

— see Kenawy, M. R. [968], 158, *340*

Bartelstone, H. J., Scherlag, B. J., Cranefield, P. F., Hoffman, B. F. [97], 70, *324*

Barthel, W., Markwardt, F. [98], 166, *324*

Bartolomei, G., see Donato, L. [437, 438], 82, *331*

Bartsch, W., Knopf, K. W. [18c], 232, *364*

— see Schaumann, W. [1661], 165, 174, *353*

Barzin, J. [99], 91, *324*

— Freson, A. [100], 278, 281, 282, 285, 286, *324*

Bassadone, E. T., see Mehrotra, T. N. [10d], 298, *371*

Bastenie, P. A., Vanhaelst, L., Neve, P. [101], 16, *324*

Bateman, F. J. A. [102], 174, 180, *324*

Batlouni, M., Betolami, V., Duprat, R. [103], 202, *324*

Batson, G. A., see Szekely, P. [1867], 221, *356*

Batterman, R. C. [104, 105], 95, 96, 109, 110, *325*

— Grossman, A. J., Schwimmer, J., Blackman, A. L. [106], 154, 155, *325*

— Mouratoff, C. J. [107], 149, *325*

Batterman, R. C., see Grossman, A. J. [747], 154, *336*

Battock, D. J., Alvarez, H., Chidsey, C. A. [108, 109], 213, 214, *325*

Bau, G., see Vettori, G. [1940], 228, *358*

Baubkus, H., see Rudolph, W. [276c], 194, *369*

Baudine, A., Chaillet, F., Charlier, R., Hosslet, A. [110], 257, 261, *325*

— see Charlier, R. [309, 310, 316, 317, 319], 168, 169, 256, 258, 259, 262, 263, 266, 269, 271, 272, *328*

Baue, A. [111], 11, *325*

Bauer, E., see Kraut, H. [1044], 309, *342*

Bauer, G. E., Michell, G. [19c], 228, *364*

Baum, W. S., see Russek, H. I. [1614], 104, 135, 151, 300, *352*

Baumann, P. C., see Lichtlen, P. [1136], 125, *343*

Baumgarten, A. [112], 168, *325*

Bauthier, J., see Charlier, R. [311, 312], 276, *328*

— see Delaunois, G. [78c], 266, *365*

Baxley, W. A., see Rackley, C. E. [264c], 35, *369*

Bay, G., Larsen, L. P., Lorentsen, E., Sivertssen, E. [113], 218, *325*

Bayley, R. H., La Due, J. S., York, D. J. [114], 154, *325*

Beanlands, D. S., see Zsoter, T. T. [141a], 212, *362*

Bear, E. S., see James, T. N. [160c], 218, *367*

Beard, O. W., see Talley, R. W. [1872], 141, *356*

Beaumont, J. L., Coblentz, B., Maurice, P., Chevalier, H., Lenegre, J. [115], 311, *325*

Bebenburg, W. von, see Thiele, K. [1881], 198, *357*

Bec, P., see Deodati, F. [80c], 287, *365*

Beck, C., see Leighninger, D. S. [1095], 122, *343*

Beck, C. S., Leighninger, D. S. [116], 169, *325*

— see Salwan, F. A. [278c], 21, *369*

Becker, A. [117], 305, *325*

Becker, H. J., see Kaltenbach, M. [169c], 247, *367*

Becker, L., Fortuin, N. J., Pitt, B. [9a], 134, *360*

— see Pitt, B. [251c], 134, *369*

Becker, M., see Abrams, W. B. [7], 163, *323*

Becker, M. C. [118], 187, *325*

— see Abrams, W. B. [6], 163, *323*

— see Shoskes, M. [1748], 162, *354*

Becker, W. H., see Schilling, F. J. [1668], 14, *353*

Beckman, H. [119], 313, *325*

Beckschäfer, W. [120], 196, *325*

Becsei, J., see Lammerant, J. [193c], 306, *367*

Beecher, H. K. [121, 122], 109, 110, *325*

Beezy, R., see Frisch, R. A. [604], 152, *334*

Beghin, B., see Linquette, M. [1157], 190, 191, *344*

Behar, V. S., see Whalen, R. E. [1982], 207, 272, 274, *358*

Behr, D. J., see Gubner, R. S. [752,] 295, *336*

Beisenherz, G., see Koss, F. W. [1021], 185, *341*

Beiser, G. D., see Epstein, S. E. [500, 501, 94c], 37, 315, 316, *332*, *365*

— see Goldstein, R. E. [54a, 55a, 118c], 147, *361*, *366*

— see Redwood, D. R. [266c], 106, *369*

— see Robinson, B. F. [1545], 207, 284, *351*

— see Stampfer, M. [1816], 38, *355*

Bekaert, J. [123] ,284, *325*

— Aubert, P. [124, 125], 169, 170, 171, 172, *325*

— Deltour, G., Broekhuysen, J. [126], 169, 171, 172, *325*

— see Deltour, G. [408], 169, *330*

Bell, H., Azarnoff, D. L., Dunn, M. [127], 190, *325*

Bellet, S., see West, J. W. [1977, 1978], 71, 181, 182, *358*

Belliveau, R. E., Covino, B. G. [128], 230, *325*

Belluardo, C., see Molino, N. [1311], 164, *346*

Ben, M., Warren, M., Drinnon, V., Scott, C. [129], 163, *325*

Benaim, S., Dixon, M. F. [130], 162, *325*

Benchimol, A., see Dimond, E. G. [431], 30, *330*

Benda, L., Doneff, D., Lujf, A., Moser, K. [131], 179, *325*

Bender, A. D., see Sullivan, F. J. [1853], 141, *356*

Bender, F., Diekmann, L., Hilgenberg, F., Dotterweich, W. [20c], 246, *364*

— Schmidt, E. [132], 226, *325*

— Sieger, W., Dotterweich, K. [10a], 226, 233, 245, *360*

Bender, S. R. [21c], 16, *364*

Bendikov, E. A., see Kaverina, N. V. [171c], 134, *367*

Benfey, B. G., Greeff, K., Heeg, E. [133], 172, 174, 177, 178, 245, 263, *325*

— see Melville, K. I. [1270], 174, *346*

Benichoux, R., Marchal, C., Royer, R. [22c], 70, *364*

Benjamin, Z. H., see Greiner, T. [738], 110, 111, 112, 113, 116, 158, 308, *336*

— see Rinzler, S. H. [1528, 1529], 305, 311, *350*

Bennett, A., see Robbins, S. L. [1539], 53, *350*

Bennett, M. A., Pentecost, B. L. [23c], 3, *364*

Bennish, A., see Bing, R. J. [165], 82, 101, 130, 151, *326*

Bensaid, J., Castan, R., Sozutek, Y., Scebat, L., Lenegre, J. [24c], 227, *364*

— Sozutek, Y., Castan, R., Scebat, L., Lenegre, J. [25c] 227, *364*

— see Scebat, L. [1652], 215, 221, *352*

Benthe, H. F., ChenPanich, K. [134], 182, *325*

Benyamine, R., see Gerard, R. [637], 192, *334*

— see Jouve, A. [919, 920, 165c, 7d], 29, 279, 298, *339*, *367*, *371*

Bergen, S. S., jr., Van Itallie, T. B., Sebrell, W. H. [135], 15, *325*

Bergman, H., see Varnauskas, E. [1922], 9, *357*

Bergogne, C., see Kaufmann, H. [961], 164, *340*

Berk, M. S., see Haight, C. [764], 121, *337*

Berkesy, L. [136], 152, *325*

Berkowitz, W. D., Wit, A. L., Lau, S. H., Steiner, C., Damato, A. N. [11a], 220, *360*

— see Damato, A. N. [387, 388, 389], 3, *330*

— see Lau, S. H. [1081], 3, *342*

— see Rosenblum, A. J. [1555], 218, *351*

— see Scherlag, B. J. [1665], 3, *353*

Berlin, D. D., see Blumgart, H. L. [189], 20, *326*

Berman, B., see Scott, R. C. [1708], 158, *353*

Berman, E. R., see Zeller, E. A. [2046], 160, *360*

Berman, J. K., Fields, D. C., Judy, H., Mori, V., Parker, R. J. [137], 90, *325*

Bermudez, G. A., see Goldborg, A. N. [52a, 53a], 5, 148, 213, *361*

Bernal, P., Abiteboul, J. [138], 279, 280, *325*

Bernard, U., see Bretschneider, H. J. [227], 181, 183, *327*

— see Frank, A. [579], 156, *333*

Bernard-Brunel, J., see Macrez, C. [1205], 191, *344*

Berne, R. M. [139—142], 60, 74, *325*

— Blackmon, J. R., Gardner, T. H. [143], 59, 74, *325*

— Rubio, R. [26c, 27c], 45, 61, *364*

— see Bunag, R. D. [256], 62, 185, *327*

— see Driscol, T. E. [450], 60, *331*

— see Jacob, M. I. [883], 60, *339*

— see Katori, M. [945], 60, *340*

— see Rubio, R. [1581, 109a], 61, *351, 362*

— see Wolff, M. M. [2028], 60, 306, 309, *359*

Bernecker, C., Roetscher, I. [28c], 244, *364*

Bernhard, P., see Fölsch, E. [569], 198, *333*

Bernhardt, D., see Hohl, O. [62a], 290, *361*

Bernsmeier, A., Rudolph, W. [144], 267, *325*

— see Rudolph, W. [1582], 186, 187, *351*

Bernstein, A., Somon, F. [145], 115, *325*

— see Di Carlo, F. J. [427], *330*

Bernstein, H., see Enescu, V. [493], 83, *332*

— see Vyden, J. K. [330c], 134, *370*

Bernstein, L., Friesinger, G. C., Lichtlen, P. R., Ross, R. S. [146], 28, 83, 123, 130, 133, *325*

— Hawker, R., Catchlove, B. [29c], *364*

Berrettoni, J. N., see Page, I. H. [241c], 15, *368*

Berry, J. W., Carney, R., Lankford, H. [147], 147, *325*

Bertaccini, G., Impicciatore, M., Visioli, O., Malagnino, G. [148], 252, *325*

Berteau, P. [149], 279, 285, *325*

Bertrand, M., see Houdas, Y. [152c], 72, *366*

— see Warembourg, H. [1958, 14d], 163, 298, *358, 371*

Bertrand, M. E., see Warembourg, H. [335c], 211, *371*

Best, C. H., see Solandt, D. Y. [1771, 1772], 310, *355*

Best, M. M., Coe, W. S. [150, 151], 152, 158, *325*

— Duncan, Ch. H. [152], 15, *325*

Besterman, E. M. M., Friedlander, D. H. [153], 221, *325*

Betolami, V., see Batlouni, M. [103], 202, *324*

Betz, E., Braasch, D., Hensel, H. [154], 181, *325*

— Schmahl, F. W., Hensel, H. [155], 169, *325*

— see Schmall, F. W. [1676], 172, *353*

Beumer, H. M. [156, 157], 217, 229, 234, 244, 287, *325*

Beyer, E., see Gersmeyer, E. F. [646], 215, *334*

Beyer, J., see Enos, W. F. [497], 7, *332*

Bianchi, C., Lucchelli, P. E., Starcich, R. [159], 227, *325*

— Starcich, R., Lucchelli, P. E. [158], 227, *325*

Bianchi, G., see Visioli, O. [1944], 252, *358*

Bigger, J. T., Weinberg, D. I., Kovalik, A. T. W., Harris, P. D., Cranefield, P. C., Hoffman, B. F. [31c], 303, *364*

— see Goldreyer, B. N. [116c, 117c], 3, *366*

— see Strauss, H. C. [303c], 250, 251, *370*

Bijlsma, U. G., see Akker, S. van den [17], 308, *323*

Bijlsma, V. G., Funcke, A. B. H., Tersteege, H. M., Rekker, R. F., Ernsting, M. J. E., Nauta, W. T. [160], 308, *326*

Billiottet, J., Ferrand, J. [161], 309, *326*

Binak, K., see Regan, T. J. [1512], 310, *350*

Binder, M. J., Kalmanson, G. M., Drenick, E. J., Rosove, J. [162], 311, *326*

— see Kalmanson, F. M. [932], 141, *340*

Binet, L., Burstein, M. [163], 72, *326*

Bing, R. J. [164], 101, *326*

— Bennish, A., Bluemchen, G., Cohen, A., Gallagher, J. P., Zaleski, E. J. [165], 82, 101, 130, 151, *326*

— Cowan, C., Bottcher, D., Corsini, G., Daniels, C. G. [167], 22, 82, 84, 93, 123, 125, 126, 127, 130, *326*

Bing, R. J., see Cohen, A. [339], 130, 151, *329*

— see Cowan, C. [27a, 28a], 22, 28, 83, 122, 125, 126, 130, 134, *360*

— see Eckenhoff, J. E. [469], 79, *331*

— see Lombardo, T. A. [1171], 55, *344*

— see Luebs, E. D. [1192], 130, 133, 151, 178, 190, *344*

— see Mack, R. E. [1203], 82, *344*

— see Madeira, R. G. [1206], 2, *345*

— see Ogawa, K. [1386], 127, 135, *348*

— see Puri, P. S. [1475, 260c], 126, 127, 251, *349, 369*

— see Robin, E. [1543], 93, 126, 130, 131, 208, *350*

— see Stock, T. B. [1842], 24, 275, *356*

— see Wendt, V. E. [1976], 181, 186, *358*

— see Zaleski, E. J. [2042], 101, 178, 190, *359*

Binon, F., see Charlier, R. [318], 255, *328*

— see Deltour, G. [409], 255, *330*

Biörck, G. [168], 96, *326*

— Pannier, R. [169], 96, *326*

Birkett, D. A., Chamberlain, D. A. [170], 211, *326*

Birkhead, N. C., see Barry, A. J. [95], 10, *324*

Bisiani, M., Fresia, P., Genovese, E., Mortari, A. [171], 161, *326*

Bisteni, A., see Sodi-Pallares, D. [1767, 1768, 1769, 1770, 115a], 295, 296, *355, 362*

Bittar, N., Pauly, T. J. [12a], 185, *360*

— Sosa, J. A., Cronin, R. F. P. [172], 21, *326*

Bjerlov, H. [173], 311, *326*

Björk, L., Cullhed, I., Hallen, A. [174], 10, *326*

Björntorp, P. [175, 176], 233, *326*

— Ek, L., Olsson, S., Schröder, G. [177], 232, *326*

— Wallentin, I. [32c], 233, *364*

— see Varnauskas, E. [1922], 9, *357*

Black, A., see Gensini, G. G. [635], 124, *334*

Black, J. W., Crowther, A. F., Shanks, R. G., Smith, L. H., Dornhorst, A. C. [178], 205, 206, *326*

— Duncan, W. A. M., Shanks, R. G. [179], 205, *326*

Black, J. W., Stephenson, J. S. [180], 42, 175, 205, *326*

Black, S. [181], 304, *326*

Blackburn, C. H., Byrne, L. J., Cullum, V. A., Farmer, J. B., Levy, G. P. [182], 253, *326*

Blackman, A. L., see Batterman, R. C. [106], 154, 155, *325*

— see Grossman, A. J. [747], 155, *336*

Blackmon, J. R., see Berne, R. M. [143], 59, 74, *325*

Blalock, A., see Anrep, G. V. [43], 68, *323*

Blatter, K., see Imhof, P. R. [64a], 227, *361*

Blinks, J. R., [183, 13a] 206, 230, *326, 360*

— see McInerny, T. K. [1255], 215, 216, *345*

Block, P., see Demey, D. [412], 115, 202, *330*

— see Vastesaeger, M. [1925], 115, 202, *357*

Blömer, H., Schimert, G. [184], 309, *326*

Blomqvist, G., see Atkins, J. M. [13c], 252, *363*

Bloom, H. S., see Donoso, E. [441], 211, *331*

Bloom, N. [185], 163, *326*

Bloomfield, D. A., Sowton, E. [186], 211, *326*

Bluemchen, C., see Cohen, A. [339], 130, 151, *329*

Blümchen, G., Landry, F., Schlosser, V. [33c], 156, *364*

— see Bing, R. J. [165], 82, 101, 130, 151, *326*

Blum, K., see Peel, A. A. [1428], 187, *348*

Blumgart, H. L., Freedberg, A. S., Kurland, G. S. [187, 188], 20, *326*

— Riseman, J. E. F., Davis, D., Berlin, D. D. [189], 20, *326*

— Schlesinger, M. J., Zoll, P. M. [190], 137, *326*

— Zoll, P. M. [191], 19, 21, 53, *326*

— see Ellis, L. B. [489], 20, 96, *331*

Boake, W. C., see Rowe, G. G. [1573], 294, *351*

Boas, E. P., see Levy, H. [1122] 305, *343*

Bobb, A. L., see Greiner, T. [738], 110, 111, 112, 113, 116, 158, 308, *336*

— see Rinzler, S. H. [1528], 305, *350*

Bobb, J. R. R., Green, H. D. [192], 313, *326*

Boblitt, D. E., see Haight, C. [764], 121, *337*

Bodem, R., see Schaumann, W. [1661], 165, 174, *353*

Bodo, R. [193], 303, 304, *326*

Bögelmann, G., see Hockerts, T. [844], 181, 185, *338*

Boehm, G. [194], 151, *326*

Boerth, R. C., Covell, J. W., Pool, P. E., Ross, J. [195], 97, 246, *326*

Bogaert, M. G., Herman, A. G., De Schaepdryver, A. F. [34c], 136, *364*

— Rosseel, M. T., De Schaepdryver, A. F. [35c, 36c], 136, *364*

Bohning, A., see Katz, L. N. [954], 55, 68, 69, *340*

Bohr, D. F. [197], 63, *326*

— see Zuberbuhler, R. C. [2053], 44, *360*

Boissier, J. R., Giudicelli, J. F., Mouille, P. [37c], 242, 246, *364*

— Schmitt, H., Giudicelli, J. J., Viars, P. [198], 167, *326*

— see Giudicelli, J.-F. [669], *335*

Bolene-Williams, C., see Katz, L. N. [960], 264, *340*

Bollinger, A. [199], 218, *326*

Bonneau, H., see Audier, M. [63], 310, *324*

Bopp, P., see Gorlin, R. [698], 22, 100, 123, 129, 130, 133, *335*

Borroni, G. [38c], 253, *364*

Bory, M., see Audier, M. [61], 279, 287, *324*

Bosmans, P., Vercruyssen, J., Clerckx, A., Verselder, R., Van Hoorickx, G., Brugmans, J., Schuermans, V. [39c], 47, 114, 203, 204, *364*

Bosse, J. [200], 288, *326*

Bosse, J. A., Schaum, E. [14a], 175, 198, *360*

Bossoney, C., see Garrone, G. [626], 15, *334*

Boswood, J., see Armitage, A. K. [55], 156, *324*

Boszormenyi, E., see Enescu, V. [493], 83, *332*

Boszormenyi, F., see Vyden, J. K. [330c], 134, *370*

Bottcher, D., see Bing, R. J. [167], 22, 82, 84, 93, 123, 125, 126, 127, 130, *326*

Botteri, L., see Chiche, P. [325], 190, *328*

Botti, G., Visioli, O., Ambanelli, U. [201], 253, *326*

Botti, G., see Visioli, O. [1944, 1945], 252, *358*

Boucek, R. J., Takeshita, R., Brady, A. H. [4b], 20, *362*

Boufas, D., see Moret, P. R. [1322], 257, 268, 269, 286, *347*

Boulard, C., see Meriel, P. [1285], 170, *346*

Bounhoure, F., see Meriel, P. [1285], 170, *346*

Bounhoure, J., see Meriel, P. [1285], 170, *346*

Bourel, M., Lenoir, P. [202], *326*

Bourgault, P., see Karczmar, A. G. [939], 313, *340*

Bourne, G., see Evans, A. [510], 96, *332*

Bousvaros, G. A., see Hoeschen, R. J. [845], 126, *338*

Bouvrain, Y., Roudy, G., Marineaud, J.-P. [40c], 297, *364*

Bowers, D. L., see Singh, R. [294c], 91, *369*

Bovet, D., Bovet-Nitti, F. [203], 138, 148, *326*

Bovet-Nitti, F., see Bovet, D. [203], 138, 148, *326*

Boyd, L. J., see Huppert, V. F. [874], 137, *339*

Boyer, N. H. [204], 154, *326*

— Green, H. D. [205], 120, 122, 145, 152, 153, *326*

Boyle, A., see Fisch, S. [552], 146, *333*

Boyles, C. M., Sieber, H. A., Orgain, E. S. [206], 111, *326*

Boyles, S., see Adam, K. R. [1e], 239, 240, *371*

Bozeman, R. F., see Woods, E. F. [2036], 101, *359*

Bozer, J., see Brachfeld, N. [208], 122, 125, 126, 129, 130, 131, 169, *326*

Braasch, D., see Betz, E. [154], 181, *325*

Braasch, W., Buchhold, R. [41c], 138, *364*

— Fleck, D. [207], 165, *326*

Brachfeld, N., Bozer, J., Gorlin, R. [208], 122, 125, 126, 129, 130, 131, 169, *326*

— Scheuer, J. [209], 25, *326*

— see Case, R. B. [279], 52, *328*

— see Gorlin, R. [698, 699], 22, 100, 123, 129, 130, 133, *335*

Bradess, V. A., see Spain, D. M. [1802], *355*

Bradlow, B. A., see Zion, M. M. [2051], 187, *360*

Brady, A. H., see Boucek, R. J. [4b], 20, *362*

Brändström, A., Corrodi, H., Junggren, U., Jönsson, T. E. [210], 229, *326*

Brandfonbrener, M., see Geller, H. M. [634], 69, 75, 80, *334*

Brandi, G., see Torres, E. C. [1894], 63, *357*

Brandt, J. L., Caccese, A., Dock, W. [211], 121, 128, 131, 132, 136, *326*

Brasseur, L., see Piette, F. [249c], 93, *369*

Brasseur, L. A., see Detry, J. M. R. [81c], 21, *365*

Braun, C., see Guzman, F. [754], 21, *336*

Braunsteiner, H., Herbst, M., Sailer, S., Sandhofer, F. [212], 14, *326*

Braunwald, E. [213, 42c], 132, 221, *326, 364*

— Cohen, L. S. [214], 218, *326*

— Covell, J. W., Maroko, P. R., Ross, J. [15a], 41, *360*

— Epstein, S. E., Glick, G., Wechsler, A. S., Braunwald, N. [215], 37, *326*

— Frye, R. L., Aygen, M. M. [43c], 33, *364*

— Vatner, S. F., Braunwald, N. S., Sobel, B. E. [44c], 315, 316, *364*

— see Chidsey, E. A. [326], 199, *328*

— see Cohen, L. S. [342, 343], 218, *329*

— see Epstein, S. E. [500 to 505, 94c], 37, 173, 206, 207, 208, 214, 215, 217, 221, 222, 250, 315, 316, *332, 365*

— see Gaffney, T. E. [620], 43, 229, 286, *334*

— see Gleason, W. L. [671], 2, *335*

— see Klocke, F. J. [999, 1000] 63, 206, 264, *341*

— see Linhart, J. W. [1151], 3, 219, *344*

— see Mason, D. T. [86a], 130, 144, *361*

— see Robinson, B. F. [1545], 207, 284, *351*

— see Sarnoff, S. J. [1644], 29, 55, 92, 93, 132, 267, *352*

— see Sonnenblick, E. H. [1789, 1790, 1791], 31, 33, 92, 93, 132, 208, 268, *355*

— see Stampfer, M. [1816], 38, *355*

— see Vatner, S. F. [321c, 322], 316, *370*

— see Williams, J. F. [2002], 128, 131, 132, *359*

Braunwald, N., see Braunwald, E. [215], 37, *326*

Braunwald, N., see Epstein, S. E. [501], 37, 332

Braunwald, N. S., see Braunwald, E. [44c], 315, 316, *364*

— see Epstein, S. E. [94c], 315, 316, *365*

Bray, C. L., Dinda, P., Ojo, S. A., Riding, W. D., Sethna, D. S. [45c], 243, *364*

Brechtel, see Doll, E. [436], 186, *331*

Bredmose, P. [216], 171, *326*

Bregani, P., see Cova, N. [374], 187, *329*

Bremond, C., see Armand, P. [53], 279, *324*

Brenes, C., see Cardenas, M. [54c], 249, *364*

Brest, A. N., see Corman, A. [365], 14, *329*

Bretschneider, H. J. [217 to 225], 19, 52, 53, 58, 61, 62, 63, 71, 133, 183, 184, 185, 268, 269, *327*

— Eberlein, H. J., Kabus, H. M., Nelle, G., Reichmann, W. [226], 52, 62, 189, 190, 269, *327*

— Frank, A., Bernard, U., Kochsiek, K., Scheler, F. [227], 181, 183, *327*

— see Frank, A. [579], 156, *333*

— see Kubler, W. [190c], 185, *367*

— see Kübler, W. [1049, 1050, 1051], 62, 185, 186, *342*

— see Strauer, B. E. [302c], 94, *370*

Brichard, G., Zimmermann, P. E. [16a], 179, *360*

Brick, I., Hutchinson, K. J., McDevitt, D. G., Roddie, I. C., Shanks, R. G. [228], 243, *327*

— — Roddie, I. C., Shanks, R. G. [229], 240, *327*

Briggs, F. N., see Hess, M. H. [824], 216, *338*

Brink, A. J., see Lewis, C. M. [1132], 208, *343*

Briquemont, F. [230], *327*

Briscoe, W. A., see Enson, Y. [92c], 91, *365*

Bristow, J. D., Van Zee, B. E., Judkins, M. P. [46c], 34, *364*

Bristow, M., Green, R. D. [47c], 230, *364*

Brockington, I. M., see Cherian, G. [322], 218, *328*

Brodbin, P., O'Connor, C. A. [1d], 298, *371*

Brody, A. J. [231], 96, *327*

Broekhuysen, J. [232], 273, *327*

— Charlier, R. [48c], 270, *364*

— Debrucq-Larucl, A., Deltour, G. [235], 268, *327*

— — Sion, R. [236], 287, *327*

— Deltour, G., Ghislain, M. [233], 268, 272, *327*

— — — Delbruyere, M. [234], 268, *327*

— see Bekaert, J. [126], 169, 171, 172, *325*

— see Deltour, G. [408, 410, 411], 169, 268, 319, *330*

Brofman, B. L. [237], 7, *327*

Brogard, M., see Ablad, B. [3], 216, 230, 231, 234, *323*

Brondyk, H. D., see Schoepke, H. G. [1691], 189, *353*

Brook, C. G. D., see Gent, A. E. [636, 109c], 51, 187, *334, 366*

Brooke, O. G., see Wilson, A. G. [135a], 241, *362*

Brooks, A. M., see Grossman, A. J. [747], 155, *336*

Brooks, H., Banas, J., Meister, S., Szucs, M., Dalen, J., Dexter, L. [49c], 252, *364*

Brooks, H. L., Banas, J. S., Dalen, J. E., Dexter, L. [17a], 249, *360*

— — Meister, S., Szucs, M., Dalen, J., Dexter, L. [18a], 251, *360*

— see Stein, P. D. [1828, 1829], 209, *356*

Brooks, R. H., see Harris, W. S. [785], 207, *337*

Brotslow, J., Alexander, M., Gaines, M., McAllister, E. [50c], 316, *364*

Broustet, P. [238], 279, *327*

— Laporte, G. [239], 279, *327*

Brown, E. M., see Wegria, R. [1970], 157, 299, *358*

Brown, G. B., see Clarke, D. A. [332], 306, *329*

Brown, J. F., see Rowe, G. G. [1576], 304, *351*

Brown, J. H., Riggilo, D. A. [241], *327*

Brown, H. R., Hoffman, M. J., De Lalla, V. [240], 95, *327*

Brown, M. G., Riseman, J. E. F. [242], 154, *327*

— see Riseman, J. E. F. [1532, 1533, 1536], 106, 140, 141, 146, 304, *350*

Brown, N. L., see Lucchesi, B. R. [1189], 220, *344*

Brown, R. C., see Master, A. M. [1233], 95, 96, 103, 104, *345*

Brown, T. G., Green, T. J. [243], 313, *327*

— — Green, R. L. [244], 313, *327*

Browse, N. L., Hall, J. H. [51c], 50, 51, *364*

Brozek, J., see Taylor, H. L. [1875], 9, *356*

Bru, A., see Lesbre, J. P. [81a], 181, 186, *361*

Bruce, R. A., see Conn, R. D. [354], 212, *329*

— see Kasser, I. S. [944], 27, *340*

Bruce, T. A., see Stock, T. B. [1842], 24, 275, *356*

Brücke, F., Hertting, G., Lindner, A., Loudon, M. [245], 307, *327*

Brücknerova, O. [246], 309, *327*

Bruenn, H. G., see Levy, R. L. [1126, 1127, 1128, 1129], 96, 106, 136, 140, 154, *343*

— see Williams, N. E. [2003], 106, 154, *359*

Brugger, A., Salva, J. A., Sopena, M. [247], 193, *327*

Brugmans, J. [248], 47, 202, 204, *327*

— see Bosmans, P. [39c], 47, 114, 203, 204, *364*

— see Jageneau, A. [886], 203, *339*

Brunner, H., Hedwall, P. R., Meier, M. [249], 222, *327*

Brunton, T. L. [250], 131, 143, *327*

Bryant, H. H., see Krantz, J. C. [1027], 128, *341*

Buchhold, R., see Braasch, W. [41c], 138, *364*

Buckley, J. P., Aceto, M. D. G., Kinnard, W. J. [251], 146, *327*

— see Aceto, M. D. [8, 9], 146, *323*

— see Kelliher, G. J. [173c], 206, *367*

— see Kinnard, W. J. [985], 149, *341*

Budde, H., see Witzleb, E. [2023], 302, 303, *359*

Büchner, C., see Gebhardt, W. [633], 207, *334*

Bürgin, D. [260], 226, *327*

Buisson, P. [252], 190, *327*

Bulle, P. H. [254], 302, 308, *327*

Bulpitt, C. J. [255], 311, *327*

Bunag, R. D., Douglas, C. R., Imai, S., Berne, R. M. [256], 62, 185, *327*

Bunde, C. A., Grupp, I. L., Grupp, G. [19a], 294, *360*

— see Grupp, I. L. [130c], 294, *366*

Bunnell, I. L., see Falsetti, H. L. [96c], 35, *365*

— see Klocke, F. J. [181c], 23, *367*

Burch, G. E., De Pasquale, N. P. [258], 135, 137, *327*

— see Love, W. D. [1179], 82, *344*

— see De Pasquale, N. P. [415], 281, *330*

— see Shen, Y. [1738], 210, 215, *354*

— see Sun, S. C. [1856], 215, *356*

Burch, Ray [257], 21, *327*

Burchell, H. B., Pruitt, R. D., Barnes, A. R. [259], 96, *327*

— see Klakeg, C. H. [990], 96, *341*

— see Pruitt, R. D. [1474], 96, *349*

Burckhardt, D., see Straessle, B. [1848], 179, *356*

Burgess, P. A., see Jewitt, D. E. [162c], 241, *367*

Burgison, R. M., Lu, G. G., Krantz, J. C., jr. [261], 149, *327*

— see Hensala, J. C. [812], 156, *338*

Burkard, W. P., see Pletscher, A. [1455], 161, *349*

Burkart, F., Barold, S., Sowton, E. [262], 109, *327*

— see Schweizer, W. [1704], 16, *353*

Burkhart, K., see Kirchhoff, H. W. [987], 196, *341*

Burks, J. W., see De Pasquale, N. P. [415], 281, *330*

Burstein, M., see Binet, L. [163], 72, *326*

Busch, E. [263—265], 71, 88, 89, 314, *327*

— see Haas, H. [757, 758], 173, 178, *336*

Bussmann, W. D., Krayenbuehl, H. P. [266], 235, 237, 239, *327*

— Lochner, W. [267], 189, *327*

— Rauh, M., Krayenbuehl, H. P. [5b], 237, *363*

— see Scholtholt, J. [1694], 62, 63, 189, *353*

Butkus, A., see Page, I. H. [241c], 15, *368*

Butterfield, T. K., see Goldbarg, A. N. [52a, 53a], 5, 148, 213, *361*

Buyanov, V. V. [268], 139, 141, 146, *327*

Buyck, J., see Marion, J. [1220], 171, *345*

Buzzo, H. J., see Lands, A. M. [76a], 237, *361*

Bygdeman, S., see Eliasson, R. [87c], 50, *365*

Byrne, L. J., see Blackburn, C. H. [182], 253, *326*

Caccese, A., see Brandt, J. L. [211], 121, 128, 131, 132, 136, *326*

Caesar, K., see Jeschke, D. [898], 179, *339*

Cahen, P., Finas, C., Froment, R. [269], 162, *327*

Calazel, P., see Lesbre, J. P. [81a], 181, 186, *361*

Calder, R. M. [270], 313, *327*

Callsen, H. [271], 180, *327*

Calva, E., see Sodi-Pallares, D. [1767], 295, *355*

Cameron, A., Craver, B. N. [272], 66, *327*

— see Anderson, F. F. [31], 66, *323*

Campion, B., Frye, R., Zitnik, R. [20a], 130, *360*

Campus, S., Fabris, F., Rappelli, A., Mathis, I. [273], 135, *327*

— see Feruglio, F. S. [541, 542], 222, 248, *333*

Candaele, G., Vastesaeger, M. [274], 298, *327*

Candiani, C., see Fauda, C. [532], 162, *332*

— see Maggi, G. C. [1208], 162, *345*

Cannon, P. J., Dell, R. B., Dwyer, E. M. [52c], 318, *364*

Cannon, R., see Letac, B. [1111], 2, *343*

Cantor, S. A. [275], 180, 299, *327*

Cantwell, J. D., Fletcher, G. F. [21a], 10, *360*

Cappelen, C. [53c], 78, *364*

Caraffa Braga, E., see Granata, L. [123c], 206, *366*

Cardenas, M., Nadal, B., Sanz, G., Brenes, C. [54c], 249, *364*

Cardinael, Y., see Deshayes, P. [417], 172, *330*

Cardoe, N. [276], 168, *328*

Carlier, J. [55c, 2e], 16, 199, *364, 371*

Carlotti, J., see Soulie, P. [1797], 160, *355*

Carlsson, A., Hillarp, N. A., Waldeck, B. [277], 166, *328*

Carmichael, E., see Allmark, M. G. [22], 161, *323*

Carmichael, E. J., see Lu, F. C. [1182], 72, 151, 158, 310, *344*

Carney, R., see Berry, J. W. [147], 147, *325*

Carr, C. J., see Krantz, J. C. [1026, 1027, 1028, 1029, 1030], 128, 140, 144, 146, 311, *341*

Carr, H. A., see Levy, R. L. [1129], 96, 106, *343*

Carr, H. A., see Williams, N. E. [2003], 106, 154, *359*

Carr, W., see Cumming, G. R. [378, 379], 207, 208, 211, *329*

Carrol, J., see Reeves, T. J. [1511], 2, 268, *350*

Carson, R. P., Wilson, W. S., Nemiroff, M. J., Weber, W. J. [278], 125, 134, *328*

Carson, V., see Nayler, W. [1346, 1347, 1348, 1349, 1352], 174, 177, 179, 208, 216, 222, 245, 246, *347*

Carvalho, M., see Vyden, J. K. [330c], 134, *370*

Casalonga, J., see Pieri, J. [1443], *349*

Casalonga, L., see Pieri, J. [1442], 190, 309, *349*

Case, R. B., Brachfeld, N. [279], 52, *328*

— Nasser, M. G., Crampton, R. S. [56c], 27, *364*

— Roven, R. B. [280, 281], 22, 55, *328*

— see Parker, J. O. [1414, 1416, 1417, 242c, 243c], 25, 26, 27, 31, 32, 33, 131, 132, *348*, *368*

— see Sarnoff, S. J. [1644, 1645], 29, 55, 92, 93, 122, 132, 267, *352*

— see Wegria, R. [1969], 121, *356*

Cassin, S., see Zoll, P. M. [2052], 145, *360*

Castan, R., see Bensaid, J. [24c, 25c], 227, *364*

Castellanos, A., see Castillo, C. A. [58c], 3, *364*

— see Lemberg, L. [1099], 221, *343*

Castenholz, A. [282], 192, *328*

Castillo, C., see Rowe, G. G. [1576], 304, *351*

Castillo, C. A. [57c], 3, *364*

— Castellanos, A. [58c], 3, *364*

— see Maxwell, G. M. [1242, 1243], 153, *345*

— see Rowe, G. G. [1573, 1574], 81, 294, *351*

Castro De, B., Parchi, C. [283], 187, *328*

Catchlove, B., see Bernstein, L. [29c], *364*

Catinat, J., Sauvan, R. [285], 299, *328*

Catley, P. F., see Livesley, B. [207c], 25, *368*

Cattel, M. K., see Greiner, T. [738], 110, 111, 112, 113, 116, 158, 308, *336*

Caughey, D. E., see Norris, R. M. [1377], 217, *348*

Cazes, D., see Cesarman, T. [290], 139, *328*

Ceremuzynski, L., Staszewska-Barczak, J., Herbaczynska-Cedro, K. [286], 242, *328*

Cesarman, T. [287—289], 41, 160, 161, 162, *328*

— Cazes, D. [290], 139, *328*

Cevese, A., see Granata, L. [123c], 206, *366*

Ceyssens, W., see Vercruyssen, J. [1937], 170, *357*

Chaillet, F., see Baudine, A. [110], 257, 261, *325*

— see Charlier, R. [309, 310, 317], 256, 258, 259, 263, 266, 269, 271, 272, *328*

Chalmers, G. L., see Peel, A. A. [1428], 187, *348*

Chamberlain, D. A. [291], 207, *328*

— Davis, W. G., Mason, D. F. J. [292], 208, *328*

— Turner, P., Sneddon, J. M. [293], 207, 284, *328*

— see Apthorp, G. H. [48], 275, *323*

— see Birkett, D. A. [170], 211, *326*

Chambers, R. J., see Spracklen, F. H. [297c], 301, *370*

Chambliss, J., see Eckstein, R. W. [474], 306, *331*

Chamla, J. [294], 191, *328*

Chan, G. K., see Somani, P. [1782], 250, *355*

Chan, J., see Nayler, W. G. [1344], 242, *347*

Chandler, H. L., Mann, G. V. [295], 311, *328*

Chapman, D. W., Peterson, P. K., Morris, G. C., Howell, J., Liston Beazley, H., Winters, L. [59c], 12, *364*

Chari, R. S., see Vineberg, A. M. [1942], 182, *358*

Charlier, R. [296—308], 39, 42, 44, 66, 67, 121, 145, 150, 153, 156, 159, 161, 168, 169, 170, 197, 266, 269, 272, 273, 287, 308, *328*

— Baudine, A., Chaillet, F. [309], 259, 263, 269, 271, 272, *328*

— — Deltour, G. [310], 256, 266, *328*

— Delaunois, G., Bauthier, J. [311], 276, *328*

— — Deltour, G. [312], 276, *328*

— Deltour, G. [313, 313bis, 314, 315], 44, 170, 266, 269, 271, 276, *328*

— — Baudine, A. [316], 262, *328*

Charlier, R., Deltour, G., Baudine, A., Chaillet, F. [317], 258, 272, *328*

— — Tondeur, R., Binon, F. [318], 255, *328*

— Hosslet, A., Baudine, A. [319], 168, 169, *328*

— see Baudine, A. [110], 257, 261, *325*

— see Broekhuysen, J. [48c], 270, *364*

— see Delaunois, G. [78c], 266, *365*

— see Deltour, G. [408, 409, 411], 169, 255, *330*

— see Vastesaeger, M. [1926], 170, *357*

Chatillon, J. [320], 95, *328*

Chavez, I. [321], 7, *328*

Chelius, C. J., see Rowe, G. G. [1575], 140, *351*

Chen, K. K., see Henderson, F. G. [810], 151, *338*

ChenPanich, K., see Benthe, H. F. [134], 182, *325*

Cherian, G., Brockington, I. M., Shah, P. M., Oakley, G. M., Goodwin, J. F. [322], 218, *328*

Chesky, R., see Friedberg, C. K. [598], 96, *333*

Chesluck, H. M., see Aronow, W. S. [11c, 12c], 5, 110, 147, 148, *363*

Chessin, M., Dubnick, B., Leeson, G., Scott, C. C. [323], 163, *328*

Chevalier, H., Simon, J. [324], 160, *328*

— see Beaumont, J. L. [115], 311, *325*

Chevalier-Cholat, A. M. [166c], 316, *367*

— see Torresani, J. [313c], 316, *370*

Cheymol, J., see Bacq, Z. M. [67], 173, *324*

Chiche, P., Botteri, L., Derrida, J. [325], 190, *328*

— see Kalmanson, D. [168c], 78, *367*

— see Soulie, P. [1797], 160, *355*

Chidsey, E. A., Braunwald, E. [326], 199, *328*

— see Battock, D. J. [108, 109], 213, 214, *325*

— see Vogel, J. H. K. [127a], 43, *362*

Childers, R. W., see Goldborg, A. N. [52a], 148, 213, *361*

Chiong, M. A., see Parker, J. O. [1414, 1417, 243c], 25, 26, 27, 31, 33, 131, *348*, *368*

Chipperfield, D., see Nayler, W. G. [1345], 223, 245, *347*

Chirikdjian, J. J., see Kraupp, O. [1040, 1042], 192, 194, *342*
— see Niessner, H. [1368], 194, *347*
— see Raberger, G. [263c], 61, *369*
Chiti, E. [60c], 253, *364*
Cho, Y. W., Matsuo, S., Aviado, D. M. [22a], 294, *360*
— see Feinsilver, O. [39a], 294, *360*
Chobanian, A. V., see Hollander, W. [850, 851], 130, 314, *338*
Chou, C. C., Radawski, D., Gazitua, S., Scott, J. B. [23a], 235, *360*
Christakis, G., Rinzler, S. H., Archer, M., Winslow, G., Jampel, S., Stephenson, J., Friedman, G., Fein, H., Kraus, A., James, G. [327], 14, *328*
— see Schilling, F. J. [1668], 14, *353*
Christensen, R. C., see Hellems, H. K. [805], 59, *337*
Christensson, B., Karlefors, T., Westling, H. [328], 130, *329*
Christman, W. [329], 164, *329*
Cisneros, F., see Sodi-Pallares, D. [1769, 115a], 295, 296, *355, 362*
Clark, J. P., Kilmore, M. A., Victor, M., Terry, W. H., Orcutt, J. A. [61c], 237, *364*
Clark, L. C., jr., Wolf, R., Granger, D., Taylor, Z. [331], 74, *329*
Clark, M. L., see Shanks, R. G. [1730], 245, *354*
Clark, T. E., see Conn, J. J. [353], 158, *329*
Clarke, D. A., Davoll, J., Philips, F. S., Brown, G. B. [332], 306, *329*
Claeys, H., see Verstraete, M. [1939], 287, *357*
Clausen, J., Jorgensen, F. S., Roin, J., Felsby, M., Nielsen, B. L., Strange, B. [333], 217, 218, 221, *329*
Clausen, J. P., Larsen, O. A., Trap-Jensen, J. [334], 9, *329*
— Trap-Jensen, J. [62c, 63c], 9, *365*
Clayton, G. A., see Sandler, G. [1640, 1641, 280c], 138, 180, 241, *352, 369*
Cleempoel, H., see Lequime, J. [1103], 90, *343*
Clement, M., see Fourneau, J. P. [12b], 295, *363*

Clerckx, A., see Bosmans, P. [39c], 47, 114, 203, 204, *364*
Cloarec, M. [335, 2d], 165, 168, 187, *329, 371*
— Grosgogeat, Y. [6b], 293, *363*
Cobb, F., Bache, R., Ebert, P., Rembert, B., Greenfield, J. [336], 208, *329*
Cobb, F. R., Bache, R. J., Ebert, P. A., Rembert, B. S., Greenfield, J. C. [337, 24a], 208, *329, 360*
Cobbin, L. B., see Thorp, R. H. [1890], 306, *357*
Coblentz, B., see Beaumont, J. L. [115], 311, *325*
Code, C. F., Evans, C. L., Gregory, R. A. [338], 60, *329*
Coe, W. S., see Best, M. M. [150, 151], 152, 158, *325*
Cohen, A., Gallacher, J. P., Luebs, E. D., Varga, Z., Yamanaka, J., Zaleski, E. J., Bluemchen, C., Bing, R. J. [339], 130, 151, *329*
— see Bing, R. J. [165], 82, 101, 130, 151, *326*
— see Luebs, E. D. [1192], 130, 133, 151, 178, 190, *344*
— see Zaleski, E. J. [2042], 101, 178, 190, *359*
Cohen, B. M. [340, 64c], 15, *329, 365*
Cohen, E. I. [341], 20, *329*
Cohen, L. S., Braunwald, E. [342, 343], 218, *329*
— Elliott, W. C., Gorlin, R. [344], 83, 84, *329*
— Klein, M. D., Gorlin, R. [345], 4, 25, 275, *329*
— Rolett, E. L., Gorlin, R. [346], 25, 26, 30, 33, 38, *329*
— Vastagh, G. F., McLaughlin, E., Mitchell, J. H. [25a], 249, *360*
— see Atkins, J. M. [13c], 252, *363*
— see Braunwald, E. [214], 218, *326*
— see Epstein, S. E. [501, 94c], 37, 315, 316, *332, 365*
— see Gorlin, R. [700], 93, *335*
— see Yurchak, P. M. [2037], 36, *359*
Cohen, S. I., see Damato, A. N. [387], 3, *330*
— see Lau, S. H. [1080, 1082], 100, *342*
Cohn, L. J., see Donoso, E. [441], 211, *331*
Cole, R. E., Goldberg, R. I. [347], 143, *329*
Cole, S. L. [348], 111, *329*

Cole, S. L., Kaye, H., Griffith, G. C. [349, 350], 110, 111, 139, 141, 156, 302, *329*
Collard, M., see Faucon, G. [528], 298, *332*
Collier, J. G., Dornhorst, A. C. [26a], 237, *360*
Colman, R. W., see Pitt, B. [98a], 63, *362*
Coltart, D. J. [65c], 241, *365*
— Meldrum, S. J. [66c], 219, *365*
Cook, D. L., see Winbury, M. M. [2015], 67, *359*
Cooke, R., see Conway, E. J. [358], 185, *329*
Condorelli, L. [352], 37, 43, 275, *329*
Conn, J. J., Kissane, R. W., Koons, R. A., Clark, T. E. [353], 158, *329*
Conn, R. D., Bruce, R. A. [354], 212, *329*
Conolly, M. E., see Dollery, C. T. [36a], 205, *360*
Conti, C. R., Pitt, B., Gundel, W. D. [67c], 27, *365*
— — — Friesinger, G. C., Ross, R. S. [3d], 24, 28, *371*
— see Pitt, B. [98a], 63, *362*
Contro, S., Haring, O. M., Goldstein, W. [356], 144, *329*
Constantin, B., Ardisson, J. L., Gasparini, J. J. [355], *329*
Conway, C. M. [357], 309, *329*
Conway, E. J., Cooke, R. [358], 185, *329*
Conway, N. [359], 300, 301, *329*
— Gupta, G. D., Sowton, E. [360], 191, *329*
— Seymour, J., Gelson, A. [361], 215, 221, *329*
Corbascio, A. N., see Pedersen, E. [1824], 95, *356*
Corbetta, F., see Tartara, A. [1873], 160, *356*
Corcondilas, A., Roubelakis, G., Ioannidis, P., Koroxenidis, G., Tsitouris, G., Michaelides, G. [362], 228, *329*
— see Koroxenidis, G. [1019], 223, *341*
— see Lekos, D. [1098], 226, *343*
Corcoran, A. C., Zimmermann, H. A., Cuturelli, R. [363], 228, 314, *329*
Corday, E., see Enescu, V. [493], 83, *332*
— see Vera, L. B. de [1936], 74, *357*
— see Vyden, J. K. [330c], 134, *370*

Corliss, R. J., see McKenna, D. H. [1258], 42, 207, 209, 272, 274, *345*
— see Rowe, G. G. [1578], 22, *351*
— see Thomsen, J. H. [1888], 200, 201, *357*
Corman, A., Brest, A. N. [365], 14, *329*
Correia Ralha, A., see Moniz de Bettencourt, J. [1314], 159, *347*
Correll, H. L., see Meyer, J. M. [1293], 152, *346*
Corrodi, H., see Brändström, A. [210], 229, *326*
Corsini, G., see Bing, R. J. [167], 22, 82, 84, 93, 123, 125, 126, 127, 130, *326*
— see Cowan, C. [27a], 22, 28, 82, 83, 125, 126, 130, 134, *360*
Cova, N., Bregani, P. [374], 187, *329*
Covell, J. W., see Boerth, R. C. [195], 97, 246, *326*
— see Braunwald, E. [15a], 41, *360*
— see Sonnenblick, E. H. [1791], 93, 132, 268, *355*
Covino, B. G., see Belliveau, R. E. [128], 230, *325*
Cosby, R. S., Mayo, M. [366], 97, *329*
Coscia, L., see Marmo, E. [1223, 1224], 208, 245, 250, *345*
Cosnier, D., see Duchene-Marullaz, P. [456, 457, 8b], 164, 178, 200, 268, 292, 295, *331, 363*
Cossio, P. [367], 160, 161, *329*
Cott, L., see Strauer, B. E. [302c], 94, *370*
Cotterill, J. A., Hughes, J. P., Jones, R., Paulley, J. W., Robertson, P. D. [69c], 295, *365*
Cottet, J. [368, 369], 15, 16, *329*
— Mathivat, A., Redel, J. [370], 15, *329*
— Vittu, C. [371], 172, *329*
— see Mathivat, A. [1238], 15, *345*
— see Richet, G. [1525], 172, *350*
Cottier, P., see Strausak, A. [1849], 160, *356*
Coulshed, N. [372], 96, *329*
Courbier, R., see Torresani, J. [313c], 316, *370*
Cournand, A., see Enson, Y. [92c, 93c], 91, *365*
Courtadaon, M., see Alix, B. [6c], 279, 286, 288, *363*

Courvoisier, S., Fournel, J., Ducrot, R., Kolsky, M., Koetschet, P. [373], 302, *329*
Coutinho, C. B., see Di Carlo, F. J. [427], *330*
Cowan, C., Duran, P. V. M., Corsini, G., Goldschlager, N., Bing, R. J. [27a], 22, 28, 82, 83, 125, 126, 130, 134, *360*
— Rival, J., Mathes, P., Bing, R. [28a], 122, *360*
— see Bing, R. J. [167], 22, 82, 84, 93, 123, 125, 126, 127, 130, *326*
— see Robin, E. [1543], 93, 126, 130, 131, 208, *350*
Cowan, M., Friedman, J., Feigl, E., Waldhausen, J. A. [70c], *365*
Cox, A. G. C., see Allanby, K. D. [21], 163, *323*
Cox, A. R., see Pitt, W. A. [1451], 219, *349*
Cox, J. L., McLaughlin, V. W., Flowers, N. C., Moran, L. G. [29a], 41, *360*
Cox, J. W., see Dwyer, E. M. [465, 9b], 211, 214, *331, 363*
— see Wiener, L. [1993, 1994], 33, 214, *358*
Craig, R. J., see Laraia, P. J. [196c], *367*
Crampton, R. S., see Case, R. B. [56c], 27, *364*
Cranefield, P. C., see Bigger, J. T. [31c], 303, *364*
Cranefield, P. F., see Bartelstone, H. J. [97], 70, *324*
Craven, P., Pitt, B. [375], 210, *329*
— see Pitt, B. [252c], 210, *369*
Craver, B. N., see Anderson, F. F. [32], 66, *323*
— see Cameron, A. [272], 66, *327*
Creux, G., see Schweizer, W. [1704], 16, *353*
Crew, M. C., see Di Carlo, F. J. [427], *330*
Criollos, R. L., Al-Shamma, A. M., Roe, B. B. [376], 10, *329*
Crislip, R. L., see Popovich, N. R. [1461], 123, *349*
Croce, G., see Ferrini, R. [540, 100c], 252, 254, *332, 365*
Croke, R. P., see Kot, P. A. [1022], 144, *341*
Cronin, R. F., Edelstein, M., Rose, C. [71c], 59, *365*
Cronin, R. F. P., see Bittar, N. [172], 21, *326*
Cros, L., see Kabela, E. [67a], 63, *361*

Cross, D., see Frick, M. H. [592], 4, 30, 34, 93, 100, 109, 128, 130, 133, *333*
— see Sowton, E. [1798, 1799], 4, 93, 100, 128, 240, *355*
Cross, D. F. [68c], 30, 34, *365*
Crowther, A. F., see Barrett, A. M. [93], 235, 236, 242, *324*
— see Black, J. W. [178], 205, 206, *326*
Crumpton, C. W., see Afonso, S. [13, 2a], 186, 201, 202, *323, 360*
— see Maxwell, G. M. [1242, 1243], 153, *345*
— see McKenna, D. H. [1257, 1258], 4, 42, 207, 209, 272, 274, *345*
— see Rowe, G. G. [1573 to 1576], 81, 140, 294, 304, *351*
Cuellar, A., Medrano, G., Arriaga, J., Hernandez, A. [72c], 295, *365*
Cugurra, F., Echinard-Garin, P. [377], 156, *329*
Cullhed, I., see Björk, L. [174], 10, *326*
Cullum, V. A., see Blackburn, C. H. [182], 253, *326*
Cumler, W., see Hellerstein, H. K. [807], 10, *337*
Cumming, G. R., Carr, W. [378, 379], 207, 208, 211, *329*
Cundey, P. E., Leet, C. J., Field, D. E., Frank, M. J. [73c], 174, 175, *365*
Cuq, G., see Deodati, F. [80c], 287, *365*
Cureton, T. K., see Holloszy, J. O. [854], 10, *338*
Curry, C. L., see Zeft, H. J. [345c], 303, *371*
Curwen, M. P., see Davies, P. [392], 171, *330*
Cuturelli, R., see Corcoran, A. C. [363], 314, *329*
Czerwonka, L. J., see Gregg, D. E. [729], *336*

Dack, S., see Master, A. M. [1231, 1232], 110, 111, 136, 154, *345*
Dagenais, G., see Pitt, B. [1450] 100, *349*
Dagenais, G. R., Pitt, B., Mason, R. E., Friesinger, G. C., Ross, R. S. [74c], 140, 143, 233, *365*
D'Agostino, L., see Scaffidi, V. [1648], 313, *352*
Dailey, R. A., see Fellows, E. J. [534], 157, *332*

Dailheu-Geoffroy, O. [380, 381, 382, 383], 139, 141, 164, 170, *330*
— Nataf, J. [384, 385], 170, *330*
Dale, N., see Stock, J. P. P. [1841], 207, 217, *356*
Dalen, J., see Brooks, H. [49c], 252, *364*
Dalen, J. E., see Brooks, H. L. [17a, 18a], 249, 251, *360*
Dall, J. L., see Peel, A. A. [1428], 187, *348*
Dallavalle, L., see Visioli, O. [1944, 1945], 252, *358*
Dalle, X., Meltzer, L. E. [386], 8, *330*
Dallemagne, M. J., see Bacq, Z. M. [67], 173, *324*
Daly, J. W., see Barry, A. J. [95], 10, *324*
Damato, A. N. [75c], 3, *365*
— Lau, S. H. [30a], 3, *360*
— — Helfant, R. H., Stein, E., Berkowitz, W. D., Cohen, S. I. [387], 3, *330*
— — — Patton, R. D., Scherlag, B. J., Berkowitz, W. D. [388], 3, *330*
— — Patton, R. D., Steiner, C., Berkowitz, W. D. [389], 3, *330*
— see Berkowitz, W. D. [11a], 220, *360*
— see Lau, S. H. [1080, 1081, 1082], 3, 100, *342*
— see Scherlag, B. J. [1665], 3, *353*
— see Steiner, C. [1831], 273, *356*
Dammann, J. F., see Singh, R. [294c], 91, *369*
Daniels, C. G., see Bing, R. J. [167], 22, 82, 84, 93, 123, 125, 126, 127, 130, *326*
Danowski, T. S., see Vester, J. W. [324c], 16, *370*
Danta, G., see Acheson, J. [2c], 51, *363*
Darby, T. D., Aldinger, E. E. [390], 129, *330*
— see Schoepke, H. G. [1691], 189, *353*
Dart, C. H., Scott, S., Fish, R., Takaro, T. [76c], 11, *365*
Data, P. G., see Granata, L. [123c], 206, *366*
D'Avanza, F. B., see Marmo, E. [1225], 223, *345*
Davies, D. F., Gropper, A. L., Schroder, H. A. [391], 21, *330*
Davies, J. P. H., see Balcon, R. [79], 217, 218, 221, *324*
Davies, P., Oram, S., Curwen, M. P. [392], 171, *330*

Davies, R. O., Mizgala, H. F., Khan, A. S. [31a], 148, 213, *360*
— see Harley, B. J. S. [783], 211, *337*
— see Mizgala, H. F. [89a, 90a] 212, *361*
Davis, D., see Blumgart, H. L. [189], 20, *326*
Davis, F. W., see Scarborough, W. R. [1651], 95, *352*
Davis, J. A., Wiesel, B. H. [393], 138, *330*
Davis, L. D., Temte, J. V. [7b], 219, *363*
Davis, R. O., see Mizgala, H. F. [1303, 1304], 211, 215, *346*
Davis, T. C., see Gent, G. [47a], 243, *361*
Davis, W. G., Macdonald, D. C., Mason, D. F. J. [394], 42, 209, *330*
— see Chamberlain, D. A. [292], 208, *328*
Davoll, J., see Clarke, D. A. [332], 306, *329*
Davy, M., see Fourneau, J. P. [12b], 295, *363*
Dawber, T. R., see Kannel, W. B. [935, 20b], 14, 16, *340*, *363*
Dawes, G. S. [395], 60, *330*
— Mott, J. C., Vane, J. R. [396], 72, *330*
Dawson, P. M. [397], 9, *330*
Dayton, S., Pearce, M. L. [398], 15, *330*
— — Hashimoto, S., Dixon, W. J., Tomiyasu, U. [399], 15, *330*
De Boyrie, E., see Robin, E. [1543], 93, 126, 130, 131, 208, *350*
De Caro, L., Baldrighi, V., Baldrighi, G., Gorini, M. [77c], 247, *365*
De Champlain, J. A., see Tremblay, G. M. [315c], 250, *370*
De Fazio, V., see Nylin, G. [1380], 96, *348*
De Geest, H., Piessens, J. [400], 115, 202, 203, *330*
— see Dotremont, G. [445], 217, 221, *332*
— see Piessens, J. [31b], 204, *363*
De Graff, A. C., Lyon, A. F. [401], 187, *330*
— see Gagliani, J. [621], 155, *334*
De Lalla, V., see Brown, H. R. [240], 95, *327*
De Micheli, A., see Sodi-Pallares, D. [1767—1770], 295, *355*

De Pasquale, N. P., Burks, J. W., Burch, G. E. [415], 281, *330*
— see Shen, Y. [1738], 210, 215, *354*
— see Sun, S. C. [1856], 215, *356*
De Schaepdryver, A. F., Tasson, J., Lamont, H. [416], 167, *330*
— see Bogaert, M. G. [34c to 36c], 136, *364*
De Schryver, C., see Lammerant, J. [193c], 306, *367*
De Soldati, L. [418], 95, *330*
— Navarro-Viola, R., Mejia, R. H. [419], 95, *330*
De Sousa Borges, A., see Silva Maltez, J. [1753], 171, *354*
De Vernejoul, P., see Di Matteo, J. [83c], 23, *365*
Dear, H. D., see Rackley, C. E. [264c], 35, *369*
Debreceni, L., see Szentivanyi, M. [1869, 1870], 64, *356*
Debrucq-Laruel, A., see Broekhuysen, J. [235], 268, *327*
Decalf, A., see Desruelles, J. [420], 164, *330*
Defazio, V., see Regan, T. J. [1512], 310, *350*
Degraff, A. C., see Fisch, S. [552, 553], 117, *333*
— see Wax, D. S. [1963], 302, *358*
Degré, S., see Messin, R. [1290], 98, *346*
Dejouhannet, S., see Pieri, J. [1442], 190, 309, *349*
Delaunois, A. L. [402], 91, *330*
Delaunois, G., Bauthier, J., Charlier, R. [78c], 266, *365*
— see Charlier, R. [311, 312], 276, *328*
Delbarre, F., Auscher, C., Olivier, J. L., Rose, A. [403], 172, *330*
Delbianco, P. L., see Sicuteri, F. [1750], 249, *354*
Delbruyere, M., see Broekhuysen, J. [234], 268, *327*
Deleixhe, A., Delrée, G. [404], 279, 280, *330*
Delius, W. [405], 218, *330*
Dell, H. D., see Lorenz, D. [83a], 182, 189, 193, *361*
Dell, R. B., see Cannon, P. J. [52c], 318, *364*
Della Bella, D., see Teotino, U. M. [1877], 248, *356*
Delle, M., see Rice, A. J. [106a], 251, *362*
Delman, A. J., see Rosenblum, R. [1554, 1555, 108a], 218, *351*, *362*

Delomez, M., see Warembourg, H. [1959], 164, *358*

Delrée, G., see Deleixhe, A. [404], 279, 280, *330*

Deltour, G. [406, 407, 79c], 6, 169, 172, 319, *330, 365*

— Bekaert, J., Broekhuysen, J., Charlier, R. [408], 169, *330*

— Binon, F., Tondeur, R., Goldenberg, C., Henaux, F., Sion, R., Deray, E., Charlier, R. [409], 255, *330*

— Broekhuysen, J. [410], 268, 319, *330*

— Charlier, R., Broekhuysen, J. [411], 169, *330*

— see Bekaert, J. [126], 169, 171, 172, *325*

— see Broekhuysen, J. [233, 234, 235], 268, 272, *327*

— see Charlier, R. [310, 312, 313, 313 bis, 314—318], 44, 170, 255, 256, 258, 262, 266, 269, 271, 272, 276, *328*

— see Michel, R. [1297], 268, *346*

Demart, F., see Gerard, R. [111c], 315, *366*

Demey, D., Dernier, J., Block, P., Paesmans, M. [412], 115, 202, *330*

Demming, J., see Eckstein, R. W. [474, 475], 74, 306, *331*

Den Bakker, P. B., see Wendt, V. E. [1976], 181, 186, *358*

Denis, B., Grunwald, D., Rival, M. A., Mallion, J. M., Avezou, F., Lanney, E., Martin-Noel, P. [32a], 279, *360*

Denis, J.-C., see Libermann, D. [1135], 163, *343*

Denison, A. B., Bardhanabaedya, S., Green, H. D. [413], 312, *330*

— Spencer, M. P., Green, H. D. [414], 74, *330*

— see Richardson, A. W. [1522], 74, *350*

Denolin, H., see Messin, R. [1290], 98, *346*

Deodati, F., Bec, P., Cuq, G., Vergnes, R. [80c], 287, *365*

Derai, C., see Kalmanson, D. [168c], 78, *367*

Deray, E., see Deltour, G. [409], 255, *330*

Dernier, J., see Demey, D. [412], 115, 202, *330*

Derowsne, C., see Gautier, J. C. [107c], 51, *366*

Derrida, J., see Chiche, P. [325], 190, *328*

Deryagina, G. P., see Ganelina, J. E. [623], 295, *334*

Desauctis, R. W., see Kastor, J. A. [68a], 4, *361*

Deshayes, P., Cardinael, Y. [417], 172, *330*

Desruelles, J., Decalf, A., Waucampt, J. J. [420], 164, *330*

Dessen, E., see Wolffe, J. B. [2029], 309, *359*

Dessy, P., see Feruglio, F. S. [541, 542], 222, 248, *333*

Detry, J. M., see Piette, F. [249c], 93, *369*

Detry, J. M. R., Piette, F., Brasseur, L. A. [81c], 21, *365*

Detry, R., Lachieze-Rey, E., Raymond, J., Pont, M. [421], 279, *330*

Deuticke, B., Gerlach, E. [422], 62, 185, *330*

— see Gerlach, E. [643], 185, *334*

Devin, R., see Audier, M. [63], 310, *324*

Dewar, H. A., Grimson, T. A. [423], 136, 158, *330*

— Horler, A. R., Newell, D. J. [424], 141, 160, 162, *330*

— Newell, D. J. [425], 170, 171 *330*

— see Srivastava, S. C. [1812], 211, *355*

Dexter, D., see Hale, G. [765], 100, *337*

Dexter, L., see Brooks, H. L. [17a, 18a, 49c], 249, 251, 252, *360, 364*

D'Heer, H. [426], 170, *330*

Dhall, D. P., see Arfors, K. E. [10c], 51, *363*

Dharamadhach, A., see Krug, A. [189c], 183, *367*

Diament, M. L., see Palmer, K. N. V. [93a], 244, *362*

Diane, P., see Audier, M. [61], 279, 287, *324*

Di Carlo, F. J., Crew, M. C., Sklow, N. J., Coutinho, C. B., Nonkin, P., Simon, F., Bernstein, A. [427], *330*

— Melgar, M. D. [33a], 119, *360*

Di Giorgi, S., see Gensini, G. G. [635], 124, *334*

— see Parker, J. O. [1415, 1418], 30, 36, 43, 128, 130, 131, *348*

Di Matteo, J., Vacheron, A., Lafont, H., Kellershohn, C., De Vernejoul, P., Mestan, J. [83c], 23, *365*

Di Paco, G. F., see Sorrentino, L. [1794], 158, *355*

Di Rosa, M., see Sorrentino, L. [1793, 1794], 158, 315, *355*

Didisheim, J. C., Uebersax, R. [428], 179, *330*

Didisheim, P. [82c], 51, *365*

Diederen, W., see Kadatz, R. [928], 124, 151, 182, *340*

Diekmann, L., see Bender, F. [20c], 246, *364*

— see Hösemann, R. [151c], 179, *366*

Dietz, A. J. [429], 146, *330*

Dietze, G., see Lydtin, H. [1198], 220, *344*

Diewitz, M., Lange, B. M. [34a], 179, *360*

Diflumeri, A. A., see Weisse, A. B. [131a], 146, *362*

Dighiero, J., Hazan, J., Aguirre, C. V., Rudolf, J. [430], 163, *330*

Dimond, E. G., Benchimol, A. [431], 30, *330*

Dinda, P., see Bray, C. L. [45c], 243, *364*

Dingle, J., see Gregg, D. E. [730], 76, *336*

D'Intino, S., see Reale, A. [1502], 226, *350*

Dittrich, W. [432], 296, *330*

Dixon, M. F., see Benaim, S. [130], 162, *325*

Dixon, W. F. [433], 300, *330*

Dixon, W. J., see Dayton, S. [399], 15, *330*

Doane, B. L., see Pyfer, H. R. [101a], 10, *362*

Dock, W. [434], 103, *330*

— see Brandt, J. L. [211], 121, 128, 131, 132, 136, *326*

Dodge, H. T., see Rackley, C. E. [264c], 35, *369*

Dodinot, B., see Faivre, G. [519], 279, *332*

Döring, H. J., see Fleckenstein, A. [561, 562], 166, 178, 216, 245, *333*

— see Grün, G. [748], 152, *336*

Doering, H. J., see Leder, O. [80a], 167, 175, *361*

Doerner, A. A., see Russek, H. I. [1613, 1615, 1616], 103, 104, 106, 135, 141, 151, 152, 154, 158, 311, 312, 313, *352*

Dörner, J., Wick, E. [443], 121, 150, 153, 156, 181, 299, 305, *331*

Dohadwalla, A. N., Freedberg, A. S., Vaughan Williams, E. M. [435], 215, 237, *331*

Doherty, J. E., see Talley, R. W. [1872], 141, *356*

Dolder, M., see Gurtner, H. P. [131c], 246, 247, *366*

Dolgin, M., see Simon, A. J. [1755], 151, *354*

Doll, E., Keul, J. [35a], 56, 186, *360*

Doll, E., Keul, J., Brechtel [436], 186, *331*
— see Keul, J. [974, 975], 187, *340*
Dollery, C. T., Paterson, J. W., Conolly, M. E. [36a], 205, *360*
Domok, L., see Karpati, E. [941, 942], 288, *340*
Donahue, D. D., see Von Oettingen, W. F. [1948], 138, 140, *358*
Donal, J. S., see Starr, I. [1823], 153, *356*
Donaldson, A., see Sloman, G. [1757], 10, *354*
Donat, K., see Witzleb, E. [2024], 309, *359*
Donato, L., Bartolomei, G., Federighi, G., Torreggiani, G. [437], 82, *331*
— — Giordani, R. [438], 82, *331*
Doneff, D., see Benda, L. [131], 179, *325*
Donnet, V., Duflot, J. C., Jacquin, M., Murisasco, A., Fornaris, M. [439], 165, *331*
— — — Peyrot, J., Pommier de Santi, P. [440], 165, *331*
Donoso, E., Cohn, L. J., Newman, B. J., Bloom, H. S., Stein, W. G., Friedberg, C. K. [441], 211, *331*
— see Master, A. M. [1229, 1230, 1236], 96, 103, *345*
— see Rosenfeld, I. [1556], 96, *351*
Dooley, J. V., see Griffith, G. C. [742], 311, *336*
Doret, J. P., see Ferrero, C. [538], 129, *332*
Dornaus, W. [442], 188, *331*
Dornhorst, A. C. [444], 212, *331*
— see Black, J. W. [178], 205, 206, *326*
— see Collier, J. G. [26a], 237, *360*
— see Shanks, R. G. [1730], 245, *354*
Dorris, E. R., see Kory, R. C. [1020], 141, *341*
Dorset, V. J., see Russek, H. I. [1619, 1620], 104, 105, 135, 137, 139, 141, 151, 152, 154, 158, 299, 311, 312, 313, *352*
Dotremont, G., De Geest, H. [445], 217, 221, *331*
Dotterweich, K., see Bender, F. [10a], 226, 233, 245, *360*
Dotterweich, W., see Bender, F. [20c], 246, *364*
Dotti, F., Piva, M., Ongari, R. [446], 249, *331*

Douglas, C. R., see Bunag, R. D. [256], 62, 185, *327*
Dow, W. I. M., see Szekely, P. [1867], 221, *356*
Dowling, C. V., see Eckstein, R. W. [478], 264, *331*
Dowling, J. T., see Vohra, J. K. [329c], 243, *370*
Downes, E. M., see Hills, E. A. [832], 178, 179, 180, *338*
Doyle, J. T., see Riff, D. P. [107a], 301, *362*
Drapeau, J. V., see Melville, K. I. [1271], 302, *346*
Draznin, N., see Hahn, N. [762, 135c], 197, *337, 366*
Drebinger, K. [84c], 192, *365*
Drechsel, U., see Raff, W. K. [103a, 265c], 122, *362, 369*
Drenick, E. J., see Binder, M. J. [162], 311, *326*
— see Kalmanson, F. M. [932], 141, *340*
Dresel, P. E. [447], 205, *331*
Dressel, J., see Gebhardt, W. [632], 181, *334*
Drews, A. [448], 196, *331*
Dreyfuss, F., see Wegria, R. [1970], 157, 299, *358*
Drill, V. A. [449], 118, *331*
Drimal, J., Aviado, D. M. [85c], 222, *365*
Drinnon, V., see Ben, M. [129], 163, *325*
Driscol, T. E., Berne, R. M. [450], 60, *331*
Drouillat, M., see Laubie, M. [1086], 58, *342*
Drumm, A. E., see Russek, H. I. [1620], 105, 137, 139, 141, 152, *352*
Drury, A. N., Szent-Gyorgyi, A. [451 bis], 305, *331*
— see Wedd, A. M. [1967], 305, *358*
Dry, T. J. [452], 96, *331*
Duarte Mantilla, G., see Balaguer-Vintro, I. [76], 279, 280, *324*
Dubinsky, A. A., see Angarskaya, M. A. [34], 304, *323*
Dubnick, B., see Chessin, M. [323], 163, *328*
Du Bois, R. [453], 217, *331*
DuBoureau, L. H., see Felix, H. [10b], 291, *363*
Duce, B. R., Garberg, L., Johansson, B. [454], 232, *331*
— — Smith, E. R. [86c], 232, *365*
Duchene-Marullaz, P., Cosnier, D., Grimald, J. [456, 457], 164, 178, 200, 268, 292, *331*
— — Perriere, J. P., Hache, J. [8b], 295, *363*

Duchene-Marullaz, P., Lavarenne, J. [455, 458], 164, 169, 298, *331*
— see Faucon, G. [528], 298, *332*
Ducrot, R., see Courvoisier, S. [373], 302, *329*
Dudik, E., see Henke, C. [811], 196, *338*
Duesel, B. F., Fand, T. I. [459], 155, *331*
Düx, A., Schaede, A. [464], 187, 190, *331*
— see Hahn, N. [762, 135c], 197, *337, 366*
Duflot, J. C., see Donnet, V. [439, 440], 165, *331*
Dulac, J. F., Many, P., Picard, P. [460], 307, *331*
Du Mesnil de Rochemont, W., see Madeira, R. G. [1206], 2, *345*
Dumke, P. R., Schmidt, C. F. [461], 74, *331*
Duncan, Ch. H., see Best, M. M. [152], 15, *325*
Duncan, W. A. M., see Black, J. W. [179], 205, *326*
Dungan, K. W., Lish, P. M. [462], 249, *331*
— see Lish, P. M. [1159], 216, 249, 250, *344*
Dunlop, D., Shanks, R. G. [463], 236, 237, *331*
— see Barrett, A. M. [93], 235, 236, 242, *324*
— see Shanks, R. G. [1729], 220, *354*
Dunn, M., see Bell, H. [127], 190, *325*
Duprat, R., see Batlouni, M. [103], 202, *324*
Duran, P. V. M., see Cowan, C. [27a], 22, 28, 82, 83, 125, 126, 130, 134, *360*
Durrer, D., see Schuilenburg, R. M. [288c], 3, *369*
Dustan, H. P., see Frohlich, E. D. [607], 218, *334*
— see Ulrych, M. [1911], 211, *357*
Dwyer, E. M. [3e], 33, 34, *371*
— Wiener, L., Cox, J. W. [465, 9b], 211, 214, *331, 363*
— see Cannon, P. J. [52c], 318, *364*
— see Wiener, L. [1993, 1994], 33, 214, *358*
Dzedin, T., see Aberg, G. [2], 249, 250, 251, *323*
Dziuba, K. [466], 202, *331*

Eakins, K. E., see Lord, C. O. [1176], 232, 235, *344*
Eberlein, H. J. [467], 60, *331*

Eberlein, H. J., see Bretschneider, H. J. [226], 52, 62, 189, 190, 269, *327*

Ebert, P., see Cobb, F. [336], 208, *329*

Ebert, P. A., see Cobb, F. R. [337, 24a], 208, *329, 360*

Echinard-Garin, P., see Cugurra, F. [377], 156, *329*

Eckel, R., see Eckstein, R. W. [478], 264, *331*

Eckenhoff, J. E., Hafkenschiel, J. H. [468], 121, 150, 153, *331*

— — Harmel, M. H., Goodale, W. T., Lubin, M., Bing, R. J., Kety, S. S. [469], 79, *331*

— — Landmesser, C. M. [470], 55, 74, *331*

— — — Harmel, M. [471], 56, *331*

— see Goodale, W. T. [691], 79, *335*

Ecker, R. R., see Keroes, J. [69a], 208, *361*

Eckhardt, W. F., see Goodyear, A. V. N. [693], 91, *335*

Eckmann, F., see Kuschke, H. J. [1062], 167, *342*

Eckstein, R. W. [472, 473], 8, *331*

— Chambliss, J., Demming, J., Wells, K. [474], 306, *331*

— McEachen, J. A., Demming, J., Newberry, W. B. [475], 74, *331*

— Newberry, W. B., McEachen, J. A., Smith, G. [476, 477], 122, 123, *331*

— Stroud, M., Eckel, R., Dowling, C. V., Pritchard, W. P. [478], 264, *331*

— see Gregg, D. E. [725, 730, 735], 73, 74, 76, *336*

Eddleman, E. E., see Hefner, L. L. [797], 138, *337*

Edelstein, M., see Cronin, R. F. [71c], 59, *365*

Edery, H., Lewis, G. P. [479], 21, *331*

Effler, D. B., see Favaloro, R. G. [533], 10, *332*

— see Fergusson, D. J. [535], 10, *332*

Eggen, D. A., see Strong, J. P. [305c], 16, *370*

Ehrenberger, W. [480], 149, *331*

Ehrlich, J. C., Shinohara, Y. [481], *331*

Eich, A. H., see Smulyan, H. [1763], 210, *354*

Eichholtz, F., see Hilton, H. [833], 20, 59, *338*

Eisel, K., Kaiser, H. [482], 180, *331*

Ejrup, B., Kumlin, T. [483], 148, *331*

Ek, L., see Ablad, B. [3], 216, 230, 231, 234, *323*

— see Björntorp, P. [177], 232, *326*

Ekstrom-Jodal, B., see Svedmyr, N. [308c], 211, 251, *370*

Elaerts, J., see Hardel, M. [58a] 279, *361*

Elek, S. R., Katz, L. N. [484, 485], 113, 151, 299, 304, *331*

Eliasson, R., Bygdeman, S. [87c], 50, *365*

Elkeles, R. S., Hampton, J. R., Honour, A. J., Mitchell, J. R. A. [88c], 51, *365*

Elliot, A. H., Nuzum, F. R. [486], 309, *331*

— see Nuzum, F. R. [1379], 309, *348*

Elliot, E. C. [487], 181, *331*

— see Pitt, B. [1449], 63, *349*

Elliott, M. S., see Lehan, P. H. [1093], 124, *343*

Elliott, W. C., Gorlin, R. [488], 25, 36, 43, 52, 58, 269, 284, *331*

— King, R. D., Ross, E., McHenry, P. L. [89c], 316, *365*

— Stone, J. M. [37a], 211, *360*

— see Cohen, L. S. [344, 345, 346], 4, 25, 26, 30, 33, 38, 83, 84, 275, *329*

— see Fallen, E. L. [521], 38, *332*

— see Gorlin, R. [700], 93, *335*

— see Herman, M. V. [817], 26, *338*

— see Kemp, H. G. [967], 48, *340*

— see Knoebel, S. B. [182c], 57, *367*

Ellis, F. W., see Krantz, J. C. [1029, 1030], 140, 146, *341*

Ellis, L. B., Blumgart, H. L., Harken, D. E., Sise, H. S., Stare, F. J. [489], 20, 96, *331*

— Hancock, E. W. [490], 142, *332*

Ellison, R. C., see Hugenholtz, P. G. [154c], 35, *367*

Ellsworth, W. J., see Haight, C. [764], 121, *337*

Elpern, B., see Karczmar, A. G. [939], 313, *340*

Emanuel, D. A., see Rowe, G. G. [1576], 304, *351*

Emele, J. F., Shanaman, J. E., Warren, M. R. [491], 161, *332*

Emmons, P. R., Harrison, M. J. G., Honour, A. J., Mitchell, J. R. A. [90c], 50, *365*

— see Mitchell, J. R. A. [223c], 51, *368*

Enescu, V., Boszormenyi, E., Bernstein, H., Corday, E. [493], 83, *332*

Endte, K. [492], 162, *332*

Engelberg, H., see Griffith, G. C. [742], 311, *336*

Engelhardt, A. [494], 245, *332*

Engelhorn, R., see Schmidt, L. [1682], 55, *353*

Engelking, H. [495], 138, *332*

Engle, E., see Starr, I. [1823], *356*

Enos, W. F. [496], 7, *332*

— Holmes, R. H., Beyer, J. [497], 7, *332*

Enright, L. P., Hannah, H. III., Reis, R. L. [91c], 30, *365*

Enselme, J. [498], 14, *332*

Enson, Y., Briscoe, W. A., Polanyi, M. L., Cournand, A. [92c], 91, *365*

— Jameson, A. G., Cournand, A. [93c], 91, *365*

Entman, M. L., Levey, G. S., Epstein, S. E. [38a], 216, *360*

Epstein, F. H. [499], 16, *332*

Epstein, S. E., Beiser, G. D., Goldstein, R. E., Redwood, D., Rosing, D. R., Glick, G., Wechsler, A. S., Stampfer, M., Cohen, L. S., Reis, R. L., Braunwald, N. S., Braunwald, E. [94c], 315, *365*

— — — Stampfer, M., Wechsler, A. S., Glick, G., Braunwald, E. [500], 37, *332*

— — Stampfer, M., Glick, G., Wechsler, A. S., Goldstein, R. E., Cohen, L. S., Braunwald, N., Braunwald, E. [501], 37, *332*

— Braunwald, E. [502, 503, 504], 173, 206, 208, 214, 215, 217, 221, 222, 250, *332*

— Robinson, B. F., Kahler, R. L., Braunwald, E. [505], 207, 208, *332*

— see Braunwald, E. [215], 37, *326*

— see Entman, M. L. [38a], 216, *360*

— see Glancy, D. L. [51a], 34, *361*

— see Goldstein, R. E. [54a, 55a, 118c], 147, *361, 366*

— see Levey, G. S. [1114], 273, *343*

Epstein, S. E., see O'Brien, K. P. [1384], 30, 34, 100, *348*
— see Redwood, D. R. [266c], 106, *369*
— see Robinson, B. F. [1545], 207, 284, *351*
— see Stampfer, M. [1816], 38, *355*
Eral, N. [506], 196, *332*
Erbring, H., Uebel, H., Vogel, G. [507], 159, *332*
Erle, G., see Vettori, G. [1940], 228, *358*
Ernould, H., see Plomteux, G. [1458], 288, *349*
Ernsting, M. J. E., see Bijlsma, V. G. [160], 308, *326*
Ersova, see Rajevskaja 191
Escobar, E., see Murray, J. F. [1333], 207, *347*
Essex, H. E., Herrick, J. F., Baldes, E. J., Mann, F. C. [508], 120, 306, *332*
— Wegria, R., Herrick, J. F., Mann, F. C. [509], 120, 150, 153, 299, 306, 307, *332*
— see Hausner, E. [791], 55, *337*
— see Leusen, I. R. [1112], 158, *343*
— see Wegria, R. [1968], 120, 150, 153, *358*
Estrellado, T., see Jablons, B. [882], 137, *339*
Etcheverry, J., see Fermoso, J. [99c], 175, 179, *365*
Evans, A., Bourne, G. [510], 96, *332*
Evans, C. L. [511], 92, *332*
— Starling, E. H. [512], 68, *332*
— see Code, C. F. [338], 60, *329*
Evans, W. [513], 7, *332*
— Hoyle, C. [514, 515], 110, 113, 136, 150, 154, 300, 309, *332*
Evreux, J. C., see Faucon, G. [529—531], 188, 189, *332*

Fabel, H., see Wettengel, R. [15d], 234, *371*
Fabris, F., see Campus, S. [273], 135, *327*
Facquet, J., Nivet, M. [516], 279, 280, *332*
— — Alhomme, P., Rahari-son, S., Grosgogeat, Y. [518], 280, 287, *332*
— — Grosgogeat, Y., Alhom-me, P., Vachon, J. [517], 286, *332*
— see Welti, J. J. [1975], 162, *358*
Fahim, I., see Samaan, K. [1634], 159, *352*

Faivre, G., Dodinot, B., Hua, G., Schmidt, C. [519], 279, *332*
— Gilgenkrantz, Lagarde, Vincent, Frenkiel [520], 97, *332*
Falicov, R. E., Resnekov, L., Kocandrle, V., King, S., Kittle, C. F. [95c], 316, *365*
Fallen, E. L., Elliott, W. C., Gorlin, R. [521], 38, *332*
Falsetti, H. L., Mates, R. E., Grant, C., Greene, D. G., Bunnell, I. L. [96c], 35, *365*
— see Klocke, F. J. [181c], 23, *367*
Fam, W. H., see McGregor, M. [1252], 48, 55, 58, 125, *345*
Fam, W. M., McGregor, M. [522, 523, 524], 53, 86, 124, 134, 182, *332*
— see Hoeschen, R. J. [845], 126, *338*
Fanciullacci, M., see Sicuteri, F. [1750], 249, *354*
Fand, T. I., see Duesel, B. F. [459], 155, *331*
Farmer, J. B., Levy, G. P. [525, 526], 249, 250, *332*
— see Blackburn, C. H. [182], 253, *326*
Farrehi, C., Perley, A., Ritz-mann, L. W., Malinow, M. R., Judkins, M. R., Gris-wold, H. E. [527], 14, *332*
Faucon, G., Duchene-Marul-laz, P., Lavarenne, J., Schaff, G., Sagols, L., Col-lard, M. [528], 298, *332*
— Evreux, J. C., Kofman, J., Perrot, E. [529], 189, *332*
— — Lavarenne, J., Kof-man, J., Perrot, E. [530], 189, *332*
— Lavarenne, J., Kofman, J., Evreux, J. C. [531], 188, 189, *332*
— see Jourdan, F. [912—917], 70, 153, 156, 157, 158, 160, 298, 313, *339*
Fauda, C., Candiani, C. [532], 162, *332*
— see Maggi, G. C. [1208], 162, *345*
Favalaro, R. G. [97c], 12, *365*
— Effler, D. B., Groves, L. K., Fergusson, D. J. G., Loza-da, J. S. [533], 10, *332*
Fawaz, G., see Simaan, J. [1754], 182, *354*
Fayard, J. M., see Barrillon, A. [17c], 163, *364*
Federighi, G., see Donato, L. [437], 82, *331*

Fedina, L., see Solti, F. [296c], 316, *370*
Feigl, E., see Cowan, M. [70c], *365*
Feigl, E. O. [98c], 316, *365*
Fein, H., see Christakis, G. [327], 14, *328*
Feinberg, H., see Gerola, A. [644, 645], 29, 264, 267, *334*
— see Katz, L. N. [960], 264, *340*
— see Lafontant, R. [1067], 68, 75, *342*
Feinsilver, O., Aviado, D. M., Cho, Y. W. [39a], 294, *360*
Feldman, A., see Marchioro, T. [213c], 81, *368*
Felix, H., DuBoureau, L. H., Saby, G. [10b], 291, *363*
Felix, R., see Hahn, N. [762, 135c], 197, *337*, *366*
Fellows, E. J., Killam, K. F., Toner, J. J., Dailey, R. A., Macko, E. [534], 157, *332*
— see Killam, K. F. [983], 157, *341*
Felsby, M., see Clausen, J. [333], 217, 218, 221, *329*
Fenn, G. K., see Gilbert, N. C. [657], 153, 300, *335*
— see Leroy, G. V. [1105], 154, *343*
Ferguson, R. K., see Rice, A. J. [106a], 251, *362*
— see Toubes, D. B. [314c], 252, *370*
Fergusson, D. J., Shirey, E. K., Sheldon, W. C., Effler, D. B., Sones, F. M. [535], 10, *332*
Fergusson, D. J. G., see Fava-loro, R. G. [533], 10, *332*
Fermoso, J., Fourcade, A., Etcheverry, J., Gobbee, R. [99c], 175, 179, *365*
Ferrand, J., see Billiottet, J. [161], 309, *326*
Ferrari, V., Finardi, G. [536], 160, *332*
Ferrero, C. [537], 162, *332*
— Arnold, E. F., Doret, J. P. [538], 129, *332*
— see Babel, J. [15c], 287, *363*
Ferrini, R. [539], *332*
— Miragoli, G., Croce, G. [540, 100c], 252, 254, *332*, *365*
Feruglio, F. S., Campus, S., Pandolfo, G., Dessy, P., Gagna, C., Uslenghi, E. [541, 542], 222, 248, *333*
Fiegel, G., Bargheer, R., Hein-dorf, M., Kukwa, D. [543], 190, *333*

Fiegel, G., Kelling, H. W., Bargheer, R., Kukwa, D. [544], 163, 190, *333*
— see Bargheer, R. [88], 159, *324*
— see Fischer, E. K. [554], 182, 187, *333*
Field, D. E., see Cundey, P. E. [73c], 174, 175, *365*
Field, L. E., see Master, A. M. [1230], 96, *345*
Fields, D. C., see Berman, J. K. [137], 90, *325*
Fierlafyn, E., Querton, M. [545] 293, *333*
Fife, R., Howitt, G., Stevenson, J. [546], 162, *333*
Figley, M. M., see Haight, C. [764], 121, *337*
Finardi, G., see Ferrari, V. [536], 160, *332*
Finas, C., see Cahen, P. [269], 162, *327*
Findlay, D., see Wolffe, J. B. [2029], 309, *359*
Finkelstein, A., see Shoshkes, M. [1748], 162, *354*
Fisch, S. [547, 548, 549, 550, 551], 117, 135, 139, 143, 164, 187, *333*
— Boyle, A., Sperber, R., Degraff, A. C. [552], 146, *333*
— Degraff, A. C. [553], 117, *333*
Fischer, E., see Szekeres, L. [1868], 150, 167, *356*
Fischer, E. K., Fiegel, C. [554], 182, 187, *333*
Fischer, G., see Kukovetz, W. R. [1056], 189, *342*
Fischer, K. [555], 179, *333*
Fish, R., see Dart, C. H. [76c], 11, *365*
Fishbein, M. [556], 163, *333*
Fisher, L. C., see Gregg, D. E. [726], 81, 92, *336*
Fishleder, B. L., see Sodi-Pallares, D. [1767, 1769, 1770], 295, *355*
Fishman, A. P., see Rosenman, R. H. [1557, 1558], 158, *351*
Fitzgerald, J. D. [557], 173, 205, 229, 251, *333*
— Barrett, A. M. [558, 559], 172, 173, 174, 177, 178, *333*
Fitzgerald, O., see Heffernan, A. [796], 16, *337*
Flament, G., see Merlen, J. F. [220c], 137, *368*
Flamm, M. D., Harrison, D. C., Hancock, E. W. [11b], 218, *363*

Flattery, K. V., Shum, A., Johnson, G. E. [560], 167, 168, *333*
Fleck, D., see Braasch, W. [207], 165, *326*
Fleckenstein, A., Döring, H. J., Kammermeier, H. [561], 166, 178, 216, 245, *333*
— Kammermeier, H., Döring, H. J., Freund, H. J. [562], 166, 178, *333*
— Tritthart, H., Fleckenstein, B., Herbst, A., Gruen, G. [563, 40a], 166, 178, *333*, *360*
— see Grün, G. [748], 152, *336*
— see Janke, J. [161c], 175, *367*
— see Leder, O. [80a], 167, 175, *361*
— see Tritthart, H. [125a], 179, 219, *362*
Fleckenstein, B., see Fleckenstein, A. [563, 40a], 166, 178, *333*, *360*
— see Tritthart, H. [125a], 179, 219, *362*
Fleming, J., Hamer, J. [564], 215, *333*
— see Hamer, J. [768, 136c], 207, *337*, *366*
— see Shinebourne, E. [1743, 1744], 211, 240, *354*
Fleming, J. G., see Somani, P. [1782], 250, *355*
Flemma, R. J., see Johnson, W. D. [164c], 12, 13, *367*
— see Walker, J. A. [333c], 13, *370*
Fletcher, G. F., Hurst, J. W., Schlant, R. C. [565, 566], 295, *333*
— see Cantwell, J. D. [21a], 10, *360*
Flowers, N. C., see Cox, J. L. [29a], 41, *360*
Fölsch, E., Bernhard, P. [569], 198, *333*
Foley, T. H., see Gent, A. E. [636, 109c], 51, 187, *334*, *366*
Folkow, B. [567], 306, *333*
Folle, L. E., Aviado, D. M. [568], 214, *333*
Foltz, E. L., Page, R. G., Sheldon, W. F., Wong, S. K., Tuddenham, W. J., Weiss, A. J. [570], 55, 81, *333*
Fontaine, J. L., Fontaine, R. [5d], 297, *371*
Fontaine, R., see Fontaine, J. L. [5d], 297, *371*
Ford, L., see Hunter, F. E. [873], 128, *339*

Forman, S. E., see Krantz, J. C. [1028—1030], 140, 144, 146, *341*
Fornaris, M., see Donnet, V. [439], 165, *331*
Forrester, J. S., see Helfant, R. H. [60a, 144c], 26, 33, *361*, *366*
Forsberg, S. A., Johnsson, G. [571], 230, 232, 233, *333*
Forsyth, R. P., see Hoffbrand, B. I. [61a], 91, *361*
Forte, I., see Schmitthenner, J. E. [1687], 300, *353*
Fortuin, N., see Pitt, B. [1450], 100, *349*
Fortuin, N. J., see Becker, L. [9a], 134, *360*
— see Pitt, B. [251c], 134, *369*
Foucault, J. F., Olivier, J. [41a], 279, 286, *360*
Foulds, R., Mac Kinnon, J. [572], 187, *333*
Fourcade, A., see Fermoso, J. [99c], 175, 179, *365*
Fourneau, J. P. [573], 158, *333*
— Davy, M., Clement, M., Lamarche, M. [12b], 295, *363*
Fournel, J., see Courvoisier, S. [373], 302, *329*
Fournet, P. C., see Moret, P. R. [1322], 257, 268, 269, 286, *347*
Fouts, J. R., see Zeller, E. A. [2047], 160, *360*
Fowler, N. O., see Scott, R. C. [1710], 152, *353*
Fowler, W. M., Hurevitz, H. M., Smith, F. M. [574], 153, *333*
Fox, R. H., Goldsmith, R., Kidd, D. J., Lewis, G. P. [575], 63, *333*
Francois, J. [576, 577, 42a], 287, *333*, *361*
Francois-Franck, C. A. [578], 143, *333*
Frank, A., Bretschneider, H. J., Kanzow, E., Bernard, U. [579], 156, *333*
— see Bretschneider, H. J. [227], 181, 183, *327*
Frank, C. W., see Wegria, R. [1970], 157, 299, *358*
Frank, M. J., Levinson, G. E. [580], 3, *333*
— see Cundey, P. E. [73c], 174, 175, *365*
Frankl, W. S., Soloff, L. A. [581], 251, *333*
Franklin, D. C., see Vatner, S. F. [321c, 322c], 316, *370*
Franklin, D. L. [582], 84, *333*

Fredenucci, P., see Gerard, R. [111c], 315, *366*

Freedberg, A. S. [583], 105, *333*
— Papp, J. G., Vaughan Williams, E. M. [101c], 270, *365*
— Riseman, J. E. F., Spiegl, E. D. [584], 106, 107, 108, 135, 140, 304, *333*
— Spiegl, E. D., Riseman, J. E. F. [585, 586], 107, 145, *333*
— see Blumgart, H. L. [187, 188], 20, *326*
— see Dohadwalla, A. N. [435], 215, 237, *331*
— see Kurland, G. S. [1060], 15, *342*

Freis, E. D. [13b], 105, 117, *363*
Fremont, R. E. [587], 148, *333*
French, G. N., see Monroe, R. G. [1316], 29, 267, *347*
Frenkiel, see Faivre, G. [520], 97, *332*
Fresia, P., Genovese, E., Mortari, A. [588], 161, *333*
— see Bisiani, M. [171], 161, *326*
Freson, A., see Barzin, J. [100], 278, 281, 282, 285, 286, *324*
Freund, H. J., see Fleckenstein, A. [562], 166, 178, *333*
Frey. E. K., Hartenbach, W., Schultz, F. [589], 309, *333*
— Kraut, H. [590, 591], 309, *333*
— see Kraut, H. [1044], 309, *342*
Friart, J., Rasson, G. [4e], 286, *371*
Frick, M. H. [43a], *361*
— Balcon, R., Cross, D., Sowton, E. [592], 4, 30, 34, 93, 100, 109, 128, 130, 133, *333*
— Katila, M. [593], 9, *333*
— — Valtonen, E. [102c], 9, *365*
— see Sowton, E. [1798, 1799], 4, 93, 100, 128, 240, *355*
Friedberg, C. K. [594, 595, 596, 597, 103c], 5, 11, 13, 17, 38, 96, 105, 113, 139, 141, 302, *333, 365*
— Jaffé, H. L., Pordy, L., Chesky, K. [598], 96, *333*
— see Donoso, E. [441], 211, *331*
Friedberg, H. D., see Walker, J. A. [333c], 13, *370*
Friedemann, M. [600], 187, *334*
— see Keul, J. [974, 975], 187, *340*
Frieden, J. [599], 218, 219, 221, *333*
— see Rosenblum, R. [1554, 1555], 218, *351*

Friedland, C., see Sodi-Pallares, D. [1770], 295, *355*
Friedlander, D. H., see Besterman, E. M. M. [153], 221, *325*
Friedman, B., see Hefner, L. L. [797], 138, *337*
Friedman, G., see Christakis, G. [327], 14, *328*
Friedman, H. F., see Mellen, H. S. [1266], 142, *346*
Friedman, J., see Cowan, M. [70c], *365*
Friedman, J. J. [601], 85, *334*
Friedman, R., see Master, A. M. [1231], 104, *345*
Frieh, P., Imbert, D. [14b], 291, *363*
Friend, D. G., O'Hare, J. P., Levine, H. D. [602], 139, *334*
Friese, G. [603], 190, 191, *334*
Friesinger, G. C., see Bernstein, L. [146], 28, 83, 123, 130, 133, *325*
— see Conti, C. R. [3d], 24, 28, *371*
— see Dagenais, G. R. [74c], 140, 143, 233, *365*
— see Pitt, A. [1447, 1450, 253c], 83, 100, 300, *349, 369*
Frink, R. J., see James, T. N. [160c], 218, *367*
Frisch, R. A., Kaufman, K. K., Beezy, R., Garry, M. W. [604], 152, *334*
Fritz, A., see Marion, J. [1220], 171, *345*
Fritz, E. [605], 168, *334*
Froer, K. L., Koenig, E., Gruenberg, G. [44a], 245, *361*
Frohlich, E. D., Scott, J. B. [606], 121, 145, 150, *334*
— Tarazi, R. C., Dustan, H. P. [607], 218, *334*
— see Ulrych, M. [1911], 211, *357*
Froment, R. [104c], 7, *365*
— see Cahen, P. [269], 162, *327*
Froněk, A., Ganz, V. [608, 609, 610], 71, 122, 150, *334*
— see Ganz, V. [624, 625], 71, 122, *334*
Fry, D. L., Griggs, D. M., Greenfield, J. G. [611], 92, *334*
Frye, R., see Campion, B. [20a], 130, *360*
Frye, R. L., see Braunwald, E. [43c], 33, *364*
— see Greenberg, B. H. [125c], 13, *366*
— see McCallister, B. D. [1245, 217c], 12, 30, 37, *345, 368*
Fuccella, L. M., Imhof, P. [612], 228, *334*

Fuccella, L. M., see Imhof, P. R. [64a], 227, *361*
Fugita, T., see Shimamato, T. [1741, 1742], 289, *354*
Fuller, H. L., Kassel, L. E. [613], 139, *334*
Fulton, W. F. M. [614, 105c], 47, 53, *334, 365*
Funcke, A. B. H., see Bijlsma, V. G. [160], 308, *326*
Funk, D. C., see Toubes, D. B. [314c], 252, *370*
Furberg, C., Jacobsson, K. A. [615], 212, *334*
Futch, E. D., see Hejtmancik, M. R. [803], 158, *337*

Gaal, P. G., Kattus, A. A., Ross, G. [616], 210, *334*
Gabel, L. P., Winbury, M. M., Rowe, H., Grandy, R. P. [617], 45, *334*
— see Winbury, M. M. [2011, 2012], 124, 134, 141, *359*
Gabel, P. V., see Honig, C. R. [857], 122, 129, *338*
Gabrielsen, Z., Myhre, J. R. [618], 112, 311, *334*
Gadd, C. W., see Madeira, R. G. [1206], 2, *345*
Gaddum, J. H., Peart, W. S., Vogt, M. [619], 72, *334*
Gadomski, M., see Rudolph, W. [276c], 194, *369*
Gaffney, T. E., Braunwald, E. [620], 43, 229, 286, *334*
Gagliani, J., De Graff, A. C., Kupperman, H. S. [621], 155, *334*
Gagna, C., see Feruglio, F. S. [541, 542], 222, 248, *333*
Gaines, M., see Brotslow, J. [50c], 316, *364*
Galinier, F., see Meriel, P. [1285], 170, *346*
Gallacher, J. P., see Cohen, A. [339], 130, 151, *329*
Gallagher, J. P., see Bing, R. J. [165], 82, 101, 130, 151, *326*
Gamba, A., see Murmann, W. [1329], 248, *347*
Gamble, C. J., see Starr, I. [1823], 153, *356*
Gamble, W. J., Hugenholtz, P. G., Monroe, R. G., Polanyi, M., Nadas, A. S. [106c], 91, *366*
— see Hugenholtz, P. G. [155c], 91, *367*
— see Wagner, H. R. [331c], 91, *370*
Gander, M., Veragut, U., Kohler, R., Luthy, E. [622], 207, *334*

Ganelina, I. E., Deryagina, G. P., Krivoruchenko, I. V. [623], 295, *334*

Ganguly, S., see Robin, E. [1543], 93, 126, 130, 131, 208, *350*

Ganz, V., Froněk, A. [624, 625], 71, 122, *334*

— see Froněk, A. [608, 609, 610], 71, 122, 150, *334*

Garberg, L., see Duce, B. R. [454, 86c], 232, *331*, *365*

Gardner, T. H., see Berne, R. M. [143], 59, 74, *325*

Garrey, W. E., see White, J. C. [1984], 19, *358*

Garrone, G., Bossoney, C. [626], 15, *334*

Garry, M. W., see Frisch, R. A. [604], 152, *334*

Garvey, H. L., Melville, K. I. [45a], 175, *361*

— see Melville, K. I. [1272], 125, 139, *346*

Garvey, L., Melville, K. I. [627], 124, *334*

— Shister, H. E., Melville, K. I. [628], 173, 174, *334*

Gasparini, J. J., see Constantin, B. [355], *329*

Gasser, P., see Jost, M. [911], 163, *339*

Gattenloehner, W., Schneider, K. W., Rost, R. [46a], 218, *361*

Gault, J. E. [629], 235, *334*

Gautier, J. C., Derouesne, C., Held, T., Lhermitte, F. [107c], 51, *366*

Gavalda, J., see Meriel, P. [1285], 170, *346*

Gavend, M., Gavend, M. R., Mercier, J. [630], 163, *334*

— see Mercier, F. [1282, 1283], 157, 161, 305, *346*

Gavend, M. R., see Gavend, M. [630], 163, *334*

— see Mercier, F. [1282, 1283], 157, 161, 305, *346*

Gavey, C. J., see Rees, J. R. [1510], 123, 125, *350*

Gazaix, M., Alzeari, J. B. [108c], 279, *366*

Gazes, P. C., Richardson, J. A., Woods, E. F. [631], 36, 101, *334*

Gazitua, S., see Chou, C. C. [23a], 235, *360*

Gebelein, H., see Kirchhoff, H. W. [987], 196, *341*

Gebhardt, W., Dressel, J., Steim, H., Reindell, H. [632], 181, *334*

— Reindell, H., König, K., Büchner, C. [633], 207, *334*

Gelb, I. J., see Sherber, D. A. [1739, 1740], 146, 147, *354*

Gelfond, D. B., see Baer, S. [69], 305, *324*

Geller, H. M., Brandfonbrener, M., Wiggers, C. J. [634], 69, 75, 80, *334*

Gelson, A., see Conway, N. [361], 215, 221, *329*

Gent, A. E., Brook, C. G. D., Foley, T. H., Miller, T. N. [636, 109c], 51, 187, *334,366*

Gent, G., Davis, T. C., McDonald, A. [47a], 243, *361*

Genovese, E., see Bisiani, M. [171], 161, *326*

— see Fresia, P. [588], 161, *333*

Gensini, G. G., DiGiorgi, S., Murad-Netto, S., Black, A. [635], 124, *334*

George, C. F., Nagle, R. E., Pentecost, B. L. [110c], 242, *366*

Gerard, J., see Hardel, M. [58a], 279, *361*

Gerard, R., Fredenucci, P., Demart, F., Jouve, A., Appaix, A. [111c], 315, *366*

— Gras, A., Benyamine, R. [637], 192, *334*

Gerbaux, A., Lenegre, J. [638, 639], 162, 163, *334*

Gerbaux, J. O. [640], 172, *334*

Gerbaux, M. A. [641], 163, *334*

Gerhard, W., Smekal, P. V., Renschler, H. E., Mueller, G. [642], 144, 227, *334*

Gerin, J., see Mercier, F. [1282], 161, *346*

Gerlach, E., Deuticke, B. [643], 185, *334*

— see Deuticke, B. [422], 62, 185, *330*

Gerola, A., Feinberg, H., Katz, L. N. [644, 645], 29, 264, 267, *334*

Gersmeyer, E. F., Beyer, E., Leicht, E., Spitzbarth, H. [646], 215, *334*

— Spitzbarth, H. [647], 218, *334*

Gerstenberg, E., see Mercker, H. [1284], 58, *346*

Gerstlauer, E. [648], 139, *334*

Gerstner, K. [649], 168, *334*

Gettes, L. S., Surawicz [650], 221, *334*

— Yoshonis, K. F. [112c], 3, 221, *366*

Gey, K. F., see Pletscher, A. [1455, 1456], 161, *349*

Ghiara, F., see Guadagno, L. [751], 179, *336*

Ghislain, M., see Broekhuysen, J. [233, 234], 268, 272, *327*

Giannelli, G., see Guadagno, L. [751], 179, *336*

Gianelly, R. E., Goldman, R. H., Treister, B., Harrison, D. C. [651], 212, *334*

— Griffin, J. R., Harrison, D. C. [652], 221, *334*

— Harrison, D. C. [113c], 221, *366*

— Treister, B. L., Harrison, D. C. [48a], 212, *361*

— see Kerber, R. E. [175c], 234, *367*

Gibson, A. [653], 187, *334*

Gibson, D., Sowton, E. [655, 49a], 222, 241, *335*, *361*

— see Rees, J. R. [1510], 123, 125, *350*

Gibson, D. G., Balcon, R., Sowton, E. [654], 243, *335*

Giese, W., Müller-Mohnssen, H. [656], 52, 193, 269, *335*

— see Hapke, H.-J. [781], 290, *337*

Gigee, W., see Raab, W. [1488], 42, *349*

Gilbert, N. C., Fenn, G. K. [657], 153, 300, *335*

— Nalefski, L. A. [658], 310, 311, *335*

— see Leroy, G. V. [1105], 154, *343*

— see Nalefski, L. A. [1339], 158, *347*

Gilfillan, J. L., see Huff, J. W. [870], 15, *339*

Gilgenkrantz, see Faivre, G. [520], 97, *332*

Gill, E. [50a], 138, *361*

Gillam, P. M. S., Prichard, B. N. C. [659, 660], 207, 211, 217, *335*

— see Prichard, B. N. C. [1467, 257c, 258c], 207, 217, 222, *349, 369*

Gille, H., Rausch, F. [661], 190, *335*

Gillilan, R. E., see Warbasse, J. R. [1956], 4, *358*

Gillis, R. A., see Melville, K. I. [1272], 125, 139, *346*

Gillot, P. [662—665], 170, 171, 276, 308, *335*

— see Vastesaeger, M. [1927, 1930], 170, 276, 278, 279, 280, 285, 319, *357*

Gillot, P. H., see Vastesaeger, M. [1923], 285, *357*

Gilman, A., see Goodman, L. S. [692, 120c], 118, 150, 151, 152, 304, *322*, *335*, *366*

Gilmour, D. P., see McInerny, T. K. [1255], 215, 216, *345*

Gimenez, J. L., see Soloff, L. A. [1773], 181, 187, *355*

Ginsberg, A. M., Stoland, O. O. [667], 70, *335*

— see Stoland, O. O. [1844], 153, 309, *356*

Ginn, W. M., Orgain, E. S. [666] 211, *335*

Ginn, W. N., see Irons, G. V. [878], 221, *339*

Gioffre, P. A., see Reale, A. [1503], 226, *350*

Giordani, R., see Donato, L. [438], 82, *331*

Giordano, G., Turrisi, E. [668], 160, *335*

Giraud, M., see Audier, M. [62], 140, 164, *324*

Giroux, R., see Vaquez, H. [1919], 309, *357*

Giudicelli, J.-F., Schmitt, H., Boissier, J. R. [669], *335*

— see Boissier, J. R. [37c], 242, 246, *364*

Giudicelli, J. J., see Boissier, J. R. [198], 167, *326*

Giusti, C. [114c], 147, *366*

Glancy, D. L., Higgs, L. M., O'Brien, K. P., Epstein, S. E. [51a], 34, *348*

— see O'Brien, K. P. [1384], 30, 34, 100, *348*

Glaviano, V. V. [670], 27, *335*

Gleason, W. L., Braunwald, E. [671], 2, *335*

Gley, P., Kisthinios, N. [672], 309, *335*

Glick, G., Parmley, W. W., Wechsler, A. S., Sonnenblick, E. H. [673], 273, *335*

— see Braunwald, E. [215], 37, *326*

— see Epstein, S. E. [500, 501, 94c], 37, 315, 316, *332*, *365*

— see Sonnenblick, E. H. [1789], 31, 33, 208, *355*

— see Williams, J. F. [2002], 128, 131, 132, *359*

Gluckman, M. I., see Yu, D. H. [139a], 186, *362*

Glynn, M. F., see Joergensen, L. [900], 4, *339*

Gobbee, R., see Fermoso, J. [99c], 175, 179, *365*

Godfraind, T., Kaba, A., Polster, P. [674], 201, *335*

Godwin, T. F., see Hebb, A. R. [794], 212, *337*

Gösswald, R., see Wirth, W. [2022], 302, *359*

Gofman, J. W., see Graham, D. M. [704], 311, *335*

— see Lyon, T. P. [1199], 311, *344*

Goghlan, C., see Reeves, T. J. [1511], 2, 268, *350*

Gokel, M., see Haas, H. [133c], 175, *366*

Goksel, F. M. [675], 313, *335*

Gold, H. [676], 110, *335*

— Kwit, N. T., Otto, H. [677], 108, 154, *335*

— Travell, J., Modell, W. [678], 154, *335*

— see Greiner, T. [738], 110, 111, 112, 113, 116, 158, 308, *336*

— see Vera, L. B. de [1936], 74, *357*

Goldbarg, A., Moran, J. F., Resnekov, L. [115c], 212, *366*

Goldbarg, A. N., Moran, J. F., Butterfield, T. K., Bermudez, G. A., Nemickas, R., Childers, R. W. [52a], 148, 213, *361*

— — — Nemickas, R., Bermudez, G. A. [53a], 5, 148, 213, *361*

Goldberg, H., see Nakhjavan, F. K. [1337, 1338], 30, 89, *347*

Goldberg, H. S., see Mellen, H. S. [1266], 142, *346*

Goldberg, L. I., see Horwitz, D. [861], 161, *338*

Goldberg, L. M. [679], 146, *335*

Goldberg, R. I., see Cole, R. E. [347], 143, *329*

Goldberg, V. A. [680], 168, *335*

Goldberger, E. [681], 136, *335*

Goldenberg, C., see Deltour, G. [409], 255, *330*

Goldie, W., see Holdsworth, C. D. [849], 163, *338*

Goldman, R. H., Kerber, R. E. [175c, 176c], 233, 234, *367*

— see Gianelly, R. E. [651], 212, *334*

Goldreyer, B. N., Bigger, J. T. [116c, 117c], 3, *366*

Goldsborough, C. E. [682], 313, *335*

Goldschlager, N., see Cowan, C. [27a], 22, 28, 82, 83, 125, 126, 130, 134, *360*

Goldsmith, R., see Fox, R. H. [575], 63, *333*

Goldstein, R. E., Beiser, G. D., Redwood, D. R., Rosing, D. R., Epstein, S. E. [118c], 147, *366*

— — — — Stampfer, M., Epstein, S. E. [54a, 55a], 147, *361*

— see Epstein, S. E. [500, 501, 94c], 37, 315, 316, *332*, *365*

— see Redwood, D. R. [266c], 106, *369*

Goldstein, R. E., see Stampfer, M. [1816], 38, *355*

Goldstein, W., see Contro, S. [356], 144, *329*

Golenhofen, K., Hensel, H., Hildebrandt, G. [683], 86, *335*

— see Hensel, H. [815], 76, *338*

Gollwitzer-Meier, K., Jungmann, H. [684], 307, *335*

— Kramer, K., Krüger, E. [685], 264, *335*

— Kroetz, C. [686], 58, 138, 139, 268, *335*

— see Witzleb, E. [2024], 309, *359*

Gomez, C. G. R. [687], 279, *335*

Gomoll, A. W. [119c], 250, *366*

Gomprecht, R. F., see Gould, L. [122c], 301, *366*

Goodale, W. T., Hackel, D. B. [688, 689], 80, *335*

— Lubin, M., Banfield, W. G. [690], 79, *335*

— — Eckenhoff, J. E., Hafkenschiel, J. H., Banfield, W. G. [691], 79, *335*

— see Eckenhoff, J. E. [469], 79, *331*

Goodell, H., see Wolff, H. G. [2027], 110, 112, *359*

Goodman, L. S., Gilman, A. [692, 120c], 118, 150, 151, 152, 304, *322*, *335*, *366*

Goodwin, J. F., see Cherian, G. [322], 218, *328*

Goodyear, A. V. N., Huvos, A., Eckhardt, W. F., Ostberg, R. H. [693], 91, *335*

Gordon, R. B., see Green, G. E. [124c], 12, *366*

Gordon, S., see Regan, T. J. [1512], 310, *350*

Gorini, M., see De Caro, L. [77c], 247, *365*

Gorlin, R. [694—697, 121c], 20, 21, 24, 25, 37, 38, 48, 53, 55, 284, 317, *335*, *366*

— Brachfeld, N., McLeod, C., Bopp, P. [698], 22, 100, 123, 129, 130, 133, *335*

— — Messer, J. V., Turner, J. D. [699], 129, *335*

— Cohen, L. S., Elliott, W. C., Klein, M. D., Lane, F. J. [700], 93, *335*

— Taylor, W. J. [701], 11, *335*

— see Amsterdam, E. A. [27, 28, 29, 30], 114, 212, 215, *323*

— see Brachfeld, N. [208], 122, 125, 126, 129, 130, 131, 169, *326*

Gorlin, R., see Cohen, L. S. [344, 345, 346], 4, 25, 26, 33, 38, 83, 84, 275, *329*
— see Elliott, W. C. [488], 25, 36, 43, 52, 58, 269, 284, *331*
— see Fallen, E. L. [521], 38, *332*
— see Hampton, J. R. [140c], 49, *366*
— see Helfant, R. H. [60a, 144c], 26, 33, *361, 366*
— see Herman, M. V. [817], 26, *338*
— see Horwitz, L. D. [150c], 126, *366*
— see Kemp, H. G. [967, 174c], 12, 48, *340, 367*
— see Krasnow, N. [1034], 4, 264, *342*
— see Levine, J. H. [1115], *343*
— see Matloff, J. M. [1239], 221, *345*
— see Messer, J. V. [1287], 38, *346*
— see Neill, W. A. [1355], 29, 55, 267, *347*
— see Smith, M. H. [1761], 122, *354*
— see Sullivan, J. M. [1854, 306c, 307c], 28, 51, *356, 370*
— see Wagman, R. J. [1953], 22, 24, 275, *358*
— see Wolfson, S. [2031, 2032, 2033, 138a], 42, 210, 211, 212, 274, *359, 362*
— see Yurchak, P. M. [2037], 36, *359*
Gould, L. [15b], 301, *363*
— Jaynal, F., Zahir, M., Gomprecht, R. F. [122c], 301, *366*
Goulet, C., see Renaud, S. [268c], 50, *369*
Gowday, C. W. [702], 312, *335*
Graber, V. C., see Smith, F. M. [1760], 153, *354*
Grabner, G., Kaindl, F., Kraupp, O. [703], 181, *335*
Graef, F., see Kaltenbach, M. [169c], 247, *367*
Graham, D. M., Lyon, T. P., Gofman, J. W., Jones, H. B., Yankley, A., Simonton, J., White, S. [704], 311, *335*
— see Lyon, T. P. [1199], 311, *344*
Graham, G. R. [705], 68, 69, *335*
— see Rodbard, S. [1548], 70, *351*
Graham, W. D., see Lu, F. C. [1183], 305, *344*
Granata, L., Caraffa Braga, E., Cevese, A., Data, P. G. [123c], 206, *366*

Granata, L., Olsson, R. A., Huvos, A., Gregg, D. E. [706], 36, *335*
Grandjean, T. [707], 228, *335*
— Rivier, J. L. [708], 226, *335*
— see Hamer, J. [769], 207, *337*
— see Rivier, J. L. [1538], 228, 229, *350*
Grandy, R. P., see Gahel, L. P. [617], 45, *334*
— see Winbury, M. M. [2012], *359*
Granger, D., see Clark, L. C., jr. [331], 74, *329*
Granjean, L., see Balatre, P. [78], 141, *324*
Grant, C., see Falsetti, H. L. [96c], 35, *365*
Grant, R. H. E., Kulan, P., Kernohan, R. J., Leonard, J. C., Nancekievill, L., Sinclair, K. [709], 217, *336*
— McDevitt, D. G., Shanks, R. G. [710], 174, 207, *336*
Grapper, A. L., see Davies, D. F. [391], 21, *330*
Gras, A., see Gerard, R. [637], 192, *334*
— see Jouve, A. [919, 7d], 298, *339, 371*
Grassi, M., see Messina, B. [1291], 249, *346*
Grauman, S. J. [711], 162, *336*
Gray, W., Riseman, J. E. F., Stearns, S. [712], 151, *336*
— see Stearns, S. [1826], 300, *356*
Grayson, J., Irvine, M., Parratt, J. R. [713, 714], 143, 144, 189, *336*
— Mendel, D. [715], 55, *336*
— see Parratt, J. R. [1423, 1424], 63, 207, 209, 210, 215, 274, *348*
Greeff, K., Greven, G. [56a], 254, *361*
— Wagner, J. [716], 130, *336*
— see Benfey, B. G. [133], 172, 174, 177, 178, 245, 263, *325*
— see Wagner, J. [1954], 206, 245, *358*
Green, G. E., Stertzer, S. H., Gordon, R. B., Tice, D. A. [124c], 12, *366*
Green, H. D. [717], 153, *336*
— Gregg, D. E. [718], 55, *336*
— see Bobb, J. R. R. [192], 313, *326*
— see Boyer, N. H. [205], 120, 122, 145, 152, 153, *326*
— see Denison, A. B. [413, 414], 74, 312, *330*
— see Gregg, D. E. [727], 56, *336*

Green, H. D., see Malindzak, G. S. [211c], 125, *368*
— see Richardson, A. W. [1522], 74, *350*
— see Wiggers, C. J. [1996], 145, 154, *359*
Green, H. L., see Pitt, B. [253c], 300, *369*
Green, L., see Pitt, B. [97a], 210, *362*
Green, P. A., see Gregg, D. E. [729], 80, *336*
Green, R. D., see Bristow, M. [47c], 230, *364*
Green, R. L., see Brown, T. G. [244], 313, *327*
Green, R. S., see Scott, R. C. [1708], 158, *353*
Green, T. J., see Brown, T. G. [243, 244], 313, *327*
Greenberg, B. H., McCallister, B. D., Frye, R. L., Wallace, R. B. [125c], 13, *366*
Greene, C. W. [719], 309, *336*
Greene, D. G., see Falsetti, H. L. [96c], 35, *365*
— see Klocke, F. J. [181c], 23, *367*
Greenfield, J., see Cobb, F. [336], 208, *329*
Greenfield, J. C., see Cobb, F. R. [337, 24a], 208, *329, 360*
— see Zeft, H. J. [345c], 303, *371*
Greenfield, J. G., see Fry, D. L. [611], 92, *334*
Gregg, D. E. [720—724, 126c, 127c], 7, 19, 36, 44, 57, 69, 75, 91, *336, 366*
— Eckstein, R. W. [725], 74, *336*
— Fisher, L. C. [726], 81, 92, *336*
— Green, H. D. [727], 56, *336*
— Khouri, E. M., Pasyk, S. [128c], 125, *366*
— — Rayford, C. R. [728], 2, 57, 77, 256, *336*
— Longino, F. H., Green, P. A., Czerwonka, L. J. [729], 80, *336*
— Pritchard, W. H., Eckstein, R. W., Shipley, R. E., Rotta, A., Dingle, J., Steege, T. W., Wearn, J. T. [730], 76, *336*
— — Shipley, R. E., Wearn, J. T. [731], 73, *336*
— Sabiston, D. C. [732], 7, 28, 57, 58, 201, 268, *336*
— Shipley, R. E. [733, 734], 69, 73, 80, 732, *336*
— — Eckstein, R. W., Rotta, A., Wearn, J. T. [735], 73, *336*

Gregg, D. E., see Granata, L. [706], 36, *335*
— see Green, H. D. [718], 55, *336*
— see Kattus, A. A. [947], 122, *340*
— see Khouri, E. M. [977, 978, 979], 29, 55, 56, 77, 90, 256, *341*
— see Mautz, F. R. [1240], 44, 85, 86, *345*
— see Olsson, R. A. [1392, 1393], 93, 268, *348*
— see Pitt, B. [1449, 32b], 63, 210, *349, 363*
— see Shipley, R. E. [1746], 76, *354*
Greggia, A., Poggioli, R. [736], 248, *336*
Gregory, R. A., see Code, C. F. [338], 60, *329*
Greif, S., Liertzer, V. [737], 198, *336*
Greiner, T., Gold, H., Cattel, M. K., Travell, J., Bakst, H., Rinzler, S. H., Benjamin, Z. H., Warshaw, L. J., Bobb, A. L., Kwit, N. T., Modell, W., Rothendler, H. H., Messeloff, C. R., Kramer, M. L. [738], 110, 111, 112, 113, 116, 158, 308, *336*
Gremels, H. [739], 264, *336*
Greven, G., see Greeff, K. [56a], 254, *361*
Griffin, J. R., see Gianelly, R. E. [652], 221, *334*
Griffith, G. C. [740, 741, 129c], 10, 163, *336, 366*
— Zinn, W. J., Engelberg, H., Dooley, J. V., Anderson, R. [742], 311, *336*
— see Cole, S. L. [349, 350], 110, 111, 139, 141, 156, 302, *329*
Griffith, L. S. C., see Schwartz, S. I. [289c], 316, *369*
Griggs, D. M., see Fry, D. L. [611], 92, *334*
— see Najmi, M. [1335], 33, 93, 131, *347*
Grimald, J., see Duchene-Marullaz, P. [456, 457], 164, 178, 200, 268, 292, *331*
Grimson, T. A., see Dewar, H. A. [423], 136, 158, *330*
Griswold, H. [743], 11, 17, *336*
Griswold, H. E., see Farrehi, C. [527], 14, *332*
Grobecker, H., Palm, D., Bak, I. J., Schmid, B. [744], 166, *336*
— — Holtz, P. [745, 746], 165, 167, *336*

Grolleau, R., see Puech, P. [259c], 3, *369*
Grollman, J. H., see Kolin, A. [1017], 78, *341*
Grosgogeat, Y., see Cloarec, M. [6b], 293, *363*
— see Facquet, J. [517, 518], 280, 286, 287, *332*
— see Mouquin, M. [1326], 307, *347*
Gross, A., see Thiele, K. [1879], *357*
Grossi, F., see Messina, B. [1291], 249, *346*
Grossman, A. J., Brooks, A. M., Blackman, A. L., Schwimmer, J., Batterman, R. C. [747], 155, *336*
— see Batterman, R. C. [106], 154, 155, *325*
Grossmann, W., see Kraupp, O. [1036], 194, *342*
Groves, L. K., see Favaloro, R. G. [533], 10, *332*
Grün, G., Haastert, H. P., Döring, H. J., Kammermeier, H., Fleckenstein, A. [748], 152, *336*
Gruen, G., see Fleckenstein, A. [563, 40a], 166, 178, *333, 360*
Gruenberg, G., see Froer, K. L. [44a], 245, *361*
Grund, G., Würzbach, K. [749], 171, *336*
Grüner, A., Hilden, T., Raaschou, F., Vogelius, H. [750], 311, *336*
Grunwald, D., see Denis, B. [32a], 279, *360*
Grupp, G., see Bunde, C. A. [19a], 294, *360*
— see Grupp, I. L. [130c], 294, *366*
Grupp, I. L., Bunde, C. A., Grupp, G. [130c], 294, *366*
— see Bunde, C. A. [19a], 294, *360*
Guadagno, L., Giannelli, G., Ghiara, F., Guadagno, P., Zucchelli, G. P. [751], 179, *336*
Guadagno, P., see Guadagno, L. [751], 179, *336*
Gubner, R. S., Behr, D. J. [752], 295, *336*
Gudbjarnason, S., see Ogawa, K. [1385, 1386], 127, 135, *348*
Guerin, R., see Hardel, M. [58a], 279, *361*
Guilleman, P. [753], 307, *336*
Guiraud, R., see Lesbre, J. P. [81a], 181, 186, *361*
Gulde, M., see Rudolph, W. [276c], 194, *369*

Gundel, W. D., see Conti, C. R. [67c, 3d], 24, 27, 28, *365, 371*
Gunton, R., see Hebb, A. R. [794], 212, *337*
Gupta, G. D., see Conway, N. [360], 191, *329*
Gurtner, H. P., Dolder, M., Kaufmann, M. [131c], 246, 247, *366*
— see Rowe, G. G. [1575], 140, *351*
Gutgesell, H. P., Tempte, J. V., Murphy, Q. R. [57a], 220, *361*
Guttmann, W., see Bargheer, R. [88], 159, *324*
Guyot, J. C., see Perrot, J. [29b], 279, 287, *363*
Guzman, F., Braun, C., Lim, R. K. S. [754], 21, *336*
Guzman, S. V., see West, J. W. [1978, 1980], 71, *358*

Haas, H. [755, 756, 16b, 132c], 159, 172, 173, 174, 175, *336, 363, 366*
— Busch, E. [757, 758], 173, 178, *336*
— Gokel, M. [133c], 175, *366*
— Hartfelder, G. [759], 172, *336*
Haastert, H. P., see Grün, G. [748], 152, *336*
Habersang, S. [134c], 197, *366*
— Leuschner, F., Schlichtegroll, A. von [760], 196, *337*
Hache, J., see Duchene-Marullaz, P. [8b], 295, *363*
Hackel, D. B., see Goodale, W. T. [688, 689], 80, *335*
Hadjigeorge, C., see Lekos, D. [1098], 226, *343*
Haefely, W., Hürlimann, A., Thoenen, H. [761], 248, *337*
Hafkenschiel, J. H., see Eckenhoff, J. E. [468, 469, 470, 471], 55, 56, 74, 79, 121, 150, 153, *331*
— see Goodale, W. T. [691], 79, *335*
— see Schmitthenner, J. E. [1687], 300, *353*
Haft, J. I., see Lau, S. H. [1080, 1082], 100, *342*
— see Helfant, R. H. [60a, 144c], 26, 33, *361, 366*
Hagfors, N., see Schwartz, S. I. [289c], 316, *369*
Haggendal, E., see Svedmyr, N. [308c, 309c], 211, 251, *370*
Hahn, N., Felix, R., Draznin, N., Meuser, H. J., Düx, A. [762], 197, *337*

Hahn, N., Felix, R., Duex, A., Draznin, N. [135c], 197, *366*
Hahn, R. A., Pendleton, R. G., Wardell, J. R. [763], 209, 248, *337*
Haiat 191
Haight, C., Figley, M. M., Sloan, H., Ellsworth, W. J., Meyer, J. A., Berk, M. S., Boblitt, D. E. [764], 121, *337*
Hakkinen, P., Relander, A., Oka, M. [5e], 199, *371*
Hale, G., Dexter, D., Jefferson, K., Leatham, A. [765], 100, *337*
Haley, T. J., see Leitch, J. L. [1096], 66, *343*
Hall, J. H., see Browse, N. L. [51c], 50, 51, *364*
Hallen, A., see Björk, L. [174], 10, *326*
Hallermann, F. J., see McCallister, B. D. [1245, 217c], 12, 30, 37, *345, 368*
Hallwachs, H., see Hensel, H. [814], *338*
Halmagyi, M., Hempel, K. J., Ockenga, T., Richter, G., Wernitsch, W., Zeitler, E. [766], 183, *337*
Halperin, M. H. [767], 314, *337*
Hamacher, J., see Schirmer, R. [284c], 293, *369*
Hambourger, W. E., see Winbury, M. M. [2015, 2016], 306, *359*
Hamer, J., Fleming, J. [768, 136c], 207, *337, 366*
— Grandjean, T., Melendez, L., Sowton, G. E. [769], 207, *337*
— Sowton, G. E. [770, 771], 208, 211, *337*
— see Fleming, J. [564], 215, *333*
— see Hess, M. H. [824], 216, *338*
— see Shinebourne, E. [1743 to 1745], 211, 220, 240, *354*
— see Sowton, E. [1800], 207, 241, 274, *355*
Hamilton, W. F., Himmelstein, A., Noble, R. P., Remington, J. W., Richards, D. W., Wheeler, N. C., Witham, A. L. [772], 91, *337*
Hamilton, W. F. D., see Palmer, K. N. V. [93a], 244, *362*
Hamm, J., Hunekohl, E., Schmidt, A. [137c], 245, *366*
— Renschler, H. E., Zack, W. J. [773], 187, *337*
Hammerl, H., Klein, K., Pichler, O. [774], 187, *337*

Hammerl, H., Kränzl, C., Pichler, O., Studlar, M. [775], *337*
— Siedek, H. [776], 187, *337*
Hammouda, M., see Anrep, G. V. [43], 68, *323*
Hampton, J. R. [138c], 50, *366*
— Harrison, M. J. G., Honour, A. J., Mitchell, J. R. A. [139c], 50, 51, *366*
— Kemp, H. G., Gorlin, R. [140c], 49, *366*
— see Elkeles, R. S. [88c], 51, *365*
— see Helfant, R. H. [60a, 144c], 26, 33, *361, 366*
Hanna, C. [777], 66, *337*
— Parker, R. C. [778], 150, *337*
— Shutt, J. H. [779], 67, *337*
— see Schmid, J. R. [1678, 33b], 174, 250, *353, 363*
Hannah, H. III., see Enright, L. P. [91c], 30, *365*
Hancock, E. W., see Ellis, L. B. [490], 142, *332*
— see Flamm, M. D. [11b], 218, *363*
Hanlon, C. R., see Kaiser, G. C. [167c], 11, *367*
Hansen, A. T., Haxholdt, B. F., Husfeldt, E., Lassen, N. A., Munck, O., Sorenson, H. R., Winkler, K. [780], 83, *337*
Hapke, H.-J., Giese, W. [781], 290, *337*
— Sterner, W. [782], 290, *337*
Hardel, U., Bajolet, A., Guerin, R., Gerard, J., Elaerts, J. [58a], 279, *361*
Hardman, H. F., see Meester, W. D. [1263], 248, *346*
— see Somani, P. [1780, 1781, 118a, 9e], 57, 134, 236, 251, *355, 362, 371*
Hardman, H. T., see Bachand, R. T. [66], 127, *324*
Hardy, J. D., see Wolff, H. G. [2027], 110, 112, *359*
Hardy, L. B., see Lumb, G. D. [1196], 90, 141, *344*
— see Malinin, T. [1212], 4, *345*
Haring, O. M., see Contro, S. [356], 144, *329*
Harken, D. E., see Ellis, L. B. [489], 20, 96, *331*
— see Matloff, J. M. [1239], 221, *345*
— see Sullivan, J. M. [306c, 307c], 51, *370*
Harley, B. J. S., Davies, R. O. [783], 211, *337*
Harmel, M. H., see Eckenhoff, J. E. [469, 471], 56, 79, *331*

Harris, P. D., see Bigger, J. T. [31c], 303, *364*
Harris, R. [784], 314, *337*
Harris, W. S., Schoenfeld, C. D., Brooks, R. H., Weissler, A. M. [785], 207, *337*
Harrison, D. C. [786], 213, *337*
— see Flamm, M. D. [11b], 218, *363*
— see Gianelly, R. E. [651, 652, 48a, 113c], 212, 221, *334, 361, 366*
— see Kerber, R. E. [176c], 233, *367*
Harrison, J., Turner, P. [787], 240, *337*
Harrison, M. J. G., see Emmons, P. R. [90c], 50, *365*
— see Hampton, J. R. [139c], 50, 51, *366*
— see Mitchell, J. R. A. [223c], 51, *368*
Harrison, T. R., see Hefner, L. L. [797], 138, *337*
— see Skinner, M. S. [1756], 129, *354*
Hartenbach, W. [788, 789], 309, *337*
— see Frey, E. K. [589], 309, *333*
Hartfelder, G., see Haas, H. [759], 172, *336*
Harthorne, J. W., see Kastor, J. A. [68a], 4, *361*
Hashimoto, K., Kumakura, S., Tanemura, I. [790], 61, 62, *337*
— see Miura, M. [1302], 62, 185, *346*
Hashimoto, S., see Dayton, S. [399], 15, *330*
Hatt, P. Y. [17b], 293, *363*
Hattori, Y., see Ikezono, E. [876], 221, *339*
Häusler, H., see Anrep, G. V. [44], 55, *323*
Hausner, E., Essex, H. E., Herrick, J. F., Baldes, E. J. [791], 55, *337*
Hauss, W. H., see Schmitt, G. [1685, 34b], 183, 193, *353, 363*
Haviano, V. V., see Masters, T. N. [88a], 208, *361*
Hawker, R., see Bernstein, L. [29c], *364*
Hawley, R. R., see Warbasse, J. R. [1956], 4, *358*
Haxholdt, B. F., see Hansen, A. T. [780], 83, *337*
Hayden, R. O., see Stock, T. B. [1842], 24, 275, *356*
Haynes, F. W., see Weiss, S. [1972], 121, 136, *358*
— see Wilkins, R. W. [2000], 121, 136, *359*

Hayward, G. W., see Apthorp, G. H. [48], 275, *323*

Hazan, J., see Dighiero, J. [430], 163, *330*

Hazard, J. [792], 311, *337*

Hazard, R., see Bacq, Z. M. [67], 173, *324*

Heathcote, R. S. A. [793], 153, *337*

Hebb, A. R., Godwin, T. F., Gunton, R. W. [794], 212, *337*

Hedbom, K. [795], 304, *337*

Hedwall, P., see Wilhelm, M. [1999], 222, *359*

Hedwall, P. R., see Brunner, H. [249], 222, *327*

Hedworth-Whitty, R. B., Housley, E., Abraham, A. S. [59a, 141c], 57, 79, *361, 366*

Heeg, E., see Benfey, B. G. [133], 172, 174, 177, 178, 245, 263, *325*

— see Wagner, J. [1954], 206, 245, *358*

Heffernan, A., Hickey, N., Mulcahy, R., Fitzgerald, O. [796], 16, *337*

Hefner, L. L., Friedman, B., Reeves, T. J., Eddleman, E. E., Harrison, T. R. [797], 138, *337*

— see Reeves, T. J. [1511], 2, 268, *350*

Hefner, M. A., see Winbury, M. M. [2013], 134, 202, 317, *359*

Hehenkamp, G. [142c], 188, *366*

Heim, F., Walter, F. [798], 174, 251, *337*

Heimann, W., Wilbrandt, W. [799], 150, 153, 157, *337*

Heimbecker, R. O. [143c], 10, *366*

Heindorf, M., see Fiegel, G. [543], 190, *333*

Heine, W. I., see Baer, S. [69], 305, *324*

Heinle, R. A., see Wolfson, S. [2032, 2033], 42, 210, 211, 274, *359*

Heinrich, F., see Tschirdewahn, B. [1903], 221, *357*

Heistracher, P., Kraupp, O., Schiefthaler, T. [802], 192, *337*

— — Spring, G. [800], 169, *337*

— see Kraupp, O. [1037], 192, *342*

Hejtmancik, M. R., Futch, E. D., Herrmann, C. R. [803], 158, *337*

Helbig, J. [804], 168, *337*

Held, T., see Gautier, J. C. [107c], 51, *366*

Helfant, R. H., Forrester, J. S., Hampton, J. R., Haft, J. I., Gorlin, R., Kemp, H. G. [60a], 26, *361*

— — — — Kemp, H. G., Gorlin, R. [144c], 33, *366*

— see Damato, A. N. [387, 388], 3, *330*

— see Lau, S. H. [1080, 1082], 100, *342*

— see Scherlag, B. J. [1665], 3, *353*

Hell, E., see Heistracher, P. [801], 193, *337*

Hellberg, K., see Spieckermann, P. G. [119a], 185, 193, *362*

Hellems, H. K., Ord, J. W., Talmers, F. N., Christensen, R. C. [805], 59, *337*

— see Regan, T. J. [1512, 1513, 1514, 1515], 301, 310, *350*

Heller, E. M. [806], 139, *337*

Hellerstein, H. K. [145c], 10, *366*

— Hirsch, E. Z., Cumler, W., Allen, L., Polster, S., Zukker, N. [807], 10, *337*

— Hornstein, T. R. [808], *337*

Hellman, L., Zumoff, B., Kessler, G., Kara, E., Rubin, I. L., Rosenfeld, R. S. [809], 16, *337*

Hellwig, H., see Hilger, H. H. [826, 827], 186, 194, *338*

Hemmer, M. L., see Winbury, M. M. [2016], 306, *359*

Hempel, K. J., see Halmagyi, M. [766], 183, *337*

Henaux, F., see Deltour, G. [409], 255, *330*

Henderson, F. G., Shipley, R. E., Chen, K. K. [810], 151, *338*

Henke, C., Dudik, E., Steim, H. [811], 196, *338*

Hennessy, D. J., see Schluger, J. [1675], 155, *353*

Hensala, J. C., Burgison, R. M., Krantz, J. C. [812], 156, *338*

Henschel, A., see Taylor, H. L. [1875], 9, *356*

Hensel, H. [813], 169, *338*

— Hallwachs, H., Schmidt-Mertens, H. H. [814], *338*

— Ruef, J., Golenhofen, K. [815], 76, *338*

— see Betz, E. [154, 155], 169, 181, *325*

— see Golenhofen, K. [683], 86, *335*

Henselmann, L., see Rudolph, W. [1582], 186, 187, *351*

Henze, H., see Kirchhoff, H. W. [987], 196, *341*

Herbaczynska-Cedro, K., see Ceremuzynski, L. [286], 242, *328*

Herbst, A., see Fleckenstein, A. [563, 40a], 166, 178, *333, 360*

— see Tritthart, H. [125a], 179, 219, *362*

Herbst, M., see Braunsteiner, H. [212], 14, *326*

Herd, J. A., Hollenberg, M., Thorburn, G. D., Kopald, H. H., Barger, A. C. [816], 83, *338*

Herman, A. G., see Bogaert, M. G. [34c], 136, *364*

Herman, M. V., Elliott, W. C., Gorlin, R. [817], 26, *338*

— see Wolfson, S. [2032], 42, 210, 211, *359*

Hermann, H., Mornex, R. [818], 161, *338*

Hermansen, K. [819, 820], 253, *338*

Hernandez, A., see Cuellar, A. [72c], 295, *365*

Herreman, F. [821], 190, *338*

Herrick, J. F., see Baldes, E. J. [81], 76, *324*

— see Essex, H. E. [508, 509], 120, 150, 153, 299, 306, 307, *332*

— see Hausner, E. [791], 55, *337*

— see Wegria, R. [1968], 120, 150, 153, *358*

Herring, D. A., see Marsh, D. F. [1226], 308, *345*

Herrlich, H. C., see Raab, W. [1491], 36, 284, *350*

Herrmann, C. R., see Hejtmancik, M. R. [803], 158, *337*

Hertting, G., see Brücke, F. [245], 307, *327*

Herschel, J. G. [822], 308, *338*

Hertault, J. [6d], 298, *371*

Herxheimer, H., Langer, I. [146c], 217, *366*

Hess, H. [823], *338*

Hess, M. H., Briggs, F. N., Shinebourne, E., Hamer, J. [824], 216, *338*

Hessel, F., see Ameur, M. [3a], 279, *360*

Heubner, W., Mancke, R. [825], 65, *338*

Heuillet, G., see Torresani, J. [313c], 316, *370*

Heusghem, C., see Plomteux, G. [1458], 288, *349*

Hickey, N., see Heffernan, A. [796], 16, *337*

Hickie, J. B. [147c], 233, *366*

Hiebert, P. E., see Stoland, O. O. [1844], 153, 309, *356*

Higgs, L. M., see Glancy, D. L. [51a], 34, *361*

— see O'Brien, K. P. [1384], 30, 34, 100, *348*

Hildebrandt, G., see Golenhofen, K. [683], 86, *335*

Hilden, T., see Grüner, A. [750], 311, *336*

Hildner, F. J., see Linhart, J. W. [1152—1154, 82a], 3, 11, 34, 126, 130, *344, 361*

Hilgenberg, F., see Bender, F. [20c], 246, *364*

— see Hösemann, R. [151c], 179, *366*

Hilger et al. 191

Hilger, H. H. [148c], 194, *366*

— Schaede, A., Wagner, J., Louven, B., Wackerbauer, J., Hellwig, H. [826], 194, *338*

— Wagner, J., Hellwig, H., Louven, B., Wackerbauer, J., Schaede, A. [827], 186, *338*

Hill, R. C., Turner, P. [828, 829], 246, 248, *338*

Hillarp, N. A., see Carlsson, A. [277], 166, *328*

Hillestad, L., Andersen, A. [830], 235, *338*

— Storstein, O. [831], 221, *338*

Hills, E. A., Downes, E. M. [832], 178, 179, 180, *338*

Hilton, R., Eichholtz, F. [833], 20, 59, *338*

Hilton, S. M., Lewis, G. P. [834, 835], 63, *338*

Himbert, J. [836], 164, *338*

— see Barrillon, A. [17c], 163, *364*

Himmelstein, A., see Hamilton, W. F. [772], 91, *337*

Hint, H. C., see Arfors, K. E. [10c], 51, *363*

Hirche, H. [837], 62, 189, *338*

— Scholtholt, J. [838], 169, *338*

— see Lochner, W. [1164], 188, 189, *344*

Hirsch, B. B., see Rinzler, S. H. [1529], 311, *350*

Hirsch, C., see Sterne, J. [1835, 1836, 38b], 164, 297, *356, 363*

Hirsch, E. Z., see Hellerstein, H. K. [807], 10, *337*

— see Macleod, C. A. [209c], 10, *368*

— see Sloman, G. [1757], 10, *354*

Hirsch, W. [839], 198, *338*

— Woschee, G. [840], 188, *338*

Hirshleifer, I. [841], 294, *338*

Hirschmann, J., see Simon, A. J. [1755], 151, *354*

Hirt, R., see Schmutz, J. [1688], 159, *353*

Hobbs, L. F. [842], 163, *338*

Hochrein, M., Keller, C. J. [843], 309, *338*

Hockerts, T., Bögelmann, G. [844], 181, 185, *338*

Hodgeman, R. J., see Lucchesi, B. R. [7e], 63, 236, *371*

Hodgemar, R. J., Lucchesi, B. R. [208c], 236, *368*

Hodges, M., see Pitt, B. [1450], 100, *349*

Hoeljes, U., see Morgenstern, C. [227c], 207, *368*

Hoeschen, R. J., Bousvaros, G. A., Klassen, G. A., Fam, W. M., McGregor, M. [845], 126, *338*

Hösemann, R., Diekmann, L., Hilgenberg, F. [151c], 179, *366*

Hofbauer, K. [846], 179, *338*

Hoffbrand, B. I., Forsyth, R. P. [61a], 91, *361*

Hoffman, B. F., see Bartelstone, H. J. [97], 70, *324*

— see Bigger, J. T. [31c], 303, *364*

— see Singer, D. H. [292c], 27, *369*

— see Strauss, H. C. [303c], 250, 251, *370*

Hoffman, M. J., see Brown, H. R. [240], 95, *327*

Hoffmann, P. [847], 179, *338*

Hoffmeister, F. S., see Regelson, W. [1516], 161, *350*

Hofmann, H., see Rudolph, W. [1582], 186, 187, *351*

Hogancamp, C. E., see Mack, R. E. [1203], 82, *344*

Hohenstein, H. [848], 192, *338*

Hohl, O., Bernhardt, D., Kentschke, G. E., Metzger, R. [62a], 290, *361*

Holdsworth, C. D., Atkinson, M., Goldie, W. [849], 163, *338*

Holen, N., see Mathisen, H. S. [1237], 149, *345*

Holland, J. F., see Wegria, R. [1969], 121, *356*

Hollander, W., Chobanian, A. V., Wilkins, R. W. [850], 314, *338*

— Madoff, I. M., Chobanian, A. V. [851], 130, *338*

— Wilkins, R. W. [852, 853], 163, *338*

Hollenberg, M., see Herd, J. A. [816], 83, *338*

Holloszy, J. O., Skinner, J. S., Barry, A. J., Cureton, T. K. [854], 10, *338*

Holmberg, S. [855], 24, *338*

— see Svedmyr, N. [308c], 211, 251, *370*

Holmes, R. H., see Enos, W. F. [497], 7, *332*

Holt, J. H., see Scheffield, L. T. [1736], 97, *354*

Holtz, P., see Grobecker, H. [745, 746], 165, 167, *336*

Holzmann, M. [856], 162, *338*

Honig, C. R., Kirk, E. S., Myers, W. W. [149c], 317, *366*

— Tenney, S. M., Gabel, P. V. [857], 122, 129, *338*

Honour, A. J., see Elkeles, R. S. [88c], 51, *365*

— see Emmons, P. R. [90c], 50, *365*

— see Hampton, J. R. [139c], 50, 51, *366*

— see Mitchell, J. R. A. [223c], 51, *368*

Hood, W. B., see Krasnow, N. [1033, 1034], 4, 25, 264, *342*

— see Letac, B. [1111], 2, *343*

Hoogerwerf, S. [858], 160, *338*

Horger, E. L., see Stewart, H. J. [1839], 96, 154, *356*

Horita, A. [859], 163, *338*

Horler, A. R., see Dewar, H. A. [424], 141, 160, 162, *330*

Horlick, L. [860], 97, *338*

Hornstein, T. R., see Hellerstein, H. K. [808], *337*

Horvath, S. M., see Sullivan, F. J. [1853], 141, *356*

Horwitz, D., Goldberg, L. I., Sjoerdsma, A. [861], 161, *338*

Horwitz, L. D., Gorlin, R., Taylor, J., Kemp, H. G. [150c], 126, *366*

Hoshikawa, K., see Miyahara, M. [26b], 204, *363*

Hossein, A. M., see Samaan, K. [1634], 159, *352*

Hosslet, A., see Baudine, A. [110], 257, 261, *325*

— see Charlier, R. [319], 168, 169, *328*

Houdas, Y., Bertrand, M., Ketelers, J. Y. [152c], 72, *366*

— see Warembourg, H. [335c], 211, *371*

Houk, P., see Varnauskas, E. [1922], 9, *357*

Housley, E., see Hedworth-Whitty, R. B. [59a, 141c], 57, 79, *361, 366*

Houtsmuller, A. J. [862, 863], 171, 172, *338*

Hovig, T., see Joergensen, L. [900], 4, *339*

Howarth, S., MacMichael, J. S., Sharpey-Schafer, E. P. [864], 153, *338*

Howe, B. B., see Winbury, M. M. [2013, 11e], 124, 134, 202, 317, *359, 371*

Howell, J., see Chapman, D. W. [59c], 12, *364*

Howitt, G., see Fife, R. [546], 162, *333*
— see Mackinnon, J. [1204], 163, *344*
— see Rowlands, D. J. [1579], 221, *351*

Hoyle, C., see Evans, W. [514, 515], 110, 113, 136, 150, 154, 300, 309, *332*

Hua, G., see Faivre, G. [519], 279, *332*

Hubner, P., see Jewitt, D. E. [163c], 243, *367*

Hudak, W. J., Kuhn, W. L., Lewis, R. E. [63a], 294, *361*
— Lewis, R. E., Kuhn, W. L. [153c], 294, *367*

Hueber, E. F. [866, 867], 163, *339*
— Kotzaurek, R. [868], 278, 280, 281, 287, *339*
— Thaler, H. [869], 137, *339*

Hüdepohl, M. [865], 198, *339*

Hürlimann, A., see Haefely, W. [761], 248, *337*

Huff, J. W., Gilfillan, J. L. [870], 15, *339*

Hugenholtz, P. G., Ellison, R. C., Urschel, C. W., Mirsky, I., Sonnenblick, E. H. [154c], 35, *367*
— Gamble, W. J., Monroe, R. G., Polanyi, M. [155c], 91, *367*
— see Gamble, W. J. [106c], 91, *366*
— see Wagner, H. R. [331c], 91, *370*

Huggins, R. A., see Ahlquist, R. P. [16], 312, *323*

Hughes, J. P., see Cotterill, J. A. [69c], 295, *365*

Hultgren, H. N., Robertson, H. S., Stevens, L. E. [871], 158, *339*

Humphreys, P., see Winsor, T. [2020], 141, *359*

Humphreys, R. J., see Raab, W. [1489], 123, 207, *349*

Hunekohl, E., see Hamm, J. [137c], 245, *366*

Hunscha, H., Kaltenbach, M., Schellhorn, W. [872], 191, *339*

Hunscha, H., see Kaltenbach, M. [169c], 247, *367*

Hunt, D., see Potanin, C. [255c], 35, *369*

Hunter, F. E., Kahana, S., Ford, L. [873], 128, *339*
— see Needleman, P. [1353], 135, *347*

Huppert, V. F., Boyd, L. J. [874], 137, *339*

Huq, S., see Melville, K. I. [1277], 174, *346*

Hurevitz, H. M., see Fowler, W. M. [574], 153, *333*

Hurst, J. W., see Fletcher, G. F. [565, 566], 295, *333*

Husfeldt, E., see Hansen, A. T. [780], 83, *337*

Hutchinson, D. L., see Wegria, R. [1970], 157, 299, *358*

Hutchinson, E. C., see Acheson, J. [2c], 51, *363*

Hutchinson, K. J., see Brick, I. [228, 229], 240, 243, *327*

Huvos, A., see Goodyear, A. V. N. [693], 91, *335*
— see Granata, L. [706], 36, *335*

Hyland, J. W., see Stein, P. D. [1828, 1829], 209, *356*

Hyman, A. L., Pearce, C. W., Barnes, G. E. [156c], 316, *367*

Iglauer, A., see Sott, R. C. [1708], 158, *353*

Igloe, M. C. [18b], 187, *363*

Iimura, O., see Miyahara, M. [26b], 204, *363*

Iisalo, E., Kallio, V. [875], 295, *339*

Ikezono, E., Yasuda, K., Hattori, Y. [876], 221, *339*

Ikkma, E., see Pyörälä, K. [1476], 171, *349*

Ikram, H., Nixon, P. G. F. [877], 217, *339*

Imai, S., see Bunag, R. D. [256] 62, 185, *327*

Imbert, D., see Frieh, P. [14b], 291, *363*

Imbs, J. L., see Spach, M. O. [36b], 229, *363*

Imhof, P., see Fuccella, L. M. [612], *334*
— see Reale, A. [1503], 226, *350*

Imhof, P. R., Blatter, K., Fuccella, L. M., Turri, M. [64a], 227, *361*

Impicciatore, M., see Bertaccini, G. [148], 252, *325*

Inamdar, A. N., see Sharma, G. V. R. K. [112a], 27, *362*

Ioannidis, P., see Corcondilas, A. [362], 228, *329*

Ioannidis, P., see Lekos, D. [1098], 226, *343*

Irons, G. V., Ginn, W. N., Orgain, E. S. [878], 221, *339*

Irvine, M., see Grayson, J. [713, 714], 143, 144, 189, *336*

Isaacs, J. H., Wilburne, M., Mills, H., Kuhn, R. [879], 101, *339*

Isokane, N., see Atsumi, T. [14c], 289, *363*

Ishinose, Y. [880], 279, *339*

Ishioka, T., see Shimamoto, T. [1741], 289, *354*

Iwai, M., Sassa, K. [881], 152, *339*

Iwami, T., see Lucchesi, B. R. [1188], 219, *344*

Izbicki, M. [157c], 279, *367*

Jablons, B., Schilero, A. J., Sicam, L., Estrellado, T. [882], 137, *339*

Jack, N. B., see Stewart, H. J. [1840], 153, *356*

Jackson, F., see Szekely, P. [1867], 221, *356*

Jacob, M. I., Berne, R. M. [883], 60, *339*

Jacobi, H., Lange, A., Pfleger, K. [884], 156, *339*

Jacobsson, K. A., Koch, G., Lindgren, M., Michaelsson, G. [885], 168, *339*
— see Furberg, C. [615], 212, *334*

Jacquin, M., see Donnet, V. [439, 440], 165, *331*

Jaedicke, W., see Janke, J. [161c], 175, *367*

Jaeger, M., see Rivier, J. L. [269c], 246, *369*

Jaffe, H. L. [158c], 17, 49, *367*
— see Friedberg, C. K. [598], 96, *333*
— see Master, A. M. [1232], 110, 111, 136, 154, *345*

Jageneau, A., Brugmans, J. [886], 203, *339*
— Schaper, W. [887, 888], 123, 165, 173, 182, 189, 200, 202, *339*
— — Van Gerven, W. [889], 202, *339*
— see Schaper, W. [111a, 282c, 283c], 47, 86, 200, 202, 204, *362, 369*

Jageneau, A. H. M., see Schaper, W. K. A. [1659, 1660], 40, 46, 47, 53, 199, 200, 203, 204, *353*

Jahn, W. [890], 306, *339*

Jaillard, J., see Warembourg, H. [1960, 129a], 279, *358, 362*

Jain, A. C., see Riff, D. P. [107a], 301, *362*
Jakobsson, B., see Svedmyr, N. [122a], 251, *362*
Jalife, J., see Kabela, E. [67a], 63, *361*
Jallut, H., see Alix, B. [6c], 279, 286, 288, *363*
James, G., see Christakis, G. [327], 14, *328*
James, T. N. [892, 159c], 19, 53, *339, 367*
— Bear, E. S., Frink, R. J., Lang, K. F., Tomlinson, J. C. [160c], 218, *367*
Jameson, A. G., see Enson, Y. [93c], 91, *365*
Jampel, S., see Christakis, G. [327], 14, *328*
Janke, J., Fleckenstein, A., Jaedicke, W. [161c], 175, *367*
Janssen, P. A. J., see Schaper, W. K. A. [1660], 40, 199, 200, 201, *353*
January, L. E., see Lewis, B. I. [1131], 308, *343*
Jaquenoud, P. [893], *339*
Jaramillo, C. V., see McKenna, D. H. [1257], 4, *345*
Jarcho, S. [894], 5, *339*
Jasinski, B. [895], 310, *339*
Jaynal, F., see Gould, L. [122c], 301, *366*
Jefferson, K., see Hale, G. [765], 100, *337*
Jellinek, M., see Kaiser, G. C. [167c], 11, *367*
Jenkins, C. D., Rosenman, R. H., Zyzanski, S. J. [896], 16, *339*
Jensen, J., see Steinberg, F. [1830], 154, *356*
Jeremias, H. [897], 170, *339*
Jeschke, D., Caesar, K., Schollmeyer, P. [898], 179, *339*
— see Scholimeyer, P. J. [1693], 186, *353*
Jetschgo, G., see Rudolph, W. [276c], 194, *369*
Jewitt, D. E., Burgess, P. A., Shillingford, J. P. [162c], 241, *367*
— Hubner, P., Maurer, B., Mills, C., Shillingford J., [163c], 243, *367*
— Mercer, C. J., Shillinford, J. P. [899], 243, *339*
— see Balcon, R. [79], 217, 218, 221, *324*
Jick, H., see Anthony, J. R. [46], *323*

Jochim, K., see Katz, L. N. [954, 955, 958, 959], 55, 66, 67, 68, 69, 121, 145, *340*
Jönsson, T. E., see Brändström, A. [210], 229, *326*
Joergensen, L., Rowsell, H. C., Hovig, T., Glynn, M. F., Mustard, J. F. [900], 4, *339*
Johansson, B., see Duce, B. R. [454], 232, *331*
Johnsen, T. S. [901], 171, *339*
Johnson, G. E., see Flattery, K. V. [560], 167, 168, *333*
Johnson, J., see Moss, A. J. [228c], 210, *368*
Johnson, J. R., Wiggers, C. J. [902], 68, 69, *339*
Johnson, P. C., Sevelius, G. [903], 22, 129, *339*
— see Sevelius, G. [1723], 81, *354*
Johnson, W. D., Flemma, R. J., Lepley, D. [164c], 12, 13, *367*
— see Walker, J. A. [333c], 13, *370*
Johnsson, G. [904], 230, *339*
— Norrby, A., Sölvell, L. [905], 232, *339*
— see Albad, B. [4], 207, 232, *323*
— see Forsberg, S. A. [571], 230, 232, 233, *333*
Jolliffe, N. [906], 15, *339*
Jolly, E. R. [907], 162, *339*
Jongebreur, G. [908], 157, 160, *339*
Jones, H. B., see Graham, D. M. [704], 311, *335*
— see Lyon, T. P. [1199], 311, *344*
Jones, N. L., see Murray, J. F. [1333], 207, *347*
Jones, R., see Cotterill, J. A. [69c], 295, *365*
Jones, W. B., see Rackley, C. E. [264c], 35, *369*
— see Reeves, T. J. [1511], 2, 268, *350*
Jorgensen, C. R., see Ross, G. [1559, 1560, 272c], 172, 174, 236, *351, 369*
Jorgensen, F. S., see Clausen, J. [333], 217, 218, 221, *329*
Joris, H., Schmetz, J. [909], 171, *339*
Joseph, L. G., Mancini, A. [910], 147, *339*
Joseph, N., see Starr, I. [1823], 153, *356*
Jost, M., Gasser, P. [911], 163, *339*
Jourdan, F., Faucon, G. [912 to 917], 70, 153, 156, 157, 158, 160, 298, 313, *339*

Jouve, A. [918], 8, 10, *339*
— Benyamine, R., Malfroy, P. [165c], 29, *367*
— Gras, A., Benyamine, R. [919, 7d], 298, *339, 371*
— Medvedowsky, J. L., Benyamine, R. [920], 279, *339*
— Torresani, J., Chevalier-Cholat, A. M. [166c], 316, *367*
— see Gerard, R. [111c], 315, *366*
— see Mercier, F. [1282], 161, *346*
— see Torresani, J. [313c], 316, *370*
Juan, H., see Kukovetz, W. R. [73a], 150, 194, *361*
Juchems, R., Wertz, U. [65a], 229, *361*
Jucznic, G., see Klensch, H. [994, 995], 136, *341*
Judkins, M. P., see Bristow, J. D. [46c], 34, *364*
Judkins, M. R., see Farrehi, C. [527], 14, *332*
Judy, H., see Berman, J. K. [137], 90, *325*
Juhasz-Nagy, A., see Szentivanyi, M. [1869, 1870], 64, *356*
Junemann, C. [921], 187, *340*
Jung, A. [19b], 297, *363*
Junge-Hülsing, G., see Schmitt, G. [1685], 193, *353*
Junggren, U., see Brändström, A. [210], 229, *326*
Jungmann, H., see Gollwitzer-Meier, K. [684], 307, *335*
Junkmann, K. [922], 138, *340*
Jury, G., see Alix, B. [6c], 279, 286, 288, *363*
Jury, G. P. M. [66a], 279, *361*

Kaba, A., see Godfraind, T. [674], 201, *335*
Kabela, E., Jalife, J., Peon, C., Cros, L., Mendez, R. [67a], 63, *361*
— Mendez, R. [923], 218, *340*
— see Mendez, R. [1280], 206, *346*
Kabus, H. M., see Bretschneider, H. J. [226], 52, 62, 189, 190, 269, *327*
Kadatz, R. [924—927], 40, 68, 181, 182, *340*
— Dieteren, W. [928], 124, 151, 182, *340*
— Pötzsch, E. [929], 181, *340*
— see Menge, H. G. [1281], 181, *346*
Kaden, F., see Schmier, J. [286c], 183, *369*
Kado, R. T., see Kolin, A. [1016], 77, 256, *341*

Kahana, S., see Hunter, F. E. [873], 128, *339*

Kahler, R. L., see Epstein, S. E. [505], 207, 208, *332*

Kahn, A. S., see Mizgala, H. F. [1303, 1304], 211, 215, *346*

Kaindl, F., Pärtan, J., Polsterer, P. [930], 307, *340*
— see Grabner, G. [703], 181, *335*

Kaiser, G. A., see Klocke, F. J. [999, 1000], 63, 206, 264, *341*
— see Sonnenblick, E. H. [1791], 93, 132, 268, *355*

Kaiser, G. C., Barner, H. B., Jellinek, M., Mudd, G., Hanlon, C. R. [167c], 11, *367*

Kaiser, H., see Eisel, K. [482], 180, *331*

Kaiser, W., Klepzig, H. [931], 138, *340*

Kallio, V., see Iisalo, E. [875], 295, *339*

Kalmanson, D., Veyrat, C., Chiche, P., Derai, C., Novikoff, N. [168c], 78, *367*

Kalmanson, F. M., Drenick, E. J., Binder, M. J., Rosove, L. [932], 141, *340*

Kalmanson, G. M., see Binder, M. J. [162], 311, *326*

Kaltenbach, M., Becker, H. J., Graef, F., Hunscha, H. [169c], 247, *367*
— Zimmermann, D. [933], 174, *340*
— see Hunscha, H. [872], 191, *339*

Kamm, O., see Winder, C. V. [2018], 152, *359*

Kammermeier, H., see Fleckenstein, A. [561, 562], 166, 178, 216, 245, *333*
— see Grün, G. [748], 152, *336*

Kandziora, J. [934], 188, *340*

Kanie, T., see Kimura, E. [984], 93, *341*

Kannel, W. B., Lebauer, E. J., Dawber, T. R., McNamara, P. M. [20b], 16, *363*
— Widmer, L. K., Dawber, T. R. [935], 14, 16, *340*

Kany, R., see Spach, M. O. [36b], 229, *363*

Kanzow, E., see Frank, A. [579], 156, *333*

Kaplan, H. R., Robson, R. D. [8d], 255, *371*
— see Robson, R. D. [11d], 255 *371*

Kaplan, M. A., see Aronow, W. S. [56], 110, 213, *324*

Kaplan, S. R., see Rosenman, R. H. [1557], 158, *351*

Kappert, A. [936—938], 168, 279, 308, *340*

Kara, E., see Hellman, L. [809], 16, *337*

Karczmar, A. G., Bourgault, P., Elpern, B. [939], 313, *340*

Karges, O. [940], 212, *340*

Karlefors, T., see Christensson, B. [328], 130, *329*

Karpati, E., Domok, L., Szporny, L. [941], 288, *340*
— Szporny, L., Domok, L., Nador, K. [942], 288, *340*

Karppinen, K. [170c], 50, *367*

Kartun, P. [943], 298, *340*

Karvonen, M. J., see Turpeinen, O. [1906], 14, *357*

Kasparian, H., see Likoff, W. [1139], 48, *343*
— see Najmi, M. [1335], 33, 93, 131, *347*
— see Wiener, L. [338c], 34, *371*

Kassel, L. E., see Fuller, H. L. [613], 139, *334*

Kasser, I. S., Bruce, R. A. [944], 27, *340*

Kastor, J. A., Desanctis, R. W., Leinbach, R. C., Harthorne, J. W., Wolfson, I. N. [68a], 4, *361*

Katila, M., see Frick, M. H. [593, 102c], 9, *333*, *365*

Kato, K., see Nimura, Y. [234c], 78, *368*

Katori, M., Berne, R. M. [945], 60, *340*

Katsu, K., see Numano, F. [238c], 289, *368*

Kattus, A. A. [946], *340*
— Gregg, D. E. [947], 122, *340*
— Mac Alpin, R. M. [948], 9, *340*
— see Alvaro, A. B. [25], 214, *323*
— see Gaal, P. G. [616], 210, *334*
— see McAlpin, R. N. [1244], 30, 136, *345*

Katz, A., Messin, R. [949], 96, *340*

Katz, A. M., Katz, L. N., Williams, F. L. [950], 55, 59, *340*

Katz, G. [951], 67, *340*

Katz, K. H., see Osher, H. L. [1397], 158, *348*
— see Ravin, I. B. [1499], 305, *350*

Katz, L. N. [952, 953], 19, 22, 109, *340*
— Jochim, K., Bohning, A. [954], 55, 68, 69, *340*
— — Weinstein, W. [955], 68, 69, *340*

Katz, L. N., Lindner, E. [956, 957], 22, 69, 121, 145, 153, *340*
— — Weinstein, W., Abramson, D. I., Jochim, K. [958], 66, 67, 121, 145, *340*
— Weinstein, W., Jochim, K. [959], 68, *340*
— Williams, F. L., Laurent, D., Bolene-Williams, C., Feinberg, H. [960], 264, *340*
— see Elek, S. R. [484, 485], 113, 151, 299, 304, *331*
— see Gerola, A. [644, 645], 29, 264, 267, *334*
— see Katz, A. M. [950], 55, 59, *340*
— see Lafontant, R. [1067], 68, 75, *342*
— see Lindner, E. [1149], 150, 153, *344*
— see Marcus, E. [1219], 88, *345*
— see Mokotoff, R. [1310], 150, 154, *346*
— see Rosenman, R. H. [1557, 1558], 158, *351*
— see Salans, A. H. [1629], 141, *352*
— see Silber, E. H. [1752], 108, 109, 110, 116, 139, *354*
— see Simon, A. J. [1755], 151, *354*

Katz, R. L., see Lord, C. O. [1176], 232, 235, *344*

Kaufman, J. W., see Scott, R. C. [1708], 158, *353*

Kaufman, K. K., see Frisch, R. A. [604], 152, *334*

Kaufmann, H., Bergogne, C., Plessis, F. [961], 164

Kaufmann, M., see Gurtner, H. P. [131c], 246, 247, *366*

Kaverina, N. V. [962, 963], 299, 303, *340*
— Bendikov, E. A., Rozonov, Y. B. [171c], 134, *367*
— Vysotskaya, N. B., Rozonov, Y. B., Shugina, T. M. [964], 134, *340*
— see Zakusov, V. V. [2040, 2041], 303, *359*

Kayaalp, S. O., see Türker, R. K. [1904, 1905], 201, *357*

Kaye, H., see Cole, S. L. [349, 350], 110, 111, 139, 141, 156, 302, *329*

Kazemi, H., Parsons, E. F., Valenca, L. M., Strieder, D. J. [172c], 35, *367*

Keefer, C. S., Resnik, W. H. [965], 19, *340*

Keelan, P. [966], 207, *340*
— see Grant, R. H. E. [709], 217, *336*

Keller, C. J., see Hochrein, M. [843], 309, *338*

Kellershohn, C., see Di Matteo, J. [83c], 23, *365*

Kelliher, G. J., Buckley, J. P. [173c], 206, *367*

Kelling, H. W., see Fiegel, G. [544], 163, 190, *333*

Kemp, H. G., Elliott, W. C., Gorlin, R. [967], 48, *340*

— Manchester, J. H., Amsterdam, E. A., Taylor, W. J., Gorlin, R. [174c], 12, *367*

— see Hampton, J. R. [140c], 49, *366*

— see Helfant, R. H. [60a, 144c], 26, 33, *361, 366*

— see Horwik, L. D. [150c], 126, *366*

— see Wolfson, S. [2032, 2033], 42, 210, 211, 274, *359*

Kemp, V. E., see Wasserman, A. J. [130a], 230, 233, 235, *362*

Kenawy, M. R., Barsoum, G. S. [968], 158, *340*

— see Anrep, G. V. [37, 38, 39, 40, 45], 67, 157, 158, 159, *323*

— see Barsoum, G. S. [96], 158, *324*

Kennamer, R., Prinzmetal, M. [969], 163, *340*

Kentschke, G. E., see Hohl, O. [62a], 290, *361*

Kerber, R. E., Gianelly, R. E., Goldman, R. H. [175c], 234, *367*

— Goldman, R. H., Alderman, E. L., Harrison, D. C. [176c], 233, *367*

Kermarec, J., see Pernod, J. [1432], 293, *348*

Kernohan, R. J. [970], 219, *340*

— see Grant, R. H. E. [709], 217, *336*

Keroes, J., Ecker, R. R., Rapaport, E. [69a], 208, *361*

Kerr, J. W., Patel, K. R. [177c], 244, *367*

Kertes, K. [971], 168, *340*

Kessler, G., see Hellman, L. [809], 16, *337*

Kesteloot, H., see Piessens, J. [31b], 204, *363*

Ketelers, J. Y., see Hondas, Y. [152c], 72, *366*

— see Warembourg, H. [335c], 211, *371*

Kettler, D., see Spieckermann, P. G. [119a], 185, 193, *362*

Kety, S. S., [972], 86, *340*

— Schmidt, C. F. [973], 79, *340*

— see Eckenhoff, J. E. [469], 79, *331*

Keul, J., Doll, E., Friedemann, M., Reindell, H. [974, 975], 187, *340*

— see Doll, E. [436, 35a], 56, 186, *331, 360*

Keulen, U. W. [178c], 248, *367*

Keys, A. [976], 14, 15, *341*

— see Taylor, H. L. [1875], 9, *356*

Khadzhai, Y. I., see Angarskaya, M. A. [34], 304, *323*

Khaja, F., Parker, J. O., Ledwich, R. J., West, R. O., Armstrong, P. W. [179c], 31, 32, *367*

— see Parker, J. O. [242c], 131, 133, *368*

Khan, A. S., see Davies, R. O. [31a], 148, 213, *360*

— see Mizgala, H. F. [89a, 90a], 212, *361*

Khanna, V. K., see Madan, B. R. [210c], 232, *368*

Khouri, E. M., Gregg, D. E. [977], 77, 256, *341*

— — Lowensohn, H. S. [978], 90, *341*

— — Rayford, C. R. [979], 29, 55, 56, 77, 256, *341*

— see Gregg, D. E. [728, 128c], 2, 57, 77, 125, 256, *336, 366*

Kidd, D. J., see Fox, R. H. [575], 63, *333*

Kienle, H., see Algan, O. [20], 188, *323*

Kiese, M., Lange, G. [980], 76, *341*

— Lange, G., Resag, K. [981], 182, *341*

Kiesewetter, E. [982], 159, *341*

Kiil, F., see Abrahamsen, A. M. [5], 136, 143, *323*

Killam, K. F., Fellows, E. J. [983], 157, *341*

— see Fellows, E. J. [534], 157, *332*

— see Lasker, N. [1077], 300, *342*

Killough, J. H., see Abrams, W. B. [6], 163, *323*

Kilmore, M. A., see Clark, J. P. [61c], 237, *364*

Kilpatrick, S. J., see Murphy, F. M. [1332], 163, *347*

Kimura, E., Ushiyama, K., Yamazaki, T., Yoshida, K., Kojima, N., Kanie, T. [984], 93, *341*

Kimura, E. T., see Schachter, R. J. [1654], 155, *352*

Kincaid-Smith, P. [180c], 51, *367*

King, M. P., see Angelakos, E. T. [8c], 63, *363*

King, R. D., see Elliott, W. C. [89c], 316, *365*

King, S., see Falicov, R. E. [95c], 316, *365*

Kinnard, W. J., Vogin, E. E., Aceto, M. D., Buckley, J. P. [985], 149, *341*

— see Aceto, M. D. [8, 9], 146, *323*

— see Buckley, J. P. [251], 146, *327*

Kinney, M. J., see Lau, S. H. [1080], 100, *342*

Kinsella, D., Troup, W., McGregor, M. [986], 187, *341*

Kipsidze et al. 191

Kirchgessner, T., see Stanton, H. C. [1818], 250, *355*

Kirchheimer, W. F., see Zeller, E. A. [2047], 160, *360*

Kirchhoff, H. W., Burkhart, K., Meyer, J., Gebelein, H., Henze, H. [987], 196, *341*

Kirk, E. S., see Honig, C. R. [149c], 317, *366*

Kirsch, U., Autenrieth, G. [70a], 198, *361*

Kisch, B. [988], 20, *341*

Kisin, I. E. [989], 315, *341*

Kissane, R. W., see Conn, J. J. [353], 158, *329*

Kissel, D., Winbury, M. M. [2014], 45, 53, 85, *359*

Kissin, M., see Bakst, H. [75], 112, 155, *324*

Kisthinios, N., see Gley, P. [672], 309, *335*

— see Vaquez, H. [1919], 309, *357*

Kitabatake, A., see Nimura, Y. [234c], 78, *368*

Kittle, C. F., see Falicov, R. E. [95c], 316, *365*

Klakeg, C. H., Pruitt, R. D., Burchell, H. B. [990], 96, *341*

Klarwein, M., Nitz, R. E. [991], *341*

Klassen, G. A., see Hoeschen, R. J. [845], 126, *338*

Kleiber, E. E. [992], 158, *341*

Klein, K., see Hammerl, H. [774], 187, *337*

Klein, M. D., see Cohen, L. S. [345], 4, 25, 275, *329*

— see Gorlin, R. [700], 93, *335*

Klensch, H. [993], 165, *341*

— Juznic, G. [994, 995], 136, *341*

— see Speckmann, K. [1804], 101, *355*

Klepzig, H., see Kaiser, W. [931], 138, *340*

— see Tschirdewahn, B. [1902] 179, *357*

Klever, R. [996], 188, *341*
Klich, R. [997], 171, *341*
Kligge, H. [998], 190, *341*
Klocke, F. J., Kaiser, G. A., Ross, J., Braunwald, E. [999, 1000], 63, 206, 264, *341*
— Wittenberg, S. M., Greene, D. G., Bunnell, I. L., Falsetti, H. L. [181c], 23, *367*
Kloster, J. H. [1001], 171, *341*
Knebel, R. [1002], 285, 286, *341*
— Ockenga, T. [1003], 196, *341*
Knick, B. [1004], 163, *341*
Knoch, G. [1005], 179, *341*
Knoche, H., Schmitt, G. [1006], 214, *341*
— see Schmitt, G. [1686], 214, *353*
Knoebel, S. B., Elliott, W. C., Ross, E., McHenry, P. L. [182c], 57, *367*
— McHenry, P. L., Roberts, D., Stein, L. [1007], 125, 130, *341*
— — Stein, L., Sonel, A. [1008], 82, 83, 92, *341*
— see McHenry, P. L. [1254], 83, *345*
Knorpp, K., see Tschirdewahn, B. [1903], 221, *357*
Knopf, K. W., see Bartsch, W. [18c], 232, *364*
Kobayashi, I., see Yamazaki, H. [341c], 289, *371*
Kobayashi, T., see West, J. W. [1979, 1980], 71, 89, *358*
Koberstein, E., see Thiele, K. [1880], 198, *357*
Kocandrle, V., see Falicov, R. E. [95c], 316, *365*
Koch, G., see Jacobsson, K. A. [885], 168, *339*
Koch-Weser, J. [1009], 220, *341*
Kochsiek, K., see Bretschneider, H. J. [227], 181, 183, *327*
— see Strauer, B. E. [302c], 94, *370*
Köhler, J. A., Sternitzke, N. [1010], 198, *341*
— see Lang, E. [77a, 194c], 156, *361*, *367*
— see Sternitzke, N. [1837], 197, *356*
Koehler, M. [183c], 246, *367*
Köhler, W. [1011], 160, *341*
Koenig, E., see Froer, K. L. [44a], 245, *361*
König, K., see Gebhardt, W. [633], 207, *334*
Koetschet, P., see Courvoisier, S. [373], 302, *329*

Kofi Ekue, J. M., Lowe, D. C., Shanks, R. G. [71a], 251, *361*
— Shanks, R. G., Zaidi, S. A. [184c], 237, *367*
Kofman, J., see Faucon, G. [529, 530, 531], 188, 189, *332*
Kohler, R., see Gander, M. [622], 207, *334*
Kojima, N., see Kimura, E. [984], 93, *341*
Kolassa, N., Pfleger, K., Rummel, W. [21b], 186, *363*
— Tram, M., Pfleger, K. [185c], 185, *367*
— see Pfleger, K. [30b], 186, 194, 202, *363*
Kolesnikov, D. G., see Angarskaya, M. A. [34], 304, *323*
Kolin, A. [1012—1014, 186c], 77, 78, 256, *341*, *367*
— Archer, J. D., Ross, G. [1015], 4, 78, *341*
— Kado, R. T. [1016], 77, 256, *341*
— Ross, G., Grollman, J. H., Archer, J. [1017], 78, *341*
Kolodzig, S. [1018], 187, *341*
Kolsky, M., see Courvoisier, S. [373], 302, *329*
Kong, Y., Morris, J. J. [187c], 318, *367*
Koons, R. A., see Conn, J. J. [353], 158, *329*
Kopald, H. H., see Herd, J. A. [816], 83, *338*
Kopitar, Z. [188c], 185, *367*
Koretsky, S., see Altman, G. E. [23], 140, *323*
— see Riseman, J. E. F. [1531], 106, 135, 137, 138, 139, 140, 142, 143, 146, *350*
Korol, B., see Melville, K. I. [1273], 120, *346*
Koroxenidis, G., Tsitouris, G., Papadopoulos, A., Vassilikos, C., Corcondilas, A., Michaelides, G. [1019], 223, *341*
— see Corcondilas, A. [362]‘ 228, *329*
— see Lekos, D. [1098], 226, *343*
— see Regan, T. J. [1513], 301, *350*
Kory, R. C., Townes, A. S., Mabe, R. E., Dorris, E. R., Meneely, G. R. [1020], 141, *341*
Koss, F. W., Beisenherz, G., Maerkisch, R. [1021], 185, *341*
Kot, P. A., Croke, R. P., Pinkerson, A. L. [1022], 144, *341*

Kotzaurek, R., see Hueber, E. F. [868], 278, 280, 281, 287, *339*
Kountz, W. B. [1023, 1024], 67, 150, 299, 304, 314, *341*
— Smith, J. R. [1025], 153, *341*
Kovalik, A. T. W., see Bigger, T. W. [31c], 303, *364*
Kracke, R. [72a], 159, *361*
Kränzl, C., see Hammerl, H. [775], *337*
Kramer, K., see Gollwitzer-Meier, K. [685], 264, *335*
Kramer, M. L., see Greiner, T. [738], 110, 111, 112, 113, 116, 158, 308, *336*
Krantz, J. C., Carr, C. J. [1026], 311, *341*
— — Bryant, H. H. [1027], 128, *341*
— — Forman, S. E. [1028], 144, *341*
— — — Ellis, F. W. [1029, 1030], 140, 146, *341*
— see Hensala, J. C. [812], 156, *338*
Krantz, J. C., jr., see Burgison, R. M. [261], 149, *327*
Krasnikov, Y. A. [1031], 211, *341*
Krasnow, N., Barbarosh, H. [1032], 221, *342*
— Hood, W. B., Rolett, E. L., Yurchak, P. M. [1033], 25, *342*
— Rolett, E. L., Yurchak, P. M., Hood, W. B., Gorlin, R. [1034], 4, 264, *342*
— see Levine, J. H. [1115], *343*
— see Wagman, R. J. [1953], 22, 24, 275, *358*
Kraupp, O., Grossmann, W., Stühlinger, W., Raberger, G. [1036], 194, *342*
— Heistracher, P., Wolner, E., Tuisl, E. [1037], 192, *342*
— Nell, G., Raberger, G., Stühlinger, W. [1038], 196, *342*
— Niessner, H. [1039], 194, *342*
— — Ploszczanski, B., Adler-Kastner, L., Springer, A., Chirikdjian, J. J. [1040], 194, *342*
— Wolner, E. [1041], 193, *342*
— — Adler-Kastner, L., Chirikdjian, J. J., Ploszczanski, B., Tuisl, E. [1042], 192, *342*
— — Suko, J. [1043], 182, 189, 194, *342*
— see Grabner, G. [703], 181, *335*

Kraupp, O., see Heistracher, P. [800, 801, 802], 169, 192, 193, *337*
— see Raberger, G. [102a, 261c, 262c, 263c], 61, 194, 196, *362, 369*
Kraupp, W. E. [1035], 59, *342*
Kraus, A., see Christakis, G. [327], 14, *328*
Krause, H., see Tritthart, H. [125a], 179, 219, *362*
Kraut, H., Frey, E. K., Bauer, E. [1044], 309, *342*
— see Frey, E. K. [590, 591], 309, *333*
Krautheim, J., Schmid, E. [1045], 198, *342*
— see Schmid, E. [1677], 167, *353*
Krayenbuehl, H. P., see Bussmann, W. D. [266, 5b], 235, 237, 239, *327, 363*
— see Wirz, P. [340c], *371*
Krivoruchenko, I. V., see Ganelina, I. E. [623], 295, *334*
Kroetz, C., see Gollwitzer-Meier, K. [686], 58, 138, 139, 268, *335*
Krüger, E., see Gollwitzer-Meier, K. [685], 264, *335*
Krueger, G. A. W. [1046], 138, *342*
Krueger, K. [1047, 1048], 168, 234, 235, *342*
Krug, A., Krug, C., Dharamadhach, A. [189c], 183, *367*
Krug, C., see Krug, A. [189a], 183, *367*
Kuba, K., see Renaud, S. [268c], 50, *369*
Kubicek, F., see Praschl, E. [1465], 290, *349*
Kubler, W., Spieckermann, P. G., Bretschneider, H. J. [190c], 185, *367*
Kübler, W., Bretschneider, H. J. [1049, 1050], 62, 185, *342*
— — Spieckermann, P. G. [1051], 186, *342*
Kühns, K. [1052], 313, *342*
Kuhn, W. L., see Hudak, W. J. [63a, 153c], 294, *361, 367*
Kuhn, R., see Isaacs, J. H. [879], 101, *339*
Kukovetz, W. R. [1053—1055], 198, 290, *342*
— Fischer, G. [1056], 189, *342*
— Juan, H., Poech, G. [73a], 150, 194, *361*
— Pöch, G. [74a, 191c, 6e], 165, 197, 198, *361, 367, 371*
Kukwa, D. [1057], 159, *342*
— see Fiegel, G. [543, 544], 163, 190, *333*

Kumakura, S., see Hashimoto, K. [790], 61, 62, *337*
Kumlin, T., see Ejrup, B. [483], 148, *331*
Kunos, G., see Szentivanyi, M. [310c], 63, *370*
Kunze, K., Lübbers, D. W., Rybak, B. [1058], *342*
Kunzig, H. J., see Rudolph, W. [1583], 190, *351*
Kupperman, H. S., see Gagliani, J. [621], 155, *334*
Kuriyama, T. [1059], 88, *342*
Kurland, G. S., Freedberg, A. S. [1060], 15, *342*
— see Blumgart, H. L. [187, 188], 20, *326*
— see Sagall, E. L. [1626], 137, *352*
Kusakari, T., see Nakano, J. [1336], 33, 207, 272, 274, *347*
Kuschke, H. J. [1061], 157, *342*
— Eckmann, F. [1062], 167, *342*
Kusus, T., see Lydtin, H. [1198], 220, *344*
Kutscha, W. [1063], 211, *342*
Kutschera, W. [1064], 137, *342*
Kutz-Echave, R. [1065], 313, *342*
Kvam, D. C., Riggilo, D. A., Lish, P. M. [1066], 251, *342*
Kwit, N. T., see Gold, H. [677], 108, 154, *335*
— see Greiner, T. [738], 110, 111, 112, 113, 116, 158, 308, *336*

Labarre, J., see Bacq, Z. M. [67], 173, *324*
Lachieze-Rey, E., see Detry, R. [421], 279, *330*
Laddu, A. R., Somani, P. [75a, 9d], 242, 246, *361, 371*
— see Somani, P. [1781, 116a to 118a, 9e], 57, 134, 236, 237, *355, 362, 371*
La Due, J. S., see Bayley, R. H. [114], 154, *325*
Lafont, H., see Di Matteo, J. [83c], 23, *365*
Lafontant, R., Feinberg, H., Katz, L. N. [1067], 68, 75, *342*
Lagarde, see Faivre, G. [520], 97, *332*
Lamarche, M., Marignac, B. [22b], 295, *363*
— Royer, R. [192c], 295, *367*
— see Fourneau, J. P. [12b], 295, *363*
Lamb, P., see Pentecost, B. L. [1430], 295, *348*

Lambert, C. J., see Adam, M. [3c], 12, *363*
Lammerant, J., Becsei, I., Mertens-Strijthagen, J., De Schryver, C. [193c], 306, *367*
Lamont, H., see De Schaepdryver, A. F. [416], 167, *330*
Lamprecht, G., Schmidt-Voigt, J. [1068], 217, *342*
Lancaster, W. M., see Peel, A. A. [1428], 187, *348*
Landmesser, C. H., see Eckenhoff, J. E. [470, 471], 55, 56, 74, *331*
Landry, F., see Blümchen, G. [33c], 156, *364*
Lands, A. M., Luduena, F. P., Buzzo, H. J. [76a], 237, *361*
Lane, F. J., see Gorlin, R. [700], 93, *335*
Lang, E., Köhler, J. A. [77a, 194c], 156, *361, 367*
— see Sternitzke, N. [1837], 197, *356*
Lang, K. F., see James, T. N. [160c], 218, *367*
Lang, O. [1071], 196, *342*
Lang, T., see Vyden, J. K. [330c], 134, *370*
Lange, A., see Jacobi, H. [884], 156, *339*
Lange, B. M., see Diewitz, M. [34a], 179, *360*
Lange, G. [1072, 1073], 170, *342*
— see Kiese, M. [980, 981], 76, 182, *341*
Langendorff, O. [1074], 65, *342*
Langer, I. [78a, 195c], 217, 290, 291, *361, 367*
— see Herxheimer, H. [146c], 217, *366*
Lankford, H., see Berry, J. W. [147], 147, *325*
Lanney, E., see Denis, B. [32a], 279, *360*
Laplace, L. B., see Wayne, E. J. [1964], 154, *358*
Laporte, G., see Broustet, P. [239], 279, *327*
Laraia, P. J., Craig, R. J., Reddy, W. J. [196c], *367*
Large, B. J., see Armitage, A. K. [55], 156, *324*
Larsen, L. P., see Bay, G. [113], 218, *325*
Larsen, O. A., see Clausen, J. P. [334], 9, *329*
Larsen, V. [1075], 67, *342*
Laruel, R., see Broekhuysen, J. [235, 236], 268, 287, *327*
Lasagna, L. [1076], 110, 116, *342*
— see Schelling, J. L. [1662], 137, 143, *353*

Lasker, N., Sherrod, T. R., Killam, K. F. [1077], 300, *342*

Lassen, N. A., Lindbjerg, J., Munck, O. [1078], 83, *342*

— see Hansen, A. T. [780], 83, *337*

Laszlo, B., Laszlo, K. [1079], 211, *342*

Laszlo, K., see Laszlo, B. [1079], 211, *342*

Latour, H., see Puech, P. [259c], 3, *369*

Lau, S. H., Cohen, S. I., Stein, E., Haft, J. I., Kinney, M. J., Young, M. W., Helfant, R. H., Damato, A. N. [1080], 100, *342*

— Damato, A. N., Berkowitz, W. D., Patton, R. D. [1081], 3, *342*

— Haft, J. I., Cohen, S. I., Helfant, R. H., Young, M. W., Damato, A. N. [1082], 100, *342*

— see Berkowitz, W. D. [11a], 220, *360*

— see Damato, A. N. [387, 388, 389, 30a], 3, *330, 360*

— see Scherlag, B. J. [1665], 3, *353*

Laubie, M., Le Douarec, J. C., Schmitt, H. [1083], 298, *342*

— Schmitt, H. [1084, 1085], 298, *342*

— — Peltier, J., Drouillat, M. [1086], 58, *342*

— — Remy, C. [1087], 62, 189, *342*

Laubry, C., Soulie, P., Laubry, P. [1088], 154, *342*

Laubry, P., see Laubry, C. [1088], 154, *342*

Lauener, H., see Schmutz, J. [1688], 159, *353*

Lauenroth, G. [1089], 168, *342*

Laurent, D., see Katz, L. N. [960], 264, *340*

Laustela, E., Tala, P. [1090], 182, *343*

Laval, G., see Ameur, M. [3a], 279, *360*

Lavallee, A., see Allmark, M. G. [22], 161, *323*

— see Lu, F. C. [1182], 72, 151, 158, 310, *344*

Lavandier, G., see Perrot, J. [29b], 279, 287, *363*

Lavarenne, J., see Duchene-Marullaz, P. [455, 458], 164, 169, 298, *331*

— see Faucon, G. [528, 530, 531,], 188, 189, 298, *332*

Lavergne, G., see Watillon, M. [1961], 287, *358*

Lavy, S., Stern, S. [197c], 205, *367*

Lawson, C. W., see Sandler, G. [1642], 171, *352*

Lawton, A. H., see Von Oettingen, W. F. [1948], 138, 140, *358*

Lazzara, R., see Singer, D. H. [292c], 27, *3*

Leatham, A., see Hale, G. [765], 100, *337*

Lebauer, E. J., see Kannel, W. B. [20b], 16, *363*

Lecerof, 298

Lecerhof, H., Malmborg, R. O. [79a], 297, *361*

— see Arborelius, M. [51], 131, *324*

Le Douarec, J. C., see Laubie, M. [1083], 298, *342*

Leder, O., Doering, H. J., Reindell, A., Fleckenstein, A. [80a], 167, 175, *361*

Ledwich, J. R. [1091], 221, *343*

— see Parker, J. O. [1416, 94a, 242c], 31, 32, 38, 131, 132, 133, *348, 362, 368*

Ledwich, R. J., see Khaja, F. [179c], 31, 32, *367*

Leeper, R. D., Mead, A. W., Money, W. L., Rawson, R. W. [1092], 15, *343*

Leeson, G., see Chessin, M. [323], 163, *328*

Leet, C. J., see Cundey, P. E. [73c], 174, 175, *365*

Leferink, B. H. G. [198c], 285, *367*

Lefevre, M., see Scebat, L. [1652], 215, 221, *352*

Legge, J. S., see Palmer, K. N. V. [93a], 244, *362*

Lehan, P. H., Oldewurtel, H. A., Weisse, A. B., Elliott, M. S., Regan, T. J. [1093], 124, *343*

— see Regan, T. J. [1513], 301, *350*

Lehtosuo, E. J., see Turpeinen, O. [1906], 14, *357*

Leibeskind, R. S., see Skinner, M. S. [1756], 129, *354*

Leibetseder, F. [1094], 196, *343*

Leibowitz, S., see Bakst, H. [75], 112, 155, *324*

Leicht, E., see Gersmeyer, E. F. [646], 215, *334*

Leighninger, D. S., see Beck, C. S. [116], 169, *325*

— Rueger, R., Beck, C. [1095], 122, *343*

— see Salwan, F. A. [278c], 21, *369*

Leinbach, R. C., see Kastor, J. A. [68a], 4, *361*

Leitch, J. L., Haley, T. J. [1096], 66, *343*

Lekieffre, J. [1097], 163, *343*

— see Warembourg, H. [41b], 291, *363*

Lekos, D., Ioannidis, P., Corcondilas, A., Hadjigeorge, C., Marnezos, E., Koroxenidis, G., Michaelides, G. [1098], 226, *343*

Leloup, A., see Vastesaeger, M. [1926, 1929, 1930], 170, 171, *357*

Lemberg, L., Castellanos, A., Arcebal, A. G. [1099], 221, *343*

Lemire, Y., see Renaud, S. [268c], 50, *369*

Lemoigne, P., see Manion, J. [1220], 171, *345*

Lenard, G., see Szekeres, L. [1867 bis] 304, *356*

Lenegre, J. [1100, 1101], 8, 10, 14, 16, 163, *343*

— see Barrillon, A. [17c], 163, *364*

— see Beaumont, J. L. [115], 311, *325*

— see Bensaid, J. [24c, 25c], 227, *364*

— see Gerbaux, A. [638, 639], 162, 163, *334*

Lenke, D. [199c], 54, *367*

Lenoir, P., see Bourel, M. [202], 308, *326*

Leon, D. F., see Thompson, M. E. [311c], 240, *370*

Leonard, J. C., see Grant, R. H. E. [709], 217, *336*

Lepeschkin, E. [1102], 19, *343*

— see Raab, W. [1490, 1491], 36, 123, 207, 284, *348, 349*

Lepley, D., see Johnson, W. D. [164c], 12, 13, *367*

— see Walker, J. A. [333c], 13, *370*

Lequime, J., Cleempoel, H., Van Thiel, E. [1103], 90, *343*

Leroux-Robert, C., see Richet, G. [1525], 172, *350*

Leroy, G. V. [1104], 154, *343*

— Fenn, G. K., Gilbert, N. C. [1105], 154, *343*

— Speer, J. H. [1106], 156, *343*

Lesbre, J. P., Calazel, P., Meriel, P., Guiraud, R., Bru, A. [81a], 181, 186, *361*

— Rumeau, M., Meriel, P. [200c], 279, *368*

Leschke, E. [1107], 309, *343*

Leshin, S. J., see Baker, L. D. [73, 74], 26, *324*

Leslie, A., Scott, W. S., Mulinos, M. G. [1108], 106, *343*

Leslie, A., see Scott, W. S. [1711], 106, *354*

Leslie, R. E. [1109], 147, *343*

Lesniak, L. J., see Regan, T. J. [1514], 301, *350*

Lesser, M. A. [1110], 305, *343*

Letac, B., Cannon, R., Hood, W. B., Lown, B. [1111], 2, *343*

Letley, E., see Thompson, R. H. [1887], 219, *357*

Leuschner, F., see Habersang, S. [760], 196, *337*

Leusen, I. R., Essex, H. E. [1112], 158, *343*

Leutenegger, A., Luthy, E. [1113], 280, 287, *343*

Levey, G. S., Epstein, S. E. [1114], 273, *343*

— see Entman, M. L. [38a], 216, *360*

Levin, H. G., see Rosenman, R. H. [1557], 158, *351*

Levin, N. W., see Rabkin, R. [1492], 211, 214, 217, *350*

Levine, H. D., see Friend, D. G. [602], 139, *334*

Levine, H. J., see Messer, J. V. [1287], 38, *346*

— see Neill, W. A. [1355], 29, 55, 267, *347*

— see Wagman, R. J. [1953], 22, 24, 275, *358*

Levine, J. H., Neill, W. A., Wagman, R. J., Krasnow, N., Gorlin, R. [1115], *343*

— Wagman, R. J. [1116], 31, 92, 128, *343*

Levine, S. A. [1117], 20, *343*

— Likoff, W. B. [1118], 305, *343*

— see Armbrust, C. A. [54], 158, *324*

Levinson, G. E., see Frank, M. J. [580], 3, *333*

Levinson, R. S., McIlduff, J. B., Regan, T. J. [201c], 295, *368*

Levitt, B., Raines, A., Moros, D., Standaert, F. G. [1119], 249, *343*

Levy, B., Ahlquist, R. P. [1120], 175, *343*

— Wasserman, M. [202c], 254, *368*

— Wilkenfeld, B. E. [1121], 235, 237, *343*

Levy, G. P., see Blackburn, C. H. [182], 253, *326*

— see Farmer, J. B. [525, 526], 249, 250, *332*

Levy, H., Boas, E. P. [1122], 305, *343*

Levy, J. V. [1123, 1124, 23b, 24b], 120, 206, 215, 245, 248, 250, *343*, *363*

Levy, J. V., Richards, V. [1125], 215, 216, *343*

Levy, R. L., Barach, A. L., Bruenn, H. G. [1126], 106, *343*

— Bruenn, H. G., Russel, N. G. [1127], 106, *343*

— — Williams, N. E. [1128], 106, 136, 140, 154, *343*

— Williams, N. E., Bruenn, H. G., Carr, H. A. [1129], 96, 106, *343*

— see Williams, N. E. [2003], 106, 154, *359*

Lew, H. T., March, H. W. [1130], 221, *343*

Lewis, B. I., Lubin, R. I., January, L. E., Wild, J. B. [1131], 308, *343*

Lewis, C. M. ,Brink, A. J. [1132], 208, *343*

Lewis, D. W., see Abrams, W. B. [6, 7], 163, *323*

Lewis, G. P. [1133], 63, *343*

— see Edery, H. [479], 21, *331*

— see Fox, R. H. [575], 63, *333*

— see Hilton, S. M. [834, 835], 63, *338*

Lewis, R. E., see Hudak, W. J. [63a, 153c], 294, *361*, *367*

Lewis, T. [1134], 19, *343*

Lhermitte, F., see Gautier, J. C. [107c], 51, *366*

Libermann, D., Denis, J.-C. [1135], 163, *343*

Lichah, E., see Armand, P. [53], 279, *324*

Lichtlen, P., Albert, H. [203c], 247, *368*

— — Moccetti, T. [204c, 205c], 247, *368*

— — Spiegel, M. [206c], 214, *368*

— Baumann, P. C. [1136], 125, *343*

Lichtlen, P. R., see Bernstein, L. [146], 28, 83, 123, 130, 133, *325*

— see Ross, R. S. [1562], 83, 84, 123, 130, *351*

Liebow, J. M., Seasohn, P. O. [1137], 48, *343*

Liertzer, V., see Greif, S. [737], 198, *336*

Liesicke, J. [1138], 138, *343*

Likoff, W., Segal, B. L., Kasparian, H. [1139], 48, *343*

Likoff, W. B., see Levine, S. A. [1118], 305, *343*

Liljedahl, J., see Sealey, B. J. [290c], 233, *369*

Lill, G. [1140], 159, *343*

Lim, H. F. [1141], 95, 96, *343*

Lim, R. K. S., see Guzman, F. [754], 21, *336*

Lindbjerg, J., see Lassen, N. A. [1078], 83, *342*

Linder, E. [1142], 85, *343*

— Seeman, T. [1143], 183, *343*

Lindert, M. C. F., see Meyer, J. M. [1293], 152, *346*

Lindgren, F. T., see Lyon, T. P. [1199], 311, *344*

Lindgren, M., see Jacobsson, K. A. [885], 168, *339*

Lindner, A., Loudon, M., Werner, G. [1150], 309, *344*

— see Brücke, F. [245], 307, *327*

Lindner, E. [1144—1148], 37, 165, 166, 167, 289, *343*

— Katz, L. N. [1149], 150, 153, *344*

— see Katz, L. N. [956, 957, 958], 22, 66, 67, 69, 121, 145, 153, *340*

— see Schöne, H. H. [1695, 1696], 166, *353*

Linhart, J. W., Braunwald, E., Ross, J. [1151], 3, 219, *344*

— Hildner, F. J., Barold, S. S., Lister, J. W., Samet, P. [82a], 34, 130, *361*

— — Samet, P. [1152 to 1154], 3, 11, 126, *344*

Linko, E., Ruosteenoja, R., Siitonen, L. [1155], 232, *344*

— Siitonen, L., Ruosteenoja, R. [1156], 235, *344*

Linquette, M., Luez, G., Beghin, B. [1157], 190, 191, *344*

Lisan, P. [1158], 314, *344*

Lish, P. M., Weikel, J. H., Dungan, K. W. [1159], 216, 249, 250, *344*

— see Dungan, K. W. [462], 249, *331*

— see Kvam, D. C. [1066], 251, *342*

Lister, J. W., see Linhart, J. W. [82a], 34, 130, *361*

Liston Beazley, H., see Chapman, D. W. [59c], 12, *364*

Littmann, D., Rodman, M. H. [1160], 96, *344*

Litvak, J., Siderides, L. E., Vineberg, A. M. [1161], 90, *344*

— see Vineberg, A. M. [1943], 90, *358*

Livesley, B., Catley, P. F., Oram, S. [207c], 25, *368*

Livingstone, W. R., see Watt, D. A. L. [337c], 221, *371*

Lloyd, H. J., see Wilson, A. G. [135a], 241, *362*

Lochner, W. [1162, 1163], 71, 261, 268, *344*

— Hirche, H. [1164], 188, 189, *344*

Lochner, W., Mercker, H., Nasseri, M. [1165], 58, *344*
— — Schürmeyer, E. [1166], 150, 153, *344*
— Nasseri, M. [1167, 1168], 58, 182, 268, *344*
— Parratt, J. R. [1169], 63, *344*
— see Bussmann, W. D. [267], 189, *327*
— see Mercker, H. [1284], 58, *346*
— see Morgenstern, C. [227c], 207, *368*
— see Raff, W. K. [103a, 265c], 122, *362, 369*
— see Scholtholt, J. [1694], 62, 63, 189, *353*
Logue, B. [1170], 14, 162, *344*
Lohmoeller, G., Lydtin, H. [84a], 229, 235, *361*
Lombardo, T. A., Rose, L., Taeschler, M., Tuluy, S., Bing, R. J. [1171], 55, *344*
Long, J., see Vineberg, A. [327c], 11, *370*
Longino, F. H., see Gregg, D. E. [729], 80, *336*
Longslet, A. [1172], 302, *344*
Longuet, D., see Marion, J. [1220], 171, *345*
Loos, H. [1173], 179, *344*
Lopes, E. C., Molenaar, M. G. [1174], 311, *344*
Lopez Salgado, A. [1175], 298, *344*
Lord, C. O., Katz, R. L., Eakins, K. E. [1176], 232, 235, *344*
Lordick, H. [1177], 192, *344*
Lore, S. A., see Scarborough, W. R. [1651], 95, *352*
Lorentsen, E., see Bay, G. [113], 218, *325*
Lorenz, D., Dell, H. D. [83a], 182, 189, 193, 201, *361*
Losada, M., see Winbury, M. M. [2014], 45, 53, 85, *359*
Loubatieres, A., Sassine, A. [1178], 309, *344*
Loudon, M., see Brücke, F. [245], 307, *327*
— see Lindner, A. [1150], 309, *344*
Louven, B., see Hilger, H. H. [826, 827], 186, 194, *338*
Love, W. D., Burch, G. E. [1179], 82, *344*
Lovell, R. H., see Nestel, P. J. [1357], 284, *347*
Lowe, D. C., see Kofi Ekue, J. M. [71a], 251, *361*
Lowe, T. E., see Nayler, W. G. [1346—1352], 174, 177, 179, 182, 208, 216, 222, 223, 242, 245, 246, *347*

Lowensohn, H. S., see Khouri, E. M. [978], 90, *341*
Lown, B., see Letac, B. [1111], 2, *343*
Loy, D. L., see Stoland, O. O. [1844], 153, 309, *356*
Lozada, J. S., see Favaloro, R. G. [533], 10, *332*
Lu, F. C. [1180, 1181], 310, *344*
— Allmark, M. G., Carmichael, E. J., MacMillan, D. B., Lavallee, A. [1182], 72, 151, 158, 310, *344*
— — Graham, W. D. [1183], 305, *344*
— Melville, K. I. [1184], 72, *344*
— see Allmark, M. G. [22], 161, *323*
— see Melville, K. I. [1274, 1275], 122, 139, 153, *346*
Lu, G. G., see Burgison, R. M. [261], 149, *327*
Lubawski, I., Wale, J. [1185], 246, *344*
Lubin, M., see Eckenhoff, J. E. [469], 79, *331*
— see Goodale, W. T. [690, 691], 79, *335*
Lubin, R. I., see Lewis, B. I. [1131], 308, *343*
Lucchelli, P. E., see Bianchi, C. [158, 159], 227, *325*
Lucchesi, B. R. [1186, 1187], 219, 221, 273, *344*
— Hodgeman, R. J. [7e], 63, 236, *371*
— Hodgemar, R. J. [208c], 236, *368*
— Iwami, T. [1188], 219, *344*
— Whitsitt, L. S., Brown, N. L. [1189], 220, *344*
— — Stickney, J. L. [1190], 219, 220, *344*
— see Whitsitt, L. S. [1989, 1990], 209, 218, *358*
Luduena, F. P., Miller, E., Wilt, W. A. [1191], 67, *344*
— see Lands, A. M. [76a], 237, *361*
Lübbers, D. W., see Kunze, K. [1058], *342*
Luebs, E. D., Cohen, A., Zaleski, E. J., Bing, R. J [1192], 130, 133, 151, 178, 190, *344*
— see Cohen, A. [339], 130, 151, *329*
Lueth, H. C., see Sutton, D. C. [1858], 19, *356*
Luez, G., see Linquette, M. [1157], 190, 191, *344*
Lugo, J. E., see Rowe, G. G. [1573], 294, *351*

Luisada, A., see Neumann, M. [1359], 174, 179, *347*
Luisada, A. A., see Aravanis, C. [50], 155, *323*
Lujf, A., Moser, K. [1193, 1194] 194, 221, *344*
— — Schwarzmeier, J. [1195], 215, *344*
— see Benda, L. [131], 179, *325*
— see Moser, K. [1323, 1324], 198, 212, *347*
— see Niessner, H. [92a, 233c], 198, 248, *361, 368*
Lum, B. K. B., see Somani, P. [1782—1784], 206, 216, 248, 249, 250, *355*
Lumb, G., see Malinin, T. [1212], 4, *345*
Lumb, G. D., Singletary, H. P., Hardy, L. B. [1196], 90, 141, *344*
Lundholm, L., see Aberg, G. [2], 249, 250, 251, *323*
Lund Larsen, G., Sivertssen, E. [85a], 235, *361*
Luthy, E., see Gander, M. [622], 207, *334*
— see Leutenegger, A. [1113], 280, 287, *343*
Lydtin, H. [1197], 218, *344*
— Kusus, T., Dietze, G., Schnelle, K. [1198], 220, *344*
— see Lohmoeller, G. [84a], 229, 235, *361*
Lyon, A. F., see De Graff, A. C. [401], 187, *330*
Lyon, T. P., Gofman, J. W., Jones, H. B., Lindgren, F. T., Graham, D. M. [1199], 311, *344*
— see Graham, D. M. [704], 311, *335*

Maassen, J. H. [1200], 190, *344*
Mabe, R. E., see Kory, R. C. [1020], 141, *341*
Mac Alpin, R. M., see Kattus, A. A. [948], 9, *340*
MacAlpin, R. N., see Alvaro, A. B. [25], 214, *323*
Mac Donald, A. G., McNeill, R. S. [1201], 244, *344*
Macdonald, D. C., see Davis, W. G. [394], 42, 209, *330*
MacDonald, H. R., see Taylor, S. H. [1876], 91, *356*
Macht, D. I. [1202], 151, *344*
Mack, R. E., Nolting, D. D., Hogancamp, C. E., Bing, R. J. [1203], 82, *344*
Mack, V., see Nayler, W. G. [1352], 216, 245, 246, *347*
MacKay, R. K. S., see Watt, D. A. L. [337c], 221, *371*

MacKinnon, J., see Foulds, R. [572], 187, *333*

Mackinnon, J., Anderson, D. E., Howitt, G. [1204], 163, *344*

Macko, E., see Fellows, E. J. [534], 157, *332*

Maclean, K. S., see Allanby, K. D. [21], 163, *323*

Macleod, C. A., Hirsch, E. Z., Schwartz, H. [209c], 10, *368*

MacMichael, J. S., see Howarth, S. [864], 153, *338*

MacMillan, D. B., see Lu, F. C. [1182], 72, 151, 158, 310, *344*

Macrez, C., Bernard-Brunel, J., Marnette-Lebrequier, H. [1205], 191, *344*

— see Mouquin, M. [1325], 159, *347*

Macruz, R., see Sarnoff, S. J. [1644, 1645], 29, 55, 92, 93, 122, 132, 267, *352*

Madan, B. R., Mishra, S. N., Khanna, V. K. [210c], 232, *368*

Madeira, R. G., Du Mesnil de Rochemont, W., Gadd, C. W., Stock, T. B., Bing, R. J. [1206], 2, *345*

Madoff, I. M., see Holander, W. [851], 130, *338*

Maerkisch, R., see Koss, F. W. [1021], 185, *341*

Maetzel, F. K., see Speckmann, K. [1804], 101, *355*

Maezawa, H., see Shimamoto, T. [1741], 289, *354*

Magaraggia, L., see Vettori, G. [1940], 228, *358*

Magendants, H., see Proger, S. H. [1469], 304, *349*

Maggi, G. C., Banno, S. [1207], 138, *345*

— Candiani, C., Fauda, C., Romeo, D. [1208], 162, *345*

Magyar, S., see Szabo, G. [1863, 1864], 302, *356*

Mahaim, I., Rothberger, C. J. [1209], 154, *345*

Mahanti, B., see Vineberg, A. M. [1943], 90, *358*

Maillot, S., see Alix, B. [6c], 279, 286, 288, *363*

Makinson, D. H., Olesky, S., Stone, R. V. [1210], 305, *345*

Malach, M. [1211], 295, *345*

Malagnino, G., see Bertaccini, G. [148], 252, *325*

— see Visioli, O. [1944], 252, *358*

Malfroy, P., see Jouve, A. [165c], 29, *367*

Malindzak, G. S., Green, H. D., Stagg, P. L. [211c], 125, *368*

Malinin, T., Stokes, J. R., Hardy, L. B., Lumb, G. [1212], 4, *345*

Malinow, M. R., see Farrehi, C. [527], 14, *332*

Mallion, J. M., see Denis, B. [32a], 279, *360*

Malm, A., see Arborelius, M. [51], 131, *324*

Malmberg, R., see Svedmyr, N. [122a, 308c, 309c], 211, 251, 362, *370*

Malmborg, R. O. [1213], 30, 298, *345*

— see Arborelius, M. [51], 131, *324*

— see Lecerhof, H. [79a], 297, *361*

Malmström, G. [1214], 96, *345*

Maloy, W. C., Sowton, E., Balcon, R. [1215], 100, *345*

— see Balcon, R. [80], 99, 100, *324*

Manchester, J. H., see Kemp, H. G. [174c], 12, *367*

Mancini, A., see Joseph, L. G. [910], 147, *339*

Mancke, R., see Heubner, W. [825], 65, *338*

Manfredi, M., see Barbaresi, F. [86], 248, 249, *324*

Mann, F. C., see Essex, H. E. [508, 509], 120, 150, 153, 299, 306, 307, *332*

— see Wegria, R. [1968], 120, 150, 153, *358*

Mann, G. V., see Chandler, H. L. [295], 311, *328*

Mann, H. [1216], 137, *345*

Manning, G. W., see McEachern, C. G. [1249], 150, *345*

Mantero, O., see Baroldi, G. [89], 53, *324*

Many, P., see Dulac, J. F. [460], 307, *331*

Manzoli, U. C., see West, J. W. [1977], 181, 182, *358*

Manzoni, A., see Strobbia, R. [304c], 164, *370*

March, H. W., see Lew, H. T. [1130], 221, *343*

Marchal, C., see Benichoux, R. [22c], 70, *364*

Marchetti, G. [212c], 252, *368*

— Merlo, L., Noseda, V. [1217, 1218], 36, 252, *345*

Marchioro, T., Feldman, A. Owens, J. C., Swan, H. [213c], 81, *368*

Marcus, E., Katz, L. N., Pick, R., Stamler, J. [1219], 88, *345*

Margolies, A., see Starr, I. [1823], 153, *356*

Marignac, B., see Lamarche, M. [22b], 295, *363*

Marinakis, P., see Voridis, E. [1950], 226, *358*

Marineaud, J.-P., see Bouvrain, Y. [40c], 297, *364*

Marion, J., Navarranne, P., Roux, M., Buyck, J., Fritz, A., Lemoigne, P., Longuet, D. [1220], 171, *345*

Markman, P., see Rowlands, D. J. [1579], 221, *351*

Marko, I., see Rudolph, W. [274c, 275c, 276c], 194, 195, *369*

Markoff, N. [1221], 160, *345*

Markwalder, J., Starling, E. H. [1222], 55, 68, *345*

Markwardt, F., see Barthel, W. [98], 166, *324*

Marmo, E., Coscia, L., Aulisio, G. A. [1223, 1224], 208, 245, 250, *345*

— Matera, A., D'Avanzo, F. B. [1225], 223, *345*

Marnette-Lebrequier, H., see Macrez, C. [1205], 191, *344*

Marnezos, E., see Lekos, D. [1098], 226, *343*

Maroko, P. R., see Braunwald, E. [15a], 41, *360*

Marrama, P., see Vecchi, G. P. [1935], 160, *357*

Marsh, D. F., Herring, D. A. [1226], 308, *345*

Marsico, F., see Nylin, G. [1380], 96, *348*

Martin-Noel, P., see Denis, B. [32a], 279, *360*

Martinez, M., see Robin, E. [1543], 93, 126, 130, 131, 208, *350*

Martinez, M. A., see Puri, P. S. [1475], 126, 127, *349*

Masironi, R. [214c], 15, *368*

Mason, D. F. J., see Chamberlain, D. A. [292], 208, *328*

— see Davis, W. G. [394], 42, 209, *330*

Mason, D. T. [215c], 33, 132, *368*

— Braunwald, E. [86a], 130, 144, *361*

— Spann, J. F., Zelis, R., Amsterdam, E. A. [87a], 39, 130, 316, *361*

— see Zelis, R. [140a], 148, *362*

Mason, G. P., see Roberts, L. N. [1542], 187, *350*

Mason, J., see Pitt, B. [98a], 63, *362*

Mason, R. E., see Dagenais, G. R. [74c], 140, 143, 233, *365*

Mason, R. E., see Scarborough, W. R. [1651], 95, *352*

Massel, H. M. [1227], 154, *345*

Massumi, R. A. [216c], 3, *368*

Master, A. M. [1228], 162, *345*
— Donoso, E., Rosenfeld, I. [1229], 103, *345*
— Field, L. E., Donoso, E. [1230], 96, *345*
— Friedman, R., Dack, S. [1231], 104, *345*
— Jaffe, H. L., Dack, S. [1232], 110, 111, 136, 154, *345*
— Nuzie, S., Brown, R. C., Parker, R. C. [1233], 95, 96, 103, 104, *345*
— Oppenheimer, E. T. [1234], 103, *345*
— Rosenfeld, I. [1235], 96, *345*
— — Donoso, E. [1236], 96, *345*
— see Rosenfeld, I., [1556], 96, *351*

Masters, T. N., Glaviano, V. V. [88a], 208, *361*

Matera, A., see Marmo, E. [1225], 223, *345*

Mates, R. E., see Falsetti, H. L. [96c], 35, *365*

Mathes, P., see Cowan, C. [28a], 122, *360*

Matheson, N. A., see Arfors, K. E. [10c], 51, *363*

Mathis, I., see Campus, S. [273], 135, *327*

Mathisen, H. S., Holen, N. [1237], 149, *345*

Mathivat, A., see Cottet, J. [370, 1238], 15, *329, 345*

Mathur, V. S., see Baker, L. D. [74], *324*

Matloff, J. M., Wolfson, S., Gorlin, R., Harken, D. E. [1239], 221, *345*

Matson, J. L., see Stein, P. D. [1828, 1829], 209, *356*

Matsuo, H., see Nimura, Y. [234c], 78, *368*

Matsuo, S., see Cho, Y. W. [22a], 294, *360*

Maurer, B., see Jewitt, D. E. [163c], 243, *367*

Maurice, M., see Scebat, L. [1653], 280, *352*

Maurice, P., see Beaumont, J. L. [115], 311, *325*

Mautz, F. R., Gregg, D. E. [1240], 44, 85, 86, *345*

Maxwell, G. M. [1241], 42, 222, *345*
— Crumpton, C. W., Rowe, G. G., White, D. H., Castillo, C. A. [1242], 153, *345*

Maxwell, G. M., White, D. H., Crumpton, C. W., Rowe, G. G., Castillo, C. A. [1243], 153, *345*
— see Rowe, G. G. [1576], 304, *351*

Mayne, N. M. C., see Pentecost, B. L. [1430], 295, *348*

Mayo, M., see Cosby, R. S. [366], 97, *329*

Mazurkiewicz, I., see Melville, K. I. [1276], 72, *346*

McAllister, E., see Brotslow, J. [50c], 316, *364*

McAlpin, R. N., Kattus, A. A., Winfield, M. E. [1244], 30, 136, *345*

McCallister, B. D., Richmond, D. R., Saltups, A., Hallermann, F. J., Wallace, R. B., Frye, R. L. [217c], 12, *368*
— Yipintsoi, T., Hallermann, F. J., Wallace, R. B., Frye, R. L. [1245], 30, 37, *345*
— see Greenberg, B. H. [125c], 13, *366*

McClish, A., Andrew, D., Noisan, A., Morin, Y. [1246, 1247], 221, *345*

McCredie, R. M. [218c], 246, *368*

McDevitt, D. G., see Brick, I. [228], 243, *327*
— see Grant, R. H. E. [710], 174, 207, *336*

McDonald, D. A. [1248], 77, *345*
— see Gent, G. [47a], 243, *361*

McDonald, I. G., see Paley, H. W. [1406], 207, 208, *348*

McDonald, R. H., see Thompson, M. E. [311c], 240, *370*

McEachen, J. A., see Eckstein, R. W. [475, 476, 477], 74, 122, 123, *331*

McEachern, C. G., Smith, F. H., Manning, G. W. [1249], 150, *345*

McGill, H. C., see Strong, J. P. [305c], 16, *370*

McGinn, J. T., see Schluger, J. [1675], 155, *353*

McGregor, M. [1250, 1251], 40, 44, 168, 182, 187, *345*
— Fam, W. H. [1252], 48, 55, 58, 125, *345*
— Palmer, W. H. [1253], 21, *345*
— see Fam, W. M. [522, 523, 524], 53, 86, 124, 134, 182, *332*
— see Hoeschen, R. J. [845], 126, *338*
— see Kinsella, D. [986], 187, *341*

McGregor, M., see Newhouse, M. T. [1360], 183, 187, *347*
— see Sosa, J. A. [1795], 168, *355*

McGuire, J., see Scott, R. C. [1708, 1710], 152, 158, *353*

McHenry, P. L., Knoebel, S. B. [1254], 83, *345*
— see Elliott, W. C. [89c], 316, *365*
— see Knoebel, S. B. [1007, 1008, 182c], 57, 82, 83, 125, 130, *341, 367*

McIlduff, J. B., see Levinson, R. S. [201c], 295, *368*

McInerny, T. K., Gilmour, D. P., Blinks, J. R. [1255], 215, 216, *345*

McInnes, L., Parratt, J. R. [1256], 192, *345*
— see Nayler, W. G. [1346 to 1352] 174, 177, 179, 208, 216, 222, 223, 245, 246, 250, *347*

McIntosh, D. A. D., see Scales, B. [1649], 216, *352*

McIntosh, H. D., see Whalen, R. E. [1982], 207, 272, 274, *358*

McKenna, D. H., Afonso, S., Jaramillo, C. V., Crumpton, C. W., Rowe, G. G. [1257], 4, *345*
— Corliss, R. J., Sialer, S., Zarnstorff, W. C., Crumpton, C. W., Rowe, G. G. [1258], 42, 207, 209, 272, 274, *345*
— see Rowe, G. G. [1578], 22, *351*

McLaughlin, E., see Cohen, L. S. [25a], 249, *360*

McLaughlin, V. W., see Cox, J. L. [29a], 41, *360*

McLeod, C., see Gorlin, R. [698], 22, 100, 123, 129, 130, 133, *335*

McMurry, M. T., see Strong, J. P. [305c], 16, *370*

McNamara, P. M., see Kannel, W. B. [20b], 16, *363*

McNeill, R. S. [219c], 217, 244, *368*
— see MacDonald, A. G. [1201], 244, *344*

McShane, W. K., see Scriabine, A. [1712], 123, 139, *354*

Mead, A. W., see Leeper, R. D. [1092], 15, *343*

Medrano, G., see Cuellar, A. [72c], 295, *365*

Medrano, G. A., see Sodi-Pallares, D. [1767—1770, 115a] 295, 296, *355, 362*

Medvedowsky, J. L. [1260], 170, *346*
— see Jouve, A. [920], 279, *339*
Meesmann, W., Bachmann, G. W. [1261, 1262], 45, 53, 86, 182, 183, *346*
Meester, W. D., Hardman, H. F., Barboriak, J. J. [1263], 248, *346*
Megyesi, K., see Szabo, G. [1865], 302, *356*
Mehmel, H., see Wirz, P. [340c], *371*
Mehrotra, T. N., Bassadone, E. T. [10d], 298, *371*
Meier, M., see Wilhelm, M. [1999], 222, *359*
— see Brunner, H. [249], 222, *327*
Meier, R., Muller, R. [1264], 312, *346*
— see Tripod, J. [1899, 1900], 66, 308, *357*
Meister, S., see Brooks, H. [18a, 49c], 251, 252, *360, 364*
Meixner, L., see Rudolph, W. [1583], 190, *351*
Mejia, R. H., see De Soldati, L. [419], 95, *330*
Meldrum, S. J., see Coltart, D. J. [66c], 219, *365*
Melendez, L., see Hamer, J. [769], 207, *337*
Melgar, M. D., see Dicarlo, F. J. [33a], 119, *360*
Melikoglu, S. [1265], 144, 310, *346*
— see Parade, G. W. [1413], 143, *348*
Mellen, H. S., Goldberg, H. S., Friedman, H. F. [1266], 142, *346*
Melon, J. M. [1267], *346*
Meltzer, L. E., see Dalle, X. [386], 8, *330*
Melville, K. I. [1268, 1269], 20, 21, 22, 299, 313, *346*
— Benfey, B. G. [1270], 174, *346*
— Drapeau, J. V. [1271], 302, *346*
— Garvey, H. L., Gillis, R. A. [1272], 125, 139, *346*
— Korol, B. [1273], 120, *346*
— Lu, F. C. [1274, 1275], 122, 139, 153, *346*
— Mazurkiewicz, I. [1276], 72, *346*
— Shister, H. E., Huq, S. [1277], 174, *346*
— see Garvey, L. [627, 628, 45a], 124, 173, 174, 175, *334, 361*
— see Lu, F. C. [1184], 72, *344*

Melville, K. I., see Varma, D. R. [1921], 89, 122, 161, 308, *357*
Mendel, D., Winterton, M. [1278], 169, *346*
— see Grayson, J. [715], 55, *336*
Mendez, R., Aceves, J., Pulido, P. [1279], 161, *346*
— Kabela, E. [1280], 63, 206, *346*
— see Kabela, E. [923, 67a], 63, 218, *340, 361*
Meneely, G. R., see Kory, R. C. [1020], 141, *341*
Menge, H. G., Kadatz, R. [1281], 181, *346*
Menges, H., see Popovich, N. R. [1461], 123, *349*
Mercer, C. J., see Jewitt, D. E. [899], 243, *339*
Mercier, C., see Vineberg, A. M. [1942], 182, *358*
Mercier, F., Jouve, A., Gavend, M., Gavend, M. R., Gerin, J., Mercier, J. [1282], 161, *346*
— see Mercier, J. [1283], 157, 305, *346*
Mercier, J., Gavend, M., Gavend, M. R., Mercier, F. [1283], 157, 305, *346*
— see Gavend, M. [630], 163, *334*
— see Mercier, F. [1282], 161, *346*
Mercker, H., Lochner, W., Gerstenberg, E. [1284], 58, *346*
— see Lochner, W. [1165, 1166], 58, 150, 153, *344*
Meriel, P., Boulard, C., Galinier, F., Bounhoure, J., Gavalda, J., Bounhoure, F. [1285], 170, *346*
— see Lesbre, J. P. [81a, 200c], 181, 186, 279, *361, 368*
Merlen, J. F. [1286], 139, *346*
— Flament, G. [220c], 137, *368*
— see Balatre, P. [77, 78], 141, 305, *324*
Merlo, L., see Marchetti, G. [1217, 1218], 36, 252, *345*
Mertens-Strijthagen, J., see Lammerant, J. [193c], 306, *367*
Messeloff, C. R., see Greiner, T. [738], 110, 111, 112, 113, 116, 158, 308, *336*
Messer, J. V., Levine, H. J., Wagman, R. J., Gorlin, R. [1287], 38, *346*
— Neill, W. A. [1288], 22, 24, 275, *346*
— see Baker, L. D. [73, 74], 26, *324*

Messer, J. V., see Gorlin, R. [699], 129, *335*
— see Pomposiello, J. C. [254c], *369*
— see Sharma, G. V. R. K. [112a], 27, *362*
— see Wagman, R. J. [1953], 22, 24, 275, *358*
Messerich, J. [1289], 187, *346*
Messin, R., see Katz, A. [949], 96, *340*
— Denolin, H., Degré, S. [1290], 98, *346*
Messina, B., Grossi, F., Grassi, M., Spada, S., Messini, R. [1291], 249, *346*
Messini, R., see Messina, B. [1291], 249, *346*
Mestan, J., see Di Matteo, J. [83c], 23, *365*
Mestdagh, C., see Wanet, J. [334c], 287, *370*
Mestern, J., see Schachter, R. J. [1654], 155, *352*
Metzger, R., see Hohl, O. [62a], 290, *361*
Meuser, H. J., see Hahn, N. [762], 197, *337*
Mewissen, A. [1292], 170, *346*
Meyer, J., see Kirchhoff, H. W. [987], 196, *341*
Meyer, J. A., see Haight, C. [764], 121, *337*
Meyer, J. D., see Speckmann, K. [1804], 101, *355*
Meyer, J. M., Correll, H. L., Peters, B. J., Lindert, M. C. F. [1293], 152, *346*
Meyler, L. 322
Meythaler, M., see Sternitzke, N. [299c, 300c], 197, *370*
Mezzasalma, G., Morpurgo, M. [1294], 305, *346*
Miazdrikova, A. A. [1295], 122, 150, 303, *346*
Michaelides, G., see Aravanis, C. [9c], *363*
— see Conway, N. [362], 228, *329*
— see Koroxenidis, G. [1019], 223, *341*
— see Lekos, D. [1098], 226, *343*
Michaelsson, G., see Jacobsson, K. A. [885], 168, *339*
Michel, D. [1296, 221c], 168, 247, *346, 368*
Michel, R., Deltour, G. [1297], 268, *346*
Micheletti, J., Renault, B. [25b], 291, *363*
Michell, G., see Bauer, G. E. [19c], 228, *364*
Michelson, A. L., see Rosenberg, H. N. [1553], *351*

Michiels, P. M., see Winbury, M. M. [2015], *359*
Miettinen, M., see Turpeinen, O. [1906], 14, *357*
Mignault, J. de L. [1298], 174, 178, *346*
Miller, B. L., see Sodi-Pallares, D. [1767], 295, *355*
Miller, E., see Luduena, F. P. [1191], 67, *344*
Miller, G. H., see Smith, F. M. [1760], 153, *354*
Miller, T. N., see Gent, A. E. [636, 109c], 51, 187, *334, 366*
Millot, J., Patrux, A. M. [1299], 164, *346*
Mills, C., see Jewitt, D. E. [163c], 243, *367*
Mills, C. J. [222c], 78, *368*
Mills, H., see Isaacs, J. H. [879], 101, *339*
Milovanovich, J. B., see Mouquin, M. [1326], 307, *347*
Minnich, W. R., see Proger, S. H. [1469], 304, *349*
Minz, B., Thuillier, J. [1300], 160, *346*
Miragoli, G., see Ferrini, R. [540, 100c], 252, 254, *332, 365*
Mirsky, I., see Hugenholtz, P. G. [154c], 35, *367*
Mishra, S. N., see Madan, B. R. [210c], 232, *368*
Misrahy, G., see Anrep, G. V. [39, 40], 157, 158, *323*
Mitchel, D. F., see Adam, M. [3c], 12, *363*
Mitchell, J. H., see McLaughlin, E. [25a], 249, *360*
Mitchell, J. R. A. [1301], 108, *346*
— Emmons, P. R., Harrison, M. J. G., Honour, A. J. [223c], 51, *368*
— see Elkeles, R. S. [88c], 51, *365*
— see Emmons, P. R. [90c], 50, *365*
— see Hampton, J. R. [139c], 50, 51, *366*
Miura, M., Tominaga, S., Hashimoto, K. [1302], 62, 185, *346*
Miyahara, M. [225c], 36, *368*
— Iimura, O., Yokoyama, M., Hoshikawa, K. [26b], 204, *363*
Mizgala, H. F., Davis, R. O., Kahn, A. S. [1303], 211, *346*
— Kahn, A. S., Davis, R. O. [1304, 89a, 90a], 212, 215, *346, 361*
— see Davies, R. O. [31a], 148, 213, *360*

Moccetti, T., see Lichtlen, P. [204c, 205c], 247, *368*
Mochizuki, S., see Nimura, Y. [234c], 78, *368*
Modell, W., [1305—1307, 226c], 5, 16, 20, 39, 144, 148, 157, 158, 164, *346, 368*
— see Gold, H. [678], 154, *335*
— see Greiner, T. [738], 110, 111, 112, 113, 116, 158, 308, *336*
Moe, G. K., Visscher, M. B. [1308], 68, *346*
Mohiuddin, S., Taskar, P. K., Morin, Y. [91a], 301, *361*
Moir, T. W. [1309], 82, *346*
Mokotoff, R., Katz, L. N. [1310], 150, 154, *346*
Molenaar, M. G., see Lopes, E. C. [1174], 311, *344*
Molino, N., Belluardo, C. [1311], 164, *346*
Moll, A., Petzel, H. [1312], 198, *346*
— see Petzel, H. [1435], 136, *349*
Molly, W. [1313], 309, *346*
Monaco, A. R., see Von Oettingen, W. F. [1948], 138, 140, *358*
Money, W. L., see Leeper, R. D. [1092], 15, *343*
Moniz de Bettencourt, J., Correia Ralha, A., Peres Gomes, F., Prista Monteiro, H. [1314], 159, *347*
— Prista Monteiro, H. [1315], 159, *347*
Monroe, R. G., French, G. N. [1316], 29, 267, *347*
— see Gamble, W. J. [106c], 91, *366*
— see Hugenholtz, P. G. [155c], 91, *367*
Morales-Anguilera, A., Vaughan-Williams, E. M. [1317, 1318], 206, 214, 215, 216, 219, *347*
Moran, J. F., see Goldbarg, A. N. [52a, 53a, 115c], 5, 148, 212, 213, *361, 366*
Moran, L. G., see Cox, J. L. [29a], 41, *360*
Moran, N. C. [1319], 173, *347*
— Perkins, M. E. [1320], 205, *347*
Morawitz, P., Zahn, A. [1321], 70, *347*
Moret, P. R., Boufas, D., Fournet, P. C. [1322], 257, 268, 269, 286, *347*
Morgenstern, C., Arnold, G., Hoeljes, U., Lochner, W. [227c], 207, *368*

Mori, V., see Berman, J. K. [137], 90, *325*
Morin, Y., see McClish, A. [1246, 1247], 221, *345*
— see Mohiuddin, S. [91a], 301, *361*
Mornex, R., see Hermann, H. [818], 161, *338*
Moros, D., see Levitt, B. [1119], 249, *343*
Morpurgo, M., see Mezzasalma, G. [1294], 305, *346*
Morris, G. C., see Chapman, D. W. [59c], 12, *364*
Morris, J. J., see Kong, Y. [187c], 318, *367*
— see Whalen, R. E. [1982], 207, 272, 274, *358*
Mortari, A., see Bisiani, M. [171], 161, *326*
— see Fresia, P. [588], 161, *333*
Moschos, C. B., see Regan, T. J. [1513, 1514], 301, *350*
Moser, K., Lujf, A. [1323, 1324], 198, 212, *347*
— see Benda, L. [131], 179, *325*
— see Lujf, A. [1193, 1194, 1195], 194, 215, 221, *344*
— see Niessner, H. [92a, 233c], 198, 248, *361, 368*
Moss, A. J., Johnson, J., Sentman, J. [228c], 210, *368*
Motolese, M., see Reale, A. [1503], 226, *350*
Motomiya, T., see Atsumi, T. [14c], 289, *363*
Mott, J. C., see Dawes, G. S. [396], 72, *330*
Mouille, P., see Boissier, J. R. [37c], 242, 246, *364*
Mouquin, M., Macrez, C. [1325], 159, *347*
— Milovanovich, J. B., Sauvan, R., Vonthron, A., Grosgogeat, Y. [1326], 307, *347*
Mouratoff, C. J., see Batterman, R. C. [107], 149, *325*
Mudd, G., see Kaiser, G. C. [167c], 11, *367*
Mueller, G., see Gerhard, W. [642], 144, 227, *334*
Müller, J., Strassburg, K. H. [1327], 170, 171, *347*
Müller, O., Rorvik, K. [1328], 30, 33, *347*
Müller, O. F., see West, J. W. [1977], 181, 182, *358*
Müller-Mohnssen, H., see Giese, W. [656], 52, 193, 269, *335*
Mulcahy, R., see Heffernan, A. [796], 16, *337*

Mulinos, M. G., see Leslie, A. [1108], 106, *343*
— see Scott, W. S. [1711], 106, *354*
Muller, R., see Meier, R. [1264], 312, *346*
Muller-Seydlitz, P., see Rudolph, W. [276c], 194, *369*
Munck, O., see Hansen, A. T. [780], 83, *337*
— see Lassen, N. A. [1078], 83, *342*
Murad-Netto, S., see Gensini, G. G. [635], 124, *334*
Murisasco, A., see Donnet, V. [439], 165, *331*
Murmann, W., Saccani-Guelfi, M.,Gamba,A.[1329],248,*347*
— see Setnikar, I. [1720], 169, *354*
Murphy, F. M., Barber, J. M. [1330, 1331], 163, *347*
— — Kilpatrick, S. J. [1332], 163, *347*
Murphy, Q. R., see Gutgesell, H. P. [57a], 220, *361*
— see Rowe, G. G. [1576], 304, *351*
Murray, J. F., Escobar, E., Jones, N. L., Rapaport, E. [1333], 207, *347*
Murrell, W. [1334], 120, *347*
Mustard, J. F., Packham, M. A. [229c], 50, *368*
— see Joergensen, L. [900], 4, *339*
Myers, W. W., see Honig, C. R. [149c], 317, *366*
Myhre, J. R., see Gabrielsen, Z. [618], 112, 311, *334*

Nadal, B., see Cardenas, M. [54c], 249, *364*
Nadas, A. S., see Gamble. W. J [106c], 91, *366*
Nadeau, R. A., see Tremblay, G. M. [315c], 250, *370*
Nadini, M., see Regan, T. J. [1514], 301, *350*
Nador, K., see Karpati, E. [942], 288, *340*
Naegele, C. F., see Russek, H.J. [1612, 1613, 1614], 104, 135, 151, 158, 300, *352*
Nagle, R. E., see George, C. F. [110c], 242, *366*
Najmi, M., Griggs, D. M., Kasparian, H., Novack, P. [1335], 33, 93, 131, *347*
Nalbantgil, I., see Yigitbasi, O. [343c], 247, *371*
Nalefski, L. A., Rudy, W. B., Gilbert,N.C.[1339],158,*347*
— see Gilbert, N. C. [658], 310, 311, *335*

Nancekievill, L., see Grant, R. H. E. [709], 217, *336*
Nakano,J.,Kusakari,T.[1336], 33, 207, 272, 274, *347*
Nakhjavan, F. K., Shedrovilzky, H., Goldberg, H. [1337], 89, *347*
— Son, R., Goldberg, H. [1338], 30, *347*
Narula, O. S., Samet, P. [230c], 3, *368*
Nash, D. T. [1340], 289, *347*
Nasser, M. G., see Case, R. B [56c], 27, *364*
Nasseri, M., see Lochner, W [1165, 1167, 1168], 58, *344*
Nassim, R., see Solandt, D. Y. [1772], 310, *355*
Nataf, J., see Dailheu-Geoffroy, P. [384, 385], 170, *330*
Nathan, D. J., see Spain, D. M. [1803], 15, *355*
Nau, P., see Salle, J. [1631], 159, *352*
Naughton, J., Balke, B. [1341], 10, *347*
Nauta, W. T., see Bijlsma, V. G. [160], 308, *326*
Navarranne, P., see Marion, J. [1220], 171, *345*
Navarro-Viola, R., see De Soldati, L. [419], 95, *330*
Nayler, W. G. [1342, 1343], 216, 223, 246, *347*
— Chan, J., Lowe, T. E.[1344], 242, *347*
— Chipperfield, D., Lowe, T. E. [1345], 223, 245, *347*
— McInnes, I., Carson, V., Swann, J., Lowe, T. E. [1346], 222, *347*
— — Swann, J. B., Carson, V., Lowe, T. E. [1347], 208, *347*
— — Price, J. M., Carson, V., Race, D., Lowe, T. E. [1348], 174, 177, 179, *347*
— — — Race, D., Carson, V., Lowe, T. E. [1349], 208, *347*
— — — Lowe, T. E. [1350], 223, 245, 250, *347*
— Price, J. M., Lowe, T. E. [1351], 182, *347*
— Stone, J., Carson, V., McInnes, I., Mack, V., Lowe, T. E. [1352], 216, 245, 246, *347*
Needleman, P., Hunter, F. E. [1353], 135, *347*
Neel, J. L. [27b], 291, *363*
Neill, W. A. [1354], 26, *347*
— Levine, H. J., Wagman, R. J., Gorlin, R. [1355], 29, 55, 267, *347*

Neill, W. A., see Levine, J. H. [1115], *343*
— see Messer, J. V. [1288], 22, 24, 275, *346*
— see Wagman, R. J. [1953], 22, 24, 275, *358*
Neilson, G. H., Seldon, W. A. [1356], 211, *347*
Neistadt, A., see Schwartz, S. I. [289c], 316, *369*
Nell, G., see Kraupp, O. [1038], 196, *342*
— see Raberger, G. [102a, 263c], 61, 196, *362*, *369*
Nelle, G., see Bretschneider, H. J. [?26], 52, 62, 189, 190, 269, *327*
Nemickas, R., see Goldbarg, A. N. [52a, 53a], 5, 148, 213, *361*
Nemiroff, M. J., see Carson, R. P. [278], 125, 134, *328*
Nestel, P. J., Verghese, A., Lovell, R. H. [1357], 284, *347*
Neumann, H. [1358], 187, *347*
Neumann, M., Luisada, A. [1359], 174, 179, *347*
Neve, P., see Bastenie, P. A. [101], 16, *324*
Newberry, W. B., see Eckstein, R. W. [475, 476, 477], 74, 122, 123, *331*
Newburger, R. A., see Segal, R. L. [1713], 20, *354*
Newell, D. J. [231c], 142, *368*
— see Dewar, H. A. [424, 425], 141, 160, 162, 170, 171, *330*
— see Srivastava [1812], 211, *355*
Newhouse, M. T., McGregor, M. [1360], 182, 187, *347*
Newman, B. J., see Donoso, E. [441], 211, *331*
Newman, E. V., see Roughgarden, J. W. [1568], 30, 33, *351*
Nickerson, E. [1362], 173, *347*
Nickerson, J. L., see Wegria, R. [1969], 121, *356*
Nickerson, M. [1361, 232c], 43, 148, *347*, *368*
Nidegger, J. C. [1363], 310,*347*
Niederau, D., see Pfleger, K. [96a], 184, *362*
Niedergerke, R. [1364], 216, *347*
Nielsen, B. L., see Clausen, J. [333], 217, 218, 221, *329*
Nielsen, K. C., Owman, C. [1365, 1366), 166, 167, 249, *347*
Nieschulz, O., Popendiker, K., Sack, K. H. [1367], 303, *347*
Niessner, H., Chirikdjian, J. J. [1368], 194, *347*

Niessner, H., Lujf, A., Moser, K. [92a, 233c], 198, 248, *361, 368*
— see Kraupp, O. [1039, 1040], 194, *342*
Nimura, Y., Mochizuki, S., Matsuo, H., Kitabatake, A., Kato, K., Abe, H. [234c], 78, *368*
Nissiotis, E., see Rivier, J. L. [269c], 246, *369*
Nitz, R. E., Pötzsch, E. [1369], 188, 190, *347*
— Resag, K. [1370, 1371], 189, *347*
— Schraven, E., Trottnow, D. [1372], 190, *347*
— see Klarwein, M. [991], *341*
— see Schraven, E. [1697], 190, *353*
Nivet, M. [1373, 1374], 280, 288, *347, 348*
— see Facquet, J. [516, 517, 518], 279, 280, 286, 287, *332*
Nixon, P. G. F., see Ikram, H. [877], 217, *339*
Nobile, F., see Uhlmann, F. [1910], 66, *357*
Noble, R. P., see Hamilton, W. F. [772], *91, 337*
Noisan, A., see McClish, A. [1246, 1247], 221, *345*
Nolting, D. D., see Mack, R. E. [1203], 82, *344*
Nonkin, P., see Di Carlo, F. J. [427], *330*
Nonnenmacher, G., see Thiele, K. [1880], 198, *356*
Nordenfelt, I., Persson, S., Redfors, A. [1375], 234, *348*
— Westling, H. [1376], 126, *348*
Nordoy, A., Rodset, J. M. [236c], 50, *368*
Norman, L. R., see Zoll, P. M. [2052], 145, *360*
Norrby, A., see Ablad, B. [4], 207, 232, *323*
— see Johnsson, G. [905], 232, *339*
Norris, R. M., Caughey, D. E., Scott, P. J. [1377], 217, *348*
Noseda, V., see Marchetti, G. [1217, 1218], 36, 252, *345*
Nott, M. W. [237c], 185, *368*
Novikoff, N., see Kalmanson, D. [168c], 78, *367*
Nowack, P., see Najmi, M. [1335], 33, 93, 131, *347*
Nowarra, G. M., see Schachter, R. J. [1654], 155, *352*
Numano, F., Takenobu, M., Katsu, K., Shimamoto, T. [238c], 289, *368*
— see Shimamoto, T. [1742], 289, *354*

Nuzie, S., see Master, A. M. [1233], 95, 96, 103, 104, *345*
Nuzum, F. R., Elliott, A. H. [1379], 309, *348*
— see Elliot, A. H. [486], 309, *331*
Nyberg, G., see Aubert, A. [8a], 233, *360*
— see Sealey, B. J. [290c], 233, *369*
Nylin, G., De Fazio, V., Marsico, F. [1380], 96, *348*

Oakley, G. M., see Cherian, G. [322], 218, *328*
Obianwu, H. [1381, 1382], 167, *348*
Obineche, E. N., see Watt, D. A. L. [337c], 221, *371*
Oblath, R. W. [1383], 163, *348*
O'Brien, G. S., see Afonso, S. [12, 13, 2a], 185, 186, 201, 202, *323, 360*
O'Brien, K. P., Higgs, L. M., Glancy, D. L., Epstein, S. E. [1384], 30, 34, 100, *348*
— see Glancy, D. L. [51a], 34, *361*
Ockenga, T., see Halmagyi, M. [766], 183, *337*
— see Knebel, R. [1003], 196, *341*
— see Rahn, K. H. [1493], 211, 245, 249, *350*
O'Connor, C. A., see Brodbin, P. [1d], 298, *371*
Odakura, T., see Yamazaki, H. [342c], 289, *371*
Oettingen, W. F. von, Donahue, D. D., Lawton, A. H., Monaco, A. R., Yagoda, H., Valaer, P. J. [1948], 138, 140, *358*
Özer, A., see Türker, R. K. [1905], 201, *357*
Ogawa, K., Gudbjarnason, S. [1385], 127, *348*
— — Bing, R. J. [1386], 127, 135, *348*
— see Puri, P. S. [1475], 126, 127, *349*
O'Hare, J. P., see Friend, D. G. [602], 139, *334*
Ohler, T., see Parade, G. W. [1413], 143, *348*
Ojo, S. A., see Bray, C. L. [45c], 243, *364*
Oka, M., see Hakkinen, P. [5e], 199, *371*
Oldewurtel, H. A., see Lehan, P. H. [1093], 124, *343*
— see Regan, T. J. [1513, 1515], 301, *350*
Olesky, S., see Makinson, D. H. [1210], 305, *345*

Oliver, M. F. [1387—1389], 16, 137, 142, *348*
Olivier, J., see Foucalt, J. F. [41a], 279, 286, *360*
Olivier, J. L., see Delbarre, F. [403], 172, *330*
Olleon, J. [1390], 70, 153, 156, 157, 158, 160, 313, *348*
Olson, R. E. [1391], 15, *348*
Olsson, L., see Aberg, G. [2], 249, 250, 251, *323*
Olsson, R. A. [28b], 61, *363*
— Gregg, D. E. [1392, 1393], 93, 268, *348*
— see Granata, L. [706], 36, *335*
— see Snow, J. A. [295c], 61, *370*
Olsson, S., see Björntorp, P. [177], 232, *326*
Ongari, R., see Dotti, F. [446], 249, *331*
— see Piva, M. [1452], 249, *349*
Opie, L., see Owen, P. [240c], 318, *368*
Opie, L. H. [239c], 296, *368*
— Thomas, M. [1394], 25, *348*
Oppenheimer, E. T., see Master, A. M. [1234], 103, *345*
Oram, S., Sowton, E. [1395], 141, 149, *348*
— see Balcon, R. [79], 217, 218, 221, *324*
— see Davies, P. [392], 171, *330*
— see Livesley, B. [207c], 25, *368*
— see Sowton, E. [1801], 149, *355*
Orcutt, J. A., see Clark, J. P. [61c], 237, *364*
Ord, J. W., see Hellems, H. K. [805], 59, *337*
Orgain, E. S., see Boyles, C. M. [206], 111, *326*
— see Ginn, W. M. [666], 211, *335*
— see Irons, G. V. [878], 221, *339*
— see Zeft, H. J. [2044], 213, 215, *359*
Oscharoff, G. [1396], 142, *348*
Osher, H. L., Katz, K. H., Wagner, D. J. [1397], 158, *348*
Osher, W. J. [1398], 55, *348*
Ostberg, R. H., see Goodyear, A. V. N. [693], 91, *335*
Oter Rodriguez, R., see Balaguer-Vintro, I. [76], 279, 280, *324*
Otto, H., see Gold, H. [677], 108, 154, *335*
Overkamp, H. [1399], 168, *348*

Owen, P., Thomas, M., Young, V., Opie, L. [240c], 318, *368*

Owens, J. C., see Marchioro, T. [213c], 81, *368*

Owman, C., see Nielsen, K. C. [1365, 1366], 166, 167, 249, *347*

Owren, P. A. [1400], 311, *348*

Packham, M. A., see Mustard, J. F. [229c], 50, *368*

Paecht, A., see Armand, P. [53], 279, *324*

Pärtan, J., see Kaindl, F. [930], 307, *340*

Paesmans, M., see Demey, D. [412], 115, 202, *330*

Page, I. H. [1401], 15, *348*

— Berrettoni, J. N., Butkus, A., Sones, F. M. [241c], 15, *368*

— Schneckloth, R. E. [1402], 15, *348*

— Stamler, J. [1403], 15, *348*

— see Ulrych, M. [1911], 211, *357*

Page, R. G., see Foltz, E. L. [570], 55, 81, *333*

Paget, G. E. [1404], 205, *348*

Pairard, J., see Perrin, A. [1433], 299, *349*

Pal, J. [1405], 151, *348*

Paley, H. W., McDonald, I. G., Peters, F. W. [1406], 207, 208, *348*

Paliard, P., Perrot, E. [1407], 191, *348*

Palm, D., see Grobecker, H. [744, 745, 746], 165, 166, 167, *336*

Palmer, D. W. [1408], 142, *348*

Palmer, J. A., Ramsey, C. G. [1409], 139, *348*

Palmer, J. H. [1410], 135, *348*

Palmer, K. N. V., Hamilton, W. F. D., Legge, J. S., Diament, M. L. [93a], 244, *362*

Palmer, W. H., see McGregor, M. [1253], 21, *345*

Pandolfo, G., see Feruglio, F. S. [541, 542], 222, 248, *333*

Pannier, R., see Biörck, G. [169], 96, *326*

Papadopulos, A., see Koroxenidis, G. [1019], 223, *341*

Papazoglou, N., see Voridis, E. [1950], 226, *358*

Papierski, D. H., see Winbury, M. M. [2016], 306, *359*

Papp, G., Szekeres, L., Szmolenszky, T. [1411], 220, *348*

Papp, J. G., Vaughan-Williams, E. M. [1412], 226, 242, *348*

Papp, J. G., see Freedberg, A. S. [101c], 270, *365*

— see Szekeres, L. [1868], 150, 167, *356*

Parade, G. W., Melikoglu, S., Ohler, T., Ting, K. [1413], 143, *348*

Parchi, C., see Castro De, B. [283], 187, *328*

Parker, J. O., Case, R. B., Khaja, F., Ledwich, J. R., Armstrong, P. W. [242c], 131, 133, *368*

— Chiong, M. A., West, R. O., Case, R. B. [1414, 243c], 26, 27, 31, 131, *348, 368*

— Di Giorgi, S., West, R. O. [1415], 30, 36, 43, 128, 130, 131, *348*

— Ledwich, J. R., West, R. O., Case, R. B. [1416], 31, 32, 132, *348*

— West, R. O., Case, R. B., Chiong, M. A. [1417], 25, 33, *348*

— — Di Giorgi, S. [1418], 30, 128, 130, *348*

— — Ledwich, J. R. [94a], 38, *362*

— see Khaja, F. [179c], 31, 32, *367*

Parker, R. C., see Hanna, C. [778], 150, *337*

— see Master, A. M. [1233], 95, 96, 103, 104, *345*

Parker, R. J., see Berman, J. K. [137], 90, *325*

Parmenter, K., see Stanton, H. C. [1818], 250, *355*

Parmley, W. W., see Glick, G. [673], 273, *335*

Parratt, J. R. [1419—1422, 244c, 245c], 40, 63, 77, 100, 209, 214, 215, 256, *348, 368*

— Grayson, J. [1423, 1424], 63, 207, 209, 210, 215, 274, *348*

— Wadsworth, R. M. [1425, 1426, 95a, 246c], 63, 230, 231, 236, 237, 239, 240, *348, 362, 368*

— see Grayson, J. [713, 714], 143, 144, 189, *336*

— see Lochner, W. [1169], 63, *344*

— see McInnes, L. [1256], 192, *345*

Parry, E. H. O., Wells, P. G. [1427], 137, 139, *348*

Parsons, E. F., see Kazemi, H. [172c], 35, *367*

Pasquale, N. P., see Burch, G. E. [258], 135, 137, *327*

Pasyk, S., see Gregg, D. E. [128c], 125, *366*

Patel, K. R., see Kerr, J. W. [177c], 244, *367*

Paterson, J. W., see Dollery, C. T. [36a], 205, *360*

Patney, L. N., see Sandler, G. [1642], 171, *352*

Patrux, A. M., see Millot, J. [1299], 164, *346*

Pattani, F., see Rey, C. [1519], 310, *350*

Patterson, S. D., see Zeft, H. J. [2044], 213, 215, *359*

Patton, R., D., see Damato, A. N. [388, 389], 3, *330*

— see Lau, S. H. [1081], 3, *342*

Paulley, J. W., see Cotterill, J. A. [69c], 295, *365*

Pauly, T. J., see Bittar, N. [12a], 185, *360*

Pearce, C. W., see Hyman, A. L. [156c], 316, *367*

Pearce, M. L., see Dayton, S. [398, 399], 15, *330*

Peart, W. S., see Gaddum, J. H. [619], 72, *334*

Pedersen, E., see Starr, I. [1824], 95, *356*

Peel, A. A., Blum, K., Lancaster, W. M., Dall, J. L., Chalmers, G. L. [1428], 187, *348*

Peel, J. S., see Wilson, D. F. [2006], 227, *359*

Pekkarinen, M., see Turpeinen, O. [1906], 14, *357*

Pele, M. F., see Sterne, J. [38b], 297, *363*

Pellmont, B., see Pletscher, A. [1456, 1457], 161, *349*

Peltier, J., see Laubie, M. [1086], 58, *342*

Pendleton, R. G., see Hahn, R. A. [763], 209, 248, *337*

Pensinger, R. R., see Winbury, M. M. [2017], 141, 182, *359*

Pentecost, B. L., Austen, W. G. [1429], 217, *348*

— Mayne, N. M. C., Lamb, P. [1430], 295, *348*

— see Bennett, M. A. [23c], 3, *364*

— see George, C. F. [110c], 242, *366*

Peon, C., see Kabela, E. [67a], 63, *361*

Pereira, E., see Wagner, J. [1954], 206, 245, *358*

Peres Gomes, F., see Moniz de Bettencourt, J. [1314], 159, *347*

Perez Casar, F., see Vega Diaz, F. [323c], 295, *370*

Perkins, M. E., see Moran, N. C. [1320], 205, *347*

Perley, A., see Farrehi, C. [527], 14, *332*

Perlman, A. [1431], 141, *348*

Permutti, B., see Todesco, S. [1893], 171, *357*

Pernod, J., Kermarec, J. [1432], 293, *348*

Perriere, J. P., see Duchene-Marullaz, P. [8b], 295, *363*

Perrin, A., Pairard, J. [1433], 299, *349*

Perrot, E., see Faucon, G. [529, 530], 189, *332*

— see Paliard, P. [1407], 191, *348*

Perrot, J., Lavandier, G., Guyot, J. C. [29b], 279, 287, *363*

Persson, S., see Nordenfelt, J. [1375], 234, *348*

Pescador, T. [1434], 279, *349*

Peters, B. J., see Meyer, J. M. [1293], 152, *346*

Peters, F. W., see Paley, H. W. [1406], 207, 208, *348*

Peterson, P. K., see Chapman, D. W. [59c], 12, *364*

Petritis, J., see Voridis, E. [1950], 226, *358*

Petta, J. M., Zaccheo, V. J. [8e bis], 256, *371*

Petzel, H., Moll, A. [1435], 136, *349*

— see Moll, A. [1312], 198, *346*

Peyrot, J., see Donnet, V. [440], 165, *331*

Pfeiffer, H. [1436], 138, 139, *349*

Pfleger, K., Niederau, D., Volkmer, J. [96a], 184, *362*

— Schöndorf, H. [1437], 185, *349*

— Volkmer, I., Kolassa, N. [30b], 186, 194, 202, *363*

— see Jacobi, H. [884], 156, *339*

— see Kolassa, N. [21b, 185c], 185, 186, *363, 367*

— see Schoendorf, H. [1689], 305, *353*

Phear, D., Walker, W. C. [1439], 163, *349*

Phear, D. N. [1438], 180, *349*

Philip, R. B. [247c], 50, *368*

Philips, F. S., see Clarke, D. A. [332], 306, *329*

Phillips, H. L., see Skinner, M. S. [1756], 129, *354*

Picard, P., see Dulac, J. F. [460], 307, *331*

Pichler, E., Strauss, A. [1440], 196, *349*

Pichler, O., see Hammerl, H. [774, 775], 187, *337*

Pichugin, V. V. [248c], 312, *368*

Pick, R., see Marcus, E. [1219], 88, *345*

Pieper, H. P. [1441], 74, *349*

Pieri, J., Casalonga, L., Dejouhannet, S. [1442], 190, 309, *349*

— Wahl, M., Casalonga, J. [1443], *349*

Piessens, J., Kesteloot, H., De Geest, H. [31b], 204, *363*

— see De Geest, H. [400], 115, 202, 203, *330*

Piette, F., Detry, J. M., Brasseur, L. [249c], 93, *369*

— see Detry, J. M. R. [81c], 21, *365*

Pifarre, R., see Vineberg, A. M. [1942], 182, *358*

Pilkington, T. R. E., Purves, M. J. [1444], 137, *349*

Pinkerson, A. L., see Kot, P. A. [1022], 144, *341*

Pinto, S. L., Telles, E. [1445], 228, *349*

Pippig, L., Schneider, K. W. [1446], 190, *349*

Pitt, A., Anderson, S. T. [250c], 227, *369*

— Friesinger, G. C., Ross, R. S. [1447], 83, *349*

— see Sloman, G. [1757], 10, *354*

Pitt, B. [1448], 36, *349*

— Becker, L., Zaret, B., Fortuin, N. J. [251c], 134, *369*

— Craven, P. [252c], 210, *369*

— Elliot, E. C., Gregg, D. E. [1449], 63, *349*

— Fortuin, N., Dagenais, G., Friesinger, G. C., Hodges, M. [1450], 100, *349*

— Green, L., Sugishita, Y. [97a], 210, *362*

— Gregg, D. E. [32b], 210, *363*

— Mason, J., Conti, C. R., Colman, R. W. [98a], 63, *362*

— Sugishita, Y., Green, H. L., Friesinger, G. C. [253c], 300, *369*

— see Becker, L. [9a], 134, *360*

— see Conti, C. R. [67c, 3d], 24, 27, 28, *365, 371*

— see Craven, P. [375], 210, *329*

— see Dagenais, G. R. [74c], 140, 143, 233, *365*

Pitt, W. A., Cox, A. R. [1451], 219, *349*

Piva, M., Ongari, R. [1452], 249, *349*

— see Dotti, F. [446], 249, *331*

Planta, W. von, [1949], 279, *358*

— see Schweizer, W. [1705], 162, *353*

Plavsic, C. [1453], 310, *349*

Plessis, F., see Kaufmann, H. [961], 164, *340*

Pletscher, A. [1454], 160, *349*

— Gey, K. F., Burkard, W. P. [1455], 161, *349*

— Pellmont, B. [1456], 161, *349*

— — Pellmont, B. [1457], 160, 161, *349*

Plomteux, G., Heusghem, C., Ernould, H., Vandeghen, N. [1458], 288, *349*

Ploszczanski, B., see Kraupp, O. [1040, 1042], 192, 194, *342*

Plotz, H. [1459], 142, *349*

Plotz, M. [1460], 141, *349*

Podevin, R., see Richet, G. [1525], 172, *350*

Poech, G., see Kukovetz, W. R. [73a, 74a, 191c, 6e], 150, 165, 197, 198, *361, 367, 371*

Pötzsch, E., see Kadatz, R. [929], 181, *340*

— see Nitz, R. E. [1369], 188, 190, *347*

Poggi, L., see Audier, M. [61], 279, 287, *324*

Poggioli, R., see Greggia, A. [736], 248, *336*

Pohl, S., see Toussaint, D. [124a], 287, *362*

Polansky, B. J., see Sodi-Pallares, D. [1769], 295, *355*

Polanyi, M., see Gamble, W. J. [106c], 91, *366*

— see Hugenholtz, P. G. [155c], 91, *367*

Polanyi, M. L., see Enson, Y. [92c], 91, *365*

Polo Friz, L., see Teotino, U. M. [1877], 248, *356*

Polster, P., see Godfraind, T. [674], 201, *335*

Polster, S., see Hellerstein, H. K. [807], 10, *337*

Polsterer, P., see Kaindl, F. [930], 307, *340*

Pommier, C., see Warembourg, H. [41b], 291, *363*

Pommier de Santi, P., see Donnet, V. [440], 165, *331*

Pomposiello, J. C., Baker, L. D., Snow, J. A., Sharma, G. V., Messer, J. V. [254c], *369*

— see Sharma, G. V. R. K. [112a], 27, *362*

Ponce de Leon, J., see Sodi-Pallares, D. [1767, 115a], 295, 296, *355, 362*

Pont, M., see Detry, R. [421], 279, *330*

Pool, P. E., see Boerth, R. C. [195], 97, 246, *326*

Popendiker, K., see Nieschulz, O. [1367], 303, *347*

Popovich, N. R., Roberts, F. F., Crislip, R. L., Menges, H. [1461], 123, *349*

Popper, H. [1462], 162, *349*

Pordy, L., see Friedberg, C. K. [598], 96, *333*

Porjé, G., see Atterhög, J. H. [60], 179, *324*

Porter, W. T. [1463], 65, *349*

Posse, P., see Rudolph, W. [276c], 194, *369*

Posselt, K., see Thiele, K. [1879, 1881], 198, *357*

Postanin, C., Hunt, D., Sheffield, L. T. [255c], 35, *369*

Powell, C. E., Slater, I. H. [1464], 205, *349*

Praschl, E., Kubicek, F. [1465], 290, *349*

Price, J. M., see Nayler, W. G. [1348, 1351], 174, 177, 179, 182, *347*

Price, T. M. L., see Allanby, K. D. [21], 163, *323*

Prichard, B. N. C. [1466], 212, 217, *349*

— Gillam, P. M. S. [1467, 257c, 258c], 207, 217, 222, *349, 369*

— see Aellig, W. H. [10, 4c], 227, 236, 241, 252, *323, 363*

— see Gillam, P. M. S. [659, 660], 207, 211, 217, *335*

Priest, W. S., see Soskin, S. [1796], 74, *355*

Prieto, G., see Reeves, T. J. [1511], 2, 268, *350*

Prinzmetal, M., see Kennamer, R. [969], 163, *340*

Prista Monteiro, H., see Moniz de Bettencourt, J. [1314, 1315], 159, *347*

Pritchard, W. H., see Gregg, D. E. [730, 731], 73, 76, *336*

Pritchard, W. P., see Eckstein, R. W. [478], 264, *331*

Proctor, J. D., Allen, F. J., Wasserman, A. J. [99a, 100a], 230, 231, 233, *362*

— see Wasserman, A. J. [130a], 230, 233, 235, *362*

Proger, S. H., Ayman, D. [1468], 137, *349*

— Minnich, W. R., Magendants, H. [1469], 304, *349*

Prokopenko, A. P., see Angarskaya, M. A. [34], 304, *323*

Proudfit, W. L., Shirey, E. K., Sones, F. M. [1470, 1471], 48, 84, 100, *349*

Provenza, D. V., see Scherlis, S. [1666], 20, *353*

Provenza, V., Scherlis, S. [1472, 1473], 20, *349*

Pruett, E. D. R., see Barry, A. J. [95], 10, *324*

Pruitt, R. D., Burchell, H. B., Barnes, A. R. [1474], 96, *349*

— see Burchell, H. B. [259], 96, *327*

— see Klakeg, C. H. [990], 96, *341*

Puech, P., Grolleau, R., Latour, H. [259c], 3, *369*

Pulido, P., see Mendez, R. [1279], 161, *346*

Pun, L.-Q., see Wale, J. [128a], 242, *362*

Puri, P., see Robin, E. [1543], 93, 126, 130, 131, 208, *350*

Puri, P. S., Bing, R. J. [260c], 251, *369*

— Ogawa, K., Robin, E., Martinez, M. A., Ribeilima, J., Bing, R. J. [1475], 126, 127, *349*

Purves, M. J., see Pilkington, T. R. E. [1444], 137, *349*

Pyfer, H. R., Doane, B. L. [101a], 10, *362*

Pyörälä, K., Ikkma, E., Siltanen, P. [1476], 171, *349*

Queneau, P. [1477], 191, *349*

Querimit, A. S., see Rowe, G. G. [1577], 188, 189, *351*

Querton, M., see Fierlafyn, E. [545], 293, *333*

Quiroz, A. C., see Shen, Y. [1738], 210, 215, *354*

Raab, W. [1478—1487], 20, 36, 42, 48, 207, 275, 284, *349*

— Gigee, W. [1488], 42, *349*

— Humphreys, R. J. [1489], 123, 207, *349*

— Lepeschkin, E. [1490], 123, 207, *349*

— Van Lith, P., Lepeschkin, E., Herrlich, H. C. [1491], 36, 284, *350*

Raaschou, F., see Grüner, A. [750], 311, *336*

Raberger, G., Kraupp, O. [261c, 262c], 194, *369*

— — Stuehlinger, W., Nell, G., Chirikdjian, J. J. [263c], 61, *369*

— Nell, G., Stuehlinger, W., Kraupp, O. [102a], 196, *362*

— see Kraupp, O. [1036, 1038], 194, 196, *342*

Rabkin, R., Stables, D. P., Levin, N. W., Suzman, M. M. [1492], 211, 214, 217, *350*

Race, D., see Nayler, W. G. [1348—1350], 174, 177, 179, 208, 223, 245, 250, *347*

Rackley, C. E., Dear, H. D., Baxley, W. A., Jones, W. B., Dodge, H. T. [264c], 35, *369*

Radawski, D., see Chou, C. C. [23a], 235, *360*

Raff, W. K., Drechsel, U., Scholtholt, J., Lochner, W. [103a, 265c], 122, *362, 369*

Raharison, S., see Facquet, J. [518], 280, 287, *332*

Rahn, K. H., Ockenga, T. [1493], 211, 245, 249, *350*

Raines, A., see Levitt, B. [1119], 249, *343*

Rajevskaja, Ersova 191

Ramsey, C. G., see Palmer, J. A. [1409], 139, *348*

Rand, M. J., see Wale, J. [128a], 242, *362*

Randall, L. O., Smith, T. H. [1494], 312, *350*

Ranieri, A. J., see Singh, R. [294c], 91, *369*

Rapaport, E., see Keroes, J. [69a], 208, *361*

— see Murray, J. F. [1333], 207, *347*

Raper, C., Wale, J. [1495, 104a], 219, 220, 221, 225, 226, 250, *350, 362*

Rappelli, A., see Campus, S. [273], 135, *327*

Rasmuson, T., see Areskog, N. H. [4a], 233, *360*

Rasson, G., see Friart, J. [4e], 286, *371*

— see Vastesaeger, M. [1927, 1928], 164, 276, 278, 279, 280, 285, 319, *357*

Ratschow, M., Schoop, W. [1496, 1497], 168, *350*

Rauh, M., see Bussmann, W. D. [5b], 237, *363*

Rausch, F., see Gille, H. [661], 190, *335*

Ravasi, M. T., see Setnikar, I. [1720, 1721], 161, 169, *354*

Ravera, M. [1498], 253, *350*

Ravin, I. B., Katz, K. H. [1499], 305, *350*

Rawson, R. W., see Leeper, R. D. [1092], 15, *343*

Rayford, C. R., see Gregg, D. E. [728], 2, 57, 77, 256, *336*

— see Khouri, E. M. [979], 29, 55, 56, 77, 256, *341*

Raymond, J., see Detry, R. [421], 279, *330*
Razzaboni, G., see Setti, L. [291c], 201, *369*
Reale, A. [1500, 1501], 226, *350*
— D'Intino, S., Vestri, A. [1502], 226, *350*
— Gioffre, P. A., Motolese, M., Imhof, P. [1503], 226, *350*
Redding, V. J., see Rees, J. R. [1504—1511], 2, 4, 83, 85, 123, 125, 183, *350*
Reddy, W. J., see Laraia, P. J. [196c], *367*
Redel, J., see Cottet, J. [370], 15, *329*
Redfors, A., see Nordenfelt, I. [1375], 234, *348*
Redwood, D., see Epstein, S. E. [94c], 315, 316, *365*
Redwood, D .R., Rosing, D. R., Goldstein, R. E., Beiser, G. D., Epstein, S. E. [266c], 106, *369*
— see Goldstein, R. E. [54a, 55a, 118c], 147, *361, 366*
Rees, J. R. [267c], 85, *369*
— Redding, V. J. [1504 to 1509], 2, 4, 83, 85, 183, *350*
— — Ashfield, R., Gibson, D., Gavey, C. J. [1510], 123, 125, *350*
— see Ross, R. S. [1562], 83, 84, 123, 130, *351*
Reeves, T. J., Hefner, L. L., Jones, W. B., Goghlan, C., Prieto, G., Carroll, J. [1511], 2, 268, *350*
— see Hefner, L. L. [797], 138, *337*
— see Scheffield, L. T. [1736, 1737], 97, *354*
Refi, Z., see Szabo, G. [1865], 302, *356*
Regan, F. D., see Russek, H. I. [1612—1614], 104, 135, 151, 158, 300, *352*
Regan, T. J., Binak, K., Gordon, S., Defazio, V., Hellems, H. K. [1512], 310, *350*
— Koroxenidis, G., Moschos, C. B., Oldewurtel, H. A., Lehan, P. H., Hellems, H. K. [1513], 301, *350*
— Weisse, A. B., Moschos, C. B., Lesniak, L. J., Nadini, M., Hellems, H. K. [1514], 301, *350*
— — Oldewurtel, H. A., Hellems, H. K. [1515], 301, *350*

Regan, T. J., see Lehan, P. H. [1093], 124, *343*
— see Levinson, R. S. [201c], 295, *368*
— see Weisse, A. B. [131a, 132a], 135, 146, *362*
Regelson, W., Hoffmeister, F. S., Wilkens, H. [1516], 161, *350*
Reichmann, W., see Bretschneider, H. J. [226], 52, 62, 189, 190, 269, *327*
Rein, H. [1517], 76, *350*
Reindell, A., see Leder, O. [80a], 167, 175, *361*
— see Schnellbacher, K. [287c], 217, *369*
Reindell, H., see Gebhardt, W. [632, 633], 181, 207, *334*
— see Keul, J. [974, 975], 187, *340*
— see Schnellbacher, K. [287c], 217, *369*
Reis, R. L., see Abel, R. M. [1a, 1c], 301, *360, 363*
— see Enright, L. P. [91c], 30, *365*
— see Epstein, S. E. [94c], 315, 316, *365*
Rekker, R. F., see Bijlsma, V. G. [160], 308, *326*
Relander, A., see Hakkinen, P. [5e], 199, *371*
Rembert, B., see Cobb, F. [336], 208, *329*
Rembert, B. S., see Cobb, F. R. [337], 208, *329*
Rembert, J. C., see Cobb, F. R. [24a], 208, *360*
— see Zeft, H. J. [345c], 303, *371*
Remington, J. W., see Hamilton, W. F. [772], 91, *337*
Remy, C., see Laubie, M. [1087], 62, 189, *342*
Renais, J., see Scebat, L. [1652], 215, 221, *352*
Renaud. S., Kuba, K., Goulet, C., Lemire, Y., Allard, C. [268c], 50, *369*
Renault, B., see Micheletti, J. [25b], 291, *363*
Renkin, E. M. [1518], 45, 85, *350*
Renschler, H. E., see Gerhard, W. [642], 144, 227, *334*
— see Hamm, J. [773], 187, *337*
Renyi-Vamos, F., see Solti, F. [296c], 316, *370*
Reploh, H. D., see Spieckermann, P. G. [119a], 185, 193, *362*

Requarth, W. H., see Roberg, N. B. [1540], 310, *350*
Resag, K., see Kiese, M. [981], 182, *341*
— see Nitz, R. E. [1370, 1371], 189, *347*
Resnekov, L. [105a], 10, *362*
— see Falicov, R. E. [95c], 316, *365*
— see Goldbarg, A. [115c], 212, *366*
Resnik, W. H., see Keefer, C. S. [965], 19, *340*
Reuse, J. J., see Bacq, Z. M. [67], 173, *324*
Rev, J., see Szabo, G. [1865], 302, *356*
Rey, C., Pattani, F. [1519], 310, *350*
Reymond, C. [1520], 279, 286, *350*
— see Rivier, J. L. [1538], 228, 229, *350*
Ribeilima, J., see Puri, P. S. [1475], 126, 127, *349*
Rice, A. J., Ferguson, R. K., Delle, M., Wilson, W. R. [106a], 251, *362*
— see Toubes, D. B. [314c], 252, *370*
Richards, D. W., see Hamilton, W. F. [772], 91, *337*
Richards, M. L., see Strong, J. P. [305c], 16, *370*
Richards, V., see Levy, J. V. [1125], 215, 216, *343*
Richardson, A. K., see Woods, E. F. [2036], 101, *359*
Richardson, A. T., [1521], 95, *350*
Richardson, A. W., Denison, A. B., Green, H. D. [1522], 74, *350*
Richardson, G. A., see Aellig, W. H. [10], 227, 241, 252, *323*
Richardson, J. A. [1523], 36, 275, *350*
— Woods, E. F. [1524], 101, *350*
— see Gazes, P. C. [631], 36, 101, *334*
— see Woods, E. F. [2036], 101, *359*
Richet, G., Cottet, J., Amiel, C., Leroux-Robert, C., Podevin, R. [1525], 172, *350*
Richmond, D. R., see McCallister, B. D. [217c], 12, *368*
Richmond, S., see Summers, D. N. [121a], 16, *362*
Richter, G., see Halmagyi, M. [766], 183, *337*
Riding, W. D., see Bray, C. L. [45c], 243, *364*

Riegel, C., see Schmitthenner, J. E. [1687], 300, *353*

Riff, D. P., Jain, A. C., Doyle, J. T. [107a], 301, *362*

Riggilo, D. A., see Brown, J. H. [241], *327*

— see Kvam, D. C. [1066], 251, *342*

Rinzler, S., see Bakst, H. [75], 112, 155, *324*

Rinzler, S. H. [1526, 1527], 14, 20, *350*

— Bakst, H., Benjamin, Z. H., Bobb, A. L., Travell, J. [*1528*], 305, *350*

— Travell, J., Bakst, H., Benjamin, Z. H., Rosenthal, R. L., Rosenfeld, S., Hirsch, B. B. [1529], 311, *350*

— see Christakis, G. [327], 14, *328*

— see Greiner, T. [738], 110, 111, 112, 113, 116, 158,308, *336*

Riseman, J. E. F. [1530], 19, 107, 116, 117, 142, *350*

— Altman, G. E., Koretsky, S. [1531], 106, 135, 137, 138, 139, 140, 142, 143, 146, *350*

— Brown, M. G. [1532, 1533], 140, 141, 146, 304, *350*

— Steinberg, L. A., Altman, G. E. [1534], 108, 304, *350*

— Stern, B. [1535], 107, *350*

— Waller, J. V., Brown, M. G. [1536], 106, *350*

— see Altman, G. E. [23], 140, *323*

— see Blumgart, H. L. [189], 20, *326*

— see Brown, M. G. [242], 154, *327*

— see Freedberg, A. S. [584, 585, 586], 106, 107, 108, 135, 140, 145, 304, *333*

— see Gray, W. [712], 151, *336*

— see Sagall, E. L. [1626], 137, *352*

— see Stearns, S. [1826], 300, *356*

Ritzmann, L. W., see Farrehi, C. [527], 14, *332*

Rival, J., see Cowan, C. [28a], 122, *360*

Rival, M. A., see Denis, B. [32a], 279, *360*

Rivier, J. L. [1537], 215, 227, *350*

— Nissiotis, E., Jaeger, M. [269c], 246, *369*

— Reymond, C., Grandjean, T. [1538], 228, 229, *350*

Rivier, J. L., see Grandjean, T. [708], 226, *335*

Robbins, S. L., Solomon, M., Bennet, A. [1539], 53, *350*

Roberg, N. B., Requarth, W. H. [1540], 310, *350*

Roberts, D., see Knoebel, S. B. [1007], 125, 130, *341*

Roberts, F. F., see Popovich, N. R. [1461], 123, *349*

Roberts, L. N., Mason, G. P., Villanueva, M. P., Babacan, B. C. [1542], 187, *350*

Roberts, J. T. [1541], 141, *350*

Robertson, H. S., see Hultgren, H. N. [871], 158, *339*

Robertson, P. D., see Cotterill, J. A. [69c], 295, *365*

Robin, E., Cowan, C., Puri, P., Ganguly, S., De Boyrie, E., Martinez, M., Stock, T., Bing, R. J. [1543], 93, 126, 130, 131, 208, *350*

— see Puri, P. S. [1475], 126, 127, *349*

Robinson, B. F. [1544], 29, 30, 43, 98, 282, *351*

— Epstein, S. E., Beiser, G. D., Braunwald, E. [1545], 207, 284, *351*

— see Epstein, S. E. [505], 207, 208, *332*

— see Wilson, A. G. [135a], 241, *362*

Robinson, C. R. [1546], 138, *351*

Robinson, M. C., see Taylor, S. H. [1876], 91, *356*

Robson, R. D., Kaplan, H. R. [11d], 255, *371*

— see Kaplan, H. R. [8d], 255, *371*

Rocha e Silva, M., see Antonio, A. [47], 63, *323*

Rochet, J., Vastesaeger, M. M. [1547], 211, *351*

— see Vastesaeger, M. [1929, 1930], 170, 171, *357*

Rodahl, K., see Barry, A. J. [95], 10, *324*

Rodbard, D., see Rodbard, S. [270c], 132, *369*

Rodbard, S., Graham, G. R., Williams, F. [1548], 70, *351*

— Williams, C. B., Rodbard, D. [270c], 132, *369*

— Williams, F., Williams, C. B. [271c], 132, *369*

Roddie, I. C., see Brick, I. [228, 229], 240, 243, *327*

Rodman, M. H., see Littmann, D. [1160], 96, *344*

Rodrigues-Pereira, E., Viana, A. P. [1549], 178, *351*

Rodset, J. M., see Nordoy, A. [236c], 50, *368*

Roe, B. B., see Criollos, R. L. [376], 10, *329*

Röth, G. [1564], 309, *351*

Roetscher, I., see Bernecker, C. [28c], 244, *364*

Roin, J., see Clausen, J. [333], 217, 218, 221, *329*

Roine, P., see Turpeinen, O. [1906], 14, *357*

Rojas, G. S. [1550], 228, 229, *351*

Rolett, E. L., see Cohen, L. S. [346], 25, 26, 30, 33, 38, *329*

— see Krasnow, N. [1033, 1034], 4, 25, 264, *342*

— see Yurchak, P. M. [2037], 36, *359*

Romeo, D., see Maggi, G. L. [1208], 162, *345*

Rookmaker, W. A. [1551, 1552], 99, 109, 227, 284, *351*

Rorvik, K., see Müller, O. [1328], 30, 33, *347*

Rose, A., see Delbarre, F. [403], 172, *330*

Rose, C., see Cronin, R. F. [71c], 59, *365*

Rose, L., see Lombardo, T. A. [1171], 55, *344*

Rosenberg, H. N., Michelson, A. L. [1553], *351*

Rosenblum, R., Delman, A. J. [108a], 218, *362*

— Frieden, J., Delman, A. J. [1554], 218, *351*

— — — Berkowitz, W. D. [1555], 218, *351*

Rosenfeld, I., Donoso, E., Master, A. M. [1556], 96, *351*

— see Master, A. M. [1229, 1235, 1236], 96, 103, *345*

Rosenfeld, R. S., see Hellman, L. [809], 16, *337*

Rosenfeld, S., see Rinzler, S. H. [1529], 311, *350*

Rosenman, R. H., Fishman, A. P., Kaplan, S. R., Levin, H. G., Katz, L. N. [1557], 158, *351*

— — Katz, L. N. [1558], 158, *351*

— see Jenkins, C. D. [896], 16, *339*

Rosenthal, R. L., see Rinzler, S. H. [1529], 311, *350*

Rosing, D. R., see Epstein, S. E. [94c], 315, 316, *365*

— see Goldstein, R. E. [54a, 55a, 118c], 147, *361, 366*

Rosing, D. R., see Redwood, D. R. [266c], 106, *369*
Roskamm, H., see Schnellbacher, K. [287c], 217, *369*
Rosove, L., see Binder, M. J. [162], 311, *326*
— see Kalmanson, F. M. [932], 141, *340*
Ross, E., see Elliott, W. C. [89c], 316, *365*
— see Knoebel, S. B. [182c], 57, *367*
Ross, G., Jorgensen, C. R. [1559, 1560, 272c], 172, 174, 236, *351, 369*
— see Gaal, P. G. [616], 210, *334*
— see Kolin, A. [1015, 1017], 4, 78, *341*
Ross, J., see Boerth, R. C. [195], 97, 246, *326*
— see Braunwald, E. [15a], 41, *360*
— see Klocke, F. J. [999, 1000], 63, 206, 264, *341*
— see Linhart, J. W. [1151], 3, 219, *344*
— see Sonnenblick, E. H. [1790, 1791], 92, 93, 132, 268, *355*
Ross, R. S. [1561], 84, *351*
— Ueda, K., Lichtlen, P. R., Rees, J. R. [1562], 83, 84, 123, 130, *351*
— see Bernstein, L. [146], 28, 83, 123, 130, 133, *325*
— see Conti, C. R. [3d], 24, 28, *371*
— see Dagenais, G. R. [74c], 140, 143, 233, *365*
— see Pitt, A. [1447], 83, *349*
Rosseel, M. T., see Bogaert, M. G. [35c, 36c], 136, *364*
Rossi, B. [1563], 141, *351*
Rost, R., see Gattenloehner, W. [46a], 218, *361*
Roth, O. [1565], 310, *351*
Rothberger, C. J., see Mahaim, I. [1209], 154, *345*
Rothendler, H. H., see Greiner, T. [738], 110, 111, 112, 113, 116, 158, 308, *336*
Rothfeld, E., see Abrams, W. B. [7], 163, *323*
Rothfeld, E. L., see Shoshkes, M. [1748], 162, *354*
Rothlin, E. [1566, 1567], 312, *351*
Rotta, A., see Gregg, D. E. [730, 735], 73, 76, *336*
Roubelakis, G., see Corcondilas, A. [362], 228, *329*
Roudy, G., see Bouvrain, Y. [40c], 297, *364*

Roughgarden, J. W., Newman, E. V. [1568], 30, 33, *351*
Roux, M., see Marion, J. [1220], 171, *345*
Roven, R. B., see Case, R. B. [280, 281], 22, 55, *328*
Rowe, G. G. [1569, 1570, 1571, 1572, 273c], 28, 39, 55, 81, 85, 92, 134, 267, 317, *351, 369*
— Afonso, S., Boake, W. C., Castillo, C. A., Lugo, J. E., Crumpton, C. W. [1573], 294, *351*
— Castillo, C. A., Afonso, S., Crumpton, C. W. [1574], 81, *351*
— Chelius, C. J., Afonso, S., Gurtner, H. P., Crumpton, C. W. [1575], 140, *351*
— Emanuel, D. A., Maxwell, G. M., Brown, J. F., Castillo, C., Schuster, B., Murphy, Q. R., Crumpton, C. W. [1576], 304, *351*
— Terry, W., Stenlund, R. R., Thomsen, J. H., Querimit, A. S. [1577], 188, 189, *351*
— Spring, D. A., Afonso, S. [12d], 294, *371*
— Thomsen, J. H., Stenlund, R. R., McKenna, D. H., Sialer, S., Corliss, R. J. [1578], 22, *351*
— see Maxwell, G. M. [1242, 1243], 153, *345*
— see McKenna, D. H. [1257, 1258], 4, 42, 207, 209, 272, 274, *345*
— see Thomsen, J. H. [1888], 200, 201, *357*
Rowe, H., see Gabel, L. P. [617], 45, *334*
Rowlands, D. J., Howitt, G., Markman, P. [1579], 221, *351*
Rowsell, H. C., see Joergensen, L. [900], 4, *339*
Royer, R., see Benichoux, R. [22c], 70, *364*
— see Lamarche, M. [192c], 295, *367*
Rozear, M., see Wallacw, A. G. [1955], *358*
Rozonov, Y. B., see Kaverina, N. V. [964, 171c], 134, *340, 367*
Rubin, A. A. [1580], 291, *351*
Rubin, I. L., see Hellman, L. [809], 16, *337*
Rubio, R., see Berne, R. M. [1581], 61, *351*
— see Berne, R. M. [109a, 26c, 27c], 45, 61, *362, 364*

Rudolf, J., see Dighiero, J. [430], 163, *330*
Rudolph, W., Bernsmeier, A., Henselmann, L., Baedeker, W. D., Hofmann, H. [1582], 186, 187, *351*
— Marko, J. [274c, 275c], 195, *369*
— — Baubkus, H., Muller-Seydlitz, P., Gadomski, M., Posse, P., Gulde, M., Jetschgo, G. [276c], 194, *369*
— Meixner, L., Kunzig, H. J. [1583], 190, *351*
— see Bernsmeiyer, A. [144], 267, *325*
Rudy, W. B., see Nalefski, L. A. [1339], 158, *347*
Ruef, J., see Hensel, H. [815], 76, *338*
Rueger, R., see Leighninger, D. S. [1095], 122, *343*
Ruf, G., see Audier, M. [63], 310, *324*
Rumeau, M., see Lesbre, J. P. [200c], 279, *368*
Rummel, W., see Kolassa, N. [21b], 186, *363*
— see Schoendorf, H. [1689], 305, *353*
Ruosteenoja, R., see Linko, E. [1155, 1156], 232, 235, *344*
Rushmer, R. F. [1584, 1585], 268, *351*
Ruskin, A. [1586, 1587, 1588], 140, 149, 311, 314, *351*
Russek, H. I. [1589—1611, 277c], 15, 19, 21, 96, 102, 103, 104, 116, 117, 135, 140, 142, 146, 147, 154, 155, 160, 162, 164, 213, 214, 299, 304, 307, 309, 314, *351, 352, 369*
— Naegele, C. F., Regan, F. D. [1612], 104, 300, *352*
— Regan, F. D., Anderson, W. H., Doerner, A. A., Naegele, C. F. [1613], 104, 158, *352*
— Smith, R. H., Baum, W. S., Naegele, C. F., Regan, F. D. [1614], 104, 135, 151, 300, *352*
— Urbach, K. F., Doerner, A. A. [1615], 104, 311, *352*
— — — Zohman, B. L. [1616], 103, 104, 106, 135, 141, 151, 152, 154, 158, 311, 312, 313, *352*
— — Zohman, B. L. [1617], 136, 137, *352*
— Zohman, B. L. [1618], 213, *352*

Russek, H. I., Zohman, B. L., Dorset, V. J. [1619], 104, 135, 137, 139, 141, 151, 152, 154, 158, 299, 311, 312, 313, 352
— — Drumm, A. E., Weingarten, W., Dorset, V. J., [1620], 105, 137, 139, 141, 152, 352
Russel, N. G., see Levy, R. L. [1127], 106, 136, 343
Rutishauser, W., see Wirz, P. [340c], 371
Rutlisberger, P. A., see Abaza, A. [1], 162, 323
Rybak, B., see Kunze, K. [1058], 342
Ryser, H., Wilbrandt, W. [1621], 67, 309, 352

Saameli, K. [1622, 1623], 245, 246, 352
Sabiston, D. C. [1624], 11, 352
— see Gregg, D. E. [732], 7, 28, 57, 58, 201, 268, 336
Saby, G., see Felix, H. [10b], 291, 363
Saccani-Guelfi, M., see Murmann, W. [1329], 248, 347
Sachs, B. A. [1625], 16, 352
Sack, K. H., see Nieschulz, O. [1367], 303, 347
Sagall, E. L., Kurland, G. S., Riseman, J. E. F. [1626], 137, 352
Sagols, L., see Faucon, G. [528], 298, 332
Sahm, F. [1627], 168, 352
Sailer, S., see Braunsteiner, H. [212], 14, 326
Saito, S., see Bargheer, R. [88], 159, 324
Sakai, S., Saneyoshi, S. [1628], 152, 352
Salans, A. H., Silber, E. H., Katz, L. N. [1629], 141, 352
Salazar, A. E. [1630], 89, 352
Salle, J., Nau, P. [1631], 159, 352
Saltups, A., see McCallister, B. D. [217c], 12, 368
Salva, J. A., see Brugger, A. [247], 193, 327
Salwan, F. A., Leighninger, D. S., Beck, C. S. [278c], 21, 369
Samaan, K. [1632, 1633], 157, 352
— Hossein, A. M., Fahim, I. [1634], 159, 352
Sambhi, M. P., Zimmerman, H. A. [1635], 16, 352
Samet, P., see Linhart, J. W. [1152—1154, 82a], 3, 11, 34, 126, 130, 344, 361

Samet, P., see Narula, O. S. [230c], 3, 368
Sanders, G. [1636], 15, 352
Sandhofer, F., see Braunsteiner, H. [211], 14, 326
Sandler, G. [1637—1639, 279c], 149, 163, 180, 242, 314, 352, 369
— Clayton, G. A. [1640, 280c], 138, 241, 352, 369
— — Thornicroft, S. G. [1641], 180, 352
— Patney, L. N., Lawson, C. W. [1642], 171, 352
Saner, R. [281c], 247, 369
Saner, R. P. [110a], 247, 362
Saneyoshi, S., see Sakai, S. [1628], 152, 352
Sano, T., see Yamazaki, H. [342c], 289, 371
Sanz, G., see Cardenas, M. [54c], 249, 364
Sanz, M., see Schmutz, J. [1688], 353
Sapienza, P. L. [1643], 142, 352
Sapru, R. P., see Taylor, S. H. [1876], 91, 356
Sarai, K., see Solti, F. [296c], 316, 370
Sarnoff, S. J., Braunwald, E., Welch, G. H., Case, R. B., Stainsby, W. N., Macruz, R. [1644], 29, 55, 92, 93, 132, 267, 352
— Case, R. B., Macruz, R. [1645], 122, 352
Sassa, K., see Iwai, M. [881], 152, 339
Sassine, A., see Loubatieres, A. [1178], 309, 344
Saulnier, R. [1646], 310, 352
Sauvan, R., see Catinat, J. [285], 299, 328
— see Mouquin, M. [1326], 307, 347
Savenkov et al. 191, 192
Sbar, S., Schlant, C. [1647], 187, 352
Scaffidi, V., D'Agostino, L. [1648], 313, 352
Scales, B., McIntosh, D. A. D. [1649], 216, 352
Scarborough, W. R. [1650], 95, 352
— Mason, R. E., Davis, F. W., Singewald, M. L., Baker, B. M., Lore, S. A. [1651], 95, 352
Scebat, L., Bensaid, J., Sozutek, Y., Lefevre, M., Renais, J. [1652], 215, 221, 352
— Maurice, M. [1653], 280, 352
— see Bensaid, J. [24c, 25c], 227, 364

Schaal, S. F., see Wallacw, A. G. [1955], 358
Schachter, R. J., Kimura, E. T., Nowarra, G. M., Mestern, J. [1654], 155, 352
Schaede, A., see Düx, A. [464], 187, 190, 331
— see Hilger, H. H. [826, 827], 186, 194, 338
Schaefer, L. E. [1655], 14, 16, 353
Schaefer, N., Stauch, M. [1656], 235, 353
Schaff, G., see Faucon, G. [528], 298, 332
Schaffer, A. I., see Scherf, D. [1664], 96, 353
Schairer, K., see Stauch, M. [1825], 245, 356
Schaper, J., see Schaper, W. [283c], 86, 369
— see Schaper, W. K. A. [1658], 46, 47, 353
Schaper, W., Jageneau, A. [111a], 200, 202, 362
— — Xhonneux, R. [282c], 47, 204, 369
— Xhonneux, R., Jageneau, A., Vandesteene, R., Schaper, J. [283c], 86, 369
— see Jageneau, A. [887, 888, 889], 123, 165, 173, 182, 189, 200, 202, 339
Schaper, W. K. A. [1657], 46, 86, 203, 204, 353
— Schaper, J., Xhonneux, R., Vandesteene, R. [1658], 46, 47, 353
— Xhonneux, R., Jageneau, A. H. M. [1659], 46, 47, 53, 201, 203, 204, 353
— — — Janssen, P. A. J. [1660], 40, 199, 200, 201, 353
Schapiro, A. [1731], 187, 354
Schapiro, A. K. [1732], 114, 354
Schapiro, S. [1733, 1734], 16, 146, 354
Schaum, E., see Bosse, J. A. [14a], 175, 198, 360
Schaumann, W., Bodem, R., Bartsch, W. [1661], 165, 174, 353
Scheffield, L. T., Holt, J. H., Reeves, T. J. [1736], 97, 354
— Reeves, T. J. [1737], 97, 354
Scheler, F., see Bretschneider, H. J. [227], 181, 183, 327
Schellhorn, W., see Hunscha, H. [872], 191, 339
Schelling, J. L., Lasagna, L. [1662], 137, 143, 353

Scherbel, A. L. [1663], 162, *353*
Scherf, D., Schaffer, A. I. [1664], 96, *353*
Scherlag, B. J., Lau, S. H., Helfant, R. H., Berkowitz, W. D., Stein, E., Damato, A. N. [1665], 3, *353*
— see Bartelstone, H. J. [97], 70, *324*
— see Damato, A. N. [388], 3, *330*
Scherlis, S., Provenza, D. V. [1666], 20, *353*
— see Provenza, V. [1472, 1473], 20, *349*
Scheuer, J. [1667], 25, *353*
— see Brachfeld, N. [209], 25, *326*
Schiefthaler, T., see Heistracher, P. [802], 192, *337*
Schild, H. O., see Wilson, A. [2004], 307, *359*
Schilero, A. J., see Jablons, B. [882], 137, *339*
Schilling, F. J., Becker, W. H., Christakis, G. [1668], 14, *353*
Schimassek, U., see Thiele, K. [1882], 196, *357*
Schimert, G. [1669], 122, 151, 154, 312, 313, *353*
— Schwalb, H. [1670], 115, 202, 203, *353*
— Zickgraf, H. [1671], 312, 313, *353*
— see Blömer, H. [184], 309, *326*
Schirmer, R., Hamacher, J. [289c], 293, *369*
Schlant, C., see Sbar, S. [1647], 187, *352*
Schlant, R. C., see Fletcher, G. F. [565, 566], 295, *333*
Schlepper, M., Witzleb, E. [1672], 172, 174, *353*
— see Böhm, C. [196], 165, 168, *326*
Schlesinger, M. J. [1673], 90, *353*
— Zoll, P. M. [1674], 52, *353*
— see Blumgart, H. L. [190], 137, *326*
Schlichtegroll, A. von, see Habersang, S. [760], 196, *337*
— see Thiele, A. [1882], 196, *357*
— see Thiemer, K. [1884], 198, *357*
Schlosser, V., see Blümchen, G. [33c], 156, *364*
Schluger, J., McGinn, J. T., Hennessy, D. J. [1675], 155, *353*
Schmahl, F. W., see Betz, E. [155], 169, *325*

Schmall, F. W., Betz, E. [1676], 172, *353*
Schmetz, J., see Joris, H. [909], 171, *339*
Schmid, A., Strausak, A. [1849], 160, *356*
Schmid, B., see Grobecker, H. [744], 166, *336*
Schmid, E., Krautheim, J., Weist, F. [1677], 167, *353*
— see Krautheim, J. [1045], 198, *342*
Schmid, J. R., Hanna, C. [1678c, 33b], 174, 250, *353*, *363*
Schmidt, A., see Hamm, J. [137c], 245, *366*
Schmidt, C., see Faivre, G. [519], 279, *332*
Schmidt, C. F., see Dumke, P. R. [461], 74, *331*
— see Kety, S. S. [973], 79, *340*
Schmidt, E., see Bender, F. [132], 226, *325*
Schmidt, H. D., Schmier, J. [1679, 1680, 285c], 45, 86, 183, *353*, *369*
— see Schmier, J. [286c], 183, *369*
Schmidt, L. [1681], 157, *353*
— Engelhorn, R. [1682], 55 *353*
Schmidt-Mertens, H. H., see Hensel, H. [814], *338*
Schmidt-Voigt, J. [1683], 217, *353*
— see Lamprecht, G. [1068], 217, *342*
Schmier, J., Kaden, F., Schmidt, H. D. [286c], 183, *369*
— see Schmidt, H. D. [1679, 1680, 285c], 45, 86, 183, *353*, *369*
Schmitt, G. [1684], 178, *353*
— Hauss, W. H. [34b], 183, *363*
— Junge-Hülsing, G., Wagner, H., Hauss, W. H. [1685], *353*
— Knoche, H. [1686], 214, *353*
— see Knoche, H. [1006], 214, *341*
Schmitt, H., see Boissier, J. R. [198], 167, *326*
— see Giudicelli, J.-F. [669], *335*
— see Laubie, M. [1083 to 1087], 58, 62, 189, 298, *342*
Schmitthenner, J. E., Hafkenschiel, J. H., Forte, I., Williams, A. J., Riegel, C. [1687], 300, *353*

Schmutz, J., Lauener, H., Hirt, R., Sanz, M. [1688], 159, *353*
Schneckloth, R. E., see Page, I. H. [1402], 15, *348*
Schneider, K. W., see Gattenloehner, W. [46a], 218, *361*
— see Pippig, L. [1446], 190, *349*
Schnellbacher, K., Reindell, H., Roskamm, H., Reindell, A. [287c], 217, *369*
Schnelle, K., see Lydtin, H. [1198], 220, *344*
Schönberg, A., see Anrep, G. V. [41], 160, *323*
Schöndorf, H., see Pfleger, K. [1437], 185, *349*
— Rummel, W., Pfleger, K. [1689], 305, *353*
Schöne, H. H., Lindner, E. [1695, 1696], 166, *353*
Schoenfeld, C. D., see Harris, W. S. [785], 207, *337*
Schoenmakers, J. [1690], 52, 269, *353*
Schoepke, H. G., Darby, T. D., Brondyk, H. D. [1691], 189, *353*
Schofield, B. M., Walker, J. M. [1692], 72, *353*
Scholimeyer, P. J., Jeschke, D. [1693], 186, *353*
Scholfield, P. C., see Adam, K. R. [1e], 239, 240, *371*
Schollmeyer, P., see Jeschke, D. [898], 179, *339*
Scholtholt, J., Bussmann, W. D., Lochner, W. [1694], 62, 63, 189, *353*
— see Hirche, H. [838], 169, *338*
— see Raff, W. K. [103a, 265c], 122, *362*, *369*
Schonbeck, M., see Wirz, P. [340c], *371*
Schoop, W., see Ratschow, M. [1496, 1497], 168, *350*
Schraven, E., Nitz, R. E. [1697], 190, *353*
— see Nitz, R. E. [1372], 190, *347*
Schrire, V., see Spracklen, F. H. [297c], 301, *370*
Schroder, H. A., see Davies, D. F. [391], 21, *330*
Schröder, G., see Björntorp, P. [177], 232, *326*
Schuermans, V., see Bosmans, P. [39c], 47, 114, 203, 204, *364*
Schuetterle, G., see Tschirdewahn, B. [1903], 221, *357*
Schuilenburg, R. M., Durrer, D. [288c], 3, *369*
Schuler, W., see Thiele, K. [1879], *357*

Schultz, F., see Frey, E. K. [589], 309, *333*

Schultz, W. J., see Soskin, S. [1796], 74, *355*

Schurger, R. [1698], 296, *353*

Schürmeyer, E., see Lochner, W. [1166], 150, 153, *344*

Schuster, B., see Rowe, G. G. [1576], 304, *351*

Schute, E., see Schute, W. [1749], 305, *354*

Schute, W., Schute, E., Vogelsang, A. [1749], 305, *354*

Schwalb, H. [1699], 9, *353*

— see Schimert, G. [1670], 115, 202, 203, *353*

Schwalbe, J. [1700], 196, *353*

Schwartz, H., see Macleod, C. A. [209c], 10, *368*

Schwartz, J., see Spach, M. O. [36b], 229, *363*

Schwartz, S. I., Griffith, L. S. C., Neistadt, A., Hagfors, N. [289c], 316, *369*

Schwartz, W. [1701], 142, *353*

Schwarzmeier, J., see Lujf, A. [1195], 215, *344*

Schweer, M., see Uhlenbrock, K. [1907, 1908], 156, 158, *357*

Schweitzer, F. [1702], 196, *353*

Schweizer, W. [1703], 162, *353*

— Burkart, F., Creux, G., Widmer,L.K.[1704],16,*353*

— Von Planta, P. [1705], 162, *353*

Schwimmer, J., see Batterman, R. C. [106], 154, 155, *325*

— see Grossman, A. J. [747], 155, *336*

Scomozoni, G., see Baroldi, G. [89], 53, *324*

Scott, C., see Ben, M. [129], 163, *325*

Scott, C. C., see Chessin, M. [323], 163, *328*

— see Winsor, T. [2021], 140, 141, 142, *359*

Scott, J. B., see Chou, C. C. [23a], 235, *360*

— see Frohlich, E. D. [606], 121, 145, 150, *334*

Scott, J. C. [1706, 1707], 56, 79, *353*

Scott, P. J., see Norris, R. M. [1377], 217, *348*

Scott, R. C., Iglauer, A., Green, R. S., Kaufman, J. W., Berman, B., McGuire, J. [1708], 158, *353*

— Seiwert, V. J. [1709], 158, *353*

— — Fowler, N. O., McGuire, J. [1710], 152, *353*

Scott, S., see Dart, C. H. [76c], 11, *365*

Scott, W. S., Leslie, A., Mulinos, M. G. [1711], 106, *354*

— see Leslie, A. [1108], 106, *343*

Scriabine, A., McShane, W. K. [1712], 123, 139, *354*

Sealey, B. J., Liljedahl, J., Nyberg, G., Ablad, B. [290c], 233, *369*

Seasohn, P. O., see Liebow, J. M. [1137], 48, *343*

Sebrell, W. H., see Bergen, S. S., jr. [135], 15, *325*

Segal, B. L., see Likoff, W. [1139], 48, *343*

Segal, R. L., Silver, S., Yohalem, S. B., Newburger, R. A. [1713], 20, *354*

Seeman, T., see Linder, E. [1143], 183, *343*

Seiwert, V. J., see Scott, R. C. [1709, 1710], 152, 158, *353*

Sekiya, A., Vaughan-Williams, E. M. [1714], 253, *354*

Seldon, W. A., see Neilson, G. H. [1356], 211, *347*

Selye, H. [1715, 1716], 48, 49, *354*

Selzer, A., Sudrann, R. B. [1717], 91, *354*

Semmler, F. [1718], 143, *354*

Sentman, J., see Moss, A. J. [228c], 210, *368*

Serban, M., see Teodorini, S. [123a], 279, *362*

Serradimigni, A., see Audier, M. [61], 279, 287, *324*

Sethna, D. S., see Bray, C. L. [45c], 243, *364*

Setnikar, I. [1719], 160, *354*

— Murmann, W., Ravasi, M. T. [1720], 169, *354*

— Ravasi, M. T. [1721], 161, *354*

— Zanolini, T. [1722], 160, *354*

Setti, L., Razzaboni, G. [291c], 201, *369*

Sevelius, G., Johnson, P. C. [1723], 81, *354*

— see Johnson, P. C. [903], 22, 129, *339*

Seymour, J., see Conway, N. [361], 215, 221, *329*

Shah, P. M., see Cherian, G. [322], 218, *328*

Shanaman, J. E., see Emele, J. F. [491], 161, *332*

Shanes, A. M., see Winegrad, S. [2019], 216, *359*

Shanks, R. C., see Barrett, A. M. [93], 235, 236, 242, *324*

Shanks, R. G. [1724—1728], 174, 175, 177, 206, 207, 214, 245, 249, 250, 272, *354*

— Dunlop, D. [1729], 220, *354*

— Wood, T. M., Dornhorst, A. C., Clark, M. L. [1730], 245, *354*

— see Black, J. W. [178, 179], 205, 206, *326*

— see Brick, I. [228, 229], 240, 243, *327*

— see Dunlop, D. [463], 236, 237, *331*

— see Grant, R. H. E. [710], 174, 207, *336*

— see Kofi Ekue, J. M. [71a, 184c], 237, 251, *361*, *367*

Share, N. N., see Varma, D. R. [1921], 89, 122, 161, 308, *357*

Sharma, G. V., see Pomposiello, J. C. [254c], *369*

Sharma, G. V. R. K., Pomposiello, J. C., Inamdar, A. N., Messer, J. V. [112a], 27, *362*

— see Baker, L. D. [73], 26, *324*

Sharma, P. L. [1735], 242, *354*

Sharpey-Schafer, E. P., see Howarth, S. [864], 153, *338*

Shaver, J. A., see Thompson, M. E. [311c], 240, *370*

Shedrovilzky, H., see Nakhjavan, F. K. [1337], 89, *347*

Sheffield, L. T., see Potanin, C. [255c], 35, *369*

Sheldon, W. C., see Fergusson, D. J. [535], 10, *332*

Sheldon, W. F., see Foltz, E. L. [570], 55, 81, *333*

Shen, Y., Quiroz, A. C., Burch, G. E., Depasquale, N. P. [1738], 210, 215, *354*

Sherber, D. A., Gelb, I. J. [1739, 1740], 146, 147, *354*

Sherrod, T. R., see Lasker, N. [1077], 300, *342*

Shevde, S., Spilker, B. A. [13d], 219, *371*

Shillingford, J. P., see Jewitt, D. E. [899, 162c, 163c], 241, 243, *339*, *367*

— see Valori, C. [1915], 243, *357*

Shimamoto, T. [113a], 289, *362*

— Maezawa, H., Yamazake, H., Atsumz, T., Fugita, T., Ishioka, T., Sunaga, T. [1741], 289, *354*

— Numano, F., Fugita, T. [1742], 289, *354*

— see Atsumi, T. [14c], 289, *363*

— see Numano, F. [238c], 289, *368*

Shimamoto, T., see Yamazaki, H. [342c], 289, *371*

Shinebourne, E., Fleming, J., Hamer, J. [1743, 1744], 211, 240, *354*

— White, R., Hamer, J. [1745], 220, *354*

— see Hess, M. H. [824], 216, *338*

— see White, R. [1988], 216, *358*

Shinohara, Y., see Ehrlich, J. C. [481], *331*

Shipley, R. E., Gregg, D. E., Wearn, J. T. [1746], 76, *354*

— Wilson, C. [1747], 73, 74, *354*

— see Gregg, D. E. [730, 731, 733—735], 69, 73, 76, 80, *336*

— see Henderson, F. G. [810], 151, *338*

Shirey, E. K., see Fergusson, D. J. [535], 10, *332*

— see Proudfit, W. L. [1470, 1471], 48, 84, 100, *349*

— see Sones, F. M. [1788], 4, 101, 124, *355*

Shister, H. E., see Garvey, L. [628], 173, 174, *334*

— see Melville, K. I. [1277], 174, *346*

Shoshkes, M., Rothfeld, E. L., Becker, M. C., Finkelstein, A., Smith, C. C., Wachtel, F. W. [1748], 162, *354*

— see Abrams, W. B. [7], 163, *323*

Shubin, H., see Wolffe, J. B. [2030], 163, *359*

Shubov, M. I., see Angarskaya, M. A. [34], 304, *323*

Shugina, T. M., see Kaverina, N. V. [964], 134, *340*

Shugoll, G. I., see Banks, T. [84], 48, *324*

Shum, A., see Flattery, K. V. [560], 167, 168, *333*

Shutt, J. H., see Hanna, C. [779], 67, *337*

Sialer, S., see McKenna, D. H. [1258], 42, 207, 209, 272, 274, *345*

— see Rowe, G. G. [1578], 22, *351*

— see Thomsen, J. H. [1888], 200, 201, *357*

Sicam, L., see Jablons, B. [882], 137, *339*

Sicuteri, F., Fanciullacci, M., Delbianco, P. L. [1750], 249, *354*

Siderides, L. E., see Litvak, J. [1161], 90, *344*

Sieber, H. A., see Boyles, C. M. [206], 111, *326*

Siedek, H., see Hammerl, H. [776], 187, *337*

Sieger, W., see Bender, F. [10a], 226, 233, 245, *360*

Siess, M. [1751], 185, *354*

Siitonen, L., see Linko, E. [1155, 1156], 232, 235, *344*

Silber, E. H., Katz, L. N. [1752], 108, 109, 110, 116, 139, *354*

— see Salans, A. H. [1629], 141, *352*

Siltanen, P., see Pyörälä, K. [1476], 171, *349*

Silva Maltez, J., De Sousa Borges, A. [1753], 171, *354*

Silver, S., see Segal, R. L. [1713], 20, *354*

Simaan, J., Fawaz, G. [1754], 182, *354*

Simon, A. J., Dolgin, M., Solway, A. J. L., Hirschmann, J., Katz, L. N. [1755], 151, *354*

Simon, F., see Di Carlo, F. J. [427], *330*

Simon, J., see Chevalier, H. [324], 160, *328*

Simonton, J., see Graham, D. M. [704], 311, *335*

Sinclair, K., see Grant, R. H. E. [709], 217, *336*

Singer, D. M., Lazzara, R., Hoffmann, B. F. [292c], 27, *369*

Singewald, M. L., see Scarborough, W. R. [1651], 95, *352*

Singh, B. M. [114a], 180, *362*

Singh, B. N., Vaughan-Williams, E. M. [35b, 293c], 232, 250, *363*, *369*

Singh, B. N., see Vaughan-Williams, E. M. [1934], 269, 270, 272, 276, *357*

Singh, R., Ranieri, A. J., Vest, H. R., Bowers, D. L., Dammann, J. F. [294c], 91, *369*

Singletary, H. P., see Lumb, G. D. [1196], 90, 141, *344*

Sion, R., see Broekhuysen, J. [236], 287, *327*

— see Deltour, G. [409], 255, *330*

Sise, H. S., see Ellis, L. B. [489], 20, 96, *331*

Sivertssen, E., see Bay, G. [113], 218, *325*

— see Lund Larsen, G. [85a], 235, *361*

Sjoerdsma, A., see Horwitz, D. [861], 161, *338*

Skinner, J. S., see Holloszy, J. O. [854], 10, *338*

Skinner, M. S., Leibeskind, R. S., Phillips, H. L., Harrison, T. R. [1756], 129, *354*

Sklow, N. J., see Di Carlo, F. J. [427], *330*

Slaastad, R., see Aubert, A. [8a], 233, *360*

Slater, I. H., see Powell, C. E. [1464], 205, *349*

Sloan, H., see Haight, C. [764], 121, *337*

Sloman, G., Pitt, A., Hirsch, E. Z., Donaldson, A. [1757], 10, *354*

— Stannard, M. [1758], 221, *354*

— see Vohra, J. K. [329c], 243, *370*

Smekal, P. V., see Gerhard, W. [642], 144, 227, *334*

Smith, C. C., see Shoshkes, M. [1748], 162, *354*

Smith, E. R., see Duce, B. R. [86c], 232, *365*

Smith, F. H., see McEachern, C. G. [1249], 150, *345*

Smith, F. M. [1759], 145, *354*

— Miller, G. H., Graber, V. C. [1760], 153, *354*

— see Fowler, W. M. [574], 153, *333*

Smith, G., see Eckstein, R. W. [476, 477], 122, 123, *331*

Smith, J. R., see Kountz, W. B. [1025], 153, *341*

Smith, L. H., see Barrett, A. M. [93], 235, 236, 242, *324*

— see Black, J. W. [178], 205, 206, *326*

Smith, M. H., Gorlin, R. [1761], 122, *354*

Smith, R. H., see Russek, H. I. [1614], 104, 135, 151, 300, *352*

Smith, T. H., see Randall, L. O. [1494], 312, *350*

Smith, W. G. [1762], 218, *354*

Smulyan, H., Eich, R. H. [1763], 210, *354*

Sneddon, J. M., see Chamberlain, D. A. [293], 207, 284, *328*

Snow, J. A., Olsson, R. A. [295c], 61, *370*

— see Pomposiello, J. C. [254c], *369*

Snow, P. J. D. [1764, 1765], 207, 217, *354*

— Anderson, D. E. [1766], 162, *354*

Sobel, B. E., see Braunwald, E. [44c], 315, 316, *364*

Sodi Pallares, D., Bisteni, A., Medrano, G. A., Cisneros, F., Ponce de Leon, J. [115a], 296, *362*

Sodi Pallares, D., Bisteni, A., Medrano, G. A., De Micheli, A., Ponce de Leon, J., Calva, E., Fishleder, B. L., Testelli, M. R., Miller, B. L. [1767], 295, *355*

— — Testelli, M. R., De Micheli, A. [1768], 295, *355*

— Fishleder, B. L., Cisneros, F., Vizcaino, M., Bisteni, A., Medrano, G. A., Polansky, B. J., De Micheli, A. [1769], 295, *355*

— Testelli, M. R., Fishleder, B. L., Bisteni, A., Medrano, G. A., Friedland, C., De Micheli, A. [1770], 295, *355*

Sölvell, L., see Ablad, B. [4], 207, 232, *323*

— see Johnsson, G. [905], 232, *339*

Solandt, D. Y., Best, C. H. [1771], 310, *355*

— Nassim, R., Best, C. H. [1772], 310, *355*

Soloff, L. A., Gimenez, J. L., Winters, W. L. [1773], 181, 187, *355*

— see Frankl, W. S. [581], 251, *333*

Solomon, M., see Robbins, S. L. [1539], 53, *350*

Solti, F., Szabo, Z., Fedina, L., Renyi-Vamos, F., Sarai, K. [296c], 316, *370*

— see Szabo, G. [1863—1865], 302, *356*

Solvay, H., Van Schepdael, J. [1774—1776], 27, 97, 98, 99, 108, 278, 281, 282, 285, *355*

— see Van Schepdael, J. [320c], 285, *370*

Solway, A. J. L., see Simon, A. J. [1755], 151, *354*

Somani, P. [1777 1778], 245, *355*

— Bachand, R. T. [1779], 249, 251, *355*

— — Hardman, H. F. [1780], 251, *355*

— — — Laddu, A. R. [1781], 134, *355*

— Fleming, J. G., Chan, G., K., Lum, B. K. B. [1782], 250, *355*

— Laddu, A. R. [116a, 117a], 237, *362*

— — Hardman, H. F. [118a, 9e], 57, 236, *362, 371*

— Lum, B. K. B. [1783, 1784], 206, 216, 248, 249, 250, *355*

— Watson, D. L. [1785], 250, *355*

Somani, P., see Bachand, R. T. [66] 127, *324*

— see Laddu, A. R. [75a, 9d], 242, 246, *361, 371*

Somerville, W. [1786, 1787], 7, 96, 100, *355*

Somon, F., see Bernstein, A. [145], 115, *325*

Son, R., see Nakhjavan, F. K. [1338], 30, *347*

Sonel, A., see Knoebel, S. B. [1008], 82, 83, 92, *341*

Sones, F. M., Shirey, E. K. [1788], 4, 101, 124, *355*

— see Fergusson, D. J. [535], 10, *332*

— see Page, I. H. [241c], 15, *368*

— see Proudfit, W. L. [1470, 1471], 48, 84, 100, *349*

Sonnenblick, E. H., Braunwald, E., Williams, J. F., Glick, G. [1789], 31, 33, 208, *355*

— Ross, J., Braunwald, E. [1790], 92, *355*

— — Covell, J. W., Kaiser, G. A., Braunwald, E. [1791], 93, 132, 268, *355*

— see Glick, G. [673], 273, *335*

— see Hugenholtz, P. G. [154c], 35, *367*

Sonntag, A. C. [1792], 5, 159, 201, *355*

Sopena, M., see Brugger, A. [247], 193, *327*

Sorenson, C. W., see Stewart, H. J. [1839], 96, 154, *356*

Sorenson, H. R., see Hansen, A. T. [780], 83, *337*

Sorrentino, L., Di Rosa, M. [1793], 315, *355*

— — Di Paco, G. F., Tauro, C. S. [1794], 158, *355*

Sosa, J. A., McGregor, M. [1795], 168, *355*

— see Bittar, N. [172], 21, *326*

Soskin, S., Priest, W. S., Schultz, W. J. [1796], 74, *355*

Soulie, P., Chiche, P., Carlotti, J., Baillet, J. [1797], 160, *355*

— see Laubry, C. [1088], 154, *342*

Southwell, N., see Allanby, K. D. [21], 163, *323*

Sowton, E., Balcon, R., Cross, D., Frick, M. H. [1798, 1799], 4, 93, 100, 128, 240, *355*

— Hamer, J. [1800], 207, 241, 274, *355*

— Oram, S. [1801], 149, *355*

— see Balcon, R. [80], 99, 100, *324*

Sowton, E., see Bloomfield, D. A. [186], 211, *326*

— see Burkart, F. [262], 109, *327*

— see Conway, N. [360], 191, *329*

— see Frick, M. H. [592], 4, 30, 34, 93, 100, 109, 128, 130, 133, *333*

— see Gibson, D. [654, 655, 49a], 222, 241, 243, *335, 361*

— see Maloy, W. C. [1215], 100, *345*

— see Oram, S. [1395], 141, 149, *348*

Sowton, G. E., see Hamer, J. [769, 770, 771], 207, 208, 211, *337*

Sozutek, Y., see Bensaid, J. [24c, 25c], 227, *364*

— see Scebat, L. [1652], 215, 221, *352*

Spach, M. O., Kany, R., Imbs, J. L., Schwartz, J. [36b], 229, *363*

Spada, S., see Messina, B. [1291], 249, *346*

Spain, D. M., Bradess, V. A. [1802], *355*

— Nathan, D. J. [1803], 15, *355*

Spann, J. F., see Mason, D. T. [87a], 39, 130, 316, *361*

Speckmann, K., Klensch, H., Maetzel, F. K., Meyer, J. D. [1804], 101, *355*

Speer, J. H., see Leroy, G. V. [1106]. 156, *343*

Spehn, W., see Uhlenbrock, K. [1909], 158, *357*

Spenar, F. C. [1805], 11, *355*

Spencer, M. P., see Denison, A. B. [414], 74, *330*

Sperber, R., see Fisch, S. [552], 146, *333*

Spieckermann, P. G., Hellberg, K., Kettler, D., Reploh, H. D., Strauer, B. [119a], 185, 193, *362*

— see Kübler, W. [190c], 185, *367*

— see Kubler, W. [1051], 186, *342*

Spiegel, M., see Lichtlen, P. [206c], 214, *368*

Spiegl, E. D., see Freedberg, A. S. [584—586], 106, 107, 108, 135, 140, 145, 304, *333*

Spier, C. [1806], *355*

Spilker, B. A., see Shevde, S. [13d], 219, *371*

Spitzbarth, H. [1807], 187, *355*

— see Gersmeyer, E. F. [646, 647], 215, 218, *334*

Spodick, D. H., see Anthony, J. R. [46], *323*

Spracklen, F. H., Chambers, R. J., Schrire, V. [297c], 301, *370*

Sprague, H. B. [1808], 15, *355*
— White, P. D. [1809], 137, *355*

Spring, D. A., see Rowe, G. G. [12d], 294, *371*

Spring, G., see Heistracher, P. [800], 169, *337*

Springer, A., see Kraupp, O. [1040], 194, *342*

Spühler, O. [1810, 1811], 139, 313, *355*

Srivastava, S. C., Dewar, H. A., Newell, D. J. [1812], 211, *355*

Stables, D. P., see Rabkin, R. [1492], 211, 214, 217, *350*

Stadler, R., see Thiemer, K. [1883, 1884], 197, 198, *357*

Stafford, A. [1813, 1814], 62, 185, *355*
— see Angkapindu, A. [35], 306, *323*

Stagg, P. L., see Malindzak, G. S. [211c], 125, *368*

Stainsley, W. N., see Sarnoff, S. J. [1644], 29, 55, 92, 93, 132, 267, *352*

Stamler, J., see Marcus, E. [1219], 88, *345*
— see Page, I. H. [1403], 15, *348*

Stampfer, E. [1815], 199, *355*

Stampfer, M., Epstein, S. E., Beiser, G. D., Goldstein, R. E., Braunwald, E. [1816], 38, *355*
— see Epstein, S. E. [500, 501, 94c], 37, 315, 316, *332*, 365
— see Goldstein, R. E. [54a, 55a], 147, *361*

Standaert, F. G., see Levitt, B. [1119], 249, *343*

Stangos, N., see Babel, J. [65, 15c], 287, *324*, *363*

Stannard, M., see Sloman, G. [1758], 221, *354*

Stanton, H. C. [1817], 175, 250, *355*
— Kirchgessner, T., Parmenter, K. [1818], 250, *355*

Starcich, R. [1819], 160, *355*
— Ambanelli, V. [1820], 36, *355*
— see Barbaresi, F. [86], 248, 249, *324*
— see Bianchi, C. [158, 159], 227, *325*

Stare, F. J., see Ellis, L. B. [489], 20, 96, *331*

Starey, F. [1821], 165, *355*

Starfinger, W. [1822], 192, *355*

Starling, E. H., see Evans, C. L. [512], 68, *332*
— see Markwalder, J. [1222], 55, 68, *345*

Staroscik, R. N., see Abel, R. M. [1a, 1c], 301, *360*, *363*

Starr, I., Gamble, C. J., Margolies, A., Donal, J. S., Joseph, N., Engle, E. [1823], 153, *356*
— Pedersen, E., Corbascio, A. N. [1824], 95, *356*

Staszewska-Barczak, J., see Ceremuzynski, L. [286], 242, 328

Stauch, M., Schairer, K. [1825], 245, *356*
— see Schaefer, N. [1656], 235, *353*

Stearns, S., Riseman, J. E. F., Gray, W. [1826], 300, *356*
— see Gray, W. [712], 151, *336*

Steege, T. W., see Gregg, D. E. [730], 76, *336*

Steffensen, K. A. [120a], 311, *362*

Stehle, R. L. [1827], 72, *356*

Stein, E., see Damato, A. N. [387, 388], 3, *330*
— see Lau, S. H. [1080], 100, *342*
— see Scherlag, B. J. [1665], 3, *353*

Stein, L., see Knoebel, S. B. [1007, 1008], 82, 83, 92, 125, 130, *341*

Stein, P. D., Brooks, H. L., Matson, J. L., Hyland, J. W. [1828, 1829], 209, *356*

Stein, W. G., see Donoso, E. [441], 211, *331*

Steinberg, D. [298c], 16, *370*

Steinberg, F., Jensen, J. [1830], 154, *356*

Steinberg, L. A., see Riseman, J. E. F. [1534], 108, 304, *350*

Steiner, C., Wit, A. L., Damato, A. N. [1831], 273, *356*
— see Berkowitz, W. D. [11a], 220, *360*
— see Damato, A. N. [389], 3, *330*

Steinmetz, J. R., see Barry, A. J. [95], 10, *324*

Steim, H., see Gebhardt, W. [632], 181, *334*
— see Henke, C. [811], 196, *338*

Steis, G., see Teotino, U. M. [1877], 248, *356*

Stenlund, R. R., see Rowe, G. G. [1577, 1578], 22, 188, 189, *351*
— see Thomsen, J. H. [1888], 200, 201, *357*

Stephen, S. A. [1832], 215, 217, 243, *356*

Stephenson, J., see Christakis, G. [327], 14, *328*

Stephenson, J. S., see Black, J. W. [180], 42, 175, 205, *326*

Stern, B., see Riseman, J. E. F. [1535], 107, *350*

Stern, P. [1833], 309, *356*

Stern, S. [1834], 221, *356*
— see Lavy, S. [197c], 205, *367*

Sterne, J. [37b], 297, *363*
— Hirsch, C. [1835, 1836], 164, *356*
— Pele, M. F., Hirsch, C. [38b], 297, *363*

Sterner, W., see Hapke, H.-J. [782], 290, *337*

Sternitzke, N., Koehler, J. A., Lang, E. [1837], 197, *356*
— Meythaler, M. [299c, 300c], 197, *370*
— see Köhler, J. A. [1010], 198, *341*

Stertzer, S. H., see Green, G. E. [124c], 12, *366*

Stevens, L. E., see Hultgren, H. N. [871], 158, *339*

Stevenson, F. H., Wilson, D. G. [1838], 311, *356*

Stevenson, J., see Fife, R. [546], 162, *333*

Stewart, H. J., Horger, E. L., Sorenson, C. W. [1839], 96, 154, *356*
— Jack, N. B. [1840], 153, *356*

Stickney, J. L., see Lucchesi, B. R. [1190], 219, 220, *344*

Stock, J. P. P., Dale, N. [1841], 207, 217, *356*

Stock, T., see Robin, E. [1543], 93, 126, 130, 131, 208, *350*

Stock, T. B., Wendt, V. E., Hayden, R. O., Bruce, T. A., Bing, R. J. [1842], 24, 275, *356*
— see Madeira, R. G. [1206], 2, *345*

Stockfisch, W. J., see Winbury, M. M. [2015], 67, *359*

Stoker, J. B. [1843], 168, *356*

Stokes, J. R., see Malinin, T. [1212], 4, *345*

Stoland, O. O., Ginsberg, A. M., Loy, D. L., Hiebert, P. E. [1844], 153, 309, *356*
— see Ginsberg, A. M. [667], 70, *335*

Stone, J., see Nayler, W. G.
[1352], 216, 245, 246, *347*
Stone, J. M., see Elliott, W. C.
[37a], 211, *360*
Stone, R. V., see Makinson,
D. H. [1210], 305, *345*
Storck, U. [1845], 190, *356*
Storman, H. [1846], 193, *356*
Storstein, O., see Hillestad, L.
[831], 221, *338*
Storstein-Spilker, L. [301c],
247, *370*
Storti, R. [1847], 310, *356*
Straessle, B., Burckhardt, D.
[1848], 179, *356*
Strange, B., see Clausen, J.
[333], 217, 218, 221, *329*
Strassburg, K. H., see Müller,
J. [1327], 170, 171, *347*
Strauer, B., see Spieckermann,
P. G. [119a], 185, 193,
362
Strauer, B. E., Tauchert, M.,
Cott, L., Kochsiek, K.,
Bretschneider, H. J. [302c],
94, *370*
Strausak, A., Cottier, P.,
Schmid, A. [1849], 160, *356*
Strauss, A., see Pichler, E.
[1440], 196, *349*
Strauss, H. C., Bigger, J. T.,
Hoffman, B. F. [303c], 250,
251, *370*
Strauss, L. H. [1850], 312, 313,
356
Strieder, D. J., see Kazemi, H.
[172c], 35, *367*
Strobbia, R., Manzoni, A.,
Zotto u Dal. [304c], 164,
370
Ströder, U. [1851], 313, *356*
Strong, J. P., Richards, M. L.,
McGill, H. C., Eggen, D. A.,
McMurry, M. T. [305c], 16,
370
Stroud, M., see Eckstein, R. W.
[478], 264, *331*
Studlar, M., see Hammerl, H.
[775], *337*
Stühlinger, W., see Kraupp,
O. [1036, 1038], 194, 196,
342
Stuehlinger, W., see Raberger,
G. [102a, 263c], 61, 196,
362, *369*
Sudrann, R. B., see Selzer, A.
[1717], 91, *354*
Suettinger, N. [1852], 137, *356*
Sugimoto, T., see Wallacw, A.
G. [1955], *358*
Sugishita, Y., see Pitt, B.
[97a, 253c], 210, 300, *362*,
369
Suko, J., see Kraupp, O.[1043],
182, 189, 194, *342*

Sullivan, F. J., Bender, A. D.,
Horvath, S. M. [1853], 141,
356
Sullivan, J. M., Gorlin, R.
[1854], 28, *356*
— Harken, D. E., Gorlin, R.
[306c, 307c], 51, *370*
— see Wolfson, S. [2032], 42,
210, 211, *359*
Sulzer, R. [1855], 300, *356*
Summers, D. N., Richmond,
S., Wechsler, B. M. [121a],
16, *362*
Sun, S. C., Burch, G. E., De-
pasquale, N. P. [1856], 215,
356
Sunaga, T., see Shimamoto, T.
[1741], 289, *354*
Sunder, J. H., see Vester, J. W.
[324c], 16, *370*
Sundermeyer, J. F., see Wendt,
V. E. [1976], 181, 186, *358*
Surawicz, see Gettes, L. S.
[650], 221, *334*
Suriyong, R., Vannotti, A.
[1857], 310, *356*
Sutton, D. C., Lueth, H. C.
[1858], 19, *356*
Suzman, M. M., see Rabkin,
R. [1492], 211, 214, 217, *350*
Svedmyr, N., Andersson, R.,
Ekstrom-Jodal, B., Holm-
berg, S., Haggendal, E.,
Malmberg, R. [308c], 211,
251, *370*
— Jakobsson, B., Malmberg,
R. [122a], 251, *362*
— Malmberg, R., Haggendal,
E. [309c], 251, *370*
— see Aberg, G. [2], 249, 250,
251, *323*
Swan, H., see Marchioro, T.
[213c], 81, *368*
Swann, J., see Nayler, W. G.
[1346, 1347], 208, 222, *347*
Swann, J. B., see Nayler, W. G.
[1348—1350], 174, 177, 179,
208, 223, 245, 250, *347*
Swanson, A. J., see Aronow,
W. S. [5a—7a], 16, *360*
Swanson, L. W. [1859], 151, *356*
Szabo, G. [1862], 302, *356*
— Magyar, S., Solti, F. [1863],
302, *356*
— Solti, F., Magyar, S. [1864],
302, *356*
— — — Rev, J., Refi, Z.,
Megyesi, K. [1865], 302, *356*
Szabo, Z., see Solti, F. [296c],
316, *370*
Szatmary, J. [1866], 196, *356*
Szekely, P., Jackson, F., Wyn-
ne, N. A., Vohra, J. K.,
Batson, G. A., Dow, W. I.
M. [1867], 221, *356*

Szekeres, L., Lenard, G. [1867
bis], 304, *356*
— Papp, J. G., Fischer, E.
[1868], 150, 167, *356*
— see Papp, G. [1411], 220, *348*
Szent-Gyorgyi, A., see Drury,
A. N. [451 bis], 305, *331*
Szentivanyi, M., Juhasz-Nagy,
A., Debreceni, L. [1869,
1870], 64, *356*
— Kunos, G. [310c], 63, *370*
Szirmai, E. [1871], 314, *356*
Szmolenszky, T., see Papp, G.
[1411], 220, *348*
Szporny, L., see Karpati, E.
[941, 942], 288, *340*
Szucs, M., see Brooks, H. [18a,
49c], 251, 252, *360*, *364*

Tachikawa, S., see Takenaka,
T. [39b], 199, 200, 201, *363*
Taeschler, M., see Lombardo,
T. A. [1171], 55, *344*
Takaro, T., see Dart, C. H.
[76c], 11, *365*
Takenaka, T., Tachikawa, S.
[39b], 199, 200, 201, *363*
Takenobu, M., see Numano, F.
[238c], 289, *368*
Takeshita, R., see Boucek, R.
J. [4b], 20, *362*
Takeuchi, K., see Yamazaki,
H. [342c], 289, *371*
Tala, P., see Laustela, E.
[1090], 182, *343*
Talaat, M., see Anrep, G. V.
[42], 60, *323*
Talley, R. W., Beard, O. W.,
Doherty, J. E. [1872], 141,
356
Tallone, G., see Barbi, G. L.
[87], 253, *324*
Talmers, F. N., see Hellems,
H. K. [805], 59, *337*
Tanemura, I., see Hashimoto,
K. [790], 61, 62, *337*
Tarazi, R. C., see Frohlich, R.
C. [607], 218, *334*
Tartara, A., Corbetta, F.[1873],
160, *356*
Taskar, P. K., see Mohiuddin,
S. [91a], 301, *361*
Tasson, J., see De Schaep-
dryver, A. F. [416], 167,
330
Tatibouet, L. [1874], 279, *356*
Tauchert, M., see Strauer, B.
E. [302c], 94, *370*
Tauro, C. S., see Sorrentino, L.
[1794], 158, *355*
Taylor, H. L., Henschel, A.,
Brozek, J., Keys, A. [1875],
9, *356*
Taylor, J., see Horwitz, L. D.
[150c], 126, *366*

Taylor, S. H., MacDonald, H. R., Robinson, M. C., Sapru, R. P. [1876], 91, *356*

Taylor, W. J., see Gorlin, R. [701], 11, *335*
— see Kemp, H. G. [174c], 12, *367*

Taylor, Z., see Clark, L. C., jr. [331], 74, *329*

Telles, E., see Pinto, S. L. [1445], 228, *349*

Tenney, S. M., see Honig, C. R. [857], 122, 129, *338*

Ten Thije, J. H., see Akker, S. van den [17], 308, *323*

Tempte, J. V., see Gutgesell, H. P. [57a], 220, *361*

Temte, J. V., see Davis, L. D. [7b], 219, *363*

Teodorini, S., Serban, M. [123a], 279, *362*

Teotino, U. M., Polo Friz, L., Steis, G., Della Bella, D. [1877], 248, *356*

Terry, W., see Rowe, G. G. [1577], 188, 189, *351*

Terry, W. H., see Clark, J. P. [61c], 237, *364*

Tersteege, H. M., see Bijlsma, V. G. [160], 308, *326*

Testelli, M. R., see Sodi-Pallares, D. [1767, 1768, 1770], 295, *355*

Thoenen, H., see Haefely, W. [761], 248, *337*

Thaler, H., see Hueber, E. F. [869], 137, *339*

Thiele, K., Gross, A., Posselt, K., Schuler, W. [1879], *357*
— Koberstein, E., Nonnenmacher, G. [1880], 198, *357*
— Posselt, K., von Bebenburg, W. [1881], 198, *357*
— Schimassek, U., Schlichtegroll, A. von [1882], 196, *357*

Thiemer, K., Stadler, R. [1883], 197, *357*
— — Schlichtegroll, A. von [1884], 198, *357*

Thierfelder, J. [1885], 170, *357*

Thomas, C. B. [1886], 15, *357*

Thomas, M., see Opie, L. H. [1394], 25, *348*
— see Owen, P. [240c], 318, *368*
— see Valori, C. [1915], 243, *357*

Thomas, R. W., see Winder, C. V. [2018], 152, *359*

Thompson, H. K., see Whalen, R. E. [1982], 207, 272, 274, *358*

Thompson, M. E., Leon, D. F., Shaver, J. A., McDonald, R. H. [311c], 240, *370*

Thompson, R. H., Letley, E. [1887], 219, *357*

Thomsen, J. H., Stenlund, R. R., Corliss, R. J., Sialer, S., Rowe, G. G. [1888], 200, 201, *357*
— see Rowe, G. G. [1577, 1578], 22, 188, 189, *351*

Thorburn, G. D., see Herd, J. A. [816], 83, *338*

Thornicroft, S. G., see Sandler, G. [1641], 180, *352*

Thorp, R. H. [1889], 306, *357*
— Cobbin, L. B. [1890], 306, *357*
— see Angkapindu, A. [35], 306, *323*

Thuillier, J., see Minz, B. [1300], 160, *346*

Tice, D. A., see Green, G. E. [124c], 12, *366*

Tilsner, V. [1891], 141, *357*

Ting, K., see Parade, G. W. [1413], 143, *348*

Tjeldflaat, L., see Aubert, A. [8a], 233, *360*

Todesco, S., Permutti, B. [1893], 171, *357*

Toker, Y., [312c], 297, *370*

Tominaga, S., see Miura, M. [1302], 62, 185, *346*

Tomiyasu, U., see Dayton, S. [399], 15, *330*

Tomlinson, J. C., see James, T. N. [160c], 218, *367*

Tondeur, R., see Charlier, R. [318], 255, *328*
— see Deltour, G. [409], 255, *330*

Toner, J. J., see Fellows, E. J. [534], 157, *332*

Torreggiani, G., see Donato, L. [437], 82, *331*

Torres, E. C., Brandi, G. [1894], 63, *357*

Torresani, J., Chevalier Cholat, A. M., Courbier, R., Heuillet, G., Jouve, A. [313c], 316, *370*
— see Jouve, A. [166c], 316, *367*

Toubes, D. B., Ferguson, R. K., Rice, A. J., Aoki, V. S., Funk, D. C., Wilson, W. R. [314c], 252, *370*

Toussaint, D., Pohl, S. [124a], 287, *362*

Towers, M. K., Wood, P. [1895], 161, 162, *357*

Townes, A. S., see Kory, R. C. [1020], 141, *341*

Tram, M., see Kolassa, N. [185c], 185, *367*

Tranchesi, J. [1896], 162, *357*

Trap-Jensen, J., see Clausen, J. P. [334, 62c, 63c], 9, *329, 365*

Travell, J., see Gold, H. [678], 154, *335*
— see Greiner, T. [738], 110, 111, 112, 113, 116, 158, 308, *336*
— see Rinzler, S. H. [1528, 1529], 305, 311, *350*

Treister, B., see Gianelly, R. E. [651], 212, *334*

Treister, B. L., see Gianelly, R. E. [48a], 212, *361*

Tremblay, G. M., De Champlain, J. A., Nadeau, R. A. [315c], 250, *370*

Trimborn, H. [1898], 289, *357*

Tripod, J., Meier, R. [1899, 1900], 66, 308, *357*

Tritthart, H., Fleckenstein, A., Fleckenstein, B., Herbst, A., Krause, H. [125a], 179, 219, *362*
— see Fleckenstein, A. [563, 40a], 166, 178, *333, 360*

Trottnow, D., see Nitz, R. E. [1372], 190, *347*

Truitt, E. B. [1901], 66, *357*

Troup, W., see Kinsella, D. [986], 187, *341*

Tschirdewahn, B., Klepzig, H. [1902], 179, *357*
— Knorpp, K., Heinrich, F., Schuetterle, G. [1903], 221, *357*

Tsitouris, G., see Corcondilas, A. [362], 228, *329*
— see Koroxenidis, G. [1019], 223, *341*

Tuddenham, W. J., see Foltz, E. L. [570], 55, 81, *333*

Türker, R. K., Kayaalp, S. O. [1904], 201, *357*
— — Özer, A. [1905], 201, *357*

Tuisl, E., see Kraupp, O. [1037, 1042], 192, *342*

Tuluy, S., see Lombardo, T. A. [1171], 55, *344*

Tuna, N., Amplatz, K. [316c], 96, *370*

Turiella, R. G., see Barrera, J. A. [91], 162, *324*

Turner, A. S., see Wilson, D. F. [2005, 2006], 227, *359*

Turner, J. D., see Gorlin, R. [699], 129, *335*

Turner, P. [317c], 234, *370*
— see Chamberlain, D. A. [293], 207, 284, *328*
— see Harrison, J. [787], 240, *337*
— see Hill, R. C. [828, 829], 246, 248, *338*

Turpeinen, O., Miettinen, M., Karvonen, M. J., Roine, P., Pekkarinen, M., Lehtosuo, E. J., Alivirta, P. [1906], 14, *357*

Turri, M., see Imhof, P. R. [64a], 227, *361*

Turrisi, E., see Giordano, G. [668], 160, *335*

Uebel, H., see Erbring, H. [507], 159, *332*

Uebersax, R., see Didisheim, J. C. [428], 179, *330*

Ueda, K., see Ross, R. S. [1562], 83, 84, 123, 130, *351*

Uhlenbrock, K., Schweer, M. [1907, 1908], 156, 158, *357*
— Spehn, W. [1909], 158, *357*

Uhlmann, F., Nobile, F. [1910], 66, *357*

Ulrych, M., Frohlich, E. D., Dustan, H. P., Page, I. H. [1911], 211, *357*

Unna, K. [1912], 308, *357*

Urbach, K. T., see Russek, H. I. [1615, 1616, 1617], 103, 104, 106, 135, 136, 137, 141, 151, 152, 154, 158, 311, 312, 313, *352*

Urschel, C. W. [1914], 249, *357*
— see Hugenholtz, P. G. [154c], 35, *367*

Ushiyama, K., see Kimura, E. [984], 93, *341*

Uslenghi, E., see Feruglio, F. S. [541, 542], 222, 248, *333*

Uzgiris, I., see Angelakos, E. T. [8c], 63, *363*

Vacheron, A., see Di Matteo, J. [83c], 23, *365*

Vachon, J., see Facquet, J. [517], 286, *332*

Valaer, P. J., see Oettingen, W. F. von [1948], 138, 140, *358*

Valenca, L. M., see Kazemi, H. [172c], 35, *367*

Valori, C., Thomas, M., Shillingford, J. P. [1915], 243, *357*

Valtonen, E., see Frick, M. H. [102c], 9, *365*

Van Belle, H. [318, 319c], 202, *370*

Van Cauwenberge, H. [9e bis], 204, *371*

Van Citters, R. L., see Vatner, S. F. [321c, 322c], 316, *370*

Van de Berg, L. [1916], 84, *357*

Van der Straeten, P., see Vastesaeger, M. [1923], 285, *357*

Van Dongen, K., see Akker, S. van den [17], 308, *323*

Van Egmond, A. A. J. [1918], 299, *357*

Van Gerven, W., see Jageneau, A. [889], 202, *339*

Van Hoorickx, G., see Bosmans, P. [39c], 47, 114, 203, 204, *364*

Van Itallie, T. B., see Bergen, S. S., jr. [135], 15, *325*

Van Lith, P., see Raab, W. [1491], 36, 284, *350*

Van Orden, L. S., see Zeller, E. A. [2047], 160, *360*

Van Schepdael, J., Solvay, H. [320c], 285, *370*
— see Solvay, H. [1774 to 1776], 27, 97, 98, 99, 108, 278, 281, 282, 285, *355*

Van Thiel, E., see Lequime, J. [1103], 90, *343*

van Wijk, T. W. [1997], 308, *359*

Van Zee, B. E., see Bristow, J. D. [46c], 34, *364*

Vandeghen, N., see Plomteux, G. [1458], 288, *349*

Vandesteene, R., see Schaper, W. K. A. [1658, 283c], 46, 47, 86, *353, 369*

Vane, J. R. [1917], 72, *357*
— see Dawes, G. S. [396], 72, *330*

Vanhaelst, L., see Bastenie, P. A. [101], 16, *324*

Vannotti, A., see Suriyong, R. [1857], 310, *356*

Vaquez, H., Giroux, R., Kisthinios, N. [1919], 309, *357*

Varga, Z., see Cohen, A. [339], 130, 151, *329*

Varkonyi, G. [1920], 190, *357*

Varma, D. R., Share, N. N., Melville, K. I. [1921], 89, 122, 161, 308, *357*

Varnauskas, E., Bergman, H., Houk, P., Björntorp, P. [1922], 9, *357*

Vassilikos, C., see Koroxenidis, G. [1019], 223, *341*

Vastagh, G. F., see Cohen, L. S. [25a], 249, *360*

Vastesaeger, M. [1924], 286, *357*
— Block, P. [1925], 115, 202, *357*
— Charlier, R., Leloup, A. [1926], 170, *357*
— Gillot, P., Rasson, G. [1927], 276, 278, 279, 280, 285, 319, *357*
— — Van der Straeten, P. [1923], 285, *357*
— Rasson, G. [1928], 164, *357*
— Rochet, J., Leloup, A. [1929], 170, 171, *357*
— — — Gillot, P. [1930], 170, *357*

Vastesaeger, M., see Candaele, G. [274], 298, *327*
— see Wanet, J. [334c], 287, *370*

Vastesaeger, M. M., see Rochet, J. [1547], 211, *351*

Vater, W., see Wirth, W. [2022], 302, *359*

Vatner, S. F., Franklin, D. C., Van Citters, R. L., Braunwald, E. [321c, 322c], 316, *370*
— see Braunwald, E. [44c], 315, 316, *364*

Vaughan Williams, E. M. [1931—1933], 219, 220, 276, *357*
— Singh, B. N. [1934], 269, 270, 272, 276, *357*
— see Dohadwalla, A. N.[435], 215, 237, *331*
— see Freedberg, A. S. [101c], 270, *365*
— see Morales-Anguilera, A. [1317, 1318], 206, 214, 215, 216, 219, *347*
— see Papp, J. G. [1412], 226, 242, *348*
— see Sekiya, A. [1714], 253, *354*
— see Singh, B. N. [35b, 293c], 232, 250, 253, *363, 369*

Vecchi, G. P., Marrama, P. [1935], 160, *357*

Vega Diaz, F., Perez Casar, F. [323c], 295, *370*

Velena, S., see Vineberg, A. [327c], 11, *370*

Vera, L. B. de, Corday, E., Gold, H. [1936], 74, *357*

Veragut, U., see Gander, M. [622], 207, *334*

Vercruyssen, J., Ceyssens, W. [1937], 170, *357*
— see Bosmans, P. [39c], 47, 114, 203, 204, *364*

Verghese, A., see Nestel, P.J. [1357], 284, *347*

Vergnes, R., see Deodati, F. [80c], 287, *365*

Verhaeghe, L. K. [1938], 115, 202, *357*

Vermylen, J., see Verstraete, M. [1939], 287, *357*

Verstraete, M., Vermylen, J., Claeys, H. [1939], 287, *357*

Verin [126a], 287, *362*

Verselder, R., see Bosmans, P. [39c], 47, 114, 203, 204, *364*

Vest, H. R., see Singh, R. [294c], 91, *369*

Vester, J. W., Sunder, J. H., Aarons, J. H., Danowski, T. S. [324c], 16, *370*

Vestri, A., see Reale, A. [1502], 226, *350*
Vettori, G., Erle, G., Magaraggia, L., Bau, G. [1940], 228, *358*
Veyrat, C., see Kalmanson, D. [168c], 78, *367*
Viana, A. P., see Rodrigues-Pereira, E. [1549], 178, *351*
Viars, P., see Boissier, J. R. [198], 167, *326*
Victor, M., see Clark, J. P. [61c], 237, *364*
Vigne, J. [325c], 298, *370*
Vilalta Bernet, C., see Balaguer-Vintro, I. [76], 279, 280, *324*
Villanueva, M. P., see Roberts, L. N. [1542], 187, *350*
Vincent, see Faivre, G. [520], 97, *332*
Vineberg, A. M. [1941, 326c], 10, 11, *358, 370*
— Chari, R. S., Pifarre, R., Mercier, C. [1942], 182, *358*
— Mahanti, B., Litvak, J. [1943], 90, *358*
— Velena, S., Long, J. [327c], 11, *370*
— see Litvak, J. [1161], 90, *344*
Visioli, O., Dallavalle, L., Bianchi, G., Botti, G., Malagnino, G. [1944], 252, *358*
— — Botti, G. [1945], 252, *358*
— see Bertaccini, G. [148], 252, *325*
— see Botti, G. [201], 253, *326*
Visscher, M. B., see Moe, G. K. [1308], 68, *346*
Vittu, C., see Cottet, J. [371], 172, *329*
Vizcaino, M., see Sodi-Pallares, D. [1769], 295, *355*
Voemel, H. J. [40b], 179, *363*
Vogel, G., see Erbring, H. [507], 159, *332*
Vogel, J. H. K., Chidsey, C. A. [127a], 43, *362*
Vogelius, H., see Grüner, A. [750], 311, *336*
Vogelsang, A. [328c], 305, *370*
— see Schute, W. [1749], 305, *354*
Vogin, E. E., see Kinnard, W. J. [985], 149, *341*
Vogt, M., see Gaddum, J. H. [619], *334*
Vohra, J. K., Dowling, J. T., Sloman, G. [329c], 243, *370*
— see Szekely, P. [1867], 221, *356*
Volkmer, I., see Pfleger, K. [96a, 30b], 184, 186, 194, 202, *362, 363*

Vonk, J. T. C. [1947], 285, *358*
Vonthron, A., see Mouquin, M. [1326], 307, *347*
Voridis, E., Antoniadis, G., Marinakis, P., Papazoglou, N., Petritis, J. [1950], 226, *358*
Vyden, J. K., Carvalho, M., Boszormenyi, F., Lang, T., Bernstein, H., Corday, E. [330c], 134, *370*
Vysotskaya, N. B., see Kaverina, N. V. [964], 134, *340*

Waal, H. J. [1951], 229, *358*
Waaler, B. A. [1952], 311, *358*
Wachtel, F. W., see Shoshkes, M. [1748], 162, *354*
Wackerbauer, J., see Hilger, H. H. [826, 827], 186, 194, *338*
Wadsworth, R. M., see Parratt, J. R. [1425, 1426, 95a, 246c], 63, 230, 231, 236, 237, 239, 240, *348, 362, 368*
Wagman, R. J., Levine, H. J., Messer, J. V., Neill, W. A., Krasnow, N., Gorlin, R. [1953], 22, 24, 275, *358*
— see Levine, J. H. [1115, 1116], 31, 92, 128, *343*
— see Messer, J. V. [1287], 38, *346*
— see Neill, W. A. [1355], 29, 55, 267, *347*
Wagner, D. J., see Osher, H. L. [1397], 158, *348*
Wagner, H., see Schmitt, G. [1685], 193, *353*
Wagner, H. R., Gamble, W. J., Albers, W. H., Hugenholtz, P. G. [331c], 91, *370*
Wagner, J., Greeff, K., Heeg, E., Pereira, E. [1954], 206, 245, *358*
— see Greeff, K. [716], 130, *336*
— see Hilger, H. H. [826, 827], 186, 194, *338*
Wahl, M., see Pieri, J. [1443], *349*
Waldeck, B., see Carlsson, A. [277], 166, *328*
Waldhausen, J. A., see Cowan, M. [70c], *365*
Wale, J. [332c], 236, *370*
— Pun, L.-Q., Rand, M. J. [128a], 242, *362*
— see Lubawski, I. [1185], 246, *344*
— see Raper, C. [1495, 104c], 219, 220, 221, 225, 226, 250, *350, 362*
Walker, J. A., Friedberg, H. D., Johnson, W. D., Flemma, R. J., Lepley, D. [333c], 13, *370*

Walker, J. M., see Schofield, B. M. [1692], 72, *353*
Walker, W. C., see Phear, D. [1439], 163, *349*
Wallace, R. B., see Greenberg, B. H. [125c], 13, *366*
— see McCallister, B. D. [1245, 217c], 12, 30, 37, *345, 368*
Wallacw, A. G., Schaal, S. F., Sugimoto, T., Rozear, M., Alexander, J. A. [1955], *358*
Wallentin, I., see Bjorntorp, P. [32c], 233, *364*
Waller, J. V., see Riseman, J. E. F. [1536], 106, *350*
Walter, F., see Heim, F. [798], 174, 251, *337*
Wanet, J., Achten, G., Barchewitz, G., Mestdagh, C., Vastesaeger, M. [334c], 287, *370*
Warbasse, J. R., Hawley, R. R., Gillilan, R. E. [1956], 4, *358*
Ward, H. P., see Wegria, R. [1970], 157, 299, *358*
Wardell, J. R., see Hahn, R. A. [763], 209, 248, *337*
Warembourg, H. [1957], 299, *358*
— Bertrand, M. [1958, 14d], 163, 298, *358, 371*
— Delomez, M. [1959], 164, *358*
— Houdas, Y., Bertrand, M. E., Ketelers, J. Y. [335c], 211, *371*
— Jaillard, J. [1960, 129a], 279, *358, 362*
— Lekieffre, J., Pommier, M. [41b], 291, *363*
Warren, M., see Ben, M. [129], 163, *325*
Warren, M. R., see Emele, J. F. [491], 161, *332*
Warshaw, L. J., see Greiner, T. [738], 110, 111, 112, 113, 116, 158, 308, *336*
Wasserman, A. J., Proctor, J. D., Allen, F. J., Kemp, V. E. [130a], 230, 233, 235, *362*
— see Proctor, J. D. [99a, 100a], 230, 231, 233, *362*
Wasserman, M., see Levy, B. [202c], 254, *368*
Wassermann, S. [336c], 315, *371*
Watillon, M., Lavergne, G., Weekers, J. F. [1961], 287, *358*
Watson, D. L., see Somani, P. [1785], 250, *355*
Watson, O. F., see Wilson, D. F. [2006], 227, *359*
Watt, D. A. [1962], 221, *358*

Watt, D. A. L., Livingstone, W. R., MacKay, R. K. S., Obineche, E. N. [337c], 221, *371*

Waucampt, J. J., see Desruelles, J. [420], 164, *330*

Wax, D. S., Degraff, A. C. [1963], 302, *358*

Wayne, E. J., Laplace, L. B. [1964], 154, *358*

Wearn, J. T. [1965], 68, 69, *358*
— see Gregg, D. E. [730, 731, 735], 73, 76, *336*
— see Shipley, R. E. [1746], 76, *354*

Weber, W. J., see Carson, R. P. [278], 125, 134, *328*

Wechsler, A. S., see Braunwald, E. [215], 37, *326*
— see Glick, G. [673], 273, *335*
— see Epstein, S. E. [500, 501, 94c], 37, 315, 316, *332*, *365*

Wechsler, B. M., see Summers, D. N. [121a], 16, *362*

Wedd, A. M. [1966], 306, 309, *358*
— Drury, A. N. [1967], 305, *358*

Weekers, J. F., see Watillon, M. [1961], 287, *358*

Wegria, R., Essex, H. E., Herrick, J. F., Mann, F. C. [1968], 120, 150, 153, *358*
— Nickerson, J. L., Case, R. B., Holland, J. F. [1969], 121, *358*
— Ward, H. P., Frank, C. W., Dreyfuss, F., Brown, E. M., Hutchinson, D. L. [1970], 157, 299, *356*
— see Essex, H. E. [509], 120, 150, 153, 299, 306, 307, *332*

Weikel, J. H., see Lish, P. M. [1159], 216, 249, 250, *344*

Weinberg, D. I., see Bigger, J. T. [31c], 303, *364*

Weiner, M. [1971], 187, *358*

Weingarten, W., see Russek, H. I. [1620], 105, 137, 139, 141, 152, *352*

Weinstein, W., see Katz, L. N. [955, 958, 959], 66, 67, 68, 69, 121, 145, *340*

Weiss, A. J., see Foltz, E. L. [570], 55, 81, *333*

Weiss, H. R., see Winbury, M. M. [11e], 124, 317, *371*

Weiss, S., Wilkins, R. W., Haynes, F. W. [1972], 121, 136, *358*
— see Wilkins, R. W. [2000], 121, 136, *359*

Weisse, A. B., Diflumeri, A. A., Regan, T. J. [131a], 146, *362*

Weisse, A. B., Regan, T. J. [132a], 135, *362*
— see Lehan, P. H. [1093], 124, *343*
— see Regan, T. J. [1514, 1515], 301, *350*

Weissler, A. M., see Harris, W. S. [785], 207, *337*

Weist, F., see Schmid, E. [1677], 167, *353*

Weitzman, D. [1973], 141, *358*

Welch, G. H., see Sarnoff, S. J. [1644], 29, 55, 92, 93, 132, 267, *352*

Wellens, H. J. [1974], 285, *358*

Wells, K., see Eckstein, R. W. [474], 306, *331*

Wells, P. G., see Parry, E. H. O. [1427], 137, 139, *348*

Welsch, M., see Bacq, Z. M. [67], 173, *324*

Welti, J. J., Facquet, J. [1975], 162, *358*

Wendt, V. E., Sundermeyer, J. F., Den Bakker, P. B., Bing, R. J. [1976], 181, 186, *358*
— see Stock, T. B., [1842], 24, 275, *356*

Werner, G., see Lindner, A. [1150], 309, *344*

Wernitsch, W., see Halmagyi, M. [766], 183, *337*

Wertz, U., see Juchems, R. [65a], 229, *361*

West, J. W., Bellet, S., Manzoli, U. C., Müller, O. F. [1977], 181, 182, *358*
— Guzman, S. V., Bellet, S. [1978], 71, *358*
— Kobayashi, T., Anderson, F. S. [1979], 89, *358*
— — Guzman, S. V. [1980], 71, *358*

West, R. O., see Khaja, F. [179c], 31, 32, *367*
— see Parker, J. O. [1414 to 1418, 94a, 243c], 25, 26, 27, 30, 31, 32, 33, 36, 38, 43, 128, 130, 131, 132, *348*, *362*, *368*

Westling, H., see Christensson, B. [328], 130, *329*
— see Nordenfelt, I. [1376], 126, *348*

Wette, K. [1981], 179, *358*

Wettengel, R., Fabel, H. [15d], 234, *371*

Whalen, R. E., Morris, J. J., Behar, V. S., Thompson, H. K., McIntosh, H. D. [1982], 207, 272, 274, *358*

Wheeler, N. C., see Hamilton, W. F. [772], 91, *337*

White, D. H., see Maxwell, G. M. [1242, 1243], 153, *345*

White, J. C. [1983], 20, *358*
— Garrey, W. E., Atkins, J. A. [1984], 19, *358*

White, P. D. [1985—1987], 7, 15, *358*
— see Sprague, H. B. [1809], 137, *355*

White, R., Shinebourne, E. [1988], 216, *358*
— see Shinebourne, E. [1745], 220, *354*

White, S., see Graham, D. M. [704], *335*

Whitsitt, L. S., Lucchesi, B. R. [1989, 1990], 209, 218, *358*
— see Lucchesi, B. R. [1189, 1190], 219, 220, *344*

Wibell, L. [133a], 297, *362*

Wick, E., see Dörner, J. [443], 121, 150, 153, 156, 181, 299, 305, *331*

Wick, T. [134a], 296, *362*

Widmer, L. K., see Kannel, W. B. [935], 14, 16, *340*
— see Schweizer, W. [1704], 16, *353*

Wiemers, K. [1991, 1992], 307, *358*

Wiener, L., Dwyer, E. M., Cox, J. W. [1993, 1994], 33, 214, *358*
— Kasparian, H. [338c], 34, *371*
— see Dwyer, E. M. [465, 9b], 211, 214, *331*, *363*

Wiesel, B. H., see Davis, J. A. [393], 138, *330*

Wiggers, C. J. [1955], 69, 75, 80, *359*
— Green, H. D. [1996], 145, 154, *359*
— see Geller, H. M. [634], 69, 75, 80, *334*
— see Johnson, J. R. [902], 68, 69, *339*

Wilbrandt, W., see Heimann, W. [799], 150, 153, 157, *337*
— see Ryser, H. [1621], 67, 309, *352*

Wilburne, M., see Isaacs, J. H. [879], 101, *339*

Wild, J. B., see Lewis, B. I. [1131], 308, *343*

Wilde, W. [1998, 339c], 170, 288, *359*, *371*

Wilhelm, M., Hedwall, P., Meier, M. [1999], 222, *359*

Wilkenfeld, B. E., see Levy, B. [1121], 235, 237, *343*

Wilkens, H., see Regelson, W. [1516], 161, *350*

Wilkins, R. W., Haynes, F. W., Weiss, S. [2000], 121, 136, *359*

Wilkins, R. W., see Hollander, W. [850, 852, 853], 163, 314, *338*
— see Weiss, S. [1972], 121, 136, *358*
Wilkinson, J. C. M. [2001], 180, *359*
Willems, D. [2001 bis], 296, *359*
Williams, A. J., see Schmitt-henner, J. E. [1687], 300, *353*
Williams, C. B., see Rodbard, S. [270c, 271c], 132, *369*
Williams, F., see Rodbard, S. [1548, 271c], 70, 132, *351*, *369*
Williams, F. L., see Katz, A. M. [950], 55, 59, *340*
— see Katz, L. N. [960], 264, *340*
Williams, J. F., Glick, G., Braunwald, E. [2002], 128, 131, 132, *359*
— see Sonnenblick, E. H. [1789], 31, 33, 208, *355*
Williams, N. E., Carr, H. A., Bruenn, H. G., Levy, R. L. [2003], 106, 154, *359*
— see Levy, R. L. [1128, 1129], 96, 106, 136, 140, 154, *343*
Wilson, A., Schild, H. O. [2004], 307, *359*
Wilson, A. G., Brooke, O. G., Lloyd, H. J., Robinson, B. F. [135a], 241, *362*
Wilson, C., see Shipley, R. E. [1747], 73, 74, *354*
Wilson, D. F., Turner, A. S. [2005], 227, *359*
— Watson, O. F., Peel, J. S., Turner, A. S. [2006], 227, *359*
Wilson, D. G., see Stevenson, F. H. [1838], 311, *356*
Wilson, W. R., see Rice, A. J. [106a], 251, *362*
— see Toubes, D. B. [314c], 252, *370*
Wilson, W. S., see Carson, R. P. [278], 125, 134, *328*
Wilt, W. A., see Luduena, F. P. [1191], 67, *344*
Winbury, M. M. [2007—2010, 10e], 4, 45, 85, 124, 134, 141, 207, 268, 317, *359*, *371*
— Gabel, L. P. [2011], 124, 134, 141, *359*
— — Grandy, R. P. [2012], *359*
— Howe, B. B., Hefner, M. A. [2013], 134, 202, 317, *359*
— — Weiss, H. R. [11e], 124, 317, *371*

Winbury, M. M., Kissil, D., Losada, M. [2014], 45, 53, *359*
— Michiels, P. M., Ham-bourger, W. E., Stockfisch, W. J., Cook, D. L. [2015], *359*
— Papierski, D. H., Hemmer, M. L., Hambourger, W. E. [2016], 306, *359*
— Pensinger, R. R. [2017], 141, 182, *359*
— see Gabel, L. P. [617], 45, *334*
Winder, C. V., Thomas, R. W., Kamm, O. [2018], 152, *359*
Winegrad, S., Shanes, A. M. [2019], 216, *359*
Winfield, M. E., see McAlpin, R. N. [1244], 30, 136, *345*
Winkler, K., see Hansen, A. T. [780], 83, *337*
Winslow, G., see Christakis, G. [327], 14, *328*
Winsor, T. [136a], 294, *362*
— Humphreys, P. [2020], 141, *359*
— Scott, C. C. [2021], 140, 141, 142, *359*
Winters, L., see Chapman, D. W. [59c], 12, *364*
Winters, W. L., see Soloff, L. A. [1773], 181, 187, *355*
Winterton, M., see Mendel, D. [1278], 169, *346*
Wirth, W., Gösswald, R., Vater, W. [2022], 302, *359*
Wirz, P., Schonbeck, M., Meh-mel, H., Krayenbuhl, H. P., Rutishauser, W. [340c], *371*
Wit, A. L., see Berkowitz, W. D. [11a], 220, *360*
— see Steiner, C. [1831], 273, *356*
Witham, A. L., see Hamilton, W. F. [772], 91, *337*
Wittenberg, S. M., see Klocke, F. J. [181c], 23, *367*
Witzleb, E., Budde, H. [2023], 302, 303, *359*
— Gollwitzer-Meier, K., Do-nat, K. [2024], 309, *359*
— see Böhm, C. [196], 165, 168, *326*
— see Schlepper, M. [1672], 172, 174, *353*
Woelke, F. [137a], 298, *362*
Wolf, H. [2025], 187, *359*
Wolf, R., see Clark, L. C., jr. [331], 74, *329*
Wolf, S. [2026], 110, *359*
Wolff, H. G., Hardy, J. D., Goodell, H. [2027], 110, 112, *359*

Wolff, M. M., Berne, R. M. [2028], 60, 306, 309, *359*
Wolffe, J. B., Findlay, D., Dessen, E. [2029], 309, *359*
— Shubin, H. [2030], 163, *359*
Wolfson, I. N., see Kastor, J. A. [68a], 4, *361*
Wolfson, S., Amsterdam, E. A., Gorlin, R. [2031], 212, *359*
— Gorlin, R. [138a], 210, *362*
— Heinle, R. A., Herman, M. V., Kemp, H. G., Sullivan, J. M., Gorlin, R. [2032], 42, 210, 211, *359*
— — Kemp, H. G., Gorlin, R. [2033], 210, 274, *359*
— see Amsterdam, E. A. [27, 28, 29, 30], 114, 212, 215, *323*
— see Matloff, J. M. [1239], 221, *345*
Wolkerstorfer, H. [2034], 196, *359*
Wollheim, E. [2035], 229, *359*
Wolner, E., see Kraupp, O. [1037, 1041, 1042, 1043], 182, 189, 192, 193, 194, *342*
Wong, S. K., see Foltz, E. L. [570], 55, 81, *333*
Wood, P., see Towers, M. K. [1895], 161, 162, *357*
Wood, T. M., see Shanks, R. G. [1730], 245, *354*
Woodbury, R. A., see Ahl-quist, R. P. [16], 312, *323*
Woods, E. F., Richardson, J. A., Richardson, A. K., Bozeman, R. F. [2036], 101, *359*
— see Gazes, P. C. [631], 36, 101, *334*
— see Richardson, J. A. [1524], 101, *350*
Woschee, G., see Hirsch, W. [840], 188, *338*
Würzbach, K., see Grund, G. [749], 171, *336*
Wynne, N. A., see Szekely, P. [1867], 221, *356*

Xhonneux, R., see Schaper, W. K. A. [1658, 1659, 1660, 282c, 283c], 40, 46, 47, 53, 86, 199, 200, 201, 203, 204, *353*, *369*

Yagoda, H., see Oettingen, W. F. von [1948], 138, 140, *358*
Yamanaka, J., see Cohen, A. [339], 130, 151, *329*
Yamazake, H., see Shimamo-to, T. [1741], 289, *354*

Yamazaki, H., Koboyashi, I. [341c], 289, *371*
— Sano, T., Odakura, T., Takeuchi, K., Shimamoto, T. [342c],289, *371*
Yamazaki, T., see Kimura, E. [984], 93, *341*
Yankley, A., see Graham, D. M. [704], 311, *335*
Yasuda, K., see Ikezono, E. [876], 221, *339*
Yigitbasi, O., Nalbantgil, I. [343c], 247, *371*
Yipintsoi, T., see McCallister, B. D. [1245], 30, 37, *345*
Yohalem, S. B., see Segal, R. L. [1713], 20, *354*
Yokoyama, M., see Miyahara, M. [26b], 204, *363*
York, D. J., see Bayley, R. H. [114], 154, *325*
Yoshida, K., see Kimura, E. [984], 93, *341*
Yoshonis, K. F., see Gettes, L. S. [112c], 3, 221, *366*
Young, M. W., see Lau, S. H. [1080, 1082], 100, *342*
Young, V., see Owen, P. [240c], 318, *368*
Yu, D. H., Gluckman, M. I. [139a], 186, *362*
Yurchak, P. M., Rolett, E. L., Cohen, L. S., Gorlin, R. [2037], 36, *359*
— see Krasnow, N. [1033, 1034], 4, 25, 264, *342*

Zaccheo, V. J., see Petta, J. M. [8e bis], 256, *371*
Zacharias, F. J. [344c], 222, *371*
Zack, W. J., see Hamm, J. [773], 187, *337*
Zahir, M., see Gould, L. [122c], 301, *366*
Zahn, A., see Morawitz, P. [1321], 70, *347*

Zahnow, W., see Banse, H. J. [85], 156, *324*
Zaidi, S. A., see Kofi Ekue, J. M. [184c], 237, *367*
Zakusov, V. V. [2038, 2039], 303, *359*
— Kaverina, N. V. [2040, 2041], 303, *359*
Zaleski, E. J., Cohen, A., Bing, R. J. [2042], 101, 178, 190, *359*
— see Bing, R. J. [165], 82, 101, 130, 151, *326*
— see Cohen, A. [339], 130, 151, *329*
— see Luebs, E. D. [1192], 130, 133, 151, 178, 190, *344*
Zanolini, F., see Setnikar, I. [1722], 160, *354*
Zaret, B., see Pitt, B. [251c], 134, *369*
Zarnstorff, W. C., see McKenna, D. H. [1258], 42, 207, 209, 272, 274, *345*
Zbinden, G. [2043], 163, *359*
Zeft, H. J., Curry, C. L., Rembert, J. C., Greenfield, J. C. [345c], 303, *371*
— Patterson, S. D., Orgain, E. S. [2044], 213, 215, *359*
Zelis, R., Mason, D. T. [140a], 148, *362*
— see Mason, D. T. [87a], 39, 130, *361*
Zeitler, E., see Halmagyi, M. [766], 183, *337*
Zeller, E. A., Barsky, J. [2045], 160, *360*
— — Berman, E. R. [2046], 160, *360*
— — Fouts, J. R., Kirchheimer, W. F., Van Orden, L. S. [2047], 160, *360*
Zelvelder, W. G. [2048], 280, *360*

Zickgraf, H., see Schimert, G. [1671], 312, 313, *353*
Zimmer, V. [2049], 180, *360*
Zimmerman, H. A., see Sambhi, M. P. [1635], 16, *352*
Zimmermann, D., see Kaltenbach, M. [933], 174, *340*
Zimmermann, H. A., see Corcoran, A. C. [363], 314, *329*
Zimmermann, P. E., see Brichard, G. [16a], 179, *360*
Zimmermann, W. [2050], 196, *360*
Zinn, W. J., see Griffith, G. C. [742], 311, *336*
Zion, M. M., Bradlow, B. A. [2051], 187, *360*
Zitnik, R., see Campion, B. [20a], 130, *360*
Zohman, B. L., see Russek, H. I. [1616—1620], 103, 104, 105, 106, 135, 136, 137, 139, 141, 151, 152, 154, 158, 213, 299, 311, 312, 313, *352*
Zoll, P. M., Norman, L. R., Cassin, S. [2052], 145, *360*
— see Blumgart, H. L. [190, 191], 19, 21, 53, 137, *326*
— see Schlesinger, M. J.[1674], 52, *353*
Zotto u Dal, see Strobbia, R. [304c], 164, *370*
Zuberbuhler, R. C., Bohr, D. F. [2053], 44, *360*
Zucchelli, G. P., see Guadagno, L. [751], 179, *336*
Zucker, N., see Hellerstein, H. K. [807], 10, *337*
Zuelzer, G. [2054], 310, *360*
Zumoff, B., see Hellman, L. [809], 16, *337*
Zsoter, T. T., Beanlands, D. S. [141a], 212, *362*
Zyzanski, S. J., see Jenkins, C. D. [896], 16, *339*

Subject Index

Acetyldigoxin 296
Adenine 306
Adenosine
—, deaminase 60
—, diphosphate 305
—, —, pain producing substance 21
—, —, pharmacological properties 305
—, —, platelet aggregation by 49
—, mediator of coronary autoregulation 60
—, monophosphate 305
—, pain producing substance 21
—, pharmacological properties 305
—, triphosphate 305
Adenylic acid 305
Adenylocrat 288
Adhesiveness
—, platelet 49
Adrenaline
—, effect on coronary blood flow 28
—, release in angina 36
Adrenergic receptors
—, in cardiac muscle 237
—, in coronary vessels 63
—, in peripheral vessels 237
Adrenergic stimulation in angina 35
Adumbran 188
Aggregation
—, platelet 49
AH 3474 253
Albumin
—, radioactive iodinated 81
Alcohol 300
—, in angina 300
—, effect on coronary circulation 300
—, predisposing factor to coronary atherosclerosis 15
Algocor 168
Alkyl-xanthines 156
Alpha adrenoceptors in coronary vessels 63
Alpha adrenoceptors blocking agents 42, 63
Alpha-tocopherol 305
Alprenolol 229
Ameroid ring 4, 90
Amiloride 49
Aminal 138
Aminocardol 153
Aminocetone 288
Amino-oxydase inhibitors 160
Aminophylline 153
Aminotheophylline 156
Amiodarone, see Cordarone
Ammicardine 157
Ammipuran 157
Ammivin 157
Ammivisnagen 157
Ammi visnaga 157

Amoproxan 292
Amotriphene 313
Amplivix 168
Amyl nitrite 143
Anaemia
—, angina pectoris in 20
Anaerobic cardiac metabolism in angina 25
Anastomoses
—, coronary 46, 53
Androphyllin 153
Angina pectoris
—, adrenaline release in 36
—, alcohol and 15
—, anaemia (angina pectoris in) 19
—, anticoagulants in 17
—, arteriospasm in 20
—, ballistocardiogram in 95
—, biochemical diagnosis of 101
—, cardiac dynamics in 30
—, carotid sinus nerve stimulation in 315
—, clinical diagnosis of 95
—, coronary blood flow in 24
—, cutaneous circulation in 35
—, diabetes and 16
—, diagnosis of 95
—, —, by generalized anoxaemia test 96
—, —, by two-step exercise 96
—, dietetics in 14
—, electrocardiogram in 95
—, epidemiology of 7
—, experimental reproduction of 4
—, —, by atrial pacing 4
—, —, by exercise 4
—, —, by isoprenaline 4
—, general management of 8
—, gout and 16
—, hypercholesterolaemia and 14
—, hypersympathicotony in 35
—, hypertension and 16
—, hypertension in 36
—, hyperthyroidism (angina pectoris in) 20
—, hypertriglyceridaemia and 14
—, hyperuricaemia and 16
—, hypothyroidism and 16
—, lactate production in 25
—, lethality of 7
—, metabolic diseases and 16
—, morbidity of 7
—, myocardial hypoxia in 18
—, myocardial ischaemia in 18
—, myocardial oxygen consumption in 24
—, noradrenaline release in 36
—, obesity and 16
—, oxygen content of coronary venous blood in 24

Angina pectoris
—, oxygen desaturation of coronary venous blood in 24
—, pain in 20
—, —, anatomic pathways of 20
—, —, mechanism of 20
—, —, mediators of 20
—, physical training in 8
—, pathophysiology of, see Pathophysiology of angina pectoris
—, predisposing factors to 14
—, pulmonary circulation in 35
—, surgical treatment of 10
—, tachycardia in 36
—, tobacco and 16
—, vectocardiogram in 95
—, ventricular compliance in 30
—, ventricular failure in 30
—, ventricular function in 30
—, without coronary disease 19
Anginal attack
—, pathophysiology of the, see Pathophysiology of the anginal attack
Anginin 289
Anginine 120
Angiotensine 3, 11
Angistat 316
Angitrit 138
Angoron, see Cordarone
Anoxaemia test
—, in diagnosis of angina 96
—, in clinical evaluation of antianginal drugs 106
Antianginal drugs
—, trends in pharmacological research 39
—, —, blockade of adrenergic beta-receptors 42
—, —, blockade of hypersympathicotony 42
—, —, coronary vasodilation 39
—, —, development of collateral coronary circulation 45
—, —, dilation of coronary conductance vessels 44
—, —, improvement of functional coronary microcirculation 45
—, —, inhibition of monoamineoxydase 41
—, —, inhibition of platelet aggregation and adhesiveness 49
—, —, overall inhibition of hypersympathicotony 43
—, —, potentiation of endogenous mediators of coronary autoregulation 47
—, —, prophylaxis of myocardial necrosis 48
—, —, reduction in cardiac work 40
—, clinical assessment of 170
—, clinical features of 118
—, clinical methods of evaluation of 95
—, —, objective methods 102
—, —, —, Frick method 109
—, —, —, Levy method 106
—, —, —, Riseman method 106
—, —, —, Rookmaker method 109
—, —, —, Russek method 102
—, —, —, Solvay method 108

Antianginal drugs, clinical methods of evaluation of, subjective methods 109
—, —, —, Greiner method 111
—, decreasing oxygen requirements 28
—, increasing oxygen supply 27
—, methods of clinical assessment of 101
—, pharmacological characteristics of an ideal 38
—, pharmacology of 118
—, side effects of 320
Antiatherogenic agents 15
Anticoagulants 17
Antihypercholesterolaemic agents 15
Antivitamin K 17
Aorta
—, pressure in, and coronary flow 55
Aorta-to-coronary artery vein bypass grafts 12
Appliruber 138
Aptin 229
Arlidin 307
Arterial coronary blood flow, see coronary blood flow
Arteriography
—, in diagnosis of angina 100
Arteriolar neoformation 46
Arterio-venous oxygen difference
—, coronary 57
Aspartate 296
—, magnesium 296
—, potassium 296
Atherosclerosis (coronary) 7
—, determining factors of 10
—, epidemiology of 7
—, predisposing factors of 14
—, —, diabetes 16
—, —, gout 16
—, —, hypercholesterolaemia 14
—, —, hyperglycaemia 16
—, —, hypertension 16
—, —, hypertriglyceridaemia 14
—, —, hyperuricaemia 16
—, —, hypothyroidism 16
—, —, metabolic diseases 16
—, —, obesity 16
—, —, tobacco 16
Assessment of antianginal drugs 95
Atrial pacing 4, 99
—, effect on coronary blood flow 28
—, in diagnosis of angina 99
—, in clinical evaluation of antianginal drugs 109
Atromid - S 15
Autoregulation of coronary circulation 58
Avlocardyl, see Inderal
AY 21011 235
8-Azaguanine 60

Ballistocardiography
—, in diagnosis of angina 95
Baralgin 289
Barbiturates 299
Barbonin 152
Baxacor 289

Benecardin 157
Benfurodil 291
Benign vasodilator 57
Benziodarone 168
Benzmalacene 15
Benzofuran 255
Benzylisoquinoline 150
Beta-adrenergic blocking drugs 205
—, definition of 205
—, physiological effects of 205
Beta adrenoceptors
—, in coronary vessels 63
Beta$_1$ adrenoceptors
—, in cardiac muscle 237
—, in coronary vessels 63
Beta$_2$ adrenoceptors
—, in coronary vessels 63
—, in peripheral vessels 237
Beta-blocking drugs
—, AH 3474 253
—, alprenolol 229
—, Aptin 229
—, Avlocardyl 206
—, AY 21011 235
—, butoxamine 63, 237
—, bunolol 255
—, Butidrate 253
—, butidrine 252
—, Ciba 39089-Ba 222
—, D477A 254
—, doberol 245
—, Dociton 206
—, Eraldin 235
—, Gubernal 229
—, H 56/28 229
—, ICI 45763 245
—, ICI 50172 235
—, Inderal 206
—, Inderal 80 222
—, INPEA 248
—, KÖ 592 245
—, LB46 246
—, MJ1999 249
—, oxprenolol 222
—, Ph QA33 253
—, pindolol 246
—, practolol 235
—, propranolol 206
—, Recetan 252
—, Ro3-3528 248
—, S-D/1601 254
—, Sotalol 249
—, Trasicor 222
—, USVC 6524 254
—, Visken 246
Beta-Intensaine 150 192
Bicor 297
Biochemistry
—, myocardial 317
Blockade of adrenergic a-receptors as research
    concept 42
Blockade of adrenergic β-receptors as rese-
    arch concept 42
Blockade of hypersympathicotony as rese-
    arch concept 42

Blood flow, see Coronary blood flow
Blood pressure
—, effect of, on coronary flow 55
Bradykinine
—, pain producing substance 21
—, mediator of coronary autoregulation 63
Bradykininogen 21
Bubble flowmeter 74
Bunolol 255
Butidrate 252
Butidrine 252
Butoxamine 63, 237

Caa 40 307
Caffeine 152
Calcium theophyllinate 156
Calorimetry 76
Calphyllin 156
Canula
—, of Eckstein 74
—, of Gregg 73
Capillary
—, pressure 53
—, sphincters 20
Carbochromene 188
Carbonic acid
—, vasomotor metabolite 59
Cardamist 138
Cardiac dynamics during the anginal attack
    30
Cardiac hypoxia 19
Cardiac necrosis 48
Cardiac output
—, effect of, on coronary flow 56
—, measurement of 90
Cardiac work
—, effect of, on coronary flow 55
—, measurement of 92
Cardilate 140
Cardiloid 140
Cardine 159
Cardio-green 91
Cardio-Khellin 157
Cardivix 168
Cardophyllin 153
Carduben 159
Carena 153
Carotid sinus nerve 37, 315
Cartrax 143
Carvasine 146
Catheterization
—, attainments of heart 2
—, of the coronary arteries 4
—, of the coronary sinus 2
—, of the left heart 2
—, of the right heart 2
Catron 163
Causes of the anginal syndrome 37
Cavodil 163
Chloracizine 303
Chloro-adenosine 306
Chloroglyceryl dinitrate 149
Chlorothiazide 49
Chlorphenothiazine 303
Chlorpromazine 302

Choledyl 155
Cholegyl 155
Choleretics 15
Cholesterol 15
—, accelerators of, catabolism 15
—, accelerators of, excretion 15
—, inhibitors of, biosynthesis 15
Choline theophyllinate 155
Choloxin 15
Chromocor 160
Chromonar 188
Chromone derivatives 159
Ciba 39089-Ba 222
Cinchamidine 304
Cinchona alkaloids 303
Cinchonidine 304
Cinchonine 304
Clinical assessment of antianginal
    drugs 101
—, conclusions on methods of 116
—, objective methods for the 102
—, —, Frick method 109
—, —, Levy method 106
—, —, Riseman method 106
—, —, Rookmaker method 109
—, —, Russek method 102
—, —, Solvay method 108
—, subjective methods for the 109
—, —, Greiner method 111
Clinical pharmacology 2
Clinium 199
Clofibrate 15
Collagene, platelet aggregation by 50
Collateral coronary circulation 45, 85
—, measurement by acute methods
—, —, Linder technique 85
—, —, McGregor technique 85
—, —, Rees technique 85
—, measurement by chronic methods 86
—, —, Meesmann technique 86
—, —, Schaper technique 86
—, —, Schmidt technique 86
Collateral coronary flow 44
Complamin 156
Conclusions on methods of clinical evaluation
    of antianginal drugs 116
Conductance coronary vessels 44
Conduction
—, intracardiac 3
Contractility index of myocardium 3
Corafurone 157
Coralgyl 305
Cordalin 156
Cordarone 255
—, pharmacological properties 256
—, —, action mechanisms 266
—, —, antiadrenergic effects 262
—, —, antiarrhythmic effects 276
—, —, intrinsic effects 256
—, therapeutic properties 276
—, —, clinical tolerance and side effects 286
—, —, double blind studies 279
—, —, effects on abnormal electrocardio-
    gram in angina 285
—, —, effects on cardiac arrhythmias 285

Cordarone, therapeutic properties, effects on
    symptomatology of cardiac overload tests
    280
—, —, —, cycloergometric test 280
—, —, —, hypoxia test 280
—, —, —, Master test 284
—, —, open studies 276
Cordilox 172
Coronaroarteriography
—, in diagnosis of angina 100
Coronaropathy
—, experimental 87
Coronary anastomoses 46
Coronary animals 87
Coronary arteriospasm 20
Coronary atherosclerosis
—, increase in myocardial blood flow in 28
—. —, by adrenaline 28
—, —, by atrial pacing 24, 28
—, —, by nitroglycerin 28
—, —, by physical exercise 24, 28
—, decrease in myocardial blood flow in 22
—, determining factors of 10
—, epidemiology of 7
—, predisposing factors of 14
—, —, diabetes 16
—, —, gout 16
—, —, hypercholesterolaemia 14
—, —, hyperglycaemia 16
—, —, hypertension 16
—, —, hypertriglyceridaemia 14
—, —, hyperuricaemia 16
—, —, hypothyroidism 16
—, —, metabolic diseases 16
—, —, obesity 16
—, —, tobacco 16
Coronary blood flow 64
—, and aortic pressure 55
—, arterial flow 72
—, and blood pressure 55
—, and cardiac output 56
—, and cardiac work 56
—, in coronary patient 22
—, determinants of 54
—, and heart diastole 57
—, and heart force 56
—, and heart metabolism 55
—, and heart rate 56
—, and heart systole 57
—, and heart work 56
—, and hypoxaemia 59
—, and intramyocardial oxygen 59
—, and intraventricular pressure 69
—, and myocardial oxygen consumption 55
—, and oxygen content of arterial blood 59
—, and potassium 60
—, and stroke volume 56
—, and tachycardia 57
—, and vasomotor metabolites 59
—, and vasomotor tone 52
—, arterial blood flow 72
—, —, procedures for measurement of 72
—, —, —, Berne method 74
—, —, —, calorimetry 76
—, —, —, electromagnetic flowmetry 77

Coronary blood flow, arterial blood flow, procedures for measurement of, Gregg method 73
—, —, —, Melville method 72
—, —, —, methods using radioactive substances 81
—, —, —, —, diffusible inert gases 83
—, —, —, —, diffusible substances 81
—, —, —, —, non-diffusible substances 81
—, —, —, nitrous oxide method 79
—, —, —, Pieper method 74
—, —, —, Schofield method 72
—, —, —, thermostromuhr 76
—, —, —, ultrasonic flowmetry 78
—, decrease in resting, in coronary atherosclerosis 22
—, increase in, in coronary atherosclerosis 28
—, —, by adrenaline 28
—, —, by atrial pacing 24, 28
—, —, by nitroglycerin 28
—, —, by physical exercise 24, 28
—, inequality of 317
—, procedures of measurement of 65
—, —, on isolated beating heart 65
—, —, —, method of Katz 66
—, —, —, method of Langendorff 65
—, —, —, method of Melville 72
—, —, —, method of Uhlman and Nobile 66
—, —, on isolated fibrillating heart 66
—, venous blood flow 68
—, —, procedures for measurement of 68
—, —, —, sinus flow 68
—, —, —, —, Busch method 71
—, —, —, —, Ganz method 71
—, —, —, —, heart-lung preparation 70
—, —, —, —, Morawitz method 70
—, —, —, —, Rodbard method 70
—, —, —, —, sinus catheterization 71
—, —, —, —, West method 71
—, —, —, total flow 70
Coronary
—, collaterals 45
—, degeneration 47
—, efficiency 22, 58
—, heart disease 7
—, —, epidemiology of 7
—, —, incidence of 7
—, —, mortality by 7
—, insufficiency 19
—, —, in anaemia 20
—, —, in angina 19
—, —, in coronary atherosclerosis 19
—, —, in hyperthyroidism 20
—, —, pathophysiology of 24
—, microcirculation 45
—, oxygen reserve 56
—, quotient 46
—, reserve 97
—, —, in angina 97
—, —, for clinical evaluation of antianginal drugs 108
—, reserves 52
—, resistance 52

Coronary, resistance, extrinsic resistance 68
—, —, intrinsic resistance 68
—, sinus 68
—, —, blood flow in 68
—, —, catheterization of 71
—, —, pacing of 100
—, vasodilation as research concept 39
—, vasodilators 57
—, —, of benign character 57
—, —, of malignant character 57
—, vessels
—, —, adrenergic receptors in 63
—, —, conductance 44
—, —, resistance 44
—, —, sympathetic innervation of 63
Coronin 157
Corontin 165
Corphyllamin 153
Cortico-surrenal hormones 48
Cortisol 49
Cortunon 310
Crataegus 288
Cromarile 160
Cutaneous circulation in angina 35
Cyanide 58
Cyclandelate 308
Cyclospasmol 308
Cytidine 306

D 477 A 274
Daily report card 111
Daucarine 304
Deaminase
—, adenosine 60
Degeneration
—, coronary 47
Dehydrogenase (lactic) in angina 27
Deltoside 159
Desaturation (oxygen, of coronary venous blood in angina) 24
Dethyron 15
Development of collateral coronary circulation as research concept 45
Dexpropranolol 241
Dextrothyroxine 15
Diabetes 16
Diacromone 159
Diagnosis of angina 95
Dialicor 315
Diaphyllin 153
Diathermy 76
Diazepam 301
Dibazole 315
Dichloroisoproterenol 205
Dicoumarol 311
Diet 14
Digi-Tromcardin 298
Dihydroergocornine 312
Dihydroergocristine 312
Dihydroergokryptine 312
Dihydroergotoxine 312
Dilatal 307
Dilation of the coronary conductance vessels as research concept 44
Dilatol 307

Dilatropon   307
Dilcoran   143
Dilcoran 80   143
Dinitrophenol   58
Dioxyline   151
Diphenylhydantoin   303
Diphryl   168
Dipyridamole   181
Diquinol   152
Diuretics   49
Diuretin   152
Doberol   245
Dociton, see Inderal
Double blind system   110
—, remote   114
dp/dt   2
d²p/dt²   2
Drop meter   74
DT₄   15
Duotrate   142
Duvadilan   307
Dye dilution method   91
Dynamic ECG anomaly
—, in angina   97
Dynamics (cardiac) in angina   30

Electrocardiography
—, in diagnosis of angina   95
Electrolyte balance in angina   26
Electromagnetic
—, flowmetry   77
Elixophyllin   155
Endarterectomy   11
End-diastolic pressure
—, ventricular, in angina   30
Equanitrate   143
Eraldin   235
Ergot   312
Erinitrit   145
Erythrityl tetranitrate   140
Erythrol tetranitrate   140
Eskel   157
Etafenon   289
Etaphylline   156
Ethacrynic acid   49
Ethaverine   152
Ethyl alcohol   300
Etrynit   149
Eucilat   291
Euphyllin   153
Exercise
—, effect of, in angina patients   24
—, effect of, on coronary blood flow   24
Experimental chronic coronary insufficiency   87

Factors of the anginal syndrome   37
Faraday's law   77
Fats   14
—, polyunsaturated   14
—, saturated   14
Features of an "ideal" antianginal drug   38
Fiberoptic hemoreflection method   91
Fibrillating heart   66
Fick method   90

Flavone-7-ethyl oxyacetate   160
Flow sensor   77
—, intravascular   78
Flow transducer   77
Flowmetry   77
—, electromagnetic   77
—, ultrasonic   78
Frenodosa   144
Frey hormone   309
Furanochromone   159
Furochromones   158

Gastro-intestinal resorption   54
Gina   149
Glucose, see polarising solutions
Glyceryl trinitrate   119
Glycolysis in angina   25
Glyo-6   294
Gout   16
Graded exercise test   97
—, in diagnosis of angina   97
Gradient in myocardial blood flow   317
Greiner method   111
Griseofulvine   291
Guanosine   306
Gubernal   229
Gynokhellan   157

H 56/28   229
Haemodynamic basis of coronary circulation   52
Hamilton formula   91
Heart
—, catheterization   2
—, effect of, dynamics on the coronary flow
—, —, contractile force   56
—, —, diastole   57
—, —, metabolism   55
—, —, output   56
—, —, rate   56
—, —, systole   56
—, —, tachycardia   57
—, —, work   56
—, extract   309
—, -lung preparation   70
—, monitoring   4
—, rate
—, —, effect of, on coronary flow   56
Heparin   17, 310
Heparinoids   15
Heredity
—, in coronary atherosclerosis   15
Hexabendin   192
Hexadylamine   294
Hexobendine   192
Hexoestrol   305
Hexyldimethylxanthine   156
Histamine
—, vasomotor metabolite   60
Hostaginan   165
5 HT (platelet aggregation by)   50
Hydergine   312
Hydrazine   163
—, benzyl   163
—, isonicotinyl isopropyl   163

Hydrazine, phenyl ethyl 163
—, phenyl isopropyl 163
—, pivaloyl benzyl 163
Hypercholesterolaemia 14
Hyperemine 64
Hyperglycaemia 16
Hypersympathicotony in angina 35
Hypertension
—, in anginal attack 36
—, and coronary atherosclerosis 16
Hyperthyroidism 20
Hypertriglyceridaemia 14
Hyperuricaemia 16
Hypocholesterolaemic agents 15
Hypothyroidism 16
Hypoxaemia 59
Hypoxanthine 60
Hypoxia
—, effect on coronary blood flow 59
—, effect on electrocardiogram 21
—, myocardial, in angina 19
Hypoxia test
—, in diagnosis of angina 96
—, in clinical evaluation of antianginal drugs
   106

ICI 45.763 245
ICI 50.172 235
Iditol, hexanitrate 120
Ildamen 196
Ildamen-S 199
Ilidar 312
Imolamine 164
Improvement of functional coronary microcirculation as research concept 45
Inderal 206
—, antianginal effect of 211
—, —, mechanisms of the 214
—, antiarrhythmic effect of 218
—, beta blocking effect of 206
—, combination with isosorbide dinitrate
   213
—, combination with nitroglycerin 214
—, effect on cardiac function 215
—, effect on cardiac output 210
—, effect on coronary blood flow 208
—, ineffectiveness in acute myocardial infarction 217
—, primary cardiac effect 207
—, quinidine-like effect 219
—, use in angina 217
—, use in cardiac arrhythmia 218
—, use in hyperkinetic heart syndrome 218
—, use in subaortic hypertrophic idiopathic
   stenosis 218
Inderal 80 222
Index
—, of Robinson 29
—, tension time 93
—, heart rate x blood pressure 29
—, cardiac, in angina 30
Indicator dilution method 91
Inequality of myocardial blood flow 317
Infarctectomy 10
—, myocardial 10

Inhibition of monoamineoxydase as research
   concept 41
Inhibition of platelet aggregation or adhesi-
   veness as research concept 49
Innervation
—, sympathetic, of coronary vessels 63
Inophyline 153
Inosine 60, 306
INPEA 248
Intensaine 188
Intensaine 150 192
Intensaine-Lanicor 192
Insulin, see polarising solutions
Iodine
—, radioactive 81
Iproclozide 163
Iproniazid 160
Iproveratril 172
Irrigor 164
Irrigor 3 165
Ischaemic heart disease, see coronary heart
   disease
Isocarboxazid 163
Isolated heart 65
Isomannide dinitrate 146
Isonicotinamide 163
Isoprenaline
—, haemodynamic effects of 4
—, mediator of coronary autoregulation 62
—, stimulating agent upon β-adrenoceptors
   291, 323
Isoptin 172
Isordil 146
—, Tembids 148
Isosorbide dinitrate 146
—, association with propranolol 147, 213
Itramin 148

J.B. 516 163

Kallikrein 21, 309
—, effect on coronary blood flow 309
—, inhibitor of 64
KCT 158
Kelamin 157
Kelicor 157
Kelicorin 157
Kellin 157
Keloid 157
Khelfren 157
Khellin 157
Khellinin 159
Khelloside 159
Khelloyd 158
Kinins 21
Kö 592 245
Krypton
—, radioactive 83

L 3428, see Cordarone
LA 1211 164
LA 1221 297
Lactate production in angina 25
Lactic acid
—, mediator of coronary autoregulation 59

Lactic acid, production of, in angina 25
—, stimulant of adrenal medulla 101
Lactic dehydrogenase in angina 27
Laevothyroxine 307
Langendorff method 65
Largactil 302
LB 46 246
Left ventricle
—, contractile state of 3
—, function of, in angina, see Ventricular
—, velocity of shortening of, fibres 2
Levy method 106
—, in diagnosis of angina 96
—, in clinical evaluation of antianginal drugs
    106
Lidoflazine 199
Linder technique 85
Lipoprotein modifying agents 15
Littman test 96
Liver extract 310
Local myocardial metabolic changes 318
Lynamine 157

Magnesium
—, aspartate 296
Malignant vasodilator 57
Malmstrom test 96
Mannitol hexanitrate 143
Marplan 163
Marsilid 160
Master test
—, in diagnosis of angina 96
—, in clinical evaluation of antianginal drugs
    103, 107
Maxitate 143
McGregor technique 85
Mederel 292
Mediators of coronary irrigation 58
Medibazine 298
Meesmann technique 86
Mepazine 303
Meprobamate 299
MER 29 15
Metabolic diseases 16
Metabolites
—, vasomotor 58
Metamine 138
Methaemoglobinaemia 149
Methafrone 157
Methyl-3-chromone 159
Methylxanthines 152
Microcirculation
—, myocardial 45, 85
Miltrate 143
Miscellaneous drugs 288
M.J.1999 249
Monoamineoxydase inhibitors 160
Morawitz method 70
Morphine 299
Myocardial biochemistry 317
Myocardial blood flow, see coronary blood
    flow
"Myocardial" heart disease 48
Myocardial nutritional circulation 45
Myocardial oxygen consumption 24

Myocardial oxygen consumption, during an-
    ginal attack 24
—, effect of, on coronary blood flow 55
—, measurement of 92
Myocardial performance
—, regional variations in 318
Myocardial perfusion
—, inequality of 317
—, regional variations of 317
—, study of regional 318
Myocardol 140
Myordil 313

N 1113 288
Naphtyl methyl adenosine 306
Nardil 163
Necrosis
—, cardiac 48
Necrotic electrolyte steroid cardiopathy 49
Neoformation
—, arteriolar 46
Nerves (cardiac) 20
Nialamide 163
Niamid 163
Nicotine 16
Nicotinic acid 313
Nilatil 148
Nitral 149
Nitranitol 143
Nitrates 118
Nitretamin 138
Nitrite
—, amyl 143
—, octyl 144
—, sodium 145
Nitrites 118
—, methaemoglobinaemia 149
Nitro bid Plateau 138
Nitroglycerin 120
—, aerosols 138
—, biochemical effects 127
—, depot 138
—, effect on coronary flow in dogs 123
—, effect on coronary flow in man 125
—, effect on venous circulation 130
—, generalities 120
—, haemodynamic effects in acute angina
    pectoris 128
—, haemodynamic effects in animals 120
—, haemodynamic effects in man 126
—, inactivation 137
—, mechanisms of the antianginal effect 129
—, ointment 138
— paradoxical reactions 136
—, retard 137
—, side effects 322
—, special galenic preparations 137
—, spray 137
—, therapeutic effects 135
Nitroglycerin retard 137
Nitroglyn 137
Nitrol 138
Nitrolamine tosylate 148
Nitrolingual spray 137
Nitro Mack Retard 138

Nitropol 137
Nitro Sandolanid 296
Nitrospan 138
Nitrous oxide method 79
Nokhel 158
Noradrenaline
—, release in angina 36
—, effect on coronary blood flow 36
—, platelet aggregation by 50
Norkel 157
Nutritional circulation 45, 85

Obesity 16
Objective methods
—, for clinical evaluation of antianginal drugs 102
Octyl nitrite 144
Opticardon 293
Organ extracts
—, heart extract 309
—, liver extract 310
—, pancreas extract 309
Ortin 138
Overall inhibition of hypersympathicotony as research concept 43
Oxiflavil 160
Oximetry
—, intracardiac 3, 91
Oxprenolol 222
Oxtriphylline 155
Oxyfedrin 196
Oxygen
—, consumption by the myocardium 92
—, —, effect on coronary blood flow 55
—, content of coronary venous blood 56
—, —, in angina 24
—, —, in normal subject 56
—, coronary arterio-venous difference 57
—, extraction in angina 24
—, use in angina 315
Oxypropyltheobromine 156

P factor 20
Pacatal 303
Pacemaker 4
Padutin 309
Pain (cardiac) 20
Pancreatic extract 309
Papaverine 150
—, derivatives 151
Pathophysiology
—, of angina pectoris 19
—, —, adenosine 21
—, —, ADP 21
—, —, bradykinine 21
—, —, cardiac hypoxia 19
—, —, cardiac nerves 20
—, —, coronary blood flow 22
—, —, coronary insufficiency 19
—, —, coronary vasodilation
—, —, —, by adrenaline 28
—, —, —, by atrial pacing 28
—, —, —, by nitroglycerin 28
—, —, —, by physical exercise 28
—, —, electrocardiogram 21

Pathophysiology, of angina pectoris, imbalance between oxygen demand and supply 19
—, —, kallicrein 21
—, —, kinins 21
—, —, myocardial ischaemia 19
—, —, myocardial oxygen consumption 22
—, —, pain 20
—, of the anginal attack 23
—, —, adrenaline release 36
—, —, adrenergic stimulation 36
—, —, anaerobic metabolism 25
—, —, cardiac dynamics 30
—, —, cardiac output 33
—, —, coronary blood flow 24
—, —, coronary vasoconstriction 36
—, —, coronary venous blood (oxygen content of) 24
—, —, cutaneous circulation 35
—, —, electrolyte balance 26
—, —, end-diastolic ventricular pressure 31
—, —, extraction of oxygen by the myocardium 24
—, —, glycolysis 25
—, —, hypersympathicotony 35
—, —, hypertension 36
—, —, lactate production 25
—, —, lactic dehydrogenase 27
—, —, left ventricular end-diastolic pressure 30
—, —, myocardial ischaemia 23
—, —, myocardial oxygen consumption 24
—, —, noradrenaline release 36
—, —, oxygen desaturation of coronary venous blood 24
—, —, potassium loss 26
—, —, pulmonary arterial pressure 30
—, —, pulmonary blood flow 35
—, —, Robinson index 29
—, —, stroke volume 30
—, —, stroke work 30
—, —, sympathetic stimulation 35
—, —, tachycardia 36
—, —, ventricular compliance 31
—, —, ventricular end-diastolic pressure 31
—, —, ventricular failure 30
—, —, ventricular function 30
Pavabid 150
Paveril 151
pCO_2 as mediator of coronary autoregulation 61
Pentaerythritol tetranitrate 140
Pentafin 140
Pentanitrine 140
Pentritol 140
Pentritol tempules 142
Pentrium 143
Perflavon 314
Perhexiline 293
Peripheral coronary pressure 45
Perithiazide 143
Peritrate 140
—, associations 143
Peritrate 80 142
Peritrate S. A. 142

Perparin 152
Persantine 181
Persumbran 188
Pexid 293
pH as mediator of coronary autoregulation
    59
Pharmacological research in antianginal
    medications 39
Pharmacological trends 39
Pharmacology
—, of coronary circulation 52
Phenelzine 163
Phenformine 16
Pheniprazine 163
Phenothiazines 302
Phenoxy isopropyl norsuprifen 307
Phenyl acetic acid 15
Phenyl chromone 160
Phenyl isobutyl norsuprifen 307
Phosphodiesterase 150, 165, 190, 197
PhQA 33 253
Physical training 8
Pindolol 246
Piridoxilate 294
Pituitrine
—, effect on electrocardiogram 21
Pivaloyl benzyl hydrazine 163
Placebo 110
Platelet
—, adhesiveness 49
—, aggregation 49
—, masses 51
—, rich plasma 50
Pneumatic occlusive cuff 77
pO₂ as mediator of coronary autoregulation
    61
Polarising solutions 295
Polarographic electrodes 4
Poly-methoxyphenol derivatives 313
Polyvinylpyrrolidone 66
Positons 82
Potassium
—, mediator of coronary autoregulation 60
—, constituant of polarising solutions 295
—, aspartate 296
—, loss in angina 26
—, orotate 296
—, radioactive 81
Potentiation of endogenous mediators as
    research concept 47
Practitioner attitude towards antianginal
    drugs 319
Practolol 235
Prenitron 138
Prenylamine 165
Priscol 312
Privine 66
Promethazine 302
Pronethalol 205
Propanediol dinitrate 149
Propatylnitrate 149
Prophylaxis of cardiac necrosis as research
    concept 48
Propranolol, see Inderal
Prospects of future research 317

Provismine 159
Pulmonary arterial pressure in angina 30
Pulmonary circulation in angina 35
Pyridinol carbamate 289
Pyrimido pyrimidines 181

Quinidine
—, effect on action potential 219
—, effect on coronary blood flow 303
—, antianginal effect 304
Quinidine-like 219
Quinine 304
Quintrate 140

Radioactive
—, iodine 81
—, krypton 83
—, potassium 81
—, rubidium 81
—, technecium 23
—, xenon 83
Radioactive tracers
—, diffusible inert gases 83
—, diffusible substances 81
—, non diffusible substances 81
Radiocardiography 81
Rapport period 111
Raubasine 308
Rauwiloid 308
Rauwolfia serpentina 308
Reactive hyperaemia 58
Receptors, see adrenergic receptors
Recetan 252
Recordil 160
Recosen 309
Reduction in cardiac work as research concept
    40
Rees technique 85
Rein technique 76
Remote double blind system 114
Reoxyl 192
Reserpine 308
Resins 15
Resistance
—, coronary 52
—, —, extrinsic 68
—, —, intrinsic 68
—, —, vessels 44
Retrangor 168
Retrograde coronary flow 44
Revascularisation
—, surgical, of the myocardium 10
—, —, aorta to coronary artery vein bypass
    grafts 12
—, —, endarterectomy 10
—, —, internal mammary artery implanta-
    tion 10
—, —, —, functional benefit 11
—, —, —, —, view of cardiologists 13
—, —, —, —, view of surgeons 13
—, —, saphenous vein bypass grafts 12
—, —, —, functional benefit 13
—, —, Vineberg procedure 10
Riseman method
—, for clinical evaluation of antianginal drugs
    106

Ro 3-3528   248
Robinson index   29
Ronicol   313
Rookmaker method
—, in diagnosis of angina   99
—, in clinical evaluation of antianginal drugs
    109
Rotameter   73
Rubidium
—, radioactive   81
Russek method
—, for clinical evaluation of antianginal drugs
    102
Rykellin   157

Sandolanid   296
Sarnoff index   55, 93
Schaper technique   86
Schmidt technique   86
S-D/1601   254
Seda nitro Mack Retard   138
Sedentarity
—, in coronary atherosclerosis
Sedo Intensaine   192
Segontin   165
Segontin 60   168
Selective coronarography   84, 100
Selye cardiopathy   49
Serumalbumin   81
Sexual hormones   305
Side effects of antianginal drugs   320
Simeskellina   157
Sinus
—, blood flow in coronary   68
—, carotid — nerve stimulation   315
—, catheterization of coronary   71
—, oxygen content in coronary blood   56
Sitosterol   15
Sodium nitrite   145
Solvay method
—, for diagnosis of angina   97
—, for clinical evaluation of antianginal drugs
    108
Sones catheter   93
Sorbitan tetranitrate   120
Sorbitrate   146
Sotalol   249
Sphincters
—, precapillary   20, 45
Steno Tromcardin   298
Steno Valocordin   138
Stereoarteriography   53
Sterols   15
Stilbene   305
Stimulator
—, carotid sinus nerve   315
Stress
—, in coronary atherosclerosis   15
Stroke volume in angina   30
Stroke work in angina   30
Subjective methods
—, for clinical evaluation of antianginal drugs
    109
Surgery
—, endarterectomy   11

Surgery, internal mammary artery implan-
    tation   10
—, saphenous vein bypass grafts   12
—, view of cardiologists   13
—, view of surgeons   13
—, Vineberg procedure   10
Surheme   297
Sursum   163
Sustac   137
Sympathetic innervation of coronary vessels,
    see innervation
Sympathetic stimulation in angina   35
Sympathine   62
Synadrin 60   168

T wave
—, asphyctic   21
Tachycardia
—, in angina   36
—, effect on coronary blood flow   57
Taluvian   180
Technecium
—, radioactive   23
Tefamin   153
Tension time index   55, 93
Terbutyl propylamine   297
Terodiline   297
Tersavid   163
Testosterone propionate   305
Tetranitrate
—, erythrityl   140
—, erythrol   140
—, pentaerythritol   140
Tetranitrin   140
Tetranitrol   140
Tetrasule Timesule   143
Thebesius vessels   68
Theobromine   152
Theophyllinate
—, calcium   156
—, choline   155
Theophylline   152
—, derivatives   155
Thermodilution method   91
Thermostromuhr   76
Thioxanthines   156
Thrombin
—, platelet aggregation by   50
Thyroid extract   307
Thyroxine   306
—, analogues   15
Tobacco   16
Tocopherol (a—)   305
Tone
—, vasomotor, of coronary vessels   58
Tracers, see radioactive tracers
Trangorex, see Cordarone
Trasicor   222
Trends in pharmacological research   39
—, blockade of adrenergic beta-receptors
    42
—, blockade of hypersympathicotony   42
—, coronary vasodilation   39
—, development of collateral coronary cir-
    culation   45

Trends in pharmacological research, dilatation of coronary conductance vessels 44
—, improvement of functional coronary circulation 45
—, inhibition of monoamineoxydase 41
—, inhibition of platelet aggregation and
adhesiveness 49
—, overall inhibition of hypersympathi-
cotony 43
—, potentiation of endogenous mediators of
coronary autoregulation 47
—, prophylaxis of myocardial necrosis 48
—, reduction in cardiac work 40
Triac 15
Triethanolamine trinitrate 138
Triglycerides 14
Triiodothyro acetic acid 15
Triiodothyro propionic acid 15
Trimanyl MG.345 305
Trimetazidine 298
Trinitrate (triethanolamine) 138
Trinitrin 120
Triopron 15
Triparanol 314
Trolnitrate phosphate 138
Tromasedan 315
Tromcardin 298
Two step exercise
—, in diagnosis of angina 96
—, in clinical evaluation of antianginal drugs
103, 107

Ultrasonic
—, flowmetry 78
Unsaturated fatty acids 15
Uridine 306
Ustimon 192
USVC 6524 254

Valium 301
Vaporol 144
Varia 314
Vasangor 149
Vasculat 308
Vasodiatol 140
Vasodilan 307
Vasokellina 157

Vasomotor
—, metabolites 58
—, tone 58
Vastarel 298
Vectocardiography 95
—, in diagnosis of angina 95
Vegetable sterols 15
Veinitrine 121
Venous coronary blood flow, see coronary
blood flow
Ventricular
—, compliance in angina 31
—, dynamics in angina 30
—, end-diastolic ventricular pressure in
angina 30
—, failure in angina 30
—, function in angina 30
—, function in coronary heart disease 34
—, volume in angina 31
Verapamil 172
Vessels, see coronary vessels
—, innervation, see innervation
Vialibran 298
Vibeline 159
Vineberg procedure 10
Visammimix 157
Visammin 157
Viscardan 157
Visken 246
Visnacorin 159
Visnadin 159
Visnagalin 157
Visnagen 157
Visnagin 159
Visnamine 159
Vitamine E 305

Win 5494 313

Xanthines 152
—, aminophylline 153
—, choline theophyllinate 155
—, theophylline derivatives 155
Xanthinol nicotinate 156
Xenon
—, radioactive 83
730 C.E.R.M. 292